CONCISE TEXTBOOK OF PAEDIATRIC NURSING

CONCISE TEXTBOOK OF PAEDIATRIC NURSING

Dr. Assuma Beevi

PhD(N), MSc(N), Dip. Med. Edn., CHPE, DHM, Cert. HRM
Acting Director, MIMS Academy
Principal, MIMS College of Nursing

ELSEVIER

ELSEVIER

RELX India Pvt. Ltd.

Registered Office: 818, Indraprakash Building, 8th Floor, 21, Barakhamba Road, New Delhi-110001
Corporate Office: 14th Floor, Building No. 10B, DLF Cyber City, Phase II, Gurgaon-122 002, Haryana, India

Notice

Practitioners and researchers must always rely on their own experience and knowledge in evaluating and using any information, methods, compounds or experiments described herein. Because of rapid advances in the medical sciences, in particular, independent verification of diagnoses and drug dosages should be made. To the fullest extent of the law, no responsibility is assumed by Elsevier, authors, editors or contributors in relation to the adaptation or for any injury and/or damage to persons or property as a matter of products liability, negligence or otherwise, or from any use or operation of any methods, products, instructions, or ideas contained in the material herein.

Content Strategist: Udita R Joseph
Content Project Manager: Fariha Nadeem
Sr Production Executive: Ravinder Sharma
Sr Graphic Designer: Milind Majgaonkar

Typeset by GW Tech

Printed in India by Thomson Press India Ltd.

This work is dedicated to my respected teachers of paediatric nursing, to all student nurses of my country and to my grandchildren Ethu and Lichu.

PREFACE

The second edition of *Textbook of Paediatric Nursing* is updated with current scientific knowledge related to paediatric nursing practice. This edition is prepared to cater the needs of all nursing students and practicing nurses in India, keeping in mind the cultural and contextual needs of Indian children. The content of the textbook covers the subject curriculum on child health nursing of Indian Nursing Council for B.Sc. Nursing. It also covers the major concepts of paediatric nursing included in postgraduate syllabus as a ready reckoner in capsular form helping postgraduate students for preparation of their examinations. The content outlines the must know, better to know and nice to know aspects of essentials of paediatric nursing practice with adequate explanations on various core areas of child health practice.

Second edition has only 8 units with 41 chapters, whereas the first edition had 21 units consisting of 47 chapters. This explains how the book is rearranged to make it more student-friendly with only necessary contents reducing redundancy. Unit 1 concentrates on concepts of paediatric nursing practice, starting with history of child health nursing. This unit has three chapters. Unit 2 comprises four chapters dealing with preventive paediatrics.

Unit 3 deals with healthy child and comprises 10 chapters dedicated to the needs of a growing child. Unit 4 deals with nutritional needs and care of children with nutritional disorders where the normal requirements of nutrients and fluids are discussed in detail with nutritional problems in three chapters. Unit 5 comprises five chapters dealing with nursing care of neonates. Within this unit, genetic issues, inborn errors of metabolism, embryological concepts, and care of normal neonates and high-risk neonates are covered. Unit 6 discusses the core issues of hospitalization and children's reactions towards hospitalization and how nurses can help children, parents and their relatives with sickness and death of children.

Unit 7 mainly deals with care of hospitalized children. The content is arranged in a format of alteration in major functions of the human organ systems and nursing process approach throughout, as far as possible. Each of the chapters of this unit concentrates on embryological development with consequences of abnormal development as essential concepts followed by the nursing management of children with common medical and surgical problems affecting organ functions. Each medical and surgical problem is presented with its description, clinical findings/assessment findings, multidisciplinary management, nursing assessment, nursing diagnoses and nursing interventions that help the students to make a quick nursing care plan and provide care for their paediatric patients.

Unit 8 has a chapter on special topics where administration of medications, life support issues, paediatric pain management and parasitic infestations in children are discussed. Another chapter discusses paediatric unit planning that deals with planning of paediatric unit, paediatric intensive care unit and neonatal intensive care unit. This unit is very special because these topics are not included in usual textbooks.

The second edition is also written as a basic textbook for beginners of paediatric nursing. But it can be useful for postgraduate students and practicing paediatric nurses. I have tried my best to include the topics that have not covered in the first edition to appear in this second edition. Certain communicable diseases such as dengue fever, H1N1 (swine flu), disorders of eye and ear, nose and throat are given special attention. Care of children with emotional disorders and childhood disability are given due importance. Developmentally supportive care and sustainable goals along with millennium development goals are also discussed. All national and international programmes dedicated to child welfare and laws related to children are also included along with status of Indian children in today's context. I hope and expect that the content of the book will be helpful for the students to assist them in their learning as a resource and to practice the care of children in a very special way with tutored compassion and honesty.

I submit this work to the student community and to the practicing professionals for your comments and reviews too.

Assuma Beevi. T.M.

PREFACE TO THE FIRST EDITION

This textbook is prepared to cater the needs of all nursing students and practicing nurses in India. Most of the books available in India are of foreign origin and depict the needs of children in their country of origin. These books are elaborate in nature, keeping basic students' needs remote to achieve. This prompted me to make a user friendly need-based Paediatric Nursing Textbook for Nursing Students of my country. This book can also be used as a reference by practicing paediatric nurses.

The content is so arranged based on syllabuses of various universities in India, keeping Indian Nursing Council standards of syllabus as criteria. The book contains 21 units consisting of 47 chapters. The content is arranged in a format of alteration in major functions of the human organ systems and nursing process approach throughout, as far as possible.

The special feature of the book is its first four units. Unit 1 of the text introduces the students to changing concepts of paediatric nursing with an overview of the evolution and historical perspective of the paediatric nursing. This unit is divided into various chapters giving all-important concepts underlying paediatric nursing practice. Chapter 3 of this unit describes the principles of paediatric nursing, roles and qualities of a paediatric nurse, which the student may not get from other books in a capsular form. Chapter 4 deals with the differences between paediatric nursing by describing the anatomical, physiological and psychological differences that a nurse needs to understand and appreciate while caring for children of different ages. Chapter 5 introduces the student to various factors affecting child health and special problems of Indian children that an Indian nurse should be cognizant with.

Unit 2 stresses the importance of child health maintenance, dealing with child welfare activities and other welfare programmes in Chapters 6 and 7. Chapter 8 provides a quick reference to child health assessment. Chapters 9 and 10 of the text deals with the importance of play in child's development, along with the common accidents and their prevention.

Unit 3 gives a brief account of various theories of development in Chapter 11 and a ready reckoner of developmental problems in Chapter 12.

Unit 4 provides a brief review of genetics, matter of facts arrangement of chromosomal anomalies and inborn errors of metabolism, including genetic counselling. This unit also stresses the embryonic concepts that a paediatric nurse should know. Units 5–8 are organized with general principles of growth and development of a child from neonatal period to adolescence with special emphasis on health maintenance role of the nurse. Each chapter gives in brief the various parameters of growth and development, health problems of each age group with special emphasis on anticipatory guidance. Unit 8 deals with the care of hospitalised child giving the impact of hospitalisation on the sick child, parents and siblings. A special emphasis is provided on the role of nurse in reducing emotional trauma of the child and family during hospitalisation, with coping strategies of parents and children.

Unit 9 is unique, and consists of the nutritional requirements in children nutritional assessment, breast feeding, complementary feeding, age-appropriate feeding techniques and special diets. This unit also describes the fluid electrolyte management in paediatric practice along with common fluid and nutritional problems in children.

Units 10–20 of the textbook deals with various alterations in organ function and the nursing management of the same, in nursing process format. Each of these units contains chapters concentrating on embryological development with consequences of abnormal development as essential concepts. Another chapter in these units describes the nursing management of children with common medical and surgical problems affecting organ functions.

Each medical and surgical problem is presented as description, clinical findings/assessment findings, multidisciplinary management, nursing assessment, nursing diagnoses and nursing interventions that helps the students to make a quick nursing care plans and provide care for their paediatric patients.

Finally, Unit 21 covers certain special topics such as administration of medications, drug calculations, paediatric pain management, paediatric trauma management and neonatal resuscitation, etc.

Though the book has been written as a basic text for beginning students of paediatric nursing, practicing nurses can use it as a ready reckoner. I hope the content of this book will assist the students and paediatric nurses in providing compassionate care to children of different ages, and also provide anticipatory guidance to parents.

I request all the renowned reviewers and students to provide me with comments about each chapter, so that the necessary changes could be done in the next edition.

Assuma Beevi. T.M. Kerala

Acknowledgements

I express my sincere gratitude to my daughter Dr Feliz Nazeer. K.E., my son-in-law Dr Titto Rahim, my daughter-in-law Sajna Nazeer and my son Shinas Nazeer for their timely support.

CONTENTS

UNIT 1

MODERN CONCEPTS OF CHILDCARE

CHANGING CONCEPTS OF PAEDIATRIC NURSING

LEARNING OBJECTIVES

At the end of the chapter, the learner will be able to:
- Discuss the historical perspective and evolution of child health practices.
- Describe the modern concepts of paediatric nursing practice.
- Describe the underlying principles of paediatric nursing practice.
- Describe the current issues and trends in paediatrics and paediatric nursing practice.
- Describe the legal and ethical concepts applied in paediatric nursing practice.

Childcare during the last decade has undergone dramatic changes in its concepts and practice. This field is one of the broadest and most challenging nursing specialties, as it includes the study of growth and development of a total person from conception through adolescence, as well as prevention, health maintenance, diagnosis and treatment of disorders affecting children during their growing years.

Paediatrics is the study and care of children in sickness and in health from conception through adolescence. Paediatrics is derived from the Greek words – pedia = pais, paidos meaning a child or denoting a relationship to a child (pedo); iatric = surgery/medicine, i.e. treatment; and ics = the suffix of a subject of science. In India

and other developing countries of the world, this care is extended to children up to the age of 10–12 years. In developed countries, paediatric care and child health programmes cater children up to adolescence.

The medical doctor who specializes in paediatrics is called a paediatrician. A paediatric team includes a host of other professionals, such as geneticists, biochemists, laboratory and prosthetic technicians, psychologists, surgeons, educationists, dentists, physical and occupational therapists, respiratory therapists, dieticians, child health nurses and aides. All of them contribute to modern childcare in a vivid and ceremonious way to prevent diseases and promote health to the next generation.

EVOLUTION OF CHILD HEALTH CARE: A HISTORICAL PERSPECTIVE

The modern childcare is part of a great historical pageantry that involved cultures of many people. A present-day child health nurse should know something about the past to fully appreciate the present and respond to the challenges of the future. Therefore, here is an attempt to heighten the enthusiasm of people who would like to learn child health nursing as their major specialty.

Prehistoric Times (Before 3000 BC)

There were no written documents to validate the practices of people. It is quite natural to assume that individuals of each generation followed the prescribed pattern of life taught by their parents without much difference until some natural catastrophe destroyed or altered their lives. Man has to live by fighting the environment to survive, and survival of the fittest was the dictum followed. Owing to this, the babies who are undesirable in any way may be allowed to die. Such babies are those born with defects and those born under undesirable climatic situations – season and weather. Strong children were considered as an asset to their parents in earning their livelihood. Such children were breastfed and taught the customs of their tribe carefully, and they developed a strong sense of security.

However, every tribe differs from the other and so do their customs. Adolescents were considered as adult. Girls are married and expected to produce children, and boys become hunters, farmers, warriors and father of future generations. This cycle repeated continuously.

In the early civilizations of Egypt, China and India, children were reared according to the traditions passed down from previous generations. Children were made to follow their parents. Girls followed their mothers, and boys followed their fathers; e.g. barber's son becomes a barber, a king's son becomes a king.

The medical practice was a combination of indigenous system of medicine and magic. Local practitioners treat adults and children with diet, rituals, magic and herbs. Old writings such as Papyrus Erbs (1500 BC) contain prescription for the treatment of urinary ailments in children. In China, herbalist's compounded complex combinations are used to treat childhood fevers and convulsions. A vaccination for small pox was first done in India and China. Mosaic Law of ancient Jews greatly affected the hygienic practices and contributed to maternal and child healthcare. Parenthood was honoured and large families were considered as blessings of God.

In ancient cultures, adoptions of orphaned children were valued high. The Babylonian code of Hammurabi included a well-defined contract between the children and their parents. In Greece, orphans of the soldiers were provided funds and free medical care. Charitable concerns for orphans were provided in Japan.

In the first century AD, Celsius was reported to be the first one to state that children require different treatment from adults. In the Western world, Soraneous (in Greece) in the second century AD wrote the first known manuscript devoted to paediatrics. In India, *Kasyapa Tantra*, which was written in 6th century BC, had a chapter on *Koumara Mritya*, i.e. service to children. Perhaps, this is the first record of paediatrics anywhere in the world. Sushruta, the Indian Hippocrates, wrote a chapter on *Koumara Mritya* in the second century AD. Soraneous also wrote his treatise about the same time.

Contrary to the above-mentioned facts of giving attention to the well-being of children, ancient cultures accepted infanticide as a means to eliminate defective children and thereby limit the size of the family. Roman law gave fathers absolute authority over their children, for punishment, imprisonment, death or sale to slavery. The humanitarian principles brought by teachings of Greek philosophers, Roman stoics and Hebrews led to the development of a new philosophical approach to the value of human life and this, in turn, affected childcare too.

Later, when Christianity became the official religion of the Western world, Roman Catholic Church took over the responsibility of scholarly work and medical care, which they continue to practice in the developing countries of the world. This motivated the medical progress.

While this was happening in the Western world, Middle East was under darkness, which is quoted as *Jahiliya* period in Islamic history. During this period, female infanticide was widely practiced. Teachings of Islam made Arabs to abandon prostitution, alcoholism and female infanticide. Rearing female children is considered as a way to heaven by Islamic teachings. Ladies were given equal status, and ownership to ancestral property declared to females proclaimed their status in the society. Taking care of orphans and widows and giving compulsory *zakah* – due for the poor – contributed to improvement in living conditions of the poor and thereby child survival.

During the medieval period (AD 450–1350), wars and epidemics swept Europe back and forth great sickness, sufferings and death in their life. One-fourth of the entire population believed to have died in the pandemic of Black Death in 1347. A 40-day detention was ordered for all vessels entering the Mediterranean Sea ports, which was known as quartana. The modern term quarantine has thus derived from this word.

The first infant asylum/hospital was founded in AD 787, which was only a shelter for abandoned children. These foundling homes were deadly due to overcrowding, poor understanding of hygiene and sanitation. No public health measures were available and death toll was very high. This period was considered as the dark ages of health.

Renaissance and Early Modern World (AD 1350–1800)

Renaissance brought tremendous changes in the course of human life. A middle class emerged, and world trade and commerce developed. The two great inventions of printing and manufacturing of papers by Chinese resulted in dissemination of knowledge. In the sixteenth century, two great medical books were published. Thomas Phaer, the Father of English Paediatrics, wrote *The Boke of Children*, and in Germany, Felix Wurtz wrote *The Children's Book*. St. Vincent de Paul, who lived from AD 1576 to 1660, is called the Patron Saint of Orphans for his work in the field of childcare.

During the period of industrial revolution, there developed a shift of small home workshops to large machine-powered factories. These factories employed large numbers of people in viciously dangerous and inhuman conditions for very low wages. Overcrowding and unsanitary living conditions took a heavy toll of human life. To survive, every member of the family had to work, including children as young as 6 years of age. This continued until the nineteenth century when the law prohibiting child labour came to effect.

Unhygienic conditions were contributed to the high incidence of morbidity and mortality in children. Epidemics and childhood illness were so common that fewer than 50% of children lived beyond the age of 5 years. Therefore, it seemed that illness and death during childhood were inevitable. Natural calamities and overwhelming poverty led to the abandonment of children. In the early seventeenth century, several children's asylums were founded for these children. By the middle of the eighteenth century, the abandonment was so severe that the asylums were overflooded with these children, which led again to poor standard of childcare and took a heavy toll on the children's lives. High mortality and morbidity among children led some physicians to look more closely at the prevailing practices of childcare. They found that there were a lot of hazardous practices in feeding, clothing and rearing. Few infants were breastfed; instead, infants received different types of soups and sugar solutions or water.

Despite these deplorable conditions, many advances in science, medicine, literature and political thought were taking place. In England, Edward Jenner developed the small pox vaccine. Harvey discovered blood circulation. Microscope, obstetrical forceps and clinical thermometers were also invented. Rousseau wrote his famous book *Emile*, which included a section on the rights of children and another on hygiene and nutrition of infants. The philosophical approach of Rousseau that 'children are not miniature adults' made revolutionary changes in the field of childcare.

Modern World (AD 1800 to the Present)

Industrial revolution brought remarkable changes in the lives of people. Mushrooming of the scientific knowledge and flourishing of humanistic social ideals entered in. During this time, people made great progress in conquering diseases, hunger, thirst, ignorance, superstition, isolation and exposure to the elements. New intellectual climate of the Renaissance made people to observe, to ask questions of what, how and why in conducting experiments and to leave their findings for others.

The humanitarian principles revolutionized the Western world and politically blossomed into democratic and socialistic forms of government. Practically, it focused attention on the need to improve a lot of the ordinary people, thus producing social advances. Knowledge about human body and the cause of diseases prompted the development of new medical interventions in treating adults and children on a wider scale.

In 1748, William Cadogan's 'Essay on Nursing' called attention to unhealthy childcare practices and identified overdressing, overfeeding and poor diet as factors contributing to childhood illness. He encouraged breastfeeding and urged parents to dress infants in loose and lightweight garments. However, in spite of the early efforts of Cadogan and others, childcare practices were too slow to change.

The study of paediatrics began in the last half of the 1800s, particularly under the influence of the Persianborn physician, Abraham Jacobi (1830–1919), who was referred being the Father of Paediatrics. In 1870, he was awarded the first professorship in paediatrics in the USA. He started paediatric departments in several New York hospitals and was one of the founders of the American Paediatric Society in 1888.

During the nineteenth century, people recognized the effects of child hood illness and injury. The bad effects of child labour, poverty and neglect on proper development of children were also recognized. The end of the nineteenth century is often regarded as the dark ages of paediatrics, and the first half of the twentieth century as the dawn of improved health care for children (T.E.Cone Jr.1979).

The recognition that childhood diseases differ from adult diseases led to the establishment of hospitals devoted solely to children. During mid-nineteenth century, a home-like atmosphere was provided where patients were encouraged to care for children during hospitalization, and children were allowed to wear their usual clothes and play with their own toys.

The recognition of the role of microbes in causation of illness during the late nineteenth century changed the style of childcare dramatically. The role of cross infection was identified, and the doors of hospitals were closed for visitors. So parents were prohibited to visit their children during hospitalization. Moreover, it was thought that parents' visit brought about emotional upset in the child when they left.

Concern about contagious diseases led to certain changes in hospital policies. Uniforms were prescribed for hospital personnel, the use of toys was restricted, and compelled to limit social contacts between children in the wards. This reduced the spread of infection; however, the emotional health of hospitalized children received little consideration.

The work of J. Bowlby (1953) stimulated research on emotional well-being of hospitalized children. Spitz (1945) conducted a study on behaviour of children in a foundling home where the staff provided competent physical care but rarely talked to or handled the children. He reported that children began to show emotional reaction even at 6 months of age.

J. Bowlby (1953) observed the effect of separation on children who were removed from their homes during World War II. Influenced by the work of Spitz and Bowlby, J. Robertson (1970) studied the effects of hospitalization on young children. Robertson observed similar behavioural patterns even during short hospitalizations. He organized these behavioural patterns into three stages – protest, despair and denial. The findings of this study helped to change the hospital policies in late twentieth century.

The rising interest in psychoanalytical theory, cognitive theory and sociocultural learning theory has brought tremendous changes in the field of paediatrics. This has stimulated intensive study of human development from conception through childbearing age. Psychoanalytic studies have shown the different needs for the children and the parents. Today, both parents are considered unique central persons in the family and having a profound influence on mental health of each of its members. Health care personnel now regard the child and the family as mutually dependent on each other and view them as a single unit. Growing recognition of the potentially unfortunate effects of hospitalization on both the child and family has stimulated a trend towards a *minimal hospital* stay and whenever possible. This promoted the concept of ambulatory treatment and home care whenever possible to avoid separation of the child from the family and local community. Recent trends, such as paediatric ambulatory care, home care and day surgery, also help to minimize the stress of illness and hospitalization on children and their families.

Now a movement towards *humanized paediatric care* has emerged out as a major source – to reduce trauma to hospitalized children. At present, children are routinely prepared emotionally for medical procedures. Along with their parents, they are fully informed about scheduled procedures, offered choices when appropriate and encouraged to participate actively in their care. The therapeutic role of play is also acknowledged. Toys from home are welcomed. Interesting toys are also available in most of the hospitals for children. Group play and occupational therapy under the supervision of trained personnel are available when isolation precautions are not in force. Awareness of the supportive effect of schoolwork for the hospitalized school child with a prolonged illness has led many hospitals in the developed countries to provide bedside teaching by qualified teachers. Paediatric super specialty has emerged for solving the complex medical/surgical problems of children.

Many advances have been made in surgical techniques in paediatric population throughout the years. For instance, paediatric cardiologists now treat children with heart problems. Children with defects previously thought to be incompatible with life are taken into special diagnostic and treatment centres – to provide expert attention.

DEVELOPMENT OF PAEDIATRICS AS A SPECIALTY

The specialties of paediatrics and paediatric nursing did not exist before the later half of the century. Hospitals for children or separate department for their care in general hospital were rare. Even six or eight children were confined to one bed in olden days. The trend towards eradicating such gross neglect of children began in 1802, where the first children's hospital was erected in Paris. The hospital for sick children, built in Great Ormond Street in London early in the nineteenth century, was the first of its kind in English-speaking country.

Today, there are many children's hospitals all over the world. The first children's hospital in India was opened in Madras. Now in all the states of India, there are many children's hospitals under the government sector as well as in private sector. Few of them in Kerala are Institute of Maternal and Child Health, Calicut; Sree Avitom Thirunal (SAT) Hospital, Thiruvananthapuram; Institute of Child Diseases, Kottayam; and many children and women hospitals in many districts. Other states also have many children's hospitals and almost all medical colleges offer specialist and super specialist training for doctors and nurses in the field of paediatrics.

DEVELOPMENT OF PAEDIATRIC MEDICINE

During the nineteenth century, for the first time some physicians of Europe, the USA and Canada began to devote the major portion of their professional interest towards the care of children.

The emphasis had previously been in the disease and not on the child. The fact that the diseases occurred in a child was having little significance to physician or adult.

Towards the middle of the nineteenth century, Dr Abraham Jacobi came to the USA, where a trend towards specialization in children's disease had already begun. Dr Jacobi was convinced that diseases in children are different from that of adults. He opened a clinic for children and began to lecture on diseases to which children are prone. In 1870, he received his first appointment in the USA from the College of Physicians and Surgeons as a professor of diseases in children; and in 1888, he played a leading role in founding the American Paediatric Society. Next remembered is Dr L. Emmet Hott, who wrote many articles on childcare, became popular among the lay and professional people. In 1888, the first Department of Paediatrics was established at Harvard University headed by Dr Thomas Morgan Rotch. In the USA, the golden age of paediatrics started with the establishment of full-time chair at John Hopkins University in 1913. Gradually super specialties were started.

Current Issues in Paediatric Practice

The term paediatrics is no more seems to be appropriate to use, as it looks to be something like doctoring children. The most appropriate term to use is child health care rather than paediatric care. According to Professor Ansely Green (UK), the philosophy of child health care giver should have a concept of **ACADEMIC** (Personal communication with Professor Ansely Green, UK):

A – Advocate for children and for their benefits
C – Communicate for children
A – Activate child health activities
D – Disseminate child health programmes
E – Educate the public about child health
M – Motivate people to participate in child health activities
I – Investigate the possible resources
C – Collaborate the activities

CURRENT TRENDS IN PAEDIATRIC MEDICINE AND A NURSE'S ROLE

In order to improve human resource and quality health care to children without any discrimination at all social and ethnic levels are essential. Futuristic models of paediatrics are based on this philosophy and utilization of **technological advancement** in the care of children. Modified key technology and its boom affect practitioner/parent/child relationship. Modern technology can even provide an electronic or digital health history on a CD or a palmtop, and the parents can view and learn more about their child's health history. Parents can even take their child to walk through a screening devise to decipher his genome and get his base biochemical parameters, get computer-based diagnosis with the help of apps-based algorithms and print out of the prescription.

Human Genome

Human behaviour and diseases are genetically determined. Human genome is a sophisticated horoscope as all life events are destined as the basis of genome. Identification and decoding of human genome is a great achievement of the twenty-first century. Human genome project had identified and sequenced 25,000 genes. Three billion DNA base pairs have been decoded by DNA probes.

About 1800 diseases have been identified to have expression through genes. With the knowledge on genome, it is now possible to plan strategies for prevention, diagnosis and treatment of disease with patient-specific drugs. Nurses have greater role in genetic counselling as a team member and also have opportunities for expanded role as nurse geneticist.

Revolution in Medical Genetics

It is now possible to detect a number of life-threatening diseases in the fetus permitting selective abortion as a part of eugenics to ensure survival of genetically normal human beings. This reduces disability and thereby improving quality of life of humans. Replacement of abnormal genes with good genes through genetic engineering technology is possible and is done. Certain conditions like severe combined immune deficiency syndrome (SCID), an adenosine deaminase deficiency (ADA), Duchenne muscular dystrophy (DMD), cystic fibrosis, haemophilia, familial hypercholesterolemia and certain cancers are now treated with the possibility of eugenics.

Genetic technology also refined various assisted reproductive technologies (ART) and feasibility to have designer babies as a part of eugenics. Now it is possible to clone babies with identical genetic make-up by artificial twinning of embryo or somatic cell nuclear transfer (SCNT). All these advancements have their own benefits and demerits. A community without diversity may remain as a question to existence of variety in the world.

Stem Cell Banking and Transplantation

Hematopoietic stem cell transplantation (HSCT) by using multi potent stem cells has revolutionized the treatment of haemolytic anaemias like thalassemia, aplastic anaemia, sickle cell anaemia, and in born errors of metabolism and auto immune disorders. Cells derived from bone marrow, peripheral blood or umbilical cord blood are stored and used for this type of treatments. The source may be autologous or allogenic. Allogenic stem cell therapy, the risk of infection, mismatching, rejection and graft-versus-host disease are high. LifeCell, Babycell, Cordlife and Stemade Biotech are companies

that provide facilities for storing and cryoprecipitating cord blood. This can be used for the donors, their parents and siblings when there are life-threatening lifestyle diseases that need treatment. Now it is possible to repair a defective organ of the body using totipotent natural or cloned stem cells. This is successfully used in many advanced tertiary and quaternary hospitals.

Diagnostic Marvels

Shift in diagnostic technology from clinical assessment and observation had made patient assessment much easy. Technological advancements like digital stethoscope, powered by iPhone or Android smart phone, head-held ultrasound device, pulse oximeter and apps-based algorithms are now used for diagnosing patient conditions. DNA and rRNA probes are increasingly used in the defective and genetic disorders, microsampling of blood for biochemical investigations, electronic devices like smart biometric wrist watch are now in pipeline for monitoring vitals, biochemical parameters, hydration status and oxygen saturation that works with noninvasive pulse wave data collector. Paediatric practitioners are waiting for the development of sensors for assessing kidney functions and add-on displays for ECG and EEG. Cutting-edge wireless smart scales for weight, BMI, body water, bone mass and daily caloric intake are underway. Japan is developing intelligent toilets for smart bottom hygiene and to assess certain body parameters. It is believed that genometers may come to the markets shortly. These technological advancements make nurses training more technology oriented, and the new-generation nurse should also be a technological wizard. Age-old training needs to be changed and every nurse educator also should undergo technological training to equip themselves as trainers. Today's paediatric nurse should be a smart nurse abreast with newer technology in the provision of quality care to children and their families. They should not forget about the compassion and humane care a human being can impart even when technological advancement is revolutionizing child health care.

Nutritional Nuances

Hippocrates, 2500 years ago, said, 'Let thy food be thy medicine and thy medicine be thy food'. Fortification of food with vitamins and micro-elements are now used to treat deficiency disorders. Protein hydrolysates and hypoallergenic foods are now available to treat and prevent food allergies. Functional food concepts are widely used to prevent illness, promote health and improve the quality of life. The phytonutrients, antioxidants, soluble and insoluble fibres and probiotics present in food promote positive health and reduce the risk of developing certain illnesses. So one should remember that *triad of quality life* and sound health are sound genetic constitution, safe environment and intake of wholesome balanced food. But one must remember that genetically modified foods are associated with greater risk for allergies and immune suppression. So now there is a worldwide movement of rejecting genetically modified foods and promoting bio-agricultural practices (organic farming) and avoiding chemical insecticides that are harmful to health. Child health nurses must be cognizant of these issues and must impart education to parents and public on these aspects as a part of health promotion practices.

Therapeutics

Needless pen-shaped device developed for vaccine administration had led to painless vaccination. Oral and mucous vaccines are developed for rotavirus, typhoid, flu, cholera, RSV and measles. It is also believed that antigen-primed or transgenic banana, potatoes, tomatoes, lettuce, rice, wheat, soya beans and corn can be developed as child-friendly vaccines.

Pharmacogenomics help to produce specific drugs on the basis of genomic subgroups and is possible to deliver the drugs at the site of disease with the help of liposomes and carrier monoclonal antibodies.

This will help in reducing the dose, below efficiency and reduce adverse reactions. The traditional dosing of children based on age, weight and body surface area, etc. can be abolished. The traditional nursing way in medicine administration principles of same medicine, same dose, same route and same duration for every child can be changed.

Monoclonal antibodies had paved way for prevention and treatment of life-threatening infections, transport and delivery of drugs to the site of disease, destruction of cancer cells and identification of metastasis with the help of radionuclide antibodies.

Memory biochips, arrays of polymer nano wires and neurobionic intervention are developed to take over the functions of damaged neurons. Development of photo dynamic and cosmetology treatments revolutionized the treatment of various disorders of pigmentation and birth marks. Production of artificial blood or blood substitute (haemoglobin-based or perfluorocarbon-based oxygen carriers) may reduce the scarcity of blood and blood products. The identification of double-stranded RNA activated caspase oligomerizers by researchers in the USA and Cambridge are useful for developing broad-spectrum antivirals.

Surgical Developments

Fast recovery with keyhole/minimally invasive surgical procedures, robotic surgeries and imaging-guided interventions is now a reality. Replacement of defective organs through transplants or through synthetic spare parts (e.g. artificial valves) revolutionized surgical procedures and treatments. Computer-aided surgical robots help in robotic surgery that help in more precision and safety to the younger ones through smaller incision, minimal blood loss, less hospital stay and less pain. This is available now in all major centres in India.

Intelligent surgical knife is available to use for bloodless incision, vaporized smoke produces while cutting, tissue analysed by mass spectrometer help in diagnosing real-time malignancy. Smart e-parts are available to prevent bed sores. All these innovations have revolutionized the nursing care and made child health nursing more challenging.

Tele Paediatrics

Tele medicine is a reality. Tele conferencing and sending images through telephone lines are easy now. Consultation can be done globally. It is possible to have global live coverage of surgical procedures. Now in developed countries paediatric nurse practitioners are using tele paediatrics in their practice.

Emergency Health Catastrophes

Although new innovations give hope and enthusiasm, there are certain factors that cause alarming concerns. Overnutrition and lifestyle diseases are emerging as public health problems. Large nucleus of infective disorders – HIV, SARS, bird flu, swine flu, Zika, Ebola, dengue and multidrug-resistant superbug – remains as threats. Some of these diseases are pandemic in certain parts of the world. Death of children with haemorrhagic dengue is a real threat. Development of early onset of type 2 diabetes in children and environmental pollutions stands as important health issues. Natural and manmade disasters like uses of chemical weapons in war front, civil wars, refugee problems, etc. stand as catastrophes especially for the weaker sections of the population. It is very frightening to see that increasing number of children and women are becoming victims of wars and calamities leading to a large number of physically and emotionally disabled and tortured children all around the world.

DEVELOPMENT OF PAEDIATRIC NURSING

Paediatric nursing is the practice of nursing with children, adolescents and their families across the health continuum. It includes health promotion, illness management and health restoration. Paediatric nursing deals with a wide range of medical conditions, treatment options but not simply medical-surgical nursing on little people. It requires knowledge of child development, the anatomical, physiological and the psychological differences between children and adults. It is family-centred identifying the worth and role of family in the life of a child to grow as a healthy adult.

Special instruction to nurses in paediatrics parallels with the development of separate units for children in hospitals. In colonial America, most children were delivered with the help of midwives and cared by their families, sing folk medicine. Only the affluent people were attended by the physicians. The founding of 'The Children's Hospital' in the USA specifically for children in Pennsylvania in 1855 is considered as the landmark event in the history of development of paediatric nursing as a specialty in the USA. During the second half of the nineteenth century, many hospitals in major cities were started to devote to the care of children in the USA. But these hospitals did not admit children with communicable diseases due to high mortality rates. Hospital schools of nursing started and this changed the policy of admission of children with communicable diseases. Children's Hospital of Philadelphia began admitting children suffering from communicable diseases in the year 1895 when they opened their school of nursing. The school of nursing provided adequate staff to provide care for children and their families including observation, assessment and education. The nursing schools associated with some of the earliest children's hospitals – those in Philadelphia, Denver, Boston and New York for instance – were devoted to the training of nurses to the care of sick children. However, it was not until the department of paediatrics was firmly established in medical schools that paediatric became a compulsory part of the undergraduate nursing curriculum. Although supplementary course for registered nurses were given in many children's hospitals, until 1940s university graduate level study of paediatric nursing did not appear.

Nurses played a major role in the child-saving activities in the early twentieth century. Many health practitioners focused on improving the artificial feeding of infants and children to decrease their mortality rates. Public and privately funded milk depots in the USA provided pasteurized milk at low prices to those who could afford to and at no cost to the poor. Nurses were employed to educate mothers about proper handling and storage of milk. Home visitations by nurses were added and the milk depots became child health stations that stress on illness prevention.

Contributions made by Lillian Wald and Mary M. Brewster were significant in the history of paediatric nursing. They worked as visiting nurses in New York's Lower East Side in 1893. In 1895, Wald opened the Nurses Settlement House on Henry Street; and by 1909, there were 37 nurses working towards welfare of children. The additional services were also provided by these nurses as first aid, obstetrical services, treated minor injuries, illnesses, educational programmes for the community and nurses training. The Sheppard–Towner Act of 1921 in the USA provided money to improve maternal and child health services that helped to employ many nurses in infant and maternal centres in the USA for promoting the development of paediatric nursing there. In 1917, the Standard Curriculum for Schools of Nursing included a section on paediatric nursing that had component on social issues and psychology, infectious diseases, orthopaedic, information on infant feeding and child development along with medical-surgical conditions. In 1923, the committee for the study of nursing education, commissioned by Rockefeller Foundation, found that the curriculum had many lacunae especially in the area of child health. The report found inherent deficiencies in the training as the hospital schools of nursing had inherent conflict of interest considering university nursing programmes. Later in the century, paediatric nursing moved forward with advanced degrees of universities. The first nurse practitioners were paediatric nurse practitioners in the USA.

The paediatric nursing curriculum has witnessed changing attitudes and research on many issues especially the role of family in the care of children, and researches on maternal deprivation, involvement of family in the care of children. Hospitalization period of children was viewed as a chance for educating the family. Visitation policy also changed and parents were allowed to visit their children in the hospital and their presence was considered positive contrary to previous belief of unnecessary, bothersome or even harmful.

Among the leaders in paediatric nursing at that time and subsequently was Florence. G. Blake, who became world renowned for her psychological insight into child development and behaviour and for her incorporation of this knowledge into nursing practice. Through her research, she had demonstrated the positive effects of involving families in the care of children. In her text, The Child, His Parents and the Nurse, she had portrayed a clear picture of the benefits of family involvement in the care of children. She is also known for her publications, research and widespread impact on the development of undergraduate and graduate nursing programmes. The push for family-centred care (FCC) began in the 1980s and was spurred on by Everett Koops 1987 report on children with health care needs which called for community-based FCC.

Then with the advent of various theories of nursing by eminent theorists, psychoanalytic theories by psychologists and theories, models and concepts were derived from and expanded the span of knowledge in the field of paediatric nursing. Now all over the world, undergraduate, graduate and superspecialties in the field of paediatric nursing are available to equip the nurses in order to cope with the changing trend of child health care.

Many professional organizations of US paediatric nurses also helped in the development of paediatric nursing specialty and its subspecialty. Many certification programmes were started by these organizations.

In India, paediatric nursing was not given due recognition in syllabi in the earlier periods of nursing training. But with the introduction of undergraduate degree programme in Nursing in Madras University (College of Nursing, CMCH, Vellore) and in Delhi University (RAK College of Nursing, Delhi), paediatric nursing as a course was introduced. The General Nursing and Midwifery Programme is given a syllabus for Paediatric Nursing, but the theory examination is given along with another specialty. In undergraduate programmes at universities of Kerala, paediatric nursing is given as a separate course devoting due importance to the 40% children of India. At present, almost all universities in India incorporate paediatric nursing as a course in its syllabus. Though specialist nurses are not posted as such in many hospitals, but nurses working in paediatric set up had a course in paediatric nursing as a part of their generalist course. Paediatric nursing is given now as a specialty in postgraduate curriculum. Postgraduate nursing studies in paediatrics date back to 1965 in India. Postgraduate studies in paediatric nursing are available in all universities in India now. Doctoral and postdoctoral studies are now possible in this field. Nurses who are interested in children even can do post-basic diploma courses in different branches of paediatric nursing as neonatal nursing, paediatric critical care nursing, etc.

At present paediatric nurses are concerned with evidence-based nursing practice, adoption of family-centred atraumatic care. Case management models are used in certain hospitals.

PRINCIPLES OF PAEDIATRIC NURSING

Paediatric nursing deals with individuals who are going through a period of growth. In the case of adults, the body will change little during the remainder of his/her life. However, in case of a child, he or she has to accommodate more than three fold increase in length and an approximate twenty fold increase in weight between birth and adolescence. The muscular and intellectual skills along with emotional control progress from rudimentary state of newborn to the complex highly integrated level of adult. The newborn undergoes various changes from helpless state of earliest infancy to adolescence where physical and emotional maturity occurs. In order to provide expert care to children of different age group, the paediatric nurse must equip herself/himself with the fundamental principles of childcare. The following are some of the guiding principles for a paediatric nurse to function effectively in a health care delivery system.

1. **Respect the child's need to regress and help him to accept dependence on others if he resists this**

   Child is not like an adult. He is different from an adult in various ways and respects. For example, an adult coming with abdominal pain will ask for injection to get relief from pain but a child resists injection and is not ready to tolerate the pain of injection. Under this circumstance, the nurse should show sympathy and common sense in her approach to the child.

   Illness produces regression since a child cannot concentrate on self-control. He will go back to the previous stages of development. For example, a preschooler wants his mother to carry him during sickness or he asks to use potty instead of using toilets. In such situations, the nurse should understand that it is the need of the child to regress in the new situation. She should respect the need of the child. An understanding and friendly approach will help the nurse to solve this problem and enable to help the child.

2. **Have an awareness of the child's need for help in reconquering the negative counterpart of the core problem in the stages of development to which he has regressed**

   In the psychological development of a child, there are core problems (otherwise known as developmental crisis or developmental tasks) with which the child struggles at the various stages of development in life. In addition, a child has so many other tasks to accomplish. These tasks are the developmental tasks. In each core, problem or crisis has a negative as well as positive counterpart of the core problem. For example, in infancy, trust versus mistrust, the negative counterpart of the core problem (mistrust) is conquered through a mutually satisfying mother–child relationship. During early years, only members influence, but in later years, the society influences to reach a high level of maturity. An understanding of human development and needs will enable the nurse to be in a position to affect the child's solution of his problems. This will also help the nurse to

empower parents or adults concerned in the care of children as an expert.

3. **Protect the child–family interpersonal relationship**

   In order to protect the child's growth potentials to the fullest, she should take into account the situation of the child's parents because they are the most important people concerning the child. The family relationship influences the child's personality development to a great extent. How does an adult behave is just the reflection of his family bringing up.

   Any illness, even if it is very mild, has a serious impact on the parents, especially the mother. Although some of them face their children's illness with some bravery; the nurse should expect various degrees of anxiety. Mother expects some understanding behaviour and she wants some relief from tension. In such a situation, the nurse can help the mother in understanding the problem of the child, which will enable her to get relief from tension to a certain extent. If the nurse is able to listen to expression of anxiety or anger, she can notice that the mother becomes more relaxed. This will help to protect the family interpersonal relationship.

4. **Awareness of the feelings of others and readiness to respond to them so as to strengthen their resources to cope up with stress is the major principle underlying effective emotional support**

   Emotional support becomes paramount when illness occurs. It is also paramount when a child or adult faces a major change in him or in his life situation. For example, when a girl first menstruates, she needs a lot of support from an elderly female whom the girl can depend. Continuity of relationship is essential when the child wants his nurse, a total stranger will not do.

   In most of our hospitals, parents are allowed and in such cases, parents especially mothers act as the emotional supporter of the child. However, in such situation, we should not forget that mother is also anxious and she needs much help. The child may have many signals, which the parents only know. For example, certain children will take milk only when they get a particular pillow. The first approach to the child should be one that helps him to know that the nurse is friendly, honest and understanding. If the child is not responding, DO NOT threaten him. Make him aware that the nurse is a person who is much friendly.

5. **Children can tolerate discomfort if they are prepared for it, comprehend its real purpose and are adequately prepared**

   Some of the child's fears can be alleviated if prepared precedes experience. If you are preparing a child before a painful treatment, it can provide a basis for the maintenance of trust. Without preparation, the child will deeply be resentful towards all persons concerned. To an older child, each step of the procedure can be explained, and the nurse should explain why it is done.

6. **To child, play is not time out from daily living, but rather an essential part of it that enables**

him grow and mature through the various stages of the developmental process

To an adult, play is recreation; taking time out of daily routines of life is for enjoyment. However, for a child, play is essential as nourishment and treatment. Play helps the child to regain his independence gradually. As adults talk out the problem, let the children play out the problem.

CURRENT TRENDS IN PAEDIATRIC NURSING PRACTICE

Child health nursing is undergoing tremendous advancements just like paediatric medicine and surgery. Practices, once thought as normal practice, have now been replaced by newer innovative care. Nurses must read the literature to stay abreast of new practices to remain updated with it in the field. The current trends in the practice are based on researches that have taken place in the field of paediatric nursing. The common trends are as follows:

- Family-centred care (FCC)
- High technology care (HTC)
- Evidence-based practice (EBP)
- Atraumatic care
- Cost containment (CC)
- Prevention and health promotion
- Integrated management of neonatal and childhood illnesses (IMNCI)

FAMILY-CENTRED CARE

It is based on the philosophy that quality care can be provided in an environment that supports family integrity and promotes psychological and physiological health of the family. It assumes that if the family gain adequate information and support, it is capable of making health care decisions (McKay and Philips, 1984). FCC suggests that health care providers acknowledge and utilize the family's knowledge of their family member's condition and make use of the family's abilities to communicate with their family member. Furthermore, FCC advocates open communications with family members throughout the assessment and management of the child. The concept of FCC was initially introduced by Foote Hospital in Michigan and prompted former US Surgeon General C. Everett Koop's initiative for family-centred, community-based, coordinated care for children with special health care needs and their families in 1987. FCC provides a holistic approach than simply providing medical and nursing care. Parents know best about their child's needs, more aware of their child's behaviour and habits. They stay as the most important people in the care of children as they are the important people for the children. The parents' needs like right to know about the condition of their child, need to be considered while caring children. Attention must be given to parents' worries and comments. Parents must be taken into confidence as partners in the provision of care that aid in better stability to the child psychologically. The nurse should not take over the care without due

importance to the parents. Involvement of the parents in the care of their children facilitates better coping in parents and reduces separation trauma to children that aids speedy recovery.

According to Johnson, McGonial and Kauffmann (1989), the philosophy of FCC is to recognize the family as the constant in a child's life and that the service system and personnel must support, respect, encourage and enhance strength and competence of the family. Encourage the natural care giving and decision-making roles of parents by building on their unique strength as individuals and families. Not only the child's needs but also the needs of family members also are considered in FCC. When a nurse makes the parents comfortable in a care milieu that also is part of FCC.

Two basic concepts of FCC are **enabling** and **empowering**. In the process of **enabling**, all the family members are helped by the professionals to create opportunities and means to utilize their present abilities, competence and acquire new skills that are necessary to provide care to their ailing children. For example, the family members may be capable of comforting a crying child. This can be entrusted to the family members instead of the nurse taking over this responsibility. However, they may not know how to tube feed a baby who requires nutritional supplementation. This can be taught by the nurse to the competent family member and then help them to acquire the skill. **Empowering** helps to foster the strengths of family members to cope up and withstand stress related to sickness of their children.

In FCC, the nurse needs to move farther from describing what is upsetting to families to describing interventions that are helpful and providing the same to recipients of care. Nurses should help families to make responsible decisions through education. Nurses need to act as interpreter and develop mutually respectful and trusting relationship with parents. Recognizing parents as unique autonomous individuals by creating humanistic empowered environment is the responsibility of the nurse in FCC. This promotes parental support and makes parents capable of providing vital elements of care to their children. This form of empowering, parents is of supreme importance in our scenario of shortage of qualified nursing personnel and forms foundation for FCC. FCC expects the nurse should be capable to provide humane care that incorporates hopes, dreams and values, cultural preferences and concerns of children and their parents that are individualistic in nature. Nurses must remember that the nursing care provided will be same but the customer changes. The care we provided will be remembered throughout their lifetime and to nurses their work can appear to be similar day after day.

Finally, all services rendered to children should be child and family centred and they should be given privilege to voice their concerns and help them to achieve their goal of being healthy. So it is essential to partner with their care rather than doing things for them.

HIGH TECHNOLOGY CARE

Advancement in the medical field has created the care of children too technologically versatile. The nurse also needs to be technologically competent enough to meet the nursing care needs of children. The advancement in the diagnostic technology has made detection of many disorders even in the fetal period. Laboratory methods to assess fetal maturity and health of the fetus in the womb, wide use of ultra-sound in diagnosis and aggressive technology in the care of premature and sick babies have created many ethical dilemmas even in nursing practice. Nurse needs to be alert to these advances. Advanced technology and computer skills in working place challenge nurses for continuing nursing education. High technology-induced ethical dilemmas include controversial fetal surgeries, fetal blood transfusions, medical termination of pregnancy, cloning, in vitro fertilization, female foeticide, etc. Here, the nurse needs to be technically competent and must possess soft skills to cope with technological advancements. (Refer Technological advancement and practice of child health)

EVIDENCE-BASED PRACTICE

In EBP, nurses need to make decisions on the best available evidence. EBP in nursing provides a systematic approach to enable nurses to effectively use the best solutions related to nursing practice. Hence, nurses need to search the literature to analyse evidence using biostatistics rules to identify generalizability of findings. Evidence-based nursing practice is the integration of best nursing research evidence with practice expertise and the values of nurses. It is not searching for the only right answer as there is rarely one right answer for any patient problems. In Evidence Based Nursing (EBN) nurses search for the best available options for a best outcome. It is not a magic bullet. EBN includes a number of skills and the development of a process that promotes new evidence, assessed and applied to services to the care of children and their families.

Attribute Required for EBN

- Formulate a question that can be answerable from a practice situation or service issue
- Search databases and finding short cuts to good quality evidence
- Critically appraising research findings
- Interpreting the results and use findings in own practice
- Evaluate the own practice

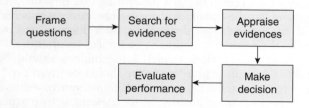

Flow chart depicting the process of using EBP in nursing.

EBP can be applied to any problem that seeks solutions. The problem-seeking solution needs to be framed as a question. A problem may have many subproblems that need to be framed as questions. After framing questions, the nurse needs to search for evidence in literature. Then appraise the evidence in terms of validity and reliability by finding out the generalizability in terms of methodology, and the type of population to find out whether it can be applied to the situation where answer is sought. After appraising the evidence make decision to use or not to use. Finally evaluate the performance.

What Kind of Research Evidence is most Useful?

1. Findings obtained from systematic review – It is a critical assessment and evaluation of research findings to address focused question using methods to minimize the likelihood of bias. It provides strong evidence when designs are good and with large samples. When statistically analysing such pools of data from different studies, it is called meta-analysis.
2. Findings from randomized control trial – An experiment in which samples are randomly allocated to receive or not receive an intervention and find out the effectiveness of interventions.
3. Quasiexperimental designs – In these type of studies, randomization is not possible and many done with naturally occurring control group who are not receiving treatment.
4. Evaluation studies with nonexperimental designs – Interventions are evaluated but without preintervention matching of groups, or with no comparison group at all.
5. Case-control studies – Individuals with a particular problem are 'matched' with controls without the problem.
6. Cohort studies – These collect information from children at intervals, often from shortly after birth into adulthood.
7. Population surveys – A sample of the population or the whole population in the case of the census is asked to provide responses to particular questions.
8. Qualitative research – It is concerned with the meanings of their experiences.
9. Practice guidelines – These consist of systematically developed guidelines for providing care to children and their families with expertise of practitioners.

Why is Evidence-based Practice Promoted in Paediatric Nursing Practice?

There are many reasons for the use of EBP in paediatric medical and nursing practice. Children and families have the right to services based on the best available evidence. EBN involves critically questioning claims coming from experts, practitioner's experience and personal experience from interest groups.

1. Improves patient care. There are evidence that use of EBP improves care of patients. A meta-analysis of 84 studies showed that 72% of patients receiving EBP had 28% better outcomes than the control group (Healer, Becker and Olson, 1998).

2. It improves quality patient care. Committee on Quality of Health Care in America, Institute of Medicine (2001) named EBP as Rule 5 of the 10 Rules for Health Care in Crossing the Quality Chasm.
3. Promotes utilization of research findings in practice. It was found that only a small percentage (21%) of health care providers are incorporating research findings into patient care decisions, though multitude of researches are done and data are published. So use of EBP promotes use of research evidences (Melnyk, Fineout-Overholt, Stone and Ackerman, 2000). It takes approximately 17 years to translate research findings into practice.
4. EBP improves nurses' and other health care professionals' job satisfaction and reduces employee turnover. This has been true in magnet hospitals where EBP is the practice frame work.
5. Without current best evidence, practice rapidly gets outdated. It took nearly 20 years for practitioners to use the research findings to keep newborns to sleep supine instead of face down to prevent sudden infant death syndrome (SIDS). Another example for delay in the use of research finding pertains to the use of antenatal steroids to prevent preterm labour saving lives of newborns.

Challenges of Using EBP in Child Health

The nurses need to be vigilant in practicing EBP in nursing children. In 1970s and 1980s, medical advice was given to nurse infants on prone position. This was based on the studies conducted in preterm babies who improved oxygenation when nursed prone and found less aspiration risk of milk. However, evidences showed that nursing term infants prone, led to more sudden infant death syndrome (SIDS). EBP is relatively less practiced in child health nursing as small number of children is nursed for long-term basis and due to ethical limitations. It is also important for nurses to find out best evidence and utilization of such evidence in practice that seems difficult due to various reasons. The following challenges are faced by practitioners in using EBP in child health practices.

Like other specialties, EBP in child health and illness faces **meta-analysis bias** in location and selection of studies. Meta-analysis has received a mixed reception in child health. Some people see this exercise as mega silliness. Some consider this calculation of weighted average as Newtonian and meta-analysis has left no place for narrative review of articles. So getting exact evidence as proposed is doubtful. Meta-analysis bias may be: **publication bias, bias in location of studies, database bias, citation bias, multiple publication biases and bias in provision of data.**

Some of the clinicians have the opinion that EBP is cook-book practice contrary to epidemiologist's belief, and it is difficult to keep track of updates and danger of progress.

Primary Nursing

The system of primary nursing provides extreme commitment to patient accountability. Twenty-four-hour responsibility and accountability by one nurse for the care of a small group of patients is possible with primary nursing. Primary nurse is the bedside nurse with few duties delegated to other nurses. When primary nurse is not working, an associate primary nurse will maintain continuity of care. This system provides better client satisfaction, and they have the privilege to get all necessary information from one person.

At this juncture, maintenance of primary core is essential. To maintain the consistency of care is to designate one primary nurse and as many associates to provide the same – standard of care. Primary nursing is promoted in paediatric care to provide consistent caregivers to care for the child. It also focuses family unit as an integral component of planning and implementing care.

Case Management

It is considered as an extension of primary nursing. It is usually used in outpatient setting by assigning a case manager to a patient or a group of patients. It utilizes time line or critical path or practice guidelines. Variations in timelines are noted to identify delay in provision of care that helps to resolve the problems related to patient system or community. Case management system is widely used in countries where health insurance paying is prevalent. In this system, care delivery needs to be balanced as per cost and quality, i.e. care delivery in a cost-effective manner.

Advantages:
- Improved patient and family satisfaction
- Decreased fragmentation of care
- Ability to describe and measure outcomes for a homogenous group of patients

Case management system utilizes set guidelines that are prepared. Many forms or models of guidelines are used, such as critical path, care maps and standardized care plan.

CHILD-ORIENTED ENVIRONMENT

A child-friendly environment should be provided to a child who is admitted to hospital. Child should be admitted to a children's ward. The outlay of the ward should be one of the child-friendly with adequate safety precautions. Education and facilities for play should be provided. Removing young children from their familiar environment to a strange ward is frightening to the child. It also disrupts family routines not only for the child but also for the siblings and others at home. Staff should be sensitive to the family's individual needs according to the social educational, cultural and religious background. Children's ward should be equipped with skilled staff. There should be a 'named nurse' responsible for planning and coordinating the care by other nurses. Ensure that families receive all information they need and the nurse need to provide a link between the team members as child health care is essentially a multidisciplinary care.

ATRAUMATIC CARE

It is the provision of therapeutic care in settings by personnel and through the use of interventions that eliminates or minimizes the psychological and physical distress experienced by children and their families in the health care system (Whaley and Wong, 1991). Therapeutic care includes the prevention, diagnosis, treatment or palliation of chronic or acute condition, and settings refer to whatever places that care is provided. The concept of atraumatic care is intended to reduce mental and physical harm and to provide an environment with minimum physical and mental trauma. There are three principles to be followed in the provision of atraumatic care – (i) **prevent or minimize the child's separation from family**, (ii) **promote sense of comfort** and (iii) **prevent or minimize bodily injury and pain.** Though there is a tremendous technological advancement in the provision of therapeutic care; the injury and pain produced with this are not reduced. A child who receives therapeutic intervention needs to be treated with tender loving care. By inculcating the above-mentioned principles, atraumatic care encompasses many aspects such as reducing separation anxiety, providing adequate information to care givers and equip them to minimize trauma of hospitalization, preparing parents to utilize positive coping and performing procedures with utmost skill and right attitude. Even the provision of child-oriented environment and skilled staff are essential components of atraumatic care.

Suggested nursing interventions are as follows:
- Foster parent–child relationship during hospitalization
- Prepare the child before any procedure
- Control pain
- Provide child privacy
- Provide play for expression fear and aggression
- Minimize loss of control
- Respect cultural and religious differences especially in Indian set-up

COST CONTAINMENT

CC is a management technique utilized to reduce the cost of hospitalization. It is achieved in many ways in hospitals either by cutting nursing positions or by improving the process of care and tightening nonlabour resources. By reducing the mortality rates, length of stay, costs and complications and by increasing family satisfaction and readiness and ability to function upon discharge, nurses make significant contribution to both the quality of hospital services and the containment of hospital costs. The case management model outlines and activates strategic management of quality patient outcomes and costs. CC strategy transforms primary nurse approach to care managers and changes the focus of nursing process to multidisciplinary outcomes. Cost-effective care will exist only in situations in which the patient is known where there is continuity of care provided by expert caregivers. Excellent results are obtained when nurses provide intuitive, scientific care to patients and families. Like FCC, enabling and empower-

ment are yet another concept followed in CC strategy too where nurses are on the position of expert caregiver helping parents to learn and provide care to their children by obtaining the necessary knowledge and skill from nurses.

HEALTH PROMOTION AND ILLNESS PREVENTION

Preventing ill health and promoting good health and early intervention for illness provide good outcome. This promotes healthy individual by 2020. The national health programmes and the national health policy 2015 emphasize on illness prevention and health promotion through various national programmes (refer Chapter 3). One should be able to provide safe and sustainable services, public–private partnership and provider–recipient partnership, etc. are very important. Workforce education training should give adequate emphasis on preventive programmes and health promotion activities, such as importance of nutrition, growth monitoring, prevention of communicable diseases, etc. They should be trained to use evidence and knowledge available and use proper technology for providing quality services to children and young people. Inequality in service provision also should be taken into consideration.

Other important practice issues requiring more attention include increased number of children requiring mental health services, increased number of children getting hospital admission due to lack of primary care facilities, increased prevalence of autism among children and increased incidence of obesity, diabetes and asthma.

LEGAL ASPECTS IN PAEDIATRIC NURSING PRACTICE

Legal requirements for paediatric nursing practice exist to assure the health, safety and welfare of children seeking health care. There are a host of legal requirement that paediatric nurse must know to provide legally acceptable care to child. The following are important points regarding legal issues in caring children in a health care facility.

Consent

Informed consent for medical care is a basic requirement that should be met in almost all practitioner–patient relationships. Section 13 of Indian Contract Act 1872 defined the consent as 'when two or more person agree upon the same thing in the same sense they are said to consent'. Consent for treatment can be given by a person who is conscious, mentally sound and older than 18 years. A conscious adult has the right to refuse treatment. Potential legal and ethical conflicts arise with consent when the patient is a **minor**. Paediatric practice deals with minors, and minors are not legally permitted to give consent for their own care based on their level of emotional maturity and cognitive development. An individual under the age of majority that is below the ages of 18 in all states of India is a minor. This definition is adopted by the Department of Health and Family Welfare and Ministry of Civil Services. The concept of informed consent has its limitation to paediatric practice. Hence two other concepts are inherently applied as parental permission and patient assent. According to the American Academy of Paediatrics, physicians have an ethical (and legal) obligation to obtain parental permission to perform medical interventions on a child. In many circumstances, physicians should also solicit an assent from children when developmentally appropriate. In cases involving emancipated or mature minors (as described in the US law) with adequate decision-making capacity, physicians should seek informed consent directly from them.

Consent for minors for any treatment is obtained from legal guardians routinely. The legal guardians are those who take care of children and are called as in loco parentis. Loco parentis includes adult relatives, foster parents, biological father of illegitimate child, persons designated by the parents or state officials designated by child welfare services of the juvenile court. **This is allowed in presumption that** they would use a 'best interest standard' and their consent for minors for treatment is accepted as valid. Parental consent generally expected when a minor seeks health care services.

Exceptions are provided to minors who seek help in the following conditions:
- Mental health services
- Pregnancy and contraceptive services
- Treatment and testing for sexually transmitted diseases and HIV/AIDS
- Drug or alcohol dependency
- Abuse of various types

Consent is not required for treatment in the following situations:
- Medical emergencies
- Notifiable diseases – This is for the best interest of public/society
- Immigrants who need medical care or need mandatory medical or health check-up and treatment
- New admission to prisons
- Court orders for examination and treatment
- Under section 53 (1) of Cr.P.C., a person can be examined on request of the police by use of force
- Members of the armed forces

Issues with Consent in Paediatric Emergency Department

Though emergency department (ED) professionals want to provide competent care in a timely manner to serve the best interest of their patient, sometimes they may get caught up with the issue of consent. They want to prevent progression of treatable disease and reduce pain and suffering. Delay in getting consent can prevent ED physicians from providing timely evaluation and care. Limitation to access of care should not be permitted. In such situation, Indian law permit professionals to provide emergency medical care to the needy even if there is no competent authority to provide consent using principles like that of Good Samaritan Law.

Act done in good faith for benefit of a person without consent is permitted by the Section 92 of Indian Penal Code. It says 'Nothing is an offence by reason of any harm which it may cause to a person for whose benefit it is done in good faith, even without that person's consent, if the circumstances are such that it is impossible for that person to signify consent, or if that person is incapable of giving consent, and has no guardian or another person in lawful charge of him from whom it is possible to obtain consent in time for the thing to be done with benefit.' But this must be ascertained.

Participation in Clinical Trial and Research

Children under 18 are not adults in the eyes of the law; therefore, legal permission for their participation must be given by their parents or guardians after going through the informed consent process on their behalf. So, many people involved in treating young people believe that the child or adolescent should be given a role in the decision to participate in a research study. It is accepted that children at age 7 and above should involve in decision-making to provide assent in participating in a clinical trial or research. It is felt that most children at this age can understand if information is tailored to their knowledge and developmental level. Children cannot give a consent as they cannot always comprehend the intent of treatment fully, they may be asked whether they agree (assent) for the treatment or disagree (dissent). The parents most of the time provide and informed permission rather than a consent.

The Assent Process

Institutional review board will usually provide the documentation process of assent or dissent in any institution. Assent may not be required if the child is not capable of participating in decision-making. In doing research , a researcher need not require an assent from the child if a study provides a treatment that is a better option than the existing one or if it is the only alternative.

MALPRACTICE IN CHILD HEALTH

When thinking about malpractice nurses must remember the following. In India, public suing nurses for malpractices is on the rise. They need to be cognizant about their professional responsibility towards their client as well as citizen responsibility in providing quality care to clients under their care whether in emergency or otherwise. Please remember that:
Nursing is a calling
Nursing is a profession
Nurses care sick whichever may be the setting
Nurses take remuneration for the care
People who take remuneration are bound to duty
If duty is not met standards, they get sued
 Adapted from (A. Beevi)
Factors in malpractice actions in the paediatric practice
- Limited communication skills of young patients
- Must rely on parents/legal guardian for history
- Family members with a different set of interpretations and concerns provide information depending on their perceptions
- Difficult physical examination

- Lack of cooperation from the children and guardians
- Issues of consent
- Long waiting time
- Lack of rapport with children, their parents and relatives
- If the nurses are performing their role as patient advocate, maintain confidentiality of the treatment and if work for the best interest of the patient malpractice litigations can be prevented. Nurses should remember that the four major elements in any malpractice are duty, breach of duty, harm and causation. They should know the implications of these four elements clearly.

THE EMERGENCY MEDICAL TREATMENT AND ACTIVE LABOR ACT 1986 (EMTALA – USA)

The Act brought legal terms and responsibilities to inter-hospital transfer. This act prevented dumping of patients in emergency to other places to avoid legal issues. In India, most of the private hospitals transfer patients to government hospitals to avoid their legal issues. Some time without any criteria also patients are transferred. The USA also had this problem. In order to overcome this situation, the US Congress passed this law in the year 1986. Interhospital transfer is allowed if the transferring facility does not have the capability to stabilize the patient and the benefits outweigh the risk of transfer. This is also done when a patient and legal guardian requests for transfer.

EMTALA Requirements for Legal Transfer

The following are some of the legal requirements for inter-hospital transfer

- The transferring hospital provides medical treatment within its capacity that minimizes the risks to the patient (and unborn child).
- The receiving hospital (a) has available space and qualified personnel for the treatment; and (b) has agreed to accept transfer and to provide appropriate treatment.
- The transferring hospital sends all medical records (history, examination findings, results of diagnostic tests, provisional diagnosis, and treatment provided) that are available at that time; the informed written consent or certification as required by EMTALA.
- The transfer is effected through qualified personnel and transportation equipment to provide life support measures during the transfer.

Hospital obligations

- Those institutions with specialized capabilities are obligated to accept transfers from hospitals who lack the capability to treat unstable emergency medical condition (EMC).
- Must report to the state survey agency any time it may have received in an unstable EMC from another hospital.

Penalties

- Hospital may be sued for personal injury in civil court under a 'private course of action'. The receiving facility can bring suit to recover damages.

- An EMTALA violation can be cited without adverse outcome to the patient.
- No EMTALA violation can be cited if the patient refuses examination and/or treatment.

EMTALA – What about the kids?

- Because the treatment of fractures, infections and other conditions may broadly be considered as the prevention of disabling complications or EMC requiring therapy, many centres currently treat all children arriving in the ED, 'even if unaccompanied by a parent or caretaker'.
- The medical examination and the stabilization of the child with an identified EMC must not be delayed.

Supreme Court Ruling, 1989: Pt Parmanand Katara *v.* The Union Government of India

According to the ruling of supreme court in the above case, 'all government hospitals, medical institutes should be asked to provide the immediate medical aid to all the cases irrespective of the fact whether they are medico legal cases or otherwise. The practice of certain Government institution to refuse even the primary medical aid to the patient and referring them to other hospitals simply because they are medico legal cases is not desirable. However after providing the primary medical aid to the patient, patient can be referred to other hospital if the expertise facilities required for the treatment are not available in the institution.'

CONSOLIDATED OMNIBUS BUDGET RECONCILIATION ACT 1986 (COBRA)

US Congress enacted this to prevent the practice of dumping of patient by private hospitals. The hospital must perform a medical screening examination of all prospective patients regardless of their ability to pay, and if the hospital must determine that a patient suffers from an emergency condition, the law requires the hospital to stabilize the condition, and the hospital cannot transfer/ discharge an un-stabilized patient unless the transfer or discharge is appropriate as defined by the Act.

CONSUMER PROTECTION ACT, GOVERNMENT OF INDIA, 1986

Supreme Court of India ruled who all are covered under the Act and held as follows:
- Service rendered for fee
- Service rendered for free to some and for fee to others
- Service rendered is paid by insurance company
- The employer bears the expenses for service rendered to an employee

CONSTITUTION OF INDIA ARTICLE 21

Every health professional must be aware of this act. It says 'No person shall be deprived of his life or personal liberty except according to procedure established by law.' Any individual whether they belong to health care profession or not they should abide to this act to save life of injured.

GUIDELINES DEALING WITH EMERGENCY CASES

i) In the hospital, the medical officer in the emergency/casualty services should admit a patient whose condition is morbid/serious in consultation with the specialist concerned on duty in the ED.

ii) In case the vacant beds are not available in the concerned department to accommodate such patient, the patient has to be given all necessary attention.

iii) Subsequently, the medical officer will make necessary arrangement to get the patient transferred to another hospital in the ambulance. The position as to whether there is vacant bed in the concerned department has to be ascertained before transferring the patient. The patient will be accompanied by the resident medical officer in the ambulance.

iv) In no case the patient will be left unattended for want of vacant beds in the emergency/casualty department.

v) The services of CATS should be utilized to the extent possible in Delhi.

vi) The efforts may be made to monitor the functioning of the ED periodically by the heads of the institution.

vii) The medical record of patient attending the emergency services should be preserved in the medical record department.

viii) The medical superintendent may coordinate with each other for providing better emergency services.

GUIDELINES FOR MAINTENANCE OF ADMISSION REGISTER OF PATIENT

a) Clear recording of the name, age, sex, address and disease of the patient by the attending medical officer.

b) Clear recording of the date and time of attendance, examination/admission of the patient.

c) Clear indication whether and where the patient has been admitted, transferred and referred

d) Safe custody of the registers.

e) Periodical inspection of the arrangement by the superintendent.

f) Fixing of responsibility of maintenance and safe custody of the registers.

GUIDELINES TO IDENTIFY THE INDIVIDUAL MEDICAL OFFICER ATTENDING TO THE INDIVIDUAL PATIENT

a) A copy of the duty roster of the medical officers/nurses should be preserved in the office of the superintendent incorporating the modifications done for unavoidable circumstances.

b) Each department shall maintain a register for recording the signature of attending medical officers denoting their arrival and departure time.

c) The attending medical officer/nurse shall write his/her full name clearly and put his/her signature in the treatment document.

d) The superintendents of the hospital shall keep all such records in safe custody.

e) A copy of the ticket issued to the patient should be maintained or the relevant date in this regard should be noted in an appropriate record for future guidance.

Refusal of Care – What Is Required?

- Competent minor/parents refusal of care can be addressed asking three questions:
- Is the treatment necessary in the foreseeable future?
  - If no, may be discharged home with appropriate, specific follow-up
  - May entail child protective services
- Is the treatment needed in the immediate future?
  - Court orders directly from judicial official or child protective services may be obtained
- Is there an immediate need for medical intervention?
  - Consider medical condition as emergency and treat
- Crucial that documentation on the medical chart indicates assessment of
  - The need for consent.
  - If indicated, determination of the parties approached for consent.
  - Measures taken to obtain an informed consent.
  - Identification and resolution of conflict.

Why Families Sue Physicians and Nurses

- Poor outcome
- Poor communication, want more information
- Seek revenge against physician and nurses
- Need to obtain financial resources
- Wish to protect society from 'bad doctor'/nurse
- Desire to relieve guilt
- Greed

Risk Management Techniques

- Listen to People
- Be nice to people
  - Consider sitting for interview
  - Address the child when age appropriate
  - Acknowledge the parents' fears
- Be careful how you say things!!! } Should not be used
  - 'He just has a virus'
  - 'Don't worry he'll be fine'
  - Address the specifics of the condition, expected progression and possible complications

Risk Management Techniques – The Chart

Documentation of all pertinent information of the patient. It should show all positive and negative information concerning assessment, treatment and diagnostic procedures. All entries should be clear, complete, free of flippant, critical or other in appropriate comments. There are particular guidelines and format for documentation in all good hospitals. Every employee should follow the guidelines of concerned documentation. They should use only approved terminology and abbreviations in documents.

All employees should treat as the most important person in the hospital; priority must be given to patient safety and satisfaction.

Remember:
- Parents' wishes are respected but not children's
- Our law does not favour children's involvement in consent
- Nurses can be influential in supporting parents during the process of consent
- Decisions may be based ethical concepts and respect towards individual and human rights.

ETHICAL PRINCIPLES

Ethics is a system of rules or principles that are used to guide human behaviour. Doing no harm and benefiting others in a loyal and truthful manner is the core of ethics. The purpose of code of ethics is to provide strong, understandable, specific and non-negotiable statement of nursing ethical obligation and duty to patients and members of the community. Respect for autonomy which is a norm of respecting the decision-making capabilities of autonomous people. Nonmaleficence is a norm of avoiding causation or harm. Beneficence which is a norm of providing the benefits, risks & cost. Justice which is a norm of fairly distributing the benefits, risks & cost

Common Ethical Issues that Nurses Face in Paediatric Nursing Practice

- End of life issues
- Organ donation with brain death
- Organ donation with cardiac death
- Abortion
- Teen pregnancy
- DNR vs Do not treat
- Quality vs quantity of life
- Family/social issues/ abuse
- Drug abuse
- Advance directives
- Suicide attempt
- Florence Nightingale's oath and its four promises have an impact on nursing practice.
- Four promises:
  - To live a pure life
  - Practice faithfully
  - Not to administer any harmful drug
  - Maintain and elevate the standard of the profession

Along with these issues, there are many questions that need to be answered when considering ethical principles applied to paediatric practice. These are as follows:
- How much information should be disclosed about child's care and treatment to parents/ relatives?
- Whether unfair share of society's resources are utilized for their care especially when there are decreased resources?

- Whose decision should be considered- Doctors, nurses or parents?
- Whether treatment needs to be provided in lethal diseases?

The common ethical principles the nurse must understand while caring children are same as that of adults and corresponds to medical ethics. The main ethical principles are as follows:
- Nonmaleficence – Do no harm.
- Beneficence – Do good.
- Justice – there are three aspects: legal justice, respect for rights and fair distribution of resources even the nurses time and attention.
- Respect for autonomy – Respect the individual's rights to make informed and thought out decisions for themselves.
- Truth telling – this is actually a subset of autonomy.

Application of Ethical Principles to Child Health Nursing

Nonmaleficence – Children are more vulnerable to harm. This includes their suffering from fear of procedures and they may not be able to express it verbally related to their developmental level. A nurse who does not have adequate training on child health nursing may not be able to identify the harm they may create to children. For example, the nurse who does not have skill in performing the technique of restraining a child for a procedure may sustain an injury to the child. Thus, lack of skill and knowledge also can cause harm.

Beneficence – Child's interest needs to be considered as the most important one. The nurse as any other health worker has to report a suspected child abuse if she/he suspect the same for the best interest of the child. This may be in conflict with parental interest. Reporting of battered child syndrome is also done as beneficence.

Justice – every child should have equal opportunity for access to health care services without creed, caste, religion, colour, etc.

Autonomy – Children under 18 years are considered minor in India. Parents are trusted to make decisions on behalf of their children as usually they act in the best interest of their children.

Truth telling–Though it is easy to reassure children falsely that procedures will not hurt. In future, when they find this to be untrue, trust will be lost. False promises also should not be given to children.

Ethical Issues Associated with Research

Research with therapeutic as well as non-therapeutic intervention in children needs to be conducted with certain safeguards as:
- Properly informed consent from responsible parent/ adults. As per the Indian Penal Code rules, informed consent of the parent (informed parental permission) and consent of the older children (assent)should be obtained for any procedure except in emergency where a Good Samaritan Rule work out. The legal age of consent to medical treatment is 18 years. Young

children should be provided with as much information as possible in language they can understand.

- With very small risks that are generally encountered and acceptable in everyday life.
- In exceptional circumstances where the benefits from research are sufficiently greater than the risk.
- The research that cannot be done in adults.

Conceptual Issues

The contemporary medical practice considers autonomy as the central principle. Since, its purpose is to allow competent patient to make their own health care decisions, e.g. refusing life-saving care for religious reasons, in children whether we can consider this as the central principle? This is very essential to have public opinion as there occurred many occasion of rejection of treatment from the part of parents.

Competence

Concept of competence is intertwined with autonomy. Only the competent patients are given the right to make decisions regarding their health care. This may be considered in the case of mature minor or emancipated minors and minors seeking medical help in exceptional cases like sexually transmitted diseases, HIV, mental illness, etc.

Beneficence

This refers to duties to avoid harm as well as to advance the welfare of others. Do no harm is the basis of this principle.

Paternalism

This is defined as interfering with the liberty of another person for his/her own benefit. This is considered as duty of parents in our country.

Truth telling

It is a requisite for any moral community. Active lying is not good. Respect of this principle is essential as children live in the present and lying with them hampers the development of trust in them.

Confidentiality

Maintaining confidentiality in treatment and other socially provoking issues are essential part of compassionate medical and nursing ethics. Certain parts of the practice need to be properly kept in confidence of the practitioners. Otherwise, there will be many social issues that may develop as the one happened recently in Kerala regarding the AIDS children.

Conflicts of interests

Child patients are usually represented by someone else, and there is a chance of conflicts of interests.

STUDY QUESTIONS

1. Briefly describe the historical development of paediatric nursing as a specialty.
2. What are the trends in paediatric nursing practice?
3. Describe the common legal issues that a paediatric nurse faces in a hospital.
4. Explain the ethical issues that may confront during child health nursing practice.
5. How does the Consumer Protection Act affect child health nursing practice?
6. What are the cultural issues that affect child health in different parts of India?
7. What are the principles of child health nursing? Describe them with suitable examples.
8. What are the risk management techniques that help a health worker to avoid suing in the court?

BIBLIOGRAPHY

1. Ahmann, E. (1994). Family Centred Care: Shifting Orientation. *Paediatric Nursing, 20*(2), 113–117.
2. Allen, M., Jacobs, S. K., & Levy, J. R. (2006). Mapping the literature of nursing. 1996-2000. *J Med Libr Assoc, 94*(2), 206–220. (PMC free article) (Pub Med)
3. Blake, F. G. (1954). *The child, his parents and the nurse.* Philadelphia, PA: JB Lippincott.
4. Cone, T. E. (1979). *History of American pediatrics.* Boston, MA: Little, Brown.
5. Cone, T.E., Jr. (1985). *History of the Care and Feeding of the Premature Infant.* Boston: Little Brown Free VD.
6. Feeg, V. D. Paediatric Nursing- not "med-surg nursing" on little people. (1995). *Pediatr Nurs, 21*(6), 500. (Pub Med)
7. Heller, R., & McKlindon, D. (1996). Families as Faculty: Parents Educating Care givers About Family Centered Care. *Pediatric Nursing, 22*(5), 428–431.
8. Kalisch, P. A., & Kalisch, B. J. (2004). *American nursing: a history.* (4th ed.). Philadelphia, PA: Lippincott Williams & Wilkins.
9. Pearson, H.A. (1988). *The Centennial History of the American Pediatrics Society.* New Haven: American Pediatric Society.
10. Roland, B. S. (1968). Observations on Current Trend in Paediatric Education and Practice". *Journal of the National Medical Association. J Natl Med Assoc.* 1968 Nov; 60(6): 500–504.
11. Spiro, H., Curnen, M. G. M., Peschel, E., & St. James, D. (1993). *Empathy and The Practice of Medicine.* New Haven, CT: Yale University.
12. Wald L.D. (1915). *The house of Henry Street.* New York, NY: H Holt.
13. Wong, D. L., Hockenberry, M. J., Wilson, D., Winkelstein, M. L. & Kline, N. E. (2003). *Wong's nursing care of infants and children.* (p. 15). St. Louis, MO: Mosby.

CHAPTER 2

DIFFERENCE BETWEEN ADULT NURSING AND CHILD NURSING

LEARNING OBJECTIVES

At the end of the chapter, the learner will be able to:
- Appreciate the difference between adult nursing and child nursing practices.
- Describe the rights of children as a special and vulnerable group.
- Explain the qualities, roles and functions of a child health nurse.

In contrast to the nursing of adults, child health nursing deals with individuals who are going through a rapid change. They include the following groups: a neonate is a baby between 0 and 28 days of age; an infant is a child up to 12 months of age; a child is 1–12 years of age; an adolescent is 13–16 years of age. For example, for a newborn, a 3-fold increase in length and 20-fold increase in weight occurs as it becomes an adult. Child nursing is entirely different from adult nursing in many respects, though the principles of nursing techniques may be the same. As is known, it is a specialty which demands the services of experienced, skilful and well-qualified personnel devoted to the care of children. Children are not miniature adults. Those who are caring for children must bear in mind that adults have completed the period of growth and development and are either in the middle of their lifespan or in a phase of the aging process.

Usually for easy understanding and for the provision of expert nursing care, the differences are classified as anatomical, physiological and psychological differences.

ANATOMICAL DIFFERENCES

Size is the outstanding difference when considering anatomical differences. It is a criterion that paediatric nurses

usually use when choosing a right method of care and equipment for child nursing. The physical set-up of a ward should be designed in a way to accommodate a number of children of various age groups. In an adult ward, we see that the cots are all of the same size and one or two of the same sizes may have side railing for nursing care of seriously ill adults or adults with altered level of consciousness. In a paediatric ward, we see different-sized cots so as to accommodate children of different sizes and various age groups. Thus, in a paediatric ward, there are cradles, cribs, cots with side rails, small pillows, weighing machines, medication cups of different sizes and shape, etc.

Another anatomical difference is the greater size and weight of the newborn's head as compared with body length and weight. This characteristic along with his/her immature motor development makes handling of an infant different from that of an older child or an adult. Because of immaturity and inadequate ossification, an injury can occur to the head of an infant from a fall more easily than in an adult. If you compare the size of the head with the total body size, the head of a newborn is one-fourth of its body size; in a 6-year-old child, it is one-sixth and in an adult, it is one-eighth.

The sutures of the skull are not united. The ossifications of the skull bones are not completed. The fontanels are not closed, and the brain is not protected at the areas of fontanels. The anterior fontanel closes only at 18 months of life. The infant's bones are neither firm nor brittle as in the case of an adult. Therefore, when the intracranial pressure increases in the infant, the head enlarges and he/she may exhibit other signs of increased intracranial pressure.

The normal shape of the head and chest of the infant can be altered by constant pressure from lying in one position. Thus, a nurse or parents who take care of the baby must be vigilant to change the position of the child frequently. This will prevent deformity of the bones and help to maintain the normal shape and configuration of the infant's body alignment. Until puberty, the percentage of cartilage in ribs is higher, making them more flexible and compliant. Until puberty, the bones are soft and can be easily bent and fractured. Muscle lack bone power and coordination during infancy. Muscles are 25% of weight in an infant, and it is 40% in an adult. There are many differences in body systems and organs. These differences determine the manner in which nursing care is given.

Mouth

The infant's tongue is large, and the nasal and oral airway passages are relatively small, making the infant more prone to airway obstruction. Infants are obligatory nose breathers up to 6 months of age; this creates further difficulty in breathing during respiratory infections. There will not be tears in the eyes of the infant in early infancy. This is related to poor functional development of the lachrymal gland and ducts. No tears when crying make the eye susceptible to infection. Nose will have milia related to blockage in the sebaceous glands.

Stomach

In adults, cardiac sphincter of the stomach is fairly tight, whereas in infants, it is relaxed. This is the reason for frequent vomiting during infancy and for adults having difficulty in vomiting even when they are nauseated. So the nurse should see the position of the infant while feeding and should burp the child after feeding to let out the swallowed gas. Abdomen offers poor protection to the liver and the spleen, making them susceptible to trauma easily.

Eustachian Tube

It is both short and straight in young children than that in the older children or adults. Air sinuses are not fully developed. Any sore throat will cause otitis media because of the structure of the Eustachian tube. This infection can lead to severe complications and infection of the brain. Therefore, frequent upper respiratory tract infections should be prevented and treated on time. Because of proximity of the Eustachian tube to the upper respiratory tract, infection in any part of the Eustachian tube will also be carried to the upper or lower respiratory tract.

Trachea

Short, narrow *trachea* in children younger than 5 years makes them susceptible to foreign body aspiration.

Height and Weight

The *height* and *weight* of a child have a greater influence on the management of the child during illness. Intravenous fluids or medicines administered in children can easily cause pedal oedema in children, especially children with congenital heart diseases. Therefore, rate flow must be adjusted appropriately. In a child, the dose of medicines and amount of fluids are calculated on the basis of body weight and surface area.

A smaller stress in an older child may lead to organ failure, and so also in an infant. However, because of the capacity of the small ones to grow and regenerate tissue, there may be little or no residual damage to a child's physiological potential. Interdependence of body systems will lead to failure in other systems. The rate of change that is seen in a severely dehydrated baby from gastroenteritis is to the extent that peripheral circulatory failure occurs within 24 hours.

Growth as a Stabilizing Mechanism

By utilizing energy substrate for the process of growth, the load presented to the excretory pathways is decreased. For example, an infant's kidney can cope with the daily excretory load, as a large proportion of the daily intake of food is used for growth of cells.

PHYSIOLOGICAL DIFFERENCES

The physiological differences are more evident between a neonate and an adult. Let us examine the important physiological differences in these age groups which will equip a paediatric nurse to deliver expert care to his/her clients.

Absolute Measurements

Rapid loss of 35 mL of blood by a newborn baby represents 10% of the blood volume. This much loss can lead to circulatory failure in an infant but of little significance when applied to an adult. Thus, loss of small volumes can also lead to a serious outcome or problem in an infant.

Basal Metabolic Rate

Basal metabolic rate (BMR) increases rapidly after delivery and is high in the newborn period. This is mainly because of the rapid consumption of energy – related to cell growth and the increased requirement for heat production. In a neonate, a value of 6–8 mL of oxygen/kg/min is normal. Then BMR decreases rapidly over the first 18 months of life to 2 years. It slowly reaches the adult value of 2–4 mL oxygen/kg/min at the time of puberty. Carbon dioxide production is increased as a consequence of the increased metabolic rate. It follows a similar course of change to oxygen consumption. Hence, a higher BMR leads to higher oxygen consumption and increases caloric demands.

Temperature Regulation

A newborn is homoeothermic and will mount an appropriate response to a thermal stress. This response is short-lived and inadequate because of the immaturity of the controlling and effecter mechanisms and the adverse physical characteristics of the small child. Poor thermoregulation is attributed to immaturity of the hypothalamus and a large body surface area to weight ratio of the infant. This leads to extremes of temperature in neonates and infants. The transient mottled appearance of the skin when an infant is cold is an outward manifestation of immaturity. Shivering and sweating mechanisms are absent in newborn babies. An infant will not normally shiver in the first few weeks of life so that involuntary heat production from the activity is also not possible.

Brown Adipose Tissue

The newborn is unique in a way that he/she has a small reserve of brown fat from which heat can be liberated by nonshivering thermogenesis. Once used, the brown fat reserve cannot be replaced. So exposure to cold climates needs to be prevented in an infant to preserve the reserve of brown fat. Brown fat is located around the scapula, the mediastinum, the kidneys and adrenal glands and constitutes about 2%–6% of the neonatal body weight.

Central Controlling Mechanisms

The central controlling mechanisms for homoeothermic control are present at birth. This process is functional even in a small premature infant. The time taken for this response is rapid, but the efficacy of the same is rapid, short and inadequate. This is attributed to poor myelination of the central nervous system. The New York skyline appearance of the temperature chart in a toddler with an infection is an example of this. The controlling negative feedback system is still not well developed, and there may be rapid peak-to-peak fluctuations of 3°C over quite short periods even with mild infection. This pattern of the underdamped response is a characteristic of paediatric physiology that will be seen in other body systems as well. The causes of febrile convulsions in infants are attributed to this phenomenon, too.

Voluntary Control

The infants have no voluntary control over the environment or activity. On a cold day, an adult can manipulate the temperature either by wearing warm clothes or by performing some exercises or even using room heaters in order to achieve a state of well-being to maintain normal body temperature. This is quite impossible in an infant. The caretaker needs to think about infants to achieve normal temperature through some manipulations.

Neutral Thermal Environment

A neutral thermal environment has to be provided to infants and children. A neutral thermal environment can be defined as an optimum zone within which a small baby can be cared for with minimum expenditure of energy by temperature regulation. The premature infant needs a higher temperature than a healthy newborn. This can be achieved by caring all premature and sick infants in an incubator which provides accurate control of the thermal environment. Use of radiant warmers in the operation theatre or blanket helps to accommodate with change in the thermal environment. Babies and infants have a large surface area to weight ratio with minimal subcutaneous fat. They have poorly developed shivering, sweating and vasoconstriction mechanisms.

Body Fluids

The fetus and fetal tissues are extremely high in water content. Towards the latter part of gestation, around 90% of the fetal body weight is water. After delivery, the body water content falls such that by the third or fourth day, the percentage reduces to approximately 80% by weight. Forty percent of weight loss is attributed to this.

Proportion of Body Water

Intracellular water changes are relatively little, being 35% by weight in a newborn and rising to 40% quite quickly. Extracellular fluid is strikingly different, being about 40% in the newborn, nearly double that of the adult figure. This large volume of readily exchangeable water is partly present as a buffer zone to protect the child from sudden fluctuations in fluid balance, and it is also readily available to leak out quickly in disease (gastroenteritis) and water conservation is a major physiological problem for the newborn. Until the later school age, the proportion of water in body weight is larger, with more and more water present in extracellular spaces. Daily water exchange rate is much higher.

Blood Volume

In a neonate, the blood volume is 85–90 mL/kg body weight and in an adult, it is 60–70 mL/kg. Looking at these figures, one may not think that there is much difference. However, a neonate weighing 3.5 kg will have a total blood volume of just 300 mL, which is 10% of the infant's total body weight. If it is not replaced, the baby experience circulatory failure. This fact is very important for a paediatric nurse, being the closest caregiver and protector of the child. Therefore, a nurse must remember to give the intravenous fluids or medicines and must record to count for fluid calculation. This will also help the nurse to protect the child from fluid overload. The blood volume of an infant 6 weeks to 2 years of age is 85 mL/kg and for those from 2 years of age to puberty is 80 mL/kg. Transfusion is recommended if there is a loss of 15% of the circulating blood volume.

Principal Sites of Loss

The maximum concentration of urine in a normal newborn period is 800 mOsmol/L. In an adult, the concentration of urine is 1400 mOsmol/L. The premature infant has less ability to concentrate urine and particularly unable to restore sodium, compounding the problems of dehydration and hyponatraemia. The glomerular filtration rate (GFR) and tubular functions are lower in the neonate than in the adult. This is owing to relatively poor blood supply to infant kidney, smaller pore size and lesser filtration power across the nephron. GFR is about 38 mL/min/1.73 m^2 in the newborn, i.e. about one-third of the adult value of 125 mL/min. Until 12–18 months of age, the kidneys do not concentrate urine effectively and do not exert optimal control over electrolyte secretion and absorption.

Alimentary Tract

The resorption of water from the alimentary canal is poorly developed. Mucosal surface of the alimentary canal is so smooth that it needs a longer length to absorb nutrients to enable growth. Even though the bowel is long, the resorption of water from the bowel is very poor and the faeces of the newborn is watery. By 1–2 years of age, the large bowel becomes fully mature. Until then, there will be a loss of water through faeces.

Immaturity of the bowel can make the absorption of certain food material difficult, the commonest being that of disaccharide intolerance. This can, in turn, lead to dehydration. This is possible during the postoperative period in children, particularly in those with bowel surgery. Infection in the gastrointestinal tract also can lead to dehydration and can progress to prerenal failure in 24 hours. If the replacement is inadequate, it will lead to circulatory failure and, in turn, lead to renal failure. A loss of 400 mL of fluid in an adult is insignificant. But a loss of the same amount in a baby of 4 kg weight represents 10% of the body weight, and this degree of dehydration can produce peripheral circulatory failure. Adequate and prompt reporting of such a loss guarantees the 'audacity and accountability of nurses to his/her commitment'.

Hypoglycaemia is a common feature in the stressed infants. So frequent monitoring of glucose is essential. Glycogen is stored in the liver and the myocardium. Hypoglycaemia may lead to a neurological damage. So 10% glucose infusion is indicated in such cases. Usually, hypoglycaemia is iatrogenic in a newborn.

Cardiovascular System

In neonates, the myocardium is less contractile, making the ventricles to be less compliant and less able to generate tension during contraction. This limits the size of stroke volume. Cardiac output is rate dependent. Infants have fixed cardiac output. Vagal parasympathetic tone is dominant, making them prone to bradycardias. Cardiac output is 300–400 mL/kg/min at birth and 200 mL/kg/min within a few months. Sinus arrhythmia is common in children, and other regular rhythms are abnormal.

During fetal life, oxygenated blood is returned from the placenta via the umbilical vein to the right side of the heart. Here, it joins deoxygenated blood returning from the various organ systems of the fetus. Most of the oxygenated blood coming from the placenta through the inferior vena cava reaches the left atrium via the foramen ovale. From there, it is pumped to the head and the neck. Most of the deoxygenated blood returning from the superior vena cava finds its way into the right ventricle and the main pulmonary artery. Approximately four-fifths of the right ventricular output is channelled away from the lungs through the patent ductus arteriosus. This is because of the high pulmonary artery pressure in the fetus. The deoxygenated blood thus returns to the placenta via the descending aorta and the umbilical arteries. After birth, this pattern changes and the lungs take up the function of oxygenation. The patent ductus arteriosus contracts within the first few weeks after birth and gets fibrosed within 2–4 weeks. Foramen ovale closes on the first day of life, as it is pressure dependent but can reopen within the next 5 years if there are pulmonary pressure differences.

Respiratory System

There are many anatomical differences in the airway and lungs that have an impact on the respiratory physiology of newborn infants. The major anatomical airway differences include the tongue that is relatively larger than the adult tongue and is prone to cause airway obstruction. The larynx is cephalad, lying at the C3–C4 level, whereas its position in adults is C4–C5. The epiglottis is narrow and omega-shaped versus the flat and 'U' shaped in the adults. The cricoid ring is the narrowest portion in infants and children up to the age of 4–6 years. After the narrowest portion is the glottis opening. The intrathoracic airways are reasonably well developed including the terminal bronchioles. But the alveolar number and development are incomplete at birth. A full-term infant will have 20–50 million terminal airspaces and are immature alveoli. Lung development occurs rapidly and reaches nearly adult numbers of 300 million alveoli by the age of 3 years. There are only 10% of alveoli at birth and develop over the first 8 years up to the adult numbers. Lung volume of the infant is relatively small compared with the body size. The functional residual capacity is only 25 mL/kg, whereas it is 40–50 mL/kg in older children and adolescents. Lung and chest wall mechanics are very different in newborns and infants. The thoracic cage is soft and compliant, and the outward recoil of the thorax is very low. Neonates use the diaphragm to produce lung expansion. The partial obstruction of the airway as a result of oedema or secretions increases resistance. Low FRC, small airway and poor elastic recoil of the airway make airway closure in neonates and infants, leading to a fatal situation.

The airway is funnel-shaped and narrowest at the level of cricoid cartilage. Trauma to the airway produce oedema, and 1 mm of oedema can narrow the baby's airway by 60%. The muscles of ventilation get easily fatigued because of the low percentage of type 1 muscle fibres in the diaphragm.

Oxygenation

In a fetus, the blood in the carotid artery has a PO_2 of 25–30 mmHg. In an adult, it is 98 mmHg. However, the fetal haemoglobin (70%–90% HbF) can accept more oxygen for a given PO_2 because of the displaced fetal oxyhaemoglobin curve that gets shifted to the left of the adult curve. The fetus also has an increased haemoglobin level of 18–21 g/100 mL of blood which has a haematocrit of 0.6. These two factors allow the fetus to receive adequate supply of oxygen for metabolic needs. Within 3 months, the levels of HbF drop to around 5% and HbA predominates.

Changes in Circulation at Birth

Separation of the placenta and the onset of air breathing lead to major changes in the intracardiac circulation. There will be a rapid fall in the right atrial pressure, as there is no placental return. Pulmonary artery pressure falls by 50% over the first few breaths, making the larger proportion of the ventricular output to go to the lungs. This, in turn, raises the left atrial pressure. The net effect of these processes is the reversal of blood flow from the right atrium to the left atrium, leading to closure of the foramen ovale. When pulmonary pressure falls and left atrial pressure rises, there is a corresponding rise in the left ventricular output and pressure. These changes cause reduction and cessation of flow in the patent ductus arteriosus. These changes take place within a few hours of delivery in a healthy newborn. The foramen ovale, although physiologically closed, may never close anatomically. Closure of patent ductus arteriosus is complete within 6 weeks of age. In a nutshell, the changes after delivery are as follows:

- Foramen ovale closes and becomes fossa ovalis.
- The umbilical vein obliterates to become ligamentum teres.
- Ductus venosus obliterates to become ligamentum teres.
- Patent ductus arteriosus obliterates to ligamentum arteriosum.
- Hypogastric arteries are known as obliterated hypogastric arteries.

Remember: As the ductus and foramen ovale are physiologically closed in the neonatal period, it is possible to reopen these channels when there is hypoxia and acidosis. Hypoxia and acidosis lower systemic arterial pressure and increase pulmonary and right atrial pressure. This can produce a right-to-left shunt in circulation.

Heart Rate

Fetal heart rate is rapid, with an average of 140 and a range of 110–160 beats/min. There is an increase in the heart rate over the first month of life, but it falls steadily over the next few years of life and reaches adult levels by puberty. Beat-to-beat variation of heart rate is marked and is normal in the fetus and young children. Wide fluctuations in the heart rate are an example of an underdeveloped feedback mechanism. Until the late school age and adolescence, cardiac output is rate dependent and not stroke volume dependent. This makes the heart rate more rapid.

Myocardial Contractility

Myocardial syncytium has a low compliance at birth and so the heart cannot respond to a fall in cardiac output by increased contractility. Because of the inelasticity of the myocardial fibre, a neonate cannot cope with a change in preload and this adds to the poor peripheral circulatory control, which, in turn, makes the neonate susceptible to blood or fluid loss.

Electrocardiogram

There is the right ventricular predominance in the electrocardiogram (ECG) at birth. By about 3 months of age, the left ventricle becomes at par with the right ventricle in size and function. Thereafter, the usual left ventricular predominance of the adult begins. It takes several years to mature the heart. So while reading an ECG, it is essential to remember the age of the child.

Functional Residual Capacity

As people think, fetal lung is not inactive, waiting for the first extrauterine breath to begin, but is an actively metabolizing organ like an exocrine gland, being distended by its own secretions – the lung fluid. The production and removal of lung liquid play a part in the maturation of the lung. At about 24 weeks of the intrauterine life, airways will reach the stage of alveolization and development of the terminal sac, which will give sufficient capacity for postnatal survival. After delivery, the lung matures rapidly but only about half of the alveoli are present at birth. This makes life difficult for the premature infant, as it has little reserve capacity. The volume of lung liquid near term is equal to the functional residual capacity (FRC) that the infant will establish after the onset of air breathing. In neonates, the FRC is small compared with total lung capacity. Thus, alveolar instability is a common problem in the newborn.

Breathing Movement

The muscles of respiration are active in utero. This occurs as a preparation for extrauterine life when the lung takes over from the placenta as the organ responsible for gas exchange. In utero, the drive to breathing movement is discontinuous and the control is rudimentary. The establishment of respiration unaided after delivery shows the testing of the system previously.

Pattern of Respiration

Neonates are obligatory nose breathers. The narrow nasal passages are easily blocked by secretions. In total, 50% of airway resistance is produced by blocked nasal passages.

The newborn breathes at a faster rate (35–40/min) than adults. The high rate is in response to the greater metabolic rate and to the immature feedback systems. Tidal volume (TV) remains constant throughout life (7 mL/kg) and is proportional to the weight. The dead space also occupies a constant proportion (one-third) of the TV from the time of delivery. Until about 10 years, there is a faster respiratory rate, fewer and smaller alveoli, and a small lung volume.

Rate versus Volume

There are good anatomical reasons why the newborn utilizes an increased rate rather than TV to meet the oxygen demand.

In the supine infant, the abdominal content invades the chest by pushing up the diaphragm. The lower ribs are more horizontal in the newborn, and the bucket handle activity of the lowermost ribs (responsible for the major portion of quite tidal respiration in adults) is not possible in infants. In older children, after chest wall strengthens and the respiratory muscles develop, recession is always abnormal. The airways are narrow in infants and children. This contributes serious respiratory problems during infections. At about 4–5 years of age, the diaphragm is the primary breathing muscle. Carbon dioxide is not effectively expired when the child is distressed, making the child susceptible to respiratory acidosis.

Renal System

Renal blood flow and glomerular filtration are low in the first 2 years of life. This results from high renal vascular resistance. Immature kidneys are unable to excrete a large sodium load. Urine output is 1–2 mL/kg/hr.

Hepatic Function

In the newborn period, the liver is still immature. The most common example of this is the physiological jaundice that is particularly associated with the premature infant owing to underdevelopment of the glucuronyl transferase system. The enzymes responsible for handling detoxification of drugs are also not at their full capacity. The systems producing albumin, clotting factors and vitamin K are also not well developed, making the newborn susceptible to various risks. Extremely premature infants have a very little reserve for glycogen and a high risk for developing hypoglycaemia. Even full-term infants can develop hypoglycaemia if they are kept starved for more than 6 hours. This is the reason why infants are not allowed to starve for a duration that is more than the normal interval between feeds. In older children, during the preoperative preparation, the period of starvation should not be so long, as the depletion of glycogen stores and lack of fluid intake combine to produce dehydration, ketosis and hypoglycaemia. Iron reserve is also less and is only sufficient to meet the demands up to 6 months of age. Then they need iron supplements to prevent iron deficiency anaemia.

Central Nervous System

Myelination within the central nervous system and the connections of the brain itself are poorly developed at birth. This is attributed to a wide variation in the respiratory rate, heart rate and temperature in a newborn. The process of myelination is not completed until the late teen years. The developmental milestones of childhood are related to the gradual maturation of the cortical connections within the brain. All brain cells are present at birth, but 90% of the brain growth takes place by 2 years of age. Nervous system immaturity accounts for a lack of genetically determined pigmentation in the eyes of a newborn. Nerve endings in the retina (rods and cones) are not fully developed. Images tend to blur and remain colourless until the vision has completed its development a few weeks later. Narcotics depress the respiratory centre. The blood–brain barrier is poorly formed, and narcotics cross the blood–brain barrier easily. The cerebral vessels in preterm infants are very fragile. They are prone to interventricular haemorrhage.

Pain Relief in Children

Children produce physiological response to pain even if there is poor myelination of the central nervous system. Myelination is incomplete; it follows that the blood–brain barrier is less efficient, at least up to 2 years of age. Fat-soluble drugs permeate more freely into cells in the brain in this age group. Particularly under the age of 6 months, analgesics of the opiate group gain ready access to the central nervous system and may produce respiratory depression at a low dosage. Because the excretory pathways in the liver and kidneys are immature, detoxification of the opiates is also delayed in infancy. Because of these reasons, the neonate/infant needs a much smaller dose than an adult. The nurse who is caring for a neonate/infant receiving opiate must institute respiratory monitoring and must be capable to intervene during respiratory failure. Remember that reduction in the dose and increase in time between doses are general rules for the administration of any drug to a neonate or young child.

Response to Trauma

About 30%–70% of paediatric deaths result from head injuries. Compared with adults, the large size of the head and relatively weak neck muscles and lax ligaments, thinner skull bones and more vascular scalp contribute to this. The infant spine has shallow facet joints, and the underdeveloped spinous process is less stiff and has a greater range of motion. Children can sustain spinal cord injuries without radiographic abnormalities. Children have a larger occiput. They are at risk of intra-abdominal injuries because of large-sized spleen, liver and greater flexibility of ribs. Children's bones are more porous, have less volumetric bone mineral density and have less compressive strength, making them prone to fractures. Trauma is one of the greatest contributors of childhood mortality.

Paediatric Differences that Affect Nursing Care Modifications with Clinical Implications in a Nutshell

Anatomical Structure	Physical Development Parameters	Clinical Implications that Affect Nursing Care
Head	Rapid growth mainly as a result of brain expansion (hypertrophy)	By the end of first year, two-thirds of adult size that makes nurses vigilant about supporting the head
	Relatively a large head compared with the body	Rapid assessment for hydration status and intracranial pressure
	Open anterior fontanel until 14–18 months of age	Nasal obstruction leads to marked respiratory distress
	Preferential nose breathing in infants <2 months of age	
Neck	Short and narrow trachea (narrowest portion is the cricoid cartilage).	Partial airway obstructions lead to marked compromise in airflow
	Soft cartilaginous larynx	Flexion and hyperextension will compress the airway
	Relatively hypermobile upper cervical spine and weak neck musculature	Upper cervical spine injuries from accelerative and torsional stresses
Chest	Intercostal muscles are poorly developed; sternum and ribs are highly elastic	Rapid fatigue to respiratory muscles
		Low risk for fractures but significant underlying injuries to the internal organs
	Primary muscle of respiration is the diaphragm	Retractions are common and lead to increased work of breathing
		Abdominal breathing is normal in an infant or a young child; pressure from above or below the hyperexpanded lungs will compromise effective respiration
Cardiovascular	Fixed stroke volume	Cardiac output is very much rate dependent
		Tachycardia increases cardiac output only marginally in the infant
		Bradycardia causes significant decrease in cardiac output
Abdomen	Comparatively large liver and spleen, poor chest and abdominal muscle protection	Increased risk of abdominal injuries owing to blunt trauma
Extremities	Open epiphysis of the long bones	When fractures develop, they are frequently at the epiphysis and may be difficult to see on the X-ray film
Skin	Large surface area to volume ratio	High risk of environmental heat loss, hyperthermia and susceptible to insensible loss of fluid and dehydration
Neurologic	Rapid changes in cognitive, language and motor skills	Age-specific assessment of the neurologic system may be conducted, and the nurse should have a thorough knowledge of milestones of development of children at each age

PSYCHOLOGICAL DIFFERENCES

Children are not miniature adults. Each child is born with his/her own instincts and unique characteristics. Normal children differ widely in behaviours. Normal expected pattern of behaviour is too narrowly defined. A child's behaviour, emotional responses and personality are the end result of interactions between genetic predisposition and environmental influences. The *temperaments* of children are also different, and depending on temperament, they are classified as easy children, difficult children and slow warm-up children. Children are unique, and they differ from each other in personality, e.g. in their physical appearance. So the nurse needs to understand that a particular framework of practice may not work with children in providing care as in adults. Below 5 years of age, a young child thinks in a way quite different from that of an adult. Children use many mental mechanisms to handle their responses to stress. All children frequently respond to their fears by trying to avoid, escape or resist intrusions of any type or any reason by strangers. Children resist procedures/treatment for any reason, too. Children in

pain may not even report pain with a fear of injections or other pain-relieving measures, as they fear the interventions more than the pain they suffer. If this fear can be blown over, then the next response will be curiosity. In a safe situation, children love to see new things, learn how things (equipment) work and explore the immediate surroundings. The nurse providing comprehensive child-centred care to his/her paediatric clients should utilize these characteristics of children.

Unlike adults, each stage of development in a child has its own characteristics and their behaviour also differ according to the age. The nurse needs to have an understanding of the psychological aspects of children at each stage of development to provide atraumatic care to them.

A child's mind works in different ways in each stage, as has been described by Piaget. He explained that cognitive ability develops in a fixed sequence of qualitatively different stages. A child's logic is different from that of an adult. Insecurity coincides with the child's increasing cognitive and motor abilities. Bear this in mind while explaining facts related to preparation of children for treatment and procedures. The nurse must be able to help parents to see an episode of problem behaviour from the child's perspective that can often improve a behaviour problem.

Understanding the psychosexual development, as explained by Freud in five stages with different parts of the body serving the focus of gratification, will help the nurse to identify the discomfort in children. It will help the nurse to resolve the discomfort by promoting the rational ego to find ways to achieve gratification.

During infancy, bonding and attachment are the two important features that decide the future reasonable psychosocial development of a child. Both these term denotes the affection and relationship between parents and infants. *Bonding* is unidirectional and occurs shortly after birth. It reflects the feelings of the parents towards the newborn. Attachment is a reciprocal feeling between the parents and the infant and develops gradually over a period of time. Attachment to a specific, stable parent figures is crucial for a child's normal mental and physical development.

Infants younger than 6 months are not usually upset by separation from their parents and will readily accept a stranger.

At about 6 months of age, the baby seeks the presence of his/her mother. By about this age, the baby shows separation anxiety. The baby may experience fear, pain and unhappiness if he/she is separated from his/her mother. The baby may not be willing to be with the nurse or repel the nurse's presence as he/she is a stranger. The sensitive responsiveness of the mother or attachment figure is essential to prevent the development of mistrust. Development of trust is essential, as it forms the prototype for future close relationships. This is the reason why rooming in is promoted when a young child is hospitalized. Absence of an attachment figure along with strange surroundings and procedures, stress of pain or illness, makes the infant double distressed. Maternal separation also causes anxiety and altered behaviours.

A 6-month-old child clings and hides his/her head in his/her mother's shoulders. It is quite common and relies on parents comforting activities or explanations for any unexpected. The infant who does not protest might be an indication of serious illness or lack of attachment to caretakers.

Infants learn to feel safe and trust the environment. This trust develops from the mother's appropriate reliable response to the infant's needs. Infant's body image is at a feeling level only in response to comfort or discomfort, hunger or satiation. Somatosensory stimulations such as touch, cuddling and play help the infant develop a healthy body image. Meeting infants' immediate needs for relief of hunger, relief of discomfort, sleep and need to suck makes them comfortable. Infants have little tolerance when these are not met. They cannot wait for these needs to be met at a later time or stage as in adults. Infants are developing senses, integrating environmental stimuli and performing purposeful movements. Older infants show signs of separation anxiety as well as stranger anxiety. Children up to 4 years of age are upset as a result of separation from parents or significant others.

Toddlers are probably the most difficult children to handle because of their negativistic feelings or behaviours. They are also the most likely group to experience short- and long-term effects of trauma because their memories of incidents are often confused and distorted.

Preschoolers often appear to have a better comprehension of the situation than toddlers. However, they may misunderstand common words and frequently distrust explanation. Preschoolers' short attention span and imagination makes them responsive to distraction. Attributing life to inanimate objects and interest in stories and fables also make them lovable and manageable. They fear separation in a stressful and strange setting and are more trusting of parents' presence. Their initiative promotes relaxation, cooperation and participation to achieve self-control. Accepting help is a means of coping and promotes emotional growth and independence. *Elementary school children* can comprehend simple situations and requests and generally cooperate with the changing situation. These children also have a fear of unknown and the nonjudgemental atmosphere. They are upset by the surgical procedures, its mutilating effects and the pain. Parental anxiety can be readily identified by children, and they react accordingly.

Adolescents are more concerned about their identity and love peers' company. They are at a period of emotional turbulence. Independence should not hamper, and more freedom must be provided with adequate guidance. These children do not welcome authority of adult figures. They fear narcosis, pain, loss of control and coping difficulties.

Providing age-appropriate care that promotes proper psychological and emotional development of children is a challenge to paediatric nurses. All-round development of children should be the motto rather than providing mere care and health promotion activities. Provision of emotional care needs to be promoted through the understanding of the emotional foods that a child needs for proper development. The nurse must see that all children under his/her care are privileged to get the emotional foods. The emotional foods are love and affection, safe motherhood, acceptance, protection, promotion of self-reliance, self-expression, trust, achievements, play, and discipline and guidance. Altogether, children live in the present and they can be easily distracted unlike adults. They will not carry grudge. Unlike adults, children are better patients to care for.

QUALITIES OF A CHILD HEALTH NURSE

A child health nurse (CHN) needs a different attitude towards a child patient. The nurse who is caring for children should be humane, compassionate, trustworthy, empathetic and a lifelong learner. The CHN should be expert in child health care and should be a competent professional with excellent knowledge of growth and development, behavioural paediatrics, health promotion strategies and models, and levels of prevention. The CHN should have good communication skills and should use therapeutic communication. The CHN should be able to provide emotional foods such as love, affection, safety and protection to all children under his/her care. She/he must be cognizant about the key strategies for meeting the survival needs of children of all age group, ranging from 0 to 18 years. The CHN should recognize the individuality, rights and resilience of children and young people. The CHN should enable children/young people and carers to be involved in the development, delivery and evaluation of services. The CHN should be flexible and responsive to current and future health and service needs. The CHN should give holistic nursing and protect children from all types of threats. The CHN is at a unique position to meet the key rights and needs of children in the four major areas such as survival, health and nutrition; education and development (including skill development); and protection and participation.

The primary issues that concern CHNs of nowadays are illness and accident prevention, health maintenance, anticipatory guidance and family counselling. Challenges for CHNs are as follows:

- Rising obesity rates among rural children and young people.
- Increasing emotional and behavioural problems.
- Children and young people with complex health care needs and support in the community.
- Increased prevalence of disabling conditions and children with long-term conditions, and children with long-term conditions requiring care closer to home.

ROLES AND FUNCTIONS OF CHILD HEALTH NURSES

CHNs are involved in all aspects of childcare. The major concern of child health is to protect children from illness and injury and assist them to attain optimum growth and development regardless of the health problem and rehabilitation. A CHN assume various roles in providing comprehensive care to children. The various roles are as follows:

Therapeutic Role/Direct Care

This role is directed to the restoration of health through caregiving activities. Nurses are intimately involved in the physical and emotional needs of children including feeding, bathing, toileting, dressing, security and socialization. They are singularly held responsible for their own actions and judgements regardless of written orders from the physicians. Primary role of the nurse is to provide direct nursing care to children and family. Nursing process provides a framework for delivery of direct care to paediatric patients. The nurse evaluates the child, identifies the nursing diagnosis, and plans and implements the care as per the responses of the child and family per the nursing diagnosis. In implementing care, special importance is given to the physical and emotional needs according to the developmental stage. In the provision of this developmentally appropriate care, the nurse attempts to minimize the physical and psychological distress experienced by children and their families. Providing support even involves listening to the concerns of children and parents and simply being present during stressful situations. In this context, a CHN must remember the concept of atraumatic care. (Atraumatic care is the provision of therapeutic care in the setting by personal actions and through the use of interventions that eliminate or minimize the psychological and physical distress experienced by children and their families in the health care system; Wong, 1989.)

Patient Advocate/Family Advocate

For a CHN, one of his/her primary responsibilities is towards the child and family who are the recipients of nursing services. The nurse works with family members and identifies their needs and problems and plans interventions that best meet their defined needs. He/she should act as a consumer advocate, by informing the health services available in the hospital and community to his/her clients. He/she must be aware of the United Nations Declaration on the Rights of Children (see the 'Rights of Children' chapter) and practice within the guidelines to ensure that every child receives optimum care. As a child advocate, the concept of atraumatic care and concern for child's total welfare must be his/her motto. Nurses must be the advocate for effective voice of all the children of the country who cannot vote, lobby or speak for themselves. The issues related to child care, child health, child welfare and mental health, violence prevention and youth development, and children of low-income family need to be addressed by nurses as their social commitment as citizens and experts in child health needs. Nurses also must consider about the environmental hazards created by adults that deny a safe world for the growing children. This is a survival need for children, and they have every right to a safe environment that nourishes and cherishes their life in this world. Hazards caused by the excessive use of pesticides in the agriculture, environmental and water pollution produced by industrial waste, and improper disposal of household and industrial wastes all pose threat to child health. Because environmental health problems are on the rise and children are the major victims of such hazards, health care professionals need to protect the health of children with regard to environmental hazards. Increased use of pesticides and insecticides in the agriculture and the chemicals that are diverted to water sources create water pollution that also leads to health hazards. Use of endosulfan in Kerala had led to many health problems in children including congenital anomalies and mental retardation. Nurses should take these aspects with social commitment and advocate for children to have a safe and healthy environment to live.

Illness Prevention and Health Promotion

Nurses have kept pace with the dictum 'Prevention is better than cure'. Paediatric nurse practitioner (PNP) role was evolved for keeping pace with this emerging trend. PNP programmes led to the emergence of several specialized ambulatory or primary care roles for nurses. These programmes have extended to prepare school health nurses to provide explicit care to school children in preventive and promotive services. Education and anticipatory guidance and disease prevention strategies such as immunization are given priority in this role of illness prevention and health promotion.

Health Education/Patient Education

Remember health education is inseparable from family advocacy and illness prevention. It improves treatment results, helps children adapt to hospital situation, prepares them for procedures and encourages parental involvement in the care. Teach parents to watch signs and symptoms and progress of treatment to increase their child's comfort. Health teaching is a direct goal of all nursing activities such as during parenting classes or may be indirect when informing parents and children about diagnosis/medical treatment, encouraging children to ask questions about their sickness, referring families to health-related professional groups and supplying appropriate literature. Direct planned teaching programme can be scheduled in paediatric wards, waiting rooms and even in outpatient departments. This will promote health promotion activities related to child survival.

Support and Counselling

Support and counselling are required when meeting emotional needs of children and their parents. The roles of a child advocate and a health educator are supportive by their very nature. Counselling is given when there is pent-up tension confronting children and parents, especially those that are concerned with stages of growth and development.

Coordination/Collaboration/Case Management

The nurse as a member of the health care team collaborates and coordinates nursing services with the activities of other professionals. Working in isolation does not serve the child's best interest. To achieve holistic care, an interdisciplinary approach is necessary. This is particularly important in the case of children suffering from debilitating, long-term illnesses and handicaps. Interdisciplinary team approach helps to meet their medical and nursing needs, as well as developmental, educational and psychological needs. A nurse being the case manager should coordinate and manage the implementation of an interdisciplinary care plan. She also should make the discharge plan to promote a smooth, rapid transition to the community.

Ethical Decision-Making

Ethical dilemmas arise with competing moral considerations that underlie various alternatives. Controversy can develop at any point. Thus, nurses should select the most beneficial or least harmful action within the framework of societal mores, professional practice standards, the law, institutional rules, religious and cultural values and the nurse's personal values.

In addition to the aforementioned usual roles, a CHN has many extended and expanded roles. Extended roles are those roles that are assumed by the nurse beyond the traditional functioning of the nurse and it is the scope of nursing outside the hospital. The common extended roles of a CHN are as follows:
- School health nurse
- Occupational health nurse
- Private duty nurse
- Home care nurse
- Hospice nurse
- Rehabilitation nurse
- Nurse epidemiologist
- Military nurse
- Aerospace nurse
- Tele nurse
- Disaster nurse
- Forensic nurse

Any of these roles can also be assumed by the paediatric nurse, as the paediatric nurse holds a basic nursing certification qualification. But among these extended roles, school health nurse is very common and most sorted out jobs by a paediatric nurse.

Expanded roles are the roles that are assumed by the CHN within the boundaries of nursing inside his/her practice areas, e.g. inside the hospital, clinic or nursing educational institutions. Some of these roles are described earlier in this chapter, as it is a part of the CHN's wider role in a paediatric set-up. These roles are nurse educator, nurse counsellor, advocate, collaborator, caregiver, etc. Other expanded roles are as follows:

Nurse as a researcher: Investigates problems to improve nursing care and to further define and expand the scope of nursing practice. May be employed in an academic setting, hospital or an independent professional or community service agency.

Nurse as a manager: Manages client care and the delivery of specific nursing services within a health care agency. Begins with positions such as the charge nurse or assistant nurse manager and then as the nurse manager of a specific patient care area.

ADVANCED PRACTICE NURSE

Advanced practice nurse (APN) is generally the most independent functioning nurse. These nurses have a master's degree in specific field of nursing, advanced education in pharmacology and physical assessment, and certification and expertise in the specialized area of practice. 'Advanced practice' is a term used to describe a health care professional (usually a nurse) who, in collaboration with a physician, provides comprehensive care for a group of patients, including tasks performed previously within the scope of nursing practice. Advanced practice nursing roles in paediatric and neonatal care encompass a variety of titles including clinical nurse specialist/neonatal nurse practitioner (CNS/NNP), APN and the expanded role of neonatal nurse (ERN). APNs may provide care in level I, II and/or III nurseries and paediatric ICUs according to their specialization. These nurses either function independently or provide in-house backup coverage.

APN Competencies

- Address infants'/children's responses to illness and treatment, parental responses and needs, and growth and development of preterm and term neonates, infants and children.
- APNs are also skilled in the application of research findings to practice, as well as the development and delivery of education to parents and other members of the health care team.

- In addition to their clinical work, APNs may participate on research teams, present at conferences and publish in peer-reviewed journals.
- The skill of the APNs in the medical and nursing management of ill neonates/children makes them excellent alternative care providers.
- Their nursing experience, knowledge and skills make them invaluable members of the health care teams whose foci are on the provision of high-quality care, as well as on education and research.
- Job description of these categories of nurses of any institution should clearly identify role/responsibilities and reporting structures. Supporting documents may include:
  - Transfer of function documents;
  - Occupational profiles;
  - Clinical practice guidelines;
  - Administrative activities;
  - Practice privileges;
  - Prescriptive authority or protocols for ordering medications; and
  - Medical directives, and mechanisms for demonstrating initial and ongoing competencies.
- **Educational Preparation**
- Master's level.
- This will permit the flexibility, versatility, professional mobility and career opportunities.
- Medicolegal considerations.
- For the advanced practice role, separate registration from the state nursing council is essential.
- It should determine the legal framework for practice.

NEONATAL ASSESSMENT NURSE AND CHILD HEALTH ASSESSMENT NURSE

Neonatal assessment nurse/child health assessment nurse (NAN/CHAN) role is a special dedicated clinical assignment of a paediatric or neonatal nurse that:
- Would positively facilitate the transition of life from the fetus to a neonate.
- Decreases mother–neonate separation.
- Increases the rate of skin-to-skin contact.
- Improves nurses' perspective of neonatal care.
- Decreases neonatal intensive care unit (NICU) admissions.
- Improves maternal satisfaction.

The NAN provides transitional care at the mother's bedside, thus changing the current practice of separating the sick infant from the mother.

Expanded Role of Neonatal/Paediatric Nurse – Importance!

- Many countries have started this programme to compact additional manpower to care for neonates.
- Current level of nursing practice lacks decision-making skills.
- Reduced content in biopsychosocial sciences to meet the current needs in the NICU.

- Technical advancement increases the survival rate of neonates, even extremely low-birth-weight neonates (less than 1000 g).
- Requires extensive supervision.
- Babies remain for extended periods in the NICU. Extended stays make daily occupancy rates very high.
- High occupancy rates continue even when neonates who are convalescent are transferred.
- Rapidly increasing level of technical skills associated with advancing technology.
- Expansion of roles through additional educational preparation helps to maintain quality of care.
- Expansion of role reduces the potential for fragmentation of care.
  - Provides an alternative to residents.
  - Improves standard of care.

CLINICAL NURSE SPECIALIST

- Nursing expertise in a specialized area of practice (medical-surgical nursing, psychiatric and mental health nursing, paediatric nursing, community health nursing, gerontological nursing) will be there with this category of nurses.
- Acts as a researcher to validate nursing observation and intervention and a change agent within the health care system.
- Provides consultant services.
- The CNS role has developed within each of the traditional specialty area, as well in subspecialties such as cardiovascular, oncology, neurology paediatrics, neonatology, etc.
- Both the CNS and the PNP are called as the advanced nurse practitioner.

Critical Care Paediatric Nurse/Neonatal Nurse

- The nurses are theoretically and technically prepared to provide effective nursing care.
- The training and education can be given in the hospital setting in the form of a certified continuous education programme.
- The programme is to prepare nurse to function as Senior Neonatal Nurse/Critical Care Neonatal Nurse.
- The post-basic specialty education will positively influence the role of SNN/CCNN.

Paediatric/Neonatal Nurse Practitioner

- Both paediatric nurse practitioner (PNP) and NNP can be created from the cadre of nurses who have passed out from the college of nursing with a BSc/MSc degree with neonatology as specialty and as any nurse with a BSc degree who has undertaken specialized training in neonatal care and has hands-on training in practical care of a newborn for a reasonable period of time.

In the NICU, it is essential to provide highly desirable quality of care with 24 hours' coverage for each of these roles.

NURSING PROCESS APPLICATION TO CHILD HEALTH NURSING

Nursing process is the framework for the practice of professional nursing. It provides a framework for evidence-based practice, as the judgements are based on evidence. Nursing process is a method of problem identification and problem solving that describes what a nurse actually does in response to a patient's problems. Hence, as in any nursing specialty, child health nursing too has adopted the nursing process as a framework of practice for its professionals.

Steps of Nursing Process

Assessment

It is the deliberate and systematic collection of data from a variety of sources such as individual health history, family members, child and significant others, observation of social interactions, growth and development assessment, physical examination and laboratory data and consultation with other professionals. A comprehensive assessment is the ideal one. If not possible, perform a screening assessment along with a focused assessment. The assessment provides cues (information) for nurses that influence their decision.

The assessment will be completed only when:
- The nurse gets adequate baseline data about the child and the family;
- Health care needs are evaluated;
- The areas that interfere with the child and family's functioning are identified; and
- A statement is made about any problem that exists.

When completed, all cues must be analysed.

Nursing Diagnosis

These are client problems that nurses by virtue of their education and experience are able and licensed to treat (Whaley and Wong, 1997). This forms the basis for selection of nursing interventions to achieve outcomes for which the nurse is accountable (Nanda, 1991). According to Nanda, three categories of nursing diagnoses exist: actual, high risk (potential) and wellness.

Once the data gathered are organized, categorized and clustered to identify significant areas, the nurse can identify whether a nursing diagnosis exists. If so, state nursing diagnosis as the naming of human responses. Nursing diagnosis does not describe all nursing activities. There are three dimensions of nursing practice: dependent activities, which are nursing activities that are required for implementation of the prescribed medical regimen; interdependent activities, which are medical and nursing responsibilities and accountabilities that overlap and require collaboration between the two disciplines; and independent activities, which are direct responsibility of the nurse. The nursing diagnoses are stated to reflect both interdependent and independent dimensions of nursing practice.

Carpenito (1995) mentioned that collaborative problems exist that require collaborative approach to prevent, treat or intervene a problem by consultation with multidisciplinary management, e.g. physiotherapist, nutritionist, etc.

The statement of nursing diagnosis has three components. They are problem (P), aetiology (E) and signs and symptoms (S). Problem statement describes the child's response to health problem in the child, family or community. This is the child's response to distribution of life processes, pattern, function or development. This first part directs to outcome development. This part can be related either to an actual problem or a risk state requiring nursing intervention. Risk state indicates a potential health problem that needs to be intervened to prevent possible hazards to the child, family or community.

The component of the aetiology is related to contributing factors that describe the physiological situation and maturational factors that cause the problem or influence its development. The aetiology can be behaviours of the patient or factors in the environment (or an interaction of both). Nurses must be careful not to use words that may imply cause and effect when linking aetiology to problems, as it may cause a legal and professional difficulty in certain places. Hence, the phrase related to aetiology is used safely to show the relationship between the problem and its aetiology. Differentiating among various aetiologies is very important, as interventions to alter the health problems are directed towards the aetiology. For example, it is also important to be specific about aetiology so that specific or particular nursing activities can be planned and implemented. (Alteration in body temperature can result from different aetiologies, such as the one in a patient with head injury as a result of a trauma associated with injury or pressure to the hypothalamus, where the fever is the central fever. The nursing interventions may be directed mainly to external cooling than to the administration of antipyretics. However, for the same diagnosis in the peripheral fever, the nursing intervention is mainly the administration of antipyretics such as the one given in infections of central nervous system or other bacterial invasion.)

Although the nursing interventions are directed towards aetiology, the problem statement also affects the nursing interventions. There are often instances in which the etiology is designated as unknown. Still the nursing care will be planned based on the presenting symptoms.

Signs and Symptoms

They are the cluster of cues or defining characteristics derived from patient evaluation, and these indicate actual health problems. The defining characteristics are observable when the health problem is present. The defining characteristics are included in nursing diagnosis only when needed for clarity. For example, in a nursing diagnosis of ineffective airway clearance, the defining characteristics are abnormal breath sounds (crackles, rhonchi, wheezes), changes in respiratory rate/depth or absent cough, hypoxia, cyanosis, dyspnoea, fever, tachycardia and orthopnoea.

Planning

When patient problems are identified with nursing diagnoses, a care plan is developed with expected outcomes (goals). The expected outcomes are the projected clinical conditions or behaviours that occur as a result of nursing activities. The expected outcomes need to be developed before the interventions are developed. It must be child-centred and individualistic, according to the capabilities of the child and the family. It should also be realistic, achievable, measurable and observable. Hence, the care plan can be evaluated. This can also facilitate setting up of long-term and short-term goals. The nurse must set up priorities of care in developing appropriate outcomes. Maslow's hierarchy of needs can be safely employed in setting priorities in care planning. Physiological needs of children must be given significant priority, as this is the most important area in saving lives of children.

Nursing Care Plan

Interventions/actions must be planned to achieve the expected outcome stated. Individualized care plan can be developed. Text usually provides standardized care plans that aids students and practitioners to prepare individualized care plans. While preparing the care plan, one must be careful to use the *framework of practice* as the base on which the plan is developed. This helps the practicing nurses to have clear picture of their theoretical base for practice. Patient *goals* must be stated as what the *patient will be expected to do* after the nursing interventions.

Nursing interventions are *specific directives for nursing care* that can be carried out to help the particular patient to move from the present state of ill health to the state described in expected outcomes. The objectives of the nursing intervention in paediatric nursing are to direct individualized care to a particular child for whom the care plan is made. In stating nursing interventions, the nurse, the child and the family are essential components in the planning process. Selected resource persons can be included as clinical experts, child life experts and psychologists. Factors that need to be considered for the patient and the family in determining nursing interventions are as follows:

- Knowledge, skill and abilities of the child and the family.
- Child's perception of health.
- Cultural and religious background.
- Access to needs, resources or support people.
- Financial resources.
- Coping mechanism usually used.

If these factors are not considered, the nursing care provided will not be individualistic and will not meet the needs of the specific client. For example, the nurse makes a care plan to give a first-class protein in the diet of a child who belongs to a class living below poverty line; this care plan is not realistic. It will not meet the needs of the child. Instead, the nurse can consult with parents, find out their financial capacity and then plan a diet with other proteins that are affordable to the family. Then the care plan is realistic.

Nursing interventions should also be selected on the basis of the direct observation and medical diagnosis. Choose only those interventions that have a greatest probability of success for which evidence can be traced from practice. It should not focus on mere symptoms of the disease or disorder. It is better to write this in terms of both child's and nurse's behaviours. The most important

nursing intervention should be placed first and carried out on the basis of priority of patient needs.

Implementation

Actual delivery of nursing care to the patient is implementation. All nursing interventions (dependent, interdependent and independent domains of nursing practices) need to be implemented again based on priority. During implementation of each intervention, the need for continued assessment is essential. Performance of reassessment to evaluate and revalidate the care too is essential. The implementation of the care needs to be documented in the patient's permanent record promptly to safeguard the nurse as well as the patient. This is also important in accounting nursing care and is useful in quality control.

Evaluation

It should be performed on the basis of the *set measurable expected outcomes*. For evaluation, there must be criteria and standards to guide observation. It also helps to determine patient progress in terms of diagnosis and goals. The nurse observes the patient to determine what skills and knowledge the child and the family have mastered. Observed data need to be compared with expected outcomes and the amount of progress achieved. Judgement is made about whether the patient outcome meets the established goal. If the patient does not achieve the expected outcome, the plan must be assessed to find out the difficulties. It also helps the nurse to set up realistic outcomes in future.

Documentation

It is an essential part for evaluation and is best performed with written evidence of progress towards outcomes.

STUDY QUESTIONS

1. Discuss the anatomical, physiological and psychological differences that affect child health nursing practice in contrast to adult nursing.
2. What are the rights of children as a vulnerable group?
3. What are the roles of a paediatric nurse?
4. How will you apply comfort theory in the practice of paediatric nursing? Illustrate with examples.
5. How will you use the nursing process as a midrange theory in the practice of paediatric nursing?

BIBLIOGRAPHY

1. Andropoulos, D. B. (2015). Pediatric Physiology: How Does It Differ from Adults?. In: Mason K (eds.), *Pediatric Sedation Outside of the Operating Room*. Springer, New York, NY.
2. Manley, L. K. (1987). Paediatric trauma: Initial assessment and management. *Journal of Emergency Nursing, 13*(2), 77–87.
3. Ojanen Thomas, D. (1988). The ABC's of Paediatric Triage. *Journal of Emergency Nursing, 14*(3), 154–159.
4. Kichuk-Chrisant, M. R. (2002). Children are not small adults: some differences between paediatric and adult cardiac transplantation. *Current Opinion in Cardiology, 17*(2), 152–159.
5. Katharine, K., DiMarco, M. A. (2005). "Comfort Theory and Its Application to Paediatric Nursing" *Pediatric Nursing, 31*(3),187–194.

CHILD WELFARE ACTIVITIES

LEARNING OBJECTIVES

At the end of the chapter, the learner will be able to:

- List various agencies and organizations involved in child welfare activities in India.
- Describe various child welfare programmes of the national and international levels.
- Explain various acts related to child welfare and children in India.
- Describe the importance of Integrated Management of Childhood Illnesses (IMCI).
- Explain Baby-Friendly Hospital Initiative (BFHI).
- Describe important activities of the National Health Policy in relation to child welfare in India.

Child welfare activities cover a broad spectrum of preventive and promotive health care activities that are aimed at promotion of child health. Children are the important asset of a country. India is a young country with 42 million children living in this subcontinent alone. So it is imperative for any health care professional to know about the various programmes available for the care and welfare of this important section of the population. In India, we have a wide range of programmes and activities that are planned and carried out by many agencies such as governmental, nongovernmental and international organizations. This chapter covers the important national and international organizations that are involved in the care of children, as well as their programmes and activities directed towards welfare of children in India.

CHILD WELFARE AGENCIES

Child welfare covers the entire spectrum of needs of children who by reason of handicap – social, economic,

physical or mental – are unable to avail of services provided by the community (Park. J & Park. K, 2003). All child welfare programmes provide services to children because of their importance in the society. These include various preventive and promotive health activities to maintain health of the children.

The important child welfare agencies in India are as follows:

1. Indian Council for Child Welfare (ICCW)
2. Central Social Welfare Board (CSWB)
3. Kasturba Gandhi Memorial Trust
4. Indian Red Cross Society
5. Child in Need Institute (CINI)

All these agencies get financial aid from the government to organize child welfare services in the country. The following are their activities in a nutshell:

- Day care services by setting *balwadies*
- Holiday homes
- Recreation facilities
- *Bal bhavans*

1. **Indian Council for Child Welfare**

   This is the first national organization formed in the country to mobilize voluntary activities in all aspects of child development. It was formulated in the year 1952. The CSWB was set up in the year 1953 to assist the voluntary organizations and mobilize their support and cooperation in the provision of social welfare activities. This national-level voluntary agency works with the following aims and objectives: to initiate, undertake and aid schemes for furtherance of child welfare in India; to organize and maintain institutions for training child welfare workers; to establish a central bureau for study, research and collection of data on child welfare work and disseminate knowledge/information; and to promote enactment of new legislation and reform in existing laws relating to children and their welfare. ICCW runs programmes directly and through states and union territories. It runs *balsevika* training programmes, *anganwadi* workers training and the *balwadi*-cum-nutrition programme.

2. **Central Social Welfare Board**
   It is an autonomous organization set up by the Government of India in August 1953 under the general administrative control of the Ministry of Education. Main functions of this organization are as follows:
   a. Surveying the needs and requirements of voluntary welfare organizations in the country;
   b. Promoting and setting up social welfare organizations on voluntary basis; and
   c. Rendering financial aid to deserving organizations/institutions.
   The board had initiated Family and Child Welfare Services under its control in the year 1968 to improve services for women and children in the rural areas. The board is involved in special education such as teaching craft, social education, literacy classes, maternity aid, distribution of milk, running *balwadies* and organization of play centres for children.
3. **Kasturba Gandhi Memorial Trust**
   It was created in memorial of Kasturba Gandhi after her death in the year 1944. Its main objective was to provide aid for women, especially of rural folk through *grama sevikas*.
4. **Indian Red Cross Society**
   Indian Red Cross Society was established in the year 1920. It has branches all over India. It is actively involved in activities related to promotion of health, prevention of illness, relief work, providing milk and medical supplies, maternal and child health (MCH) activities, etc.
5. **Child in Need Institute**
   It was established in the year 1974 in Daulatpur, West Bengal, to provide services to women and children. The institute has three main foci, namely health services, women's welfare and training of personnel. CINI has centres in West Bengal and Tamil Nadu.

International organizations concerned with child welfare are World Health Organization (WHO), UNICEF, UNFPA, World Bank, Cooperative for Assistance and Relief Everywhere (CARE) Ford Foundation, International Union for Child Welfare and FAO of the United Nations.

UNIVERSAL CHILDREN'S DAY

November 14th is observed as the Universal Children's Day. It was started by the International Union for Child Welfare and UNICEF. In 1954, the United Nations General Assembly passed a formal resolution establishing the Universal Children's Day and assigned to UNICEF the responsibility for promoting this annual day. In India, we celebrate this day along with the birthday of the first Prime Minister Sri. Jawaharlal Nehru.

Government and various voluntary agencies celebrate this day with various activities. Exceptional children are given recognition through awards by the central and state governments on this day. It is celebrated in schools; the postal department issues commemorative stamps on the occasion for sale, and the money is utilized for child welfare activities.

INTEGRATED CHILD DEVELOPMENT SERVICES

There are about 5320 Integrated Child Development Services (ICDS) projects functioning in India. The principal worker in the project is the *anganwadi* worker who provides a package of health services (supplementary nutrition, immunization, health check-up, referral, nutrition, and health education and nonformal education services) to mothers and children. The activities of ICDS are guided by the child development project officer.

BABY-FRIENDLY HOSPITAL INITIATIVE

Since 1993, WHO's efforts to improve infant and young child nutrition have focused on promoting breastfeeding. It has been calculated that breastfeeding could prevent deaths of at least 1 million children annually. BFHI is created and promoted by WHO and UNICEF and has proved highly successful in encouraging proper infant feeding practices starting at birth. BFHI is supported by major medical and nursing professional bodies in India. There are 10 steps listed in this initiative. These include the following: to help mothers to initiate breastfeeding within the first hour of birth in normal delivery and 4 hours following caesarean section; to encourage breastfeeding on demand; to allow mothers and infants to remain together 24 hours a day, except for medical reasons; to give newborn infants no food or drink, other than breast milk, unless medically indicated; to promote exclusive breastfeeding till 4–6 months of age; and to not allow advertisement, promotional material or free products for infant feeding in the facility. BFHI in India is also expected to follow all child survival activities such as antenatal care, clean delivery practices, essential newborn care, immunization and oral rehydration therapy (ORT). For further explanation on BFHI, the reader is advised to look at unit 11 on preventive paediatrics.

UNDER-FIVE CLINICS

The under-five clinics provide a whole sum of care, not only preventive paediatrics such as well-baby clinics but also a comprehensive outlook to childcare. The objectives of under-five clinics are outlined in its symbol itself.
1. Care in illness
2. Growth monitoring
3. Preventive care

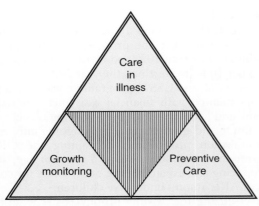

Symbol for Under-Five Clinics.

1. Care in illness comprises diagnosis and treatment of the following:
   (a) Acute illness
   (b) Chronic illness including physical, mental, congenital and acquired abnormalities
   (c) Disorders of growth and development
   (d) Use of X-rays and other laboratory and referral services
2. Preventive care includes the following:
   (a) Immunization
   (b) Nutrition surveillance
   (c) Health check-ups
   (d) Oral rehydration
   (e) Family planning/welfare
   (f) Health education

Growth monitoring includes checking weight of the child periodically at monthly intervals during the first year, every 2 months during the second year and every 3 months thereafter up to 5–6 years of age, and plotting this weight as growth charts to detect malnutrition and growth failure. Heath education will be provided after assessing the cause for growth failure by the worker if it is identified.

SCHOOL HEALTH SERVICES

School heath service is an important aspect of health promotion in school children. It is an economical and powerful means of delivering care to school children. The development of school health services in India dates back to 1909 when the first medical examination of school children took place in Baroda city. Later, the Bhore Committee recommended the need for the constitution of school health services in India. In the year 1960, the School Health Committee was constituted by the Government of India to identify and deal with the health problems of school children.

The objectives of school health services are as follows:
1. Promotion of positive health
2. Prevention of diseases
3. Early diagnosis, treatment and follow-up of defects

4. Awakening health awareness in children
5. Provision of healthful environment

The major aspects of school health services are as follows:
1. Health appraisal of school children and school personnel
2. Remedial measures and follow-up
3. Prevention of communicable diseases
4. Healthful environment
5. Nutritional services
6. First aid and emergency care
7. Mental health
8. Dental health
9. Eye health
10. Health education
11. Education of handicapped children
12. Proper maintenance and use of school health records

DIARRHOEAL DISEASE CONTROL PROGRAMME

The Diarrhoeal Disease Control Programme (DDCP) was started during the Sixth Plan with an intention to reduce diarrhoea-related mortality, including cholera, through ORT. During the Seventh Plan, this programme was integrated into primary health care. The main aim of this programme is to provide health education on prevention and home management of diarrhoea. This is achieved through free distribution of teaching materials in regional languages to all and mother's education for promotion of ORT in managing their children at home. The emphases are given on providing home-made fluids, continuing feeding during diarrhoea and recognizing early signs of dehydration. Other important methods of diarrhoea control are to promote exclusive breastfeeding for the first 4–6 months of life, proper weaning, infant immunization, especially against measles, and prophylaxis against vitamin A deficiency.

Training of health personnel on diarrhoea management has been integrated with training for control of acute respiratory infections (ARIs) and care of newborn since the year 1993. Diarrhoea Treatment and Training Units (DTUs) were established in the Department of Paediatrics at all medical colleges and district hospitals. During 1985–1992, 85 medical colleges and 100 district hospitals have established DTUs.

Since 1992–1993, the DDCP has been integrated with the Child Survival and Safe Motherhood (CSSM) programme. ORS packages are now being supplied in drug kits to subcentres. About 150 packets are given every 6 months for a population of 3000–5000 (roughly 380–630 under-five children). In this scheme, ORS packets for districts are supplied to the state.

ACUTE RESPIRATORY INFECTION CONTROL PROGRAMME

ARI control programme was taken up as a pilot project in 14 districts of the country in the year 1990. Since

1992–1993, the programme is being implemented as a part of the CSSM programme to reduce mortality rate in children as a result of ARIs by 20% by 1991 and by 40% by the year 2000.

The strategies are as follows:
- Ensure standard case management of pneumonia in children younger than 5 years by training medical and other health personnel.
- Train other peripheral health staff to recognize and treat cases of pneumonia.
- Promote timely referral of severe pneumonia by the peripheral health staff and community.
- Improve maternal knowledge about home management of cough and cold and recognition of early danger signs for seeking appropriate care.
- Promote immunization, including measles immunization, exclusive breastfeeding in the first 4–6 months of life, proper weaning and vitamin A administration.

The treatment of pneumonia by the peripheral health staff is limited only to CSSM districts. Co-trimoxazole tablets are included in the drug kits supplied to subcentres in these districts. Each kit contains 1000 paediatric tablets of co-trimoxazole supplied every 6 months.

IODINE DEFICIENCY DISORDERS PROGRAMME

Iodine Deficiency Disorders (IDD) Programme has been initiated on a nationwide scale by the use of iodized salt. It was decided as a national policy to fortify all edible salt in a phased manner by the end of the Eighth Plan. Essential activities include the following:
- Use of iodized salt in place of the common salt
- Monitoring and surveillance
- Manpower training and mass communication

With the assistance of UNICEF, an intensive IDD monitoring has been implemented in certain states (Uttar Pradesh [UP], Madhya Pradesh [MP], Himachal Pradesh [HP] and Assam) to reduce the prevalence of goitre in the age group 10–14 years to less than 5% and to reduce the number of cretins born by the year 2000.

NATIONAL PROGRAMME FOR CONTROL OF BLINDNESS

This programme was launched in the year 1976 along with the trachoma control programme started in 1968. Other agencies that help in the control of blindness include DANIDA, WHO and voluntary agencies such as Lions International and Rotary International and its branches. The programme is aimed at community health education and prevention of blindness by vitamin A prophylaxis.

CHILD SURVIVAL AND SAFE MOTHERHOOD PROGRAMME

National Health Policy (NHP) 1983 has listed 17 goals. Of the 17, nine goals are related to child health. This programme was introduced to reduce the infant mortality

rate (IMR) to below 60 per 1000 live births and the child mortality rate (CMR) to below 10 per 1000 child population, as well as to reduce the proportion of low-birth-weight babies to less than 10% and maternal mortality to below two per 1000 live birth by the year 2000.

In August 1992, the CSSM programme was launched and is implemented with financial assistance from the World Bank and UNICEF with the following objectives:
- Sustaining and strengthening the ongoing universal immunization programme, containing the ORT programme for children below 5 years of age, and introducing and expanding the programme for control of ARIs among under-five children.
- Universalizing the existing prophylaxis scheme for control of blindness as a result of deficiency of vitamin A among children up to the age of 3 years. Prophylaxis against nutritional anaemia among pregnant and lactating mothers as well as children up to 5 years of age through administration of iron and folic acid (IFA) tablets.
- Imposing newborn care and maternal care at the community level.

The two components of this programme are as follows:
- Universal Programme of Immunization (UIP) plus package includes UIP, ORT, prophylaxis scheme and ARI control programme for all states and union territories.
- Safe motherhood initiatives for six high maternal mortality rate (MMR) states (Assam, Bihar, MP, Orissa, Rajasthan and UP).

FAMILY WELFARE – MILESTONES

- 1951   Family Planning Program
- 1971   Maternal Child Health and Family Planning integrated
- 1972   Postpartum Program, Medical Termination of Pregnancy (MTP) Act
- 1977   National Family Welfare Programme
- 1983   National Health Policy
- 1985   MCH, UIP
- 1992   CSSM

The project was implemented in a phased manner. The activities include continued supply of vaccines, cold-chain equipment, needles and syringes and ORS packets. The programme includes training of peripheral-level workers for recognition of pneumonia and treatment with co-trimoxazole. The pregnant and lactating mothers and under-five children are given IFA tablets. It also aimed at blindness prophylaxis by administration of vitamin A to children from 6 months to 3 years of age (first dose 1 lakh IU). It is administered along with measles vaccine at 9 months of age, followed by another dose along with a booster dose of DPT/OPV.

Maternal Care

Training of traditional birth attendants (*dais*). Provision of delivery kits and increasing fees from Rs 3 to Rs 10 per case to birth attendants under the CSSM programme were implemented.

Training in a Phased Manner

Training of medical and paramedical workers for continuing activities (immunization, ORS and other prophylaxis schemes).

- Impart skill-based training to medical and paramedical personnel for pneumonia control activities and essential newborn care. The training for programme managers, medical officers and the paramedical staff has been integrated to include the entire range of MCH care interventions.
- First referral units (FRUs) for emergency obstetric care in all district hospitals with essential equipment and skill-based training for health personnel and appointment of medical officers (gynaecologist, paediatrician, etc.) with blood bank facilities are also provided under the scheme.

REPRODUCTIVE CHILD HEALTH

A state of health where people are able to have a responsible, satisfying and safe sex life and that they have the capability to reproduce and the freedom to decide, if when and how often to do so.

(ICPD, 1994)

Though there are improvements in health over the last 30 years, IMR and MMR still remain high in India. IMR in India is as high as 63 per 1000 live births. Most of these deaths occur in the first month of life. In total, 30% of the world's neonatal deaths occur in India. Similar is the case with MMR. Fourteen per cent of deaths among women of child-bearing age result from pregnancy or childbirth.

Children in India continue to lose their life to vaccine-preventable diseases such as measles. More than 2 million children die every year as a result of vaccine-preventable diseases.

MMR India	
NFHS (1992)	424
NFHS (1998–1999)	540
SRS (1998)	407
WHO-UNFPA	540
UNICEF (2000)	
Wide Variation among States	
Gujarat	28
Tamil Nadu	76
UP	707

High MMR – Causes in India

a. **Medical**
   Haemorrhage, puerperal sepsis, obstructed labour, eclampsia, complicated abortion
b. **Access/Utilization and Availability**
   - Home deliveries
   - Lack or limited access to: antenatal care (ANC)/postnatal care (PNC), emergency obstetric and newborn care (EmOC) and safe abortion services

c. **Maternal Deaths – Economic and social differential determinants**
   Below poverty line (BPL)
d. **Women's status**
   - Low literacy
   - Age at marriage
   - Poor nutritional status

Reproductive Rights According to RCH

- To be informed
- To have access to safe, effective, acceptable and affordable contraception
- Provide access to health services that will enable women to go safely through pregnancy and childbirth
- Provide couples the best chance of having a healthy infant

RCH Program – Characteristics

These are as follows:
- Life cycle approach, where *women's health across their life cycle is taken care of.*
- *Integrates* safe motherhood and child health with fertility regulation and reproductive health programmes for men and women.
- *Quality care* – Need-based, client-centred, demand-driven.
- *Bottom-up approach* – Decentralized participatory – Impact assessment.

MATERNAL CHILD HEALTH CARE

Priority Group

Women 15–44 years	19%
Children <15 years	40%

Vulnerable Group

High mortality as a special risk group

Reproductive Health – Milestones

1994	ICPD Cairo
1996	Target-Free Approach
1997	RCH I
2000	National Population Policy
2002	National Health Policy
2005	RCH II

RCH – Key Components

- Maternal health
- Newborn care
- Child health
- Adolescent health
  RTI/STI (reproductive tract infection/sexually transmitted infection) treatment

State-wise Differential Approach

- Community participation/public–private mix
- Urban poor/tribals
- Male participation

RCH Services – Safe Motherhood

- Essential obstetric care
- Emergency obstetric care (comprehensive/basic)
- Essential newborn care through Integrated Management of Neonatal and Childhood Illness (IMNCI)
- MTP services
- Contraceptive – delivery
- RTI/STI care
- Empowering adolescents
- Strengthening immunization – Injection safety

Reproductive Health Problems

In total, 39% had RTI/STI symptoms.
In Kerala, 42.4% had symptoms.

RCH II – Inputs

- Operationalize 2000+ FRUs in the country (Comprehensive Emergency Obstetric and Newborn Care [CEmONC]).
- Make at least 50% public health centres (PHCs) operational for 24 hours for Basic Emergency Obstetric and New Born Care (BEMONC).
- Ensure management of common obstetrical complications and management of common childhood problems.
- Provide early and safe abortion services.
- Provide RTI/STI services.
  - Train/empower medical officers (MOs)/auxiliary nurse midwives (ANMs)/lady health visitor (LHVs) as skilled birth attendants.
  - Develop referral linkages.
  - FRUs – 5 lakh population – CEmONC centres.
- Infrastructural improvements of operation theatres, labour rooms and water supply.
- Logistics – Emergency drugs/blood storage systems, kits E–P.
- Specialist – Anaesthetics/OB-Gyn/paediatrician's appointment and availability in all FRUs.

Social Mobilization

- Referral transport services – Rural ambulances
- Government/NGOs
- Janani Suraksha Yojana for BPL families
- Promote institutional delivery through panchayats
- Vande Mataram Yojna through private doctors
- Incentives
- Information Education Communication(IEC)/Behavioral Change Communication (BCC)

RCH Interventions – Child Care

- IMNCI
- Essential newborn care (at limited facilities)

- Immunization
- Diarrhoeal disease control
- ARI control
- Vitamin A prophylaxis

IMMUNIZATION

	India	Kerala
Fully immunized	54%	84%
BCG	72	97
DPT3	55	91
OPV3	63	91
Measles	51	89
Unimmunized	17.5	–

New Pneumococcal Conjugate Vaccine against Pneumonia

New pneumococcal conjugate vaccine (PCV) for pneumonia was launched on 13 May 2017 by Union Minister for Health Mr J.P. Nadda at Lal Bhadhur Shastri Medical College Hospital in Mandi district of HP. This vaccine will help reduce the childhood mortality, as more than 1 lakh children die of pneumonia every year in India. This vaccine will prevent pneumonia resulting from 13 strains of pneumococci. This is the 12th vaccine the Government of India has launched. It protects children against *Streptococcal pneumonia* and diseases like pneumonia, ear infections, sinus infections and meningitis. This vaccine is now included in the UIP.

Government of India Action on Health in RCH

- Strengthen the existing health system by increasing the number of health workers.
- Prevent newborn deaths through home-based medical visits.
- Increase children's access to immunizations, etc.
- Other initiatives.
- National Rural Health Mission (NRHM)
- ASHA (accredited social health activist)
- Indian Public Health Standards (IPHS) for PHCs and community health centres (CHCs) under preparation
- Janani Suraksha Yojana
- A comprehensive infection management and environment plan for RCH 11 is already prepared for implementation at PHCs, CHCs and sub-centers.

Making Pregnancy Safe

- Avoid teenage pregnancy
- Early identification of pregnancy
- Early registration
- All pregnancies wanted
- Monitoring health during pregnancy, childbirth and the postnatal period

- Timely referral
- Cut short the delays
- Increase participation of the mother and other family members
- Use of a skilled birth attendant where home delivery is prevalent
- Convincing advices on nutrition and immunization
- Prepare a birth plan

Matter of Concern

- India's economic growth rate is 8%, and our country has crossed a population of more than 1 billion in 2006.
- Almost 50% of the population in India is in the reproductive age group.
- Thirty per cent of Indians are illiterate.
- In India, 300 women die every day as a result of pregnancy and childbirth; and one of nine children dies before his/her first birthday.

Interventions to Reduce Maternal and Newborn Mortality Rates (MMR and NNR)

Skilled care at every birth:
- Good nutrition, especially for the girl child and prior to pregnancy.
- Protection from infectious diseases which requires, in part, a strong immunization programme.
- Quality antenatal care.
- Increased education opportunities for girls and young women.
  1. Good parenting including health education for healthy families and recognition of danger signs in neonates.
  2. Access to family planning for birth spacing and limiting the size of families.
  3. Early and exclusive breastfeeding which is still not a common practice in many countries in the region.
  4. Scheme for provision of honorarium to doctors and specialists when they are on call and paid for each maternal health service they handle.
  5. Provision of 24 hours' delivery services at PHCs and CHCs.
  6. Provision of referral transport in case of obstetric complications.
  7. Provision for safe abortion services.
  8. Prevention and management of RTI/STI.
  9. Training of dais.
  10. RCH camps to provide services to people living in remote areas.

The key characteristics of the RCH II program include:
1. Adoption of sector-wise approach.
2. Rationalization of existing budget heads and creation of a flexible funding pool.
3. Donor convergence; e.g. central as well as state projects supported by the developmental partners.
4. State ownership, and decentralizing planning and programme implementation.

Small Efforts Can Make a Big Difference

Everybody can contribute to delivery of quality post-natal services, which depend on the work of all cadres of the hospital staff.

Everyone has the same right to life. We need to value the inherent right to life of every woman and child as human beings in order to prevent maternal and neonatal deaths.

Universal Programme of Immunization

The Government of India launched its expanded programme of immunization (EPI) in 1978 with objective of reducing mortality and morbidity resulting from vaccine-preventable diseases of childhood. The UIP was started in 1985 with two components:
- Immunization of pregnant women against tetanus.
- Immunization of children in their first year of life against the six major killer diseases. Under the UIP, about 25 million infants are vaccinated every year before 1 year of age. Under this scheme, Pulse Polio immunization is introduced to eradicate poliomyelitis. It was first started as the National Immunization Days on 9 December 1995 and 20 January 1996.

CHILD WELFARE PROGRAMME FOR DISABLED CHILDREN

According to UNICEF's report on the status of Disability in India (2000), there were around 30 million children with disability. The Sixth All India Educational Survey (NCERT, 1998) reports that 20 million school-aged children (6–14 years of age) require special education. Average gross enrollment in school is more than 90% for normal children. Only less than 5% of children with disability enroll in school. That means the mainstay of children with disability are not getting enrolled in school.

The Constitution of India states that free and compulsory education should be provided to all children until they complete the age of 14 years.

Disability in Five-Year Plans

First Five-Year Plan – Launched as a small unit by the Ministry of Education for the visually impaired in 1947.

Second Five-Year Plan – Under the Ministry of Education, a National Advisory Council for the physically challenged was established.

Third Five-Year Plan – Attention was given to rural areas and facilitated training and rehabilitation of the physically challenged.

Fourth Five-Year Plan – More emphasis was given to preventive work.

Sixth 5-year plan – National policies were made for provision of community-oriented disability prevention and rehabilitation services to promote self-reliance:
- National-level institutes were set up by the Government of India.
- National Institute for Visually Handicapped – 1982 in Dehradun.

- National Institute for Orthopedically Handicapped – 1982 in Kolkata.
- Ali Yavar Jug National Institute for the Hearing Handicapped – 1983 in Mumbai.
- National Institute of Rehabilitation Training and Research – 1984 in Orissa.
- National Institute for the Mentally Handicapped – 1984 in Hyderabad.
- Institute for the Physically Handicapped – 1976 in Delhi.
- Rehabilitation Council of India – 1986 in Delhi – converted to a statutory body under the Rehabilitation Council of India Act 1992.

National-Level Practices on Education of Children with Disabilities

- Early childhood care and education (ECCE) – It is now globally recognized that systematic provision of ECCE can help in the development of children in a variety of ways. ECCE is being promoted as a holistic input for fostering health, psychosocial, nutritional and educational development of children. ECCE will be possible only when there are strong linkages with the primary health care system.

Project for Integrated Education Development and Integrated Education for the Disabled Children

The government launched the Project for Integrated Education Development (PIED) with assistance from UNICEF in 1986. In 1992, children with moderate disabilities were included in this project. This project facilitated disabled children to mingle with their normal counterpart and thus created a social awareness among all types of children. This project was found to be successful in the states of Kerala and Tamil Nadu. The success of this project resulted in the centrally sponsored scheme launched by the Ministry of Human Resource Development called Integrated Education for Disabled Children (IEDC) in 1992. IEDC has the scope for preschool training of children with disabilities and counselling for parents, and 100% financial assistance can be provided for education of these children through this project. Under IEDC, more than 120,000 children with disabilities are being educated in more than 24,000 mainstream schools. The National Council for Educational Research and Training (NCERT) acknowledges that there is a lack of clarity at different levels in the understanding regarding inclusive education in the Indian context.

Sarva Shiksha Abhiyan – A Movement to Educate All

The Sarva Shiksha Abhiyan (SSA) programme aims to achieve universalization of elementary education (UEE) for all. This project underscores effective decentralization, sustainable financing, cost-effective strategies for universalizing education, community-owned planning and implementation. It mainly focuses on girls and marginalized populations of the community.

District Primary Education Project

District Primary Education Project (DPEP) was launched in many states with World Bank assistance in the year 1994. It focuses on in-service training of general teachers to enable early detection and assessment, as well as to use aids and make individual educational plans. The integrated education for children with disabilities was formally included in this plan in the year 1997. In the initial stage, only 15 states with 176 districts were covered under DPEP, but by the year 1998, many states had carried out surveys and formal assessments for implementation. Quality improvement is the cornerstone of DPEP. It supports community mobilization and early detection of disabilities.

District Rehabilitation Centres and National Programme for Rehabilitation for Persons with Disability

The Ministry of Social Justice and Empowerment has set up 11 District Rehabilitation Centres in 10 states of India and launched National Programme for Rehabilitation for Persons with Disability (NPRPD) in 1999. Under this programme, community-based rehabilitation as a strategy is practiced and promoted. Within this scheme, community empowerment of the disabled people is done mainly as a service.

VOLUNTARY AGENCIES THAT PROVIDE SERVICES TO CHILDREN

Balkan Ji-Bari

It is a child welfare association of India, literally meaning children's own garden, founded in the year 1923. Its aim is to provide children a fuller life and development of harmonious personality. It is an all India organization, and its motto is education and entertainment. It aims to work for the physical, mental, moral and social welfare of children.
Objectives:
   Extension of relief to orphans and handicapped children.
   Establish and conduct ashrams, orphanages, child welfare centres, child guidance clinics, youth clubs, crèches, preschools, schools and training institutes.
   Prevention of cruelty towards children and securing enactment of beneficial legislation for children.
   It trains voluntary workers for carrying out their activities.

Vikaswadi Kosbad

This is a simple pattern of running *balwadies* with active involvement of community that has formed in Kosbad in

Maharashtra. It runs a large number of *balwadies* for tribal children and trains its own functionaries. It was set up by Tarabai Modak with a model of running *balwadies* in village courtyards or under trees. Her famous concept is Meadow School, where teachers went to meadows to teach students who cannot leave their cattle to attend school.

Mobile Crèches

This was formed by Mira Mahadevan in 1969 for helping children of construction workers. This organization is presently running a chain of centres in Delhi, Pune and Mumbai.

SOS Children's Village in India

Save Our Souls (SOS) Children's Village in India is dedicated to the total care of needy, orphaned and destitute children. It was established in 1964. Its main motto is to establish children's village where neglected children are given care in a near family atmosphere under the care of a mother. These children go the community and live as any other children in a family.

Ruchika

This is a school for street children and is run on the railway platform of Bhubaneswar city. It gives care to children from the age of 6 months to 14 years. It was started by the Ruchika School Society in 1985. This programme gives not only education but also regular health check-ups and nutritional inputs. This programme is run using the fund raised by the society through donations.

Beti Bachao Beti Padhao Scheme

The 2011 census in India showed a marked discrepancy in the male to female ratio in India. Child sex ratio had shown an alarming decrease in the number of females (for every 1000 males, there are 918 females). This is owing to discrimination of gender in India and the wide practice of female feticide. The government has taken a number of steps such as prohibition of sex determination in all ultrasound scanning centres, clinics and hospitals. Still the female ratio is declining and is even expanding to rural areas. Alarmed by the sharp decline, the Government of India has introduced the Beti Bachao Beti Padhao (BBBP) scheme for improving the gender ratio. The important objectives of this scheme include:
1. Prevent gender-biased sex-selective elimination.
2. Ensure survival and protection of the girl child.
3. Ensure education of the girl child.

Main activities under this scheme are mass communication campaign to ensure that the girl child is born, nurtured and educated without discrimination; and multisectoral interventions in 100 gender critical districts covering all states/union territories in close coordination with the Ministry of Health and Family Welfare and the Ministry of Human Resource Development to ensure survival and protection of the girl child. Important activities are registration of all antenatal women, monitoring of preconception and prenatal diagnosing techniques (PCP&DT) Act 1994, increase in institutional deliveries, registration of all births, strengthening Pre-Natal Diagnostic Techniques (PNDT) cells, setting up monitoring committees, universal enrolment of the girl child in schools, decrease in dropout rate, girl child-friendly school environment, strict implementation of Right to Education (RTE), construction of girl-friendly toilet facilities, etc.

Kishori Shakti Yojana

Kishori Shakti Yojana (KSY) is a programme undertaken to promote and educate young girls between 11 and 18 years of age regarding environment, social status, social problems, health, hygiene, marriage, etc. This programme also aims at providing vocational training to empower the girl child to become self-reliant and to be a useful and confident individual of the society. This programme is modification of the Adolescent Girl Scheme under ICDS. The project is financed by the Government of India. This scheme focuses on welfare of the girl child. Its objectives are as follows:
1. To provide adequate knowledge regarding nutrition, health and hygiene, development and welfare of adolescent girls, and family care.
2. To make the adolescents knowledgeable about their environment and social strata and become self-reliant.
3. To provide proper nutrition to girl child between 11 and 18 years of age.
4. To deliver training to make them capable of taking important decisions.
5. To train girls on vocational skills and home science.
6. To make them aware that a girl should be married only after 18 years of age.
7. To make them aware of the environmental and social problems that may affect their health and decent living.
8. To encourage them to take up useful projects to be productive and self-sufficient.

Facilities available under this scheme are formal and informal education, immunization, general health checkups, treatment of minor illness, deworming, prophylactic measures for anaemia, goitre, vitamin deficiencies, referral to PHCs/district hospitals and convergence of RCH.

Protection of Children from Sexual Offenses e-box (POCSO e-Box)

The Union Ministry of Women and Child Development launched a programme called POCSO e-Box on 26 August 2016. The POCSO Act was enacted in the year 2012 to protect children from offenses of sexual assault, sexual harassment and pornography and safeguarding the interest of children in all aspects of life.

POCSO e-Box is an online complaint management system for easy and direct reporting of sexual offenses against children. It is an initiative of the National Commission for

Protection of Child Rights (NCPCR) for direct reporting of child sexual abuse. This is incorporated in the home page of the National Commission for Protection of Child Rights website. The user can lodge complaint by pressing the arrow on this page that navigates to another page where he/she has to select a picture denoting the type of harassment. The user also needs to fill the form with details such as email, mobile number and description of the harassment in order to register the complaint. There is short animation movie that tells children that it is not their fault and they need not feel bad on this and they will get adequate help.

Government of India Schemes and Programmes for Children

- Integrated Child Development Scheme (ICDS, 1975)
- Swachh Bharat Mission (Total Sanitation Campaign, 1999, and Swachh Bharat Mission, 2014)
- Sarva Shiksha Abhiyan (2000)
- National Health Mission (NHM, 2005)
- Integrated Child Protection Scheme (ICPS, 2009)
- National Skill Development Mission (NSDM, 2015), etc.
- The National Nutrition Mission is soon to be relaunched to address key issues of undernutrition in a comprehensive way.
- Mahatma Gandhi National Employment Guarantee Act does not directly relate to children; however, it significantly affects children's condition.

The benefits of Mahatma Gandhi National Rural Employment Guarantee Act (MNREGA) are extended to children by developing better infrastructure at the community level through convergence and empowering vulnerable households by providing them employment in their own village.

WHO DEPARTMENT OF CHILD AND ADOLESCENT HEALTH AND DEVELOPMENT

The Department of Child and Adolescent Health and Development (CAH) is working for children's and adolescents' rights. The department believes that all children and adolescents should have the means and opportunities to develop to their full potential. According to CAH, life, survival, maximum development, access to health and health services are not just basic needs of children and adolescents but also the fundamental human rights. Other common rights of children and adolescents include the right to the following:

- Nondiscrimination
- Education and access to appropriate information
- Privacy and confidentiality
- Protection from all forms of violence
- Rest, leisure and play
- An adequate standard of living
- Freedom from all forms of exploitation
- Participation, including the right to be heard

The primary instrument for protecting and fulfilling these rights is the Convention on the Rights of the Child (CRC). This was adopted by the United Nations. The work of CRC includes the following:

- Provision of a channel for both advocacy and practical support for children's and adolescents' health.
- Provision of a guiding framework for WHO's work across the broad spectrum of children's and adolescents' health and development.

The work of CAH in the area of children's and adolescents' health includes the following:

- Development of test guidelines to prevent ill health
- Care for illness if and when they occur

For neonates (up to 1 month of age) and infants (up to 1 year of age), its work focuses mainly on the mother and other caretakers. The issues related to prevention in these groups include breastfeeding and appropriate introduction of complementary foods, hygienic practices and caring behaviours that contribute to the healthy development of young children. Care of infants and neonates during illness is also very important, as young children can die very quickly if illness is not recognized.

CAH work towards prevention and treatment of most health problems in older children such as measles, diarrhoea, malaria, ARI and malnutrition. Prevention has a greater importance in major health problems related to adolescents. The common problems that have been taken as issues by CAH are sexual and reproductive health, substance use and mental health including suicide and prevention of accident and injuries.

WHO GLOBAL SCHOOL INITIATIVE

This seeks to mobilize and strengthen health promotion and education at the local, national, regional and global levels.

As a part of the WHO Global School Initiative, in India, the Education Commission of 1996 (Kothari Commission) drew attention to the education of children with disabilities. In 1974, for the first time, the necessity of integrated education was explicatively emphasized under the IEDC scheme. The National Policy on Education (1986) follows up the actions for education for all. The World Declaration on Education for All adopted in 1990 gave further boost to the education of the disabled. The Rehabilitation Council of India Act (1992) initiated a training programme for the development of professionals to respond to the needs of students with disability. The enactment of the People with Disability Act (1996) provided legislature support. This act makes it mandatory to provide free education to children with disabilities in an appropriate environment until the age of 18 years. In 1991, the National Trust for Welfare of Persons with Autism, Cerebral Palsy, Mental Retardation and Multiple Disability Act for economic rehabilitation of people with disabilities (by the government) was instituted. Two major initiatives have been launched by the government for achieving the goals of UEE, DPEP in 1994 and SSA in 2002. All these programmes are instituted by the government with help of the World Bank and UNICEF.

The World Declaration on Education for All adopted in 1990 gave further boost to the education of the disabled. The Rehabilitation Council of India Act (1992) initiated a training programme.

INTEGRATED MANAGEMENT OF CHILDHOOD ILLNESSES

The core IMCI intervention is integrated case management of the five most important causes of childhood deaths (ARI, diarrhoea, measles, malaria and malnutrition). The strategy includes a range of other preventive and curative interventions which aim to improve practices both in health facilities and at home.

IMCI Strategy

The three strategies for IMCI programmes are as follows:
1. Improving skills of health workers – The substrategies include standard guidelines, training (preservice and in-service) and follow-up after training.
2. Strengthening health systems – The substrategies include essential drug supply and management, organization of work in health facilities, and management and supervision.
3. Improving family and community practices – Care seeking, nutrition, home case management and adherence to recommended treatment and community involvement.

The interventions currently included in the IMCI strategy include the following:
- Promotion of growth
- Prevention of disease – Community/home-based interventions to improve nutrition

Home-based care includes insecticide-treated bed nets to prevent mosquito bites, thereby preventing malaria and filariasis.
- Response to sickness (curative care) – Early case management and appropriate care seeking (For further explanation on IMNCI, see chapter 4.)

UN SUPPORT TO PRIMARY EDUCATION: COMMUNITY SCHOOL PROGRAMME

The Community School Programme is a unique multistate, multiagency initiative. UN organizations – UNDP, UNICEF, UNFPA, UNIESCO and ILO – are participants in the programme with five nodal ministries and nine state departments. The programme is a vehicle for channelling UN support for ongoing efforts towards UEE by helping to enhance and sustain community participation in effective school management and protection of child rights. The support ensures interactive, gender-sensitive and child-centred teaching methodologies in classrooms. A special emphasis is given to the girl child. The focus is on addressing the educational needs of working children, children with disabilities and adolescent girls. The UN-supported education advocates an inclusive education based on the Salamanca Principles and UNESCO guidelines.

ACTS RELATED TO CHILD WELFARE

The Children's Act of 1960

This Act provides for penalization of offenders for cruel treatment of children, employment of children in begging, giving liquor or dangerous drugs and employing a person below 14 years of age in factories or mines. This Act had some confusion, as some states considered children up to 18 years of age as children. The Act was amended in 1978 so as to meet the needs of delinquent children.

Right to Education

The Supreme Court has recognized the RTE as an implied fundamental right under Article 21. It provides provision for free education up to 14 years of age. Recently, the Government of India has made an amendment for free education to the only female child of a family in CBSE schools in India.

Child Marriage Restraint Act (1929)

Marriage of girls at unripe age is a major cause of maternal and paediatric morbidity and mortality. This Act, last amended in 1978, raised the minimum age at marriage to 21 years for males and 18 years for females. It is a preventive measure for maternal and infant mortality and morbidity.

Child Labour (Protection and Regulation Act, 1986)

This Act flows from Article 39 that the tender age of children shall not be abused and that citizen are not forced by economic necessity to enter avocations unsuited to their age or strength. This Act protects children to be employed in dangerous work and industries up to 14 years of age.

The other Acts related to children are the Central Children Act (1960) and the Juvenile Justice (Care and Protection) of Children Act (2000).

RIGHTS OF THE CHILD

Children are recognized as having their own human rights. These are laid down in UNCRC.

The Indian Constitution gives ample privilege to the child population through various Acts such as:
- Article 24 prohibits employment of children below the age of 14 years in factories.
- Article 39 prevents abuse of children of tender age.
- Article 45 provides free and compulsory education for all children until they complete the age of 14 years.

United Nations Declaration of the Rights of the Child

The General Assembly of the United Nations adopted on 20 November 1959 the Declaration of the Rights of the Child. The rights of children are as follows:

1. Right to develop in an atmosphere of affection and security and, wherever possible, in the care and under the responsibility of his/her parents.
2. Right to enjoy the benefits of social security, including nutrition, housing and medical care.
3. Right to free education.
4. Right to full opportunity for play and recreation.
5. Right to a name and nationality.
6. Right to special care, if handicapped.
7. Right to be among the first to service protection and relief in times of disaster.
8. Right to learn to be a useful member of society and to develop in a healthy and normal manner and in conditions of freedom and dignity.
9. Right to be brought up in spirit of understanding, tolerance, friendship among the people, peace and universal brotherhood.
10. Right to enjoy these rights, regardless of race, colour, sex, religion, national or social origin.

Summary of the United Nations Convention on the Rights of the Child (1989)

1. Survival rights:
   The child's right to life and to the most basic needs – food, shelter and access to health care.
2. Developmental rights:
   To achieve their full potential – education, play, freedom of thought, conscience and religion.
   Those with disabilities to receive special services.
3. Protection rights:
   Against all forms of abuse, neglect, exploration and discrimination.
4. Participation rights:
   To take an active role in their communities and nations.

Recent Child-Centric Acts and Schemes

India has passed various child-centric legislations such as:
- The Juvenile Justice Care and Protection Act (2000) and the new Act of 2015 keeping in line with standards of care and protection required in present time
- Establishment of the National Commission for the Protection of Child Rights (NCPCR, 2005)
- The Prohibition of Child Marriage Act (2006)
- The Right of Children to Free and Compulsory Education Act (2009)
- The Protection of Children from Sexual Offences (POCSO) Act (2012)

NATIONAL POLICY FOR CHILDREN

The Government of India adopted a National Policy for children in August 1974 in response to UN declaration of the rights of the child. The Policy declares:

'It shall be the policy of the state to provide adequate services to children, both before and after birth, and through the period of growth to ensure their full physical, mental and social development. The state shall progressively increase the scope of such services so that within a reasonable time, all children in the country enjoy optimum conditions for their balanced growth'.

According to this Policy, the development of children has been considered as an integral part of national development. The Policy recognizes children as the nation's supremely important asset and the nation is responsible for their nurture and solicitude. A high-level National Children's Board with Prime Minister as Chairperson was established for this purpose. As a part of the National Policy, many programmes were set up for the children's welfare. Some of these are ICDS, programmes of Supplementary Feeding, Nutrition Education and Production of Nutritious Food, constitution of the National Children's Fund under the Charitable Endowments Acts (1980), institution of National Awards for Child Welfare, Welfare of the Handicapped, CSSM programme, etc.

NHP 2017 came into existence after a long gap of 15 years to address the emerging health issues. The last NHP was launched in the year 2002. NHP 2017 was approved by the Cabinet on 16 March 2017. NHP 2017 focuses on preventive and promotive health care and universal access to good-quality health care services. Based on NHP 2017, the National Plan for Child Care 2017 was formulated.

The National Plan of Action for Children (NPAC) was drafted by the Ministry of Women and Child Welfare on the basis of the National Policy for Children in the year 2016.

According to the National Policy for Children, 26 April 2013, every person below the age of 18 years is a child in India. National Policy for Children acknowledges a multisectoral and multidimensional approach to secure the rights of children.

The National Policy for Children adheres to the constitutional mandate and guiding principles of UN CRC and reflects a paradigm shift from a 'needs-based' to a 'rights-based' approach.

For focused attention, four key priority areas were identified: **survival, health and nutrition; education and development; and protection and participation.**

The National Policy for Children, 2013, was based on the following principles in a nutshell:
- Every child has universal, inalienable and indivisible human rights that are interrelated and interdependent.
- Every child has the right to life, survival, development, education, protection and participation and also encompasses the right to identity and nationality with equal rights, and no child shall be discriminated against on grounds of religion, race, caste, sex, place of birth, class, language, and disability, social, economic or any other status.
- Mental, emotional, cognitive, social and cultural development of the child is to be addressed in totality and in the best interest of the child.
- Every child has the right to have a conducive family and a dignified life, free from exploitation. Safety

and security of all children are integral to their well-being.
- Children's views are to be heard in all matters that affect them.

Policy Framework for Children in India

1. National Policy for Children, 1974
2. Promotion and Adoption of International Year of the Child (IYC), 1979
3. National Policy for Education, 1986
4. Adoption of 1990s' World Child Survival and Development Goals, 1990
5. Accession to UN CRC, 1992
6. National Nutrition Policy, 1993
7. National Health Policy, 2002
8. National Charter for Children, 2003
9. National Plan of Action for Children, 2005
10. Adoption of Guidelines for NCPCR, 2011 and 2015
11. National Policy for Children, 2013
12. National Early Childhood Care and Education (*ECCE*) Policy, 2013
13. India Newborn Action Plan, 2014

The National Plan of Action for Children, 2016

It succeeds the Plan of Action adopted in 2005. The previous plan had identified 12 key areas, keeping in mind the following priorities:
- Reducing IMR
- Reducing MMR
- Reducing malnutrition among children
- Achieving 100% civil registration of births
- Universalization of early childhood care and development, and quality education for all children achieving 100% access and retention in schools, including ECCE
- Complete abolition of female feticide, female infanticide and child marriage and ensuring the survival, development and protection of the girl child
- Improving water and sanitation coverage in both rural and urban areas
- Addressing and upholding the rights of children in difficult circumstances
- Securing for all children all legal and social protection from all kinds of abuse, exploitation and neglect
- Complete abolition of child labour with the aim of progressively eliminating all forms of economic exploitation of children
- Monitoring, review and reform of policies, programmes and laws to ensure protection of children's interests and rights
- Ensuring child participation and choice in matters and decisions affecting their lives

Key Priority Areas Defined in NPC 2013 and NPAC 2016:

The rights of the children are categorized under four *Key Priority Areas*, which are:
1. Survival, health and nutrition

1. Beti Bachao Beti Padhao
2. Dindayal Disabled Rehabilitation Scheme
3. Integrated Child Development Services (including SABLA and Kishori Shakti Yojana)
4. Indira Gandhi Matritva Sahayog Yojana
5. Integrated Child Protection Scheme
6. Integrated Rashtriya Madhyamikd Shiksha Abhiyan
7. Janani Suraksha Yojana
8. Janani Shishu Suraksha Karyakram
9. Mid Day Meal
10. Mahatma Gandhi National Rural Employment Guarantee Scheme
11. National Health Mission
12. National Nutrition Mission
13. National Rural/Urban Drinking Water Mission
14. National Mental Health Programme
15. National AIDS Control Programme
16. Pradhanmantri Kaushal Vikas Yojana
17. Rashtriya Bal Swasthya Karyakram
18. Rajiv Gandhi National Creche Scheme
19. Rashtriya Kishor Swasthya Karyakram
20. Sarva Shiksha Mission
21. Swachh Bharat Mission
22. Scholarship Schemes
23. Schemes Under National Trust Act
24. Ujjawala

Key Programmes and Schemes in NPAC 2016

2. Education and development (including skill development)
3. Protection
4. Participation

In alignment with the National Policy for Children, 2013, NPAC 2016 has the following objectives:

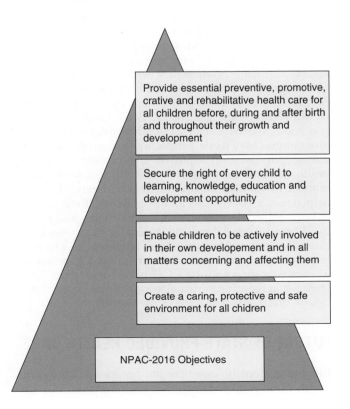

Provide essential preventive, promotive, crative and rehabilitative health care for all children before, during and after birth and throughout their growth and development

Secure the right of every child to learning, knowledge, education and development opportunity

Enable children to be actively involved in their own developement and in all matters concerning and affecting them

Create a caring, protective and safe environment for all chidren

NPAC-2016 Objectives

Key Priority Areas and Its Major Concerns

S.No.	Key Priority Area	Major Concerns
1	Survival, health and nutrition	1. High MMR and CMR, particularly neonatal mortality 2. CMR is higher for girls in rural areas 3. High rates of undernutrition and anaemia among children 4. Lack of adequate maternal and child care 5. Poor access to water and sanitation, particularly in rural areas and urban slums 6. Children from poor and marginalized communities show poor indicators for survival, health and nutrition
2	Education and development	1. ECCE accessed by very few children 2. Poor retention and high dropout rates at the elementary level, especially for schedule caste (SC) and schedule tribe (ST) children 3. A large number of children with special needs and SC/ST children are out of school 4. Lack of adequate infrastructure in primary schools 5. Poor quality of education at the elementary level 6. All children in the 15+ years age group do not have access to education/vocational training 7. Lack of adequately trained teachers at the elementary level as per the RTE norms
3	Protection	1. A large number of child labourers 2. Trafficking of children on the rise 3. Lack of comprehensive information, research and data on child migration and child trafficking 4. A large number of girls being married before the legal age 5. Rise in crimes against children, especially sexual offences 6. Poor rates of case disposal and conviction for crimes against children 7. Rise in Juveniles in Conflict with Law (JCL) cases 8. A majority of juveniles in conflict with law appear to have discontinued education after the primary level and also belong to the economically weaker section
4	Participation	1. Children lack information on their own rights, entitlements and policies and programmes concerning them. 2. Children's voices are seldom heard and their views are seldom given due respect by adult community members 3. Children's abilities and confidence to be built to enable them to express their views freely, deal with stress and trauma, and participate in meaningful activities

CURRENT STATUS OF INDIAN CHILDREN

Policies on provision of health care to all have not been successful in India owing to various reasons. India has tried to reduce inequalities in provision of health care through mitigation of poverty by various means such as BPL health insurance scheme, Nariyojana scheme, rural poverty reduction programmes, National Rural Employment Guarantee Act, Integrated Rural Development Programme/Swarnajayanti Gram Swarozgar Yojana, Wage Employment Programmes, NRHM and a host of other programmes. These programmes have made a tremendous improvement in reducing poverty and improved the capacity for paying health care and accepting responsibility for own health. A number of women empowerment programmes have also helped reduce poverty and improved female literacy, which, in turn, helped decrease childhood morbidity and mortality. These activities have made certain impact on health care as a whole and in particular to child health. The progress made on development programmes for promoting women education and the RCH programme have done a great job in reducing perinatal, neonatal and infant mortality and morbidity in all parts of the country.

FUTURE OF STATE-PROVIDED HEALTH CARE

India traditionally assumed the responsibility for the health of its people. Health has been accepted as a state responsibility in India, and free medical care to its people, whether they are able to pay or not, is considered a part of the government responsibility. These principles of the government led to three important consequences in the delivery and development of health care policies in India.

The two principles contributed to the present system of health care in the country. The first consequence of these principles *has led to inadequate priority to public health*, poor investment in safe water and sanitation and the neglect of the key role of personal hygiene in good health, culminating in the persistence of communicable diseases such as cholera in many parts of the country. The second set of consequences *pertains to substantially unrealized goals of NHP 1983* owing to funding difficulties from compression of public expenditures and from organizational inadequacies. NHP 1983 envisioned significant reduction in infant mortality, maternal mortality and childhood mortality (IMR, MMR and CMR by 2000. All the child health programmes are directed towards achieving these goals. But this could not be achieved because of failure in planning, especially in the aspect of strengthening rural health. The third set of consequences *appears to be the inability to develop and integrate plural systems of medicine and the failure to assign practical roles to the private sector and to assign public duties for private professionals.* These consequences had led to an unsatisfactory level of development in the field of public health, especially in achieving anticipated goals for child health.

A close look on the status of Indian children seven decades after independence is also not promising. Reduction in child mortality requires much attention. It should involve activities such as protecting children from infection, ensuring good nutrition and providing a holistic approach towards mother and child health services. There a number of services planned through NHP, such as antenatal services, delivery care and postpartum attention and care of low-birth-weight babies, prevention and management of childhood diarrhoea, and ARI management. But even with these programmes, the childhood mortality in many states of India is still high compared with developed countries. The programmes of immunization and childhood nutrition have shown better results in states such as Kerala. This indicates that a sustained attention to routine and complex investments into growing children as a group makes them grow into persons capable of living a long life. But unfortunately interest often fades among health care professionals in pursuing the unglamorous routine of supervised immunizations and is substituted by pulse campaigns owing to default in immunizations. Child health experts fear that in the long run this may turn out to be counterproductive. Indeed, persistence with improved routines and care for quality in immunization would also be a pathway to reduce the world's highest rates of infant and childhood mortality.

According to the National Health Survey 2005–2006, on average, 47% of children are malnourished. In the so-called prosperous states such as Gujarat and Kerala, the number of malnourished children is on the rise. According to National Family Health Survey (NFHS) 3 data, nearly three-fourths of all infants and children between 6 and 35 months of age are anaemic. These data indicate that about one-third of children up to 3 years of age are stunted and one-sixth of them are wasted; two-fifths of children are underweight. Though the proportion of wasted children has increased, the number of underweight children has marginally reduced. The number of anaemic women has risen from 49% to 54% in all underdeveloped states of India. The pregnant women who are anaemic give birth to anaemic and unhealthy infants. The real, harsh facts of Indian children can be observed in Azad Foundation's findings, which state that 'every second child under 5 years is malnourished, ¼ adolescent girls between the ages of 15–19 are married, 30% of girls entering schools will not complete primary education, and 50% of new AIDS infections are seen in the age group 15–24 years'. The findings also indicate that the worst offenders are states such as Bihar, Arunachal Pradesh, Sikkim and Rajasthan. (Azad Foundation, 2012)

The census status of India considers that any person below the age of 14 years is a child. All government data keep 14 years as the age limit for children in India. NHP 2013 and NPAC 2016 in India and UNCRC consider individuals below the age of 18 years as a child. There are 472 million children under the age of 0–18 years in India, comprising 39% of the country's total population. India is a young country with 472 million children. Children in the age group 0–18 years constitute 39% of the country's total population. An analysis of age-wise distribution reveals that 29.5% of children are aged 0–5 years, 33% are aged 6–11 years, 16.4% are aged 12–14 years and 21% are aged 15–18 years, respectively. The majority of India's children (73%) live in rural areas.

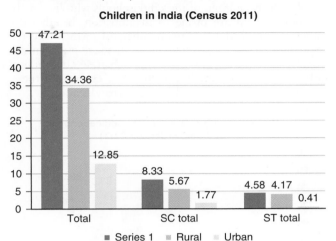

Children in India (Census 2011)

About 128.5 million children reside in urban areas, with 7.8 million children under the age of 0–6 years live in abject poverty and poor living conditions. There is a wide divide between the rich and the poor in India, though India is the third largest economy of Asia. In total, 50% of the wealth is owned by only 10% of the population in our country. A striking contrast is offered by the fact that Mumbai alone has more billionaires than all of Scandinavia, and yet about half of the population of the megapolis lives in slums. India ranks 94th out of 118 nations in the Global Hunger Index. Little children begging at traffic signals is a common sight in almost all cities of India. Several charity-funded nonprofit organizations are working alongside government agencies to bring some stability to child welfare. International aid covers only about US $1 per primary school-aged child.

In total, 54.7% of SC/ST people are landless and 75% of them earn less than Rs 5000 per month. India has 13.1% of the child population aged 0–6 years. An estimated 26 millions of children are born every year in India. According to the 2011 census, the total number of children aged 0–6 years is 158.79 million. Although India has made great progress in the health sector, the young population, especially in the age group 0–6 years, continuously lose their lives as a result of inadequate nutrition and proper care. Death related to malnutrition is still a problem in India. This is brought out by the latest 'Rapid Survey on Children – 2013–2014' by the Ministry of Women and Child Development.

Socioeconomic Status

Approximately 27.5% of children belong to the traditionally marginalized and disadvantaged communities (17.6% belong to SC and 9.7% to ST). According to the Socioeconomic and Caste Census 2011 published by the Government of India,[4] 38% of households in rural areas of the country are landless and are engaged in manual casual labour. The average monthly income of highest earning members in 75% of rural households is less than Rs 5000.00

per month. The percentage is noticeably higher for SC and ST households, depicting a higher level of economic vulnerability for these communities in terms of conditions of economic exploitation and social discrimination. This adversely affects children of these households who live in abject poverty and are prone to malnutrition, health risks, migration, trafficking and many other risks which threaten their right to survival, development, protection and meaningful participation. There are more than 449,000 households recorded as houseless in the 2011 census. Of these, 43% were in rural areas and 57% in urban locations.

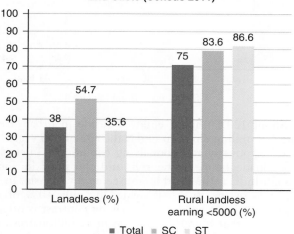

HH by Economic Deprivation, Socioeconomic and Caste (Census 2011)

Child Sex Ratio

The declining child sex ratio has been a cause of concern for India, which has steeply dropped from 945 girls per 1000 boys in 1991 to 918 girls per 1000 boys in 2011. It is attributed largely to female feticide as well as neglect of the girl child. The sex ratio is slightly better in rural areas than in urban areas. The child sex ratio has declined from 935 to 905 in urban areas between 1991 and 2011, whereas it has declined from 948 to 923 in rural areas.
(Census of India, 1991–2011).

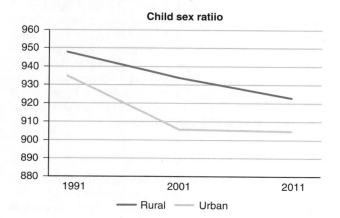

Child sex ratiio

Children with Disabilities

According to the 2011 census, there are more than 7.8 million children with disabilities, constituting

approximately 2% of the total child population. The majority of them (58%) are in the 10+ year age group. Special conditions of children in different categories are depicted in the following Figure (Type of disability) of the total number of children with disabilities, approximately 8% suffer from mental retardation.

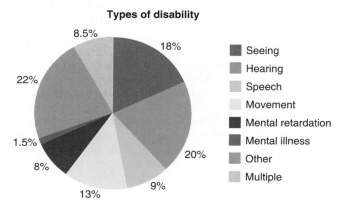

Types of disability

Children Affected by Natural Disasters

India is among the countries which at high risk of damage from natural hazards and is now increasingly facing ill effects of climate change. According to estimates of the Centre for Research on the Epidemiology of Disasters, between 2013 and 2015, more than 20 million people were affected by various natural disasters in India. Man-made disasters are also a serious concern in an already hazard-prone environment. It is estimated that a large proportion of the affected population would be children who are the worst affected population in emergency situations, as they face multiple protection and health risks.

Anaemia among Children

The prevalence of iron-deficiency anaemia among children is a major cause of concern in India. The Annual Health Survey conducted in nine states (Assam, Bihar, Chhattisgarh, Jharkhand, MP, Odisha, Rajasthan, UP and Uttarakhand) shows that a majority of children in these states are anaemic. It affects the cognitive and psychomotor development of children as well as their general health. A 1000-day approach has been instituted to improve nutrition in the period between a woman's conception and when her child turns 2 years old. The 1000-day approach has adopted 10 essential nutrition interventions:
1. Timely initiation of breastfeeding within 1 hour of birth.
2. Exclusive breastfeeding during the first 6 months of life.
3. Timely introduction of complementary foods immediately on completion of 6 months of age.
4. Age-appropriate complementary foods for children between 6 and 23 months of age, with appropriate energy and nutrient-dense, quantity, variety and frequency (including IFA supplements).
5. Safe handling of complementary foods and hygienic complementary feeding practices.

6. Full immunization and biannual vitamin A supplementation with deworming.
7. Frequent, appropriate and active feeding of children during and after illness, including oral rehydration with zinc supplements during diarrhoea.
8. Timely and quality therapeutic feeding and care of all children with severe acute malnutrition.
9. Education and improved food and nutrient intake for adolescent girls, particularly to prevent anaemia, by delaying marriage and/or pregnancy until at least 18 years of age.
10. Improved food and adequate nutrient intake for women, particularly during pregnancy and lactation and compulsory four ANC visits.

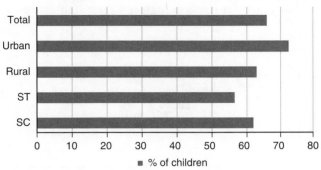

Percentage of children aged 12–23 months fully immunized

Immunization, RSOC (2013–2014).

Access to Safe Water and Sanitation:

Safe and sufficient drinking water, along with adequate sanitation and hygiene, positively impacts survival, health and nutrition status of the population. A study by the World Bank[15] (June 2010) in 70 countries shows a robust association between access to water and sanitation and child morbidity and mortality. The results show that good water and sanitation infrastructure lowers the odds of children suffering from diarrhoea by 7%–17% and reduces the mortality risk for children under the age of 5 years by approximately 5%–20%.

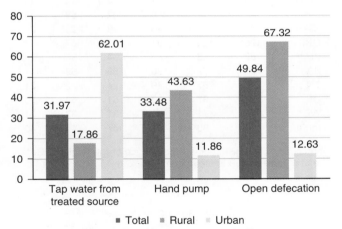

Water and sanitation, Census 2011.

According to WHO (2014), 43% of Indian children are underweight, about 38.7% of children have stunted growth and 15.1% are wasted.

Child mortality is a very sensitive indicator of socioeconomic development of a country. Infant mortality rate (IMR) and under-five mortality (U5M) rate are the most important components of child mortality. IMR is the cumulative rate of deaths among neonates (aged 0–29 days) and postneonatal mortality rate. IMR is expressed as a rate per 1000 live births. Infant mortality is defined as the number of deaths in the first year of child's life per 1000 live births in the given year.

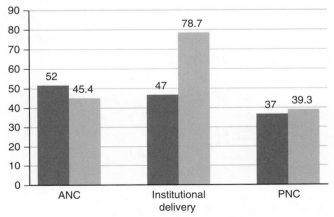

Nutrition status of children aged 0–59 months

Nutritional status of children, RSOC (2013–2014).

Access to Mother and Child Health Care and Nutrition Services

According to WHO, maternal and child deaths are preventable by providing a continuum of care through integrated service delivery for mothers and children from pre-pregnancy to delivery, the immediate postnatal period and childhood (within a period of 1000 days from conception)

Maternal and neonatal care, NFHS 3 (2005–2006), RSOC (2013–2014).

Although at the all India level IMR has declined for the last years, yet it was as high as 40 per 1000 live birth in 2013.

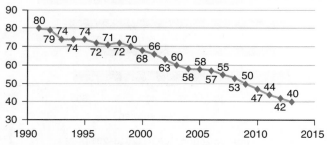

Infant Mortality Rate In India, 1990–2013.
Source: Sample registration system, Office of the Registrar General of India, 1991–2013.

Neonatal Mortality Rate

About 0.76 million newborns die every year in India. NNM of India in the year 1991 was 51 per 1000 live births. In 2012, it was 29 per 1000 live births. The major causes of NNM are preterm birth and infections during birthing. Neonatal mortality is a greater contributor to the total childhood mortality rate. Two-thirds of the infant deaths and one-half of the U5M result during the neonatal period itself.

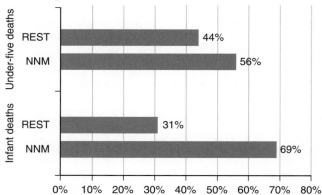

Neonatal deaths as a percentage of infant deaths and of under-five deaths. Source: SRC, statistical report, 2012.

States	1987	1991	2001	2011	2012	2013
AP	79	73	66	46	43	39
ASM	102	81	74	58	55	54
BR	101	69	62	48	44	42
GUJ	97	69	60	44	41	36
HAR	87	68	66	48	44	41
KAR	75	77	58	38	35	31
KER	28	16	11	13	12	12
MP	120	117	86	62	59	54
MAH	66	60	45	28	25	24
ORS	126	124	91	61	57	51
PUJ	62	53	52	34	30	24
RAJ	102	79	80	55	52	47
TN	76	57	49	24	22	21
UP	127	97	83	61	57	50
WB	71	71	51	31	32	31
India	95	80	66	47	44	40

Infant Mortality Rate In Various States In India From 1987 To 2013

Source: Sample registration system, Office of the Registrar General of India, CAGR is taken from Annexure-1

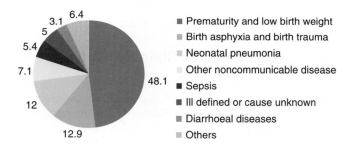

Causes of neonatal deaths

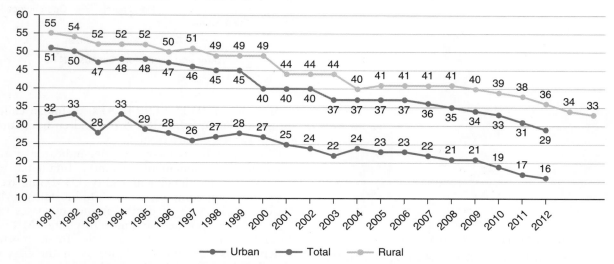

Neonatal mortality rate in India 1991–2012. Source: SRC statistical report 2012, Government of India.

Child Mortality Rate

CMR is the death of a child before completing 4 years of his/her life. This is also calculated per 1000 child population per year. A major share of childhood mortality comes from Madhya Pradesh, UP, Assam, Rajasthan and Bihar, where the majority of illiterate people of India reside. Poor socioeconomic status and illiteracy of mothers are important factors contributing to childhood mortality. Diarrhoea and malnutrition are the major medical reasons for these deaths. Childhood mortality in the year 1991 was 16.6% and had come down to 11.5% in 2012.

A wide rural–urban gap is seen in all these mortality rates. In total, 70% of U5M in India are mainly owing to six killer diseases. The leading causes of death among children under 5 years of age in 2015 were preterm birth complications, pneumonia, intrapartum-related complications, diarrhoea and congenital abnormalities. Neonatal deaths accounted for 45% of under-five deaths in 2015.

Childhood mortality is a challenge for health workers in India. Though India along with other countries of the world is committed to achieve Millennium Development Goals #4 of reducing U5M by two-thirds, between 1991 and 2015, U5M dropped to 36 per 1000 live births and IMR to 27 per 1000. Currently, our IMR is still unbearably high (58 per 1000 live births).

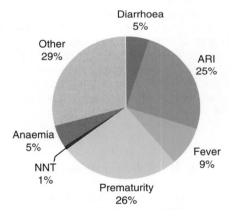

Estimated causes of U5M in India.

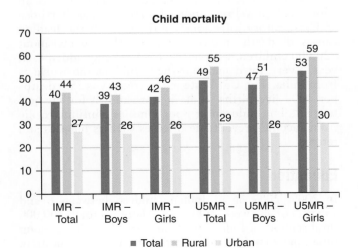

Key Indicators for Children in India:
1. Maternal mortality 167 per 100,000 live births (SRS 2011–2013)
2. Neonatal mortality 28 per 1000 live births (SRS 2013)
3. Infant mortality 40 per 1000 live births (SRS 2013)
4. U5M 49 per 1000 live births (SRS 2013)
5. 48% of neonatal deaths as a result of prematurity and low birth weight (SRS 2010–2013)
6. 45.4% of mothers received four or more ANC visits (RSOC 2013–2014)
7. 78.7% of institutional delivery (RSOC 2013–2014)
8. 39.3% of neonates received PNC within 48 hours of delivery/discharge (RSOC 2013–2014)
9. 38.7% of children aged 0–59 months have stunted growth; the percentage is higher for SC/ST (RSOC 2013–2014)
10. 15.1% of children aged 0–59 months are wasted; the percentage is higher for SC/ST (RSOC 2013–2014)
11. 29.4% of children aged 0–59 months are underweight; the percentage is higher for SC/ST (RSOC 2013–2014)
12. 44.6% of children aged 0–23 months breastfed immediately/within 1 hour of birth (RSOC 2013–2014)
13. 65.3% of children aged 12–23 months are fully immunized; the percentage is lower for SC/ST (RSOC 2013–2012)
14. 49.84% of households practice open defecation (Census 2011)
15. Net enrolment ratio at the elementary level: 88.45% (U-DISE 2014–2015)
16. Net enrolment ratio at the secondary level: 48.46% (U-DISE 2014–2015)
17. Dropout rates at the elementary level: 36.3% (Educational Statistics at a Glance, MOHRD; 2014)
18. Dropout rates for SC/ST at the elementary level: 38.8% and 48.2%, respectively (Educational Statistics at a Glance, MOHRD; 2014)
19. 33 million children in the age group 5–18 years are engaged in the labour force (Census 2011)
20. 30.3% of women in the age group 20–24 years are married before 18 years of age (RSOC 2013–2014)
21. Rise in the rate of crimes against children as well as crimes committed by children (NCRB 2014)
22. Approximately 40% of the reported offences against children are sexual offences (NCRB 2014)

Child Mortality Gender/Spatial, SRS 2013, ORGI

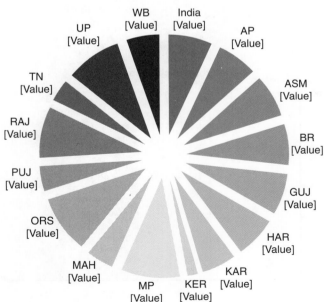

Figure: Share of neonatal mortality by major states. Source: Sample registration system, statistical report, 2012.

Children in Urban Slums

The number children in urban slums is on the rise, making a wide gap in the provision of facilities. About 7.8 million young children are growing up in slums. Requirements of these children are often neglected by urban planning. Inclusive and child-friendly cities must be developed to provide a physical environment that ensures children's health, develops their faculties and fosters their love for community and for nature. During the first 3 years of life, children need day care, health care, nutrition, and a safe and healthy environment which is accessible, equitable and affordable to all the poor and needy. Programmes such as Child-Friendly Smart Cities, AMRUT, Housing for All, Swachh Bharat mission, etc. provide hope for betterment of child life in India.

Population Percentage of Children in India, 2015

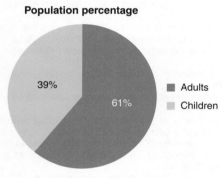

Population percentage

Total number of children.

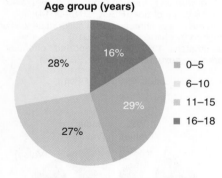

Age group (years)

Age group of children in India.

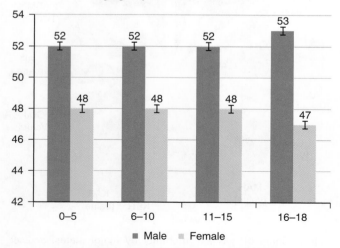

Age versus gender – Children and adolescents.

LEGAL STATUS OF INDIAN CHILDREN

According to Indian Penal Code (IPC) 1860, no the child below 7 years of age be held liable for criminal offenses; in the case of mental disability, the age is raised to 12 years. A girl should be 16 years of age to give legal consent for sexual activity unless she is married; in that case, the prescribed age is 15 years.

According to Article 21(a) of the Indian Constitution, all children between 6 and 14 years of age should be provided with free and compulsory education. Article 45 states that the state should provide early childhood education to all children below the age of 6 years. Article 51(k) directs all parents to give opportunities for education to all children between 6 and 14 years of age. The Child Labour Prohibition and Regulation Act, 1986 defines a child as person who has not completed 14 years of age. But the Factories Act, 1948, and Plantation Labour Act, 1951, define a child as an individual who has not completed 15 years of age and an adolescent as the one who has completed 15 years of age and not completed 18 years of age. According to Factories Act, 1948, adolescents are permitted to work in factories if they are medically fit for the same. The Prohibition of Child Marriage Act, 2006, states that a male who has not reached 21 years of age and a female who has not completed 18 years of age are not legally permitted to marry. The Indian Majority Act, 1875, the Guardian and Wards Act, 1890, the Hindu Minority and Guardianship Act, 1956, the Hindu Adoption and Maintenance Act, 1956, and Muslim, Christian and Zoroastrian personal laws also uphold 18 years of age as the age of majority and those below 18 years of age are considered as minors. The Juvenile Justice (Care and Protection of Children) Act, 2000, also considers a child as the one who has not completed 18 years of age.

Health

Almost half of all children in India, under the age of 5 years, suffer from stunted growth as a result of malnutrition. In total, 46% of children under the age of 3 years are too small for their age and at least 16% show signs of wasting. Anaemia affects 74% of all children under the age of 3 years and a shocking 90% of all adolescent girls. Preventable diseases such as diarrhoea and respiratory infections continue to be the leading causes of death among children. HIV infects about 220,000 children, with nearly 60,000 being added each year. Every third malnourished child in the world is from India. The U5M rate in the country is 78.6 deaths per 1000 live births. India is now known for medical tourism, but children of poor families continue to die from vaccine-preventable diseases such as measles and tetanus.

Education

In 2009, 20% of all Indian children between 6 and 14 years of age were still not in school. In total, 700,000 rural schools in India have inadequate facilities, making rural children not getting equal opportunities for education.

The gap between the haves and have-nots has increased and widened further by underqualified and untrained teachers for these rural children. One in six rural schools is equipped with some sort of toilet facilities, making the girl child not attending the school. A shocking absenteeism rate of 27% is costing the Indian government about US $2 billion per year.

Less than 25% of all enrolled children in India attend a grade commensurate with their age. Moreover, according to a 2007 survey, less than half of the children in grade 3 could read a text designed for grade 1. Furthermore, only 38% of the students in grade 4 could do subtraction or division. Higher education tells a similarly dismaying story, with only a 12% enrolment rate.

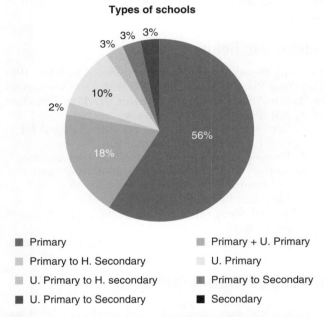

Distribution of Schools by Level; U-DISE 2014–2015, NUEPA. According to U-DISE 2014–2015, there are 56% primary schools and 18% primary and upper primary schools. The data show that India still needs a lot to reach 100% literacy.

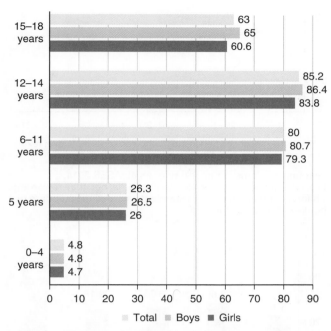

Age-specific attendance in any educational institution; Census 2011.
Age-specific attendance in any educational institutions shows that the attendance rate for girls is lower than that of boys.

The retention rate of students in the educational institution shows that girls are more retained than boys; in the SC/ST community, also girls' retention is better than boys. Gender disparities have also declined, making a significant stride towards gender parity in primary education. With sufficient help from the capable and responsible Indians in terms of financial aid and volunteering activities, it is possible to eradicate this social evil and help everyone on board the bus to true freedom.

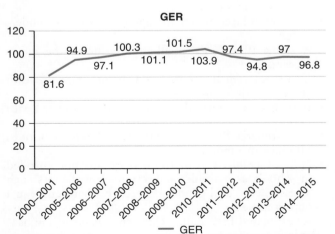

Gross enrolment ratio shows that there is an increase from 81.6% in the year 2001 to 96.8 % in the year 2015.
GER, U-DISE 2014–2015, NUEPA.

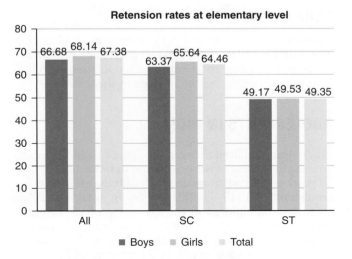

Retention rates, U-DISE 2014–2015, NUEPA.

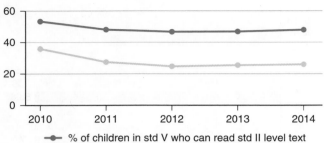

Learning outcomes at the primary level; ASER 2014.
Learning outcome at the primary level is not that rewarding. Children who are in the fifth standard can read the standard text books of the third standard.

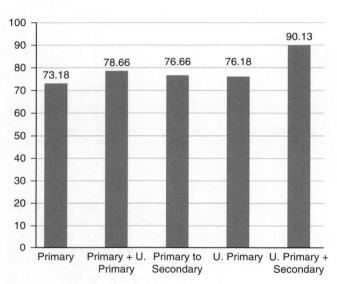

Trained teachers, U-DISE 2014–2015, NUEPA.
Availability of trained teachers in the year 2014–2015 shows that primary schools alone have 73.18% and upper primary and secondary together have 90.13%. But a high student to teacher ratio is a major problem in meeting proper learning outcomes for the children.

Child Labour

Though there are defined laws to prevent child labour, 12.6 million children engaged in hazardous occupation make India home to the largest population of child labourers under the age of 14 years in the world.

ADOLESCENTS IN INDIA

Adolescents (children between the ages of 10 and 19 years) account for 22.8% of the population in India. Girls below 19 years of age constitute one-fifth of India's fast-growing population (NFHS 3, 2005–2006). In total, there are 100.2 million children in the age group of 14–18 years, which constitute 11% of the total population. A majority of them are forced to assume the role of adults owing to various reasons such as poverty, economic and personal security.

There exist lots of exploitative environments for these children related to early marriage and a lack of education both at home and in the society, denying fundamental rights.

Adolescent Child Labour

Total workforce in India is 400 million people, and of these, 32 million are adolescents. Of the 312 million people employed as main workers, 20 million are adolescents between 14 and 18 years of age. Of the 90 million employed as marginal workers, 11 million are adolescents. According to the 2001 census, about 32 million children in the age group 14–18 years are involved in the workforce of the country.

According to the NFHS 3, 33.4% of girls and 50.4% of boys (in the 15–24 years age group) are engaged in labour.

Adolescent Health

Planning for adolescents was first initiated with the 10th Five-Year Plan in India (2002–2007). A Working Group on Youth Affairs was constituted in the 11th Five-Year Plan, and it has given following suggestions:

1. Setting up Regional Resource Centres for Adolescent Education and Development.
2. Provision of quality of education for adolescents.
3. Setting up of counselling for adolescents and special attention on substance abuse problem.
4. Life skills for students out of school.
5. Special focus on education of SC, ST and other minorities.
6. Sex and HIV/AIDS-related education for students.

ISSUES OF INDIAN CHILDREN

- IMR is still very high such as 63 deaths per 1000 live births.
- Most deaths occur in the first month of life. with up to 47 deaths in the first week of life.
- Children die with vaccine-preventable diseases such as measles and tetanus.
- 46% of children under the age of 3 years are underweight.
- Anaemia affects 74% of all children under the age of 3 years.
- Diarrhoea remains the second major cause of death among children after respiratory illnesses.
- India has an estimated 220,000 children infected with HIV.
- It is estimated that 55,000–60.000 children are born to HIV-positive mothers.
- 20% of children aged 6–14 years are not enrolled in schools as a result of discriminating factors such as caste, class and gender differences that deny equal opportunities.
- An estimated 12.6 million children are engaged in hazardous occupations.
- India has the largest number of child labourers in the world.

- Female feticide is a common problem, though there is a stringent regulation on sex determination.
- Female to male ratio is alarmingly getting lower in the northern states of India.

Status of children in India is very poor, with wide disparities among different states. It requires constant efforts from health care providers, professionals and the policy makers to be committed for a better India with lots of health promotion initiatives to safeguard our children to make them grow as better citizens for a prosperous India.

Study Questions

- List the various national and international organizations involved in the care of children in India.
- Describe the functions of ICDS programme.
- Describe various child welfare activities with its merits and demerits.
- Explain Beti Bachao Beti Padhao scheme.
- What is POCSO? Explain the use of POCSO e-box.
- Discuss the current status of Indian children.
- What measures the Government of India has taken to prevent child sexual abuse?
- What is 1000-day programme? How is it going to improve the nutritional status of children?
- Express your concern regarding gender discrimination in the light of alarming decline in the child sex ratio.
- After studying this chapter, what is your feeling about education of our children and what contribution can you make on this aspect as a citizen?
- Explain the Child Marriage Act.

BIBLIOGRAPHY

1. Farahani M, Subramanian SV. (2009). The effect of changes in health sector resources on infant mortality in the short-run and the long-run: A longitudinal econometric analysis. Soc Sci Med 68: 1918–1925.
2. Park. K. (2011). Park's Text book of Social and Preventive Medicine. M/s Banarsidas Bhanot Pub Jabalpur, India. 21st Ed; pp. 848-851.
3. Pradhan M, Sahn DE, Younger SD. (2003). Decomposing world health inequality. J Health Econ 22: 271-293.
4. Usmani G, Ahmad N. (March, 30 2017). Health Status of Children in India 3:138.doi:10.4172/2471-9870.10000138.
5. A report on current status of children in India.
6. District level household survey reports (I, II, III). (2013). Ministry of health and family welfare, New Delhi.
7. Government of India. (2006). Bulletin on rural health statistics in India. Ministry of health and family welfare, New Delhi.
8. Government of India. (2012). Universal health coverage report, New Delhi.
9. National Family Health Survey. (1992-1993). International institute for population sciences, India.
10. National Family Health Survey-2. (1998-1999). International institute for population sciences, India.
11. National Family Health Survey-3. (2005-2006). International institute for population sciences, India.
12. National Sample Survey Organization reports. Ministry of statistics and programme implementation, Government of India: New Delhi.
13. Press Information Bureau, Government of India, Ministry of Health and Family Welfare. Achievements Under Millennium Development Goals 24-July-2015 14:19 IST.
14. Rapid Survey on Children. (2013-2014). Ministry of women and child development. Government of India.
15. Rates of infant mortality, maternal mortality reducing fast: Govt to Rajya Sabha.
16. Sample registration system bulletin. (2013). Office of registrar general of India, 48: 2.
17. The National Plan of Action for Children, 2016. Ministry of Women Child Development, Govt.of India. March, 2017.
18. WHO. (2014) World health statistics. Global health observatory data.
19. 1000 Days Approach. Window of 1,000 days identified as the critical window to lay the nutritional foundation for a child's lifelong health, cognitive development, and future potential; in papers published by R.E.Black, L.H.Allen, et al, and C.G. Victoria,L. Adair, et. al, in The Lancet 2008 (Vol. 371).
20. http:1/ www.ncpcr.gov.in Email id pocsoebox-ncpcr@gov.in.
21. www.wcd.nic.in/BBBPScheme/implementingguidelinesofBBBPScheme.pdf. http:/wcd.nic.in BBBPScheme/training module. htm.
22. www.mygov.in/group_info/betibachao-beti-padhao.

SOCIAL AND PREVENTIVE PAEDIATRICS

Social and preventive paediatrics is concerned with child health maintenance for prevention and promotion of child health. It includes all the activities directed towards improving health of children aged 0–18 years. Preventive paediatrics includes all aspects of promoting health and preventing illnesses in children through surveillance, health education and accident prevention. Community paediatrics is also a part of preventive paediatrics that mainly concentrates on child abuse, adoption services, foster care and care of children with special needs. Illness prevention and health promotion are two arms of preventive paediatrics. According to the Ottawa Charter for Health Promotion, 'Health promotion is the process of enabling people to increase control over *determinants of health*, and to improve their health' (WHO, Geneva, 1986). It is a comprehensive social and political process.

It embraces actions directed at strengthening the skills and capabilities of individuals, and actions are directed towards changing social, environmental and economic conditions so as to alleviate their impact on public and individual health.

CHAPTER 4

Illness Prevention Strategies Related to Child Health

CHAPTER OUTLINE

- Causes of childhood morbidity and mortality
- Universal Immunization Programme
- Cold Chain
- Under-Five Clinics
- Well-Baby Clinics
- Child Guidance Clinics
- Integrated Management of Neonatal and Childhood Illness
- Millennium Development Goals and Sustainable Development Goals
- Baby-Friendly Hospital Initiative

LEARNING OBJECTIVES

At the end of the chapter, the learner will be able to:

- Understand the importance of illness prevention strategies in child health.
- Outline the causes of childhood morbidity and mortality.
- Describe the universal immunization schedule.
- Know the contraindications of immunization in children.
- Understand the importance of cold chain.
- Describe the functions of under-five clinics, well-baby clinics and child guidance clinics.
- Describe the importance and functions of Integrated Management of Neonatal and Childhood Illness (IMNCI).
- Explain Millennium Development Goals (MDGs).
- Describe the importance of sustainable development in child health care practices.
- Discuss the programme of Baby-Friendly Hospital Initiative (BFHI).

Illness prevention is an important part of preventive paediatrics that includes a range of approaches to reduce the risks of ill health and promote good health. Educating oneself and one's own patients, making healthy life styles changes, making behaviour modification and ensuring access to mediation or other interventions that prevent disease onset are its key factors. It focuses on prevention strategies to reduce the risk of developing chronic diseases and other morbidities such as communicable diseases.

LEVELS OF PREVENTION

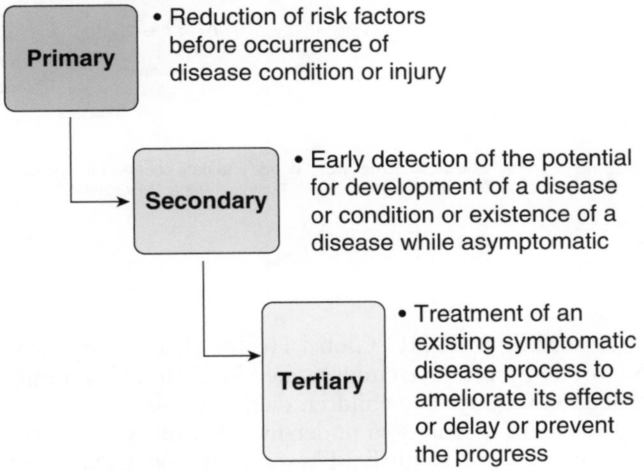
Primary
• Reduction of risk factors before occurrence of disease condition or injury
Secondary
• Early detection of the potential for development of a disease or condition or existence of a disease while asymptomatic
Tertiary
• Treatment of an existing symptomatic disease process to ameliorate its effects or delay or prevent the progress

Causes of Morbidity

There are various causes described by various researchers. In a study conducted by I.C. Verma and Santosh Kumar, 10 leading causes of morbidity were identified. They were upper respiratory tract infections, gastroenteritis, superficial infections of the skin, pyrexia of unknown origin, ulcers and injury, otitis media, anaemia, lower respiratory tract infection, pain in the abdomen and scabies.

A study conducted by B.P. Gladstone and colleagues to identify determinants of morbidity among infants in an Indian slum showed that infants experienced 12 episodes (95% confidence interval [CI], 11–13) of illness, spending about one-fifth of their infancy with illness. Respiratory and gastrointestinal symptoms were most common with incidence rates (95% CI) of 7.4 (6.9–7.9) and 3.6 (3.3–3.9) episodes per child-year, respectively. Factors independently associated with a higher incidence of respiratory and gastrointestinal illness were age (3–5 months), male sex, cold/wet season and household involved in *beedi* making. The rate (95% CI) of hospitalization, mainly for respiratory and gastrointestinal illness, was 0.28 (0.22–0.35) per child-year. **Among school children**, the major morbidity included malnutrition (10.0%–98.0%), dental ailments (4.0%–70.0%), worm infestation (2.0%–30.0%), skin diseases (5.0%–10.0%), eye diseases (4.0%–8.0%) and anaemia (4.0%–15.0%).

Causes of Mortality

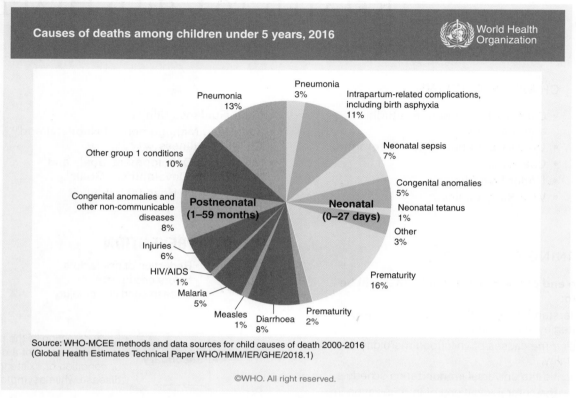

Causes of deaths among children under 5 years, 2016 — World Health Organization

Source: WHO-MCEE methods and data sources for child causes of death 2000-2016 (Global Health Estimates Technical Paper WHO/HMM/IER/GHE/2018.1)

Global Health Observatory data.

According to WHO Global Health Observatory data, 5.6 million under-five children died in 2016. This means that 15,000 under-five children died every day. The leading causes of mortality in under-five children are preterm birth complications, birth asphyxia, pneumonia, diarrhoea and malaria. Intrapartum-related complications and congenital anomalies are other leading causes. Neonatal deaths constitute 46% of the under-five deaths in 2016.

LEVELS OF HEALTH CARE

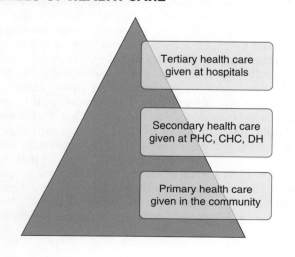

In this chapter, the major illness prevention strategy of immunization, its importance and what a health professional should do to prevent communicable diseases in children are described. This chapter also gives an account of the functions of various clinics aimed to prevent illness in children and promote their health along with certain international programmes such as IMNCI, MDGs and Sustainable Development Goals (SDGs), and BFHI that are designed specifically to suit Indian scenario.

Immunity can be defined as a state of resistance to infection owing to the presence of antibodies. The immunity may be natural immunity or artificial immunity. Natural immunity is inborn, acquired naturally by having the disease or being exposed to the organism over a period of time or by the passage of maternal antibodies via the placenta and breast milk. Artificial immunity is acquired by immunization. It can be either active immunity or passive immunity. The other type of immunity is called cell-mediated immunity or cellular immunity. This is the response by certain lymphocytes to material recognized by the body as non-self; it is one of the causes of transplanted organ or tissue rejection.

IMMUNIZATION

Immunization is the artificial means by which the state of immunity is increased. This is the most important invention that conferred the highest benefit to children in the world. It has prevented many communicable diseases such as diphtheria and polio. It has helped eradicate polio and small pox from the community. Recently, a highly successful introduction of immunization against *Haemophilus influenzae* type b (Hib) has been achieved that reduces invasive infections such as Hib meningitis.

- **Active immunization:** It is achieved by the use of vaccines containing attenuated organisms or bacterial products such as toxins, e.g. tetanus. This type of immunity results in the production of antibodies and is generally long-lasting. Active immunity is induced by:
  - A live attenuated vaccine such as measles–mumps–rubella (MMR) vaccine or bacillus Calmette–Guerin (BCG) vaccine for tuberculosis (TB);
  - An inactivated organism, e.g. inactivated poliomyelitis vaccine (IPV), pertussis;
  - A component of the organism, e.g. Hib, pneumococcal vaccine, hepatitis B and meningitis C; and
  - An inactivated toxin (toxoid), e.g. tetanus vaccine, diphtheria vaccine.
- **Passive immunization:** It is achieved by injecting antibodies. It is of short duration and gives only temporary protection. Passive immunity is conferred by the injection of human immunoglobulin. These are of two types, namely human normal immunoglobulin (HNIG) and specific immunoglobulins of tetanus, hepatitis B, rabies and varicella zoster.
- **Immunoglobulins** are antibodies. Antibodies are a group of proteins present in the blood, intestinal secretions and respiratory secretions.
- **Antigen:** A variety of foreign substances including bacteria viruses, toxins and foreign proteins that stimulate the formulation of antibodies.
- **Toxins:** A poisonous substance usually produced by the invading microorganisms.
- **Antitoxin:** Antibody formed in response to a toxin.
- **Toxoid:** A toxin that has been treated to destroy its toxic properties but retain its antigenic quality.

- **Immunization programme:** It is a routine programme of immunization offered during childhood for prevention against the killer diseases of childhood and prevent occurrence of certain dreaded diseases in the adulthood so that human resources can be maintained without hazards.

UNIVERSAL IMMUNIZATION PROGRAMME

The Universal Immunization Programme (UIP) was launched in India in 1985, extending the Expanded Programme for Immunization (EPI) that had been developed to provide recommended vaccines against six major killer diseases. The Ministry of Health and Family Welfare was responsible for the programme, with significant support from the international community. The programme has achieved some of its targets but has faced many challenges.

The evolution of the UIP and related initiatives included the following major events:

- 1978: EPI
- 1985: UIP
  - For reduction of mortality and morbidity as a result of six vaccine-preventable diseases (VPDs)
  - Indigenous vaccine production capacity enhanced
  - Cold chains established
  - Phased implementation – All districts [to be] covered by 1989–1990
  - Monitoring and evaluation of systems implemented
  - The Adverse Events Following Immunization (AEFI)
- 1986: Technology Mission on Immunization
- 1992: Child Survival and Safe Motherhood (CSSM)
- 1997: Reproductive Child Health (RCH 1)
- 2001: The National Technical Advisory Group on Immunization (NTAGI) in India
- 2005: National Rural Health Mission (NRHM)
- 2005/2006: The AEFI guidelines were revised
- 2010: Reconstituted the NTAGI

Administering Vaccines: Route, Site and Dose

To Whom	Vaccine	Number of Doses	Route	Site	To Protect	Dose
Infants	BCG	1	Intradermal	Left deltoid	Tuberculosis	0.05 mL
	OPV-liquid vaccine	5 + 1[a]	Oral	Mouth	Poliomyelitis	Two drops
	DPT-liquid vaccine	3 + 1[a]	Intramuscular	Vastus lateralis	Diphtheria, pertussis and tetanus	0.5 mL
	HBV-liquid vaccine	3	Intramuscular	Vastus lateralis	Hepatitis B	0.5 mL
	Measles lyophilized vaccine	1	Subcutaneous/ intramuscular	Do	Measles	0.5 mL
Children under 5 years of age	DT	1[b]	Intramuscular	Vastus lateralis	Diphtheria and tetanus	0.5 mL
Children older than 7 years	TT	1[b]	Intramuscular	Deltoid muscle	Tetanus	0.5 mL
Pregnant women	TT	1[b]	Intramuscular	Deltoid muscle	Neonatal tetanus in newborn	0.5 mL

[a]Booster dose.
[b]Give two doses, 6–8 weeks apart, if not vaccinated previously.
BCG (Bacillus Calmette–Guerin)

- There have been additional national efforts to improve coverage:
  - Immunization Strengthening Project (ISP)
  - Urban Measles Campaigns and that of Border Districts Cluster Strategy (BDCS)
  - Celebration of immunization week in the low-performing districts
  - Other important developments of this period include the following: NTAGI in India was constituted in 2001 and was reconstituted in 2010

Under UIP, the Government of India is now providing vaccination to seven preventable diseases.

The Vaccination Schedule under the UIP is as follows:

1. BCG one dose at birth (up to 1 year of age if not given earlier)
2. DPT (diphtheria, pertussis and tetanus toxoid) five doses; three primary doses at 6, 10 and 14 weeks and two booster doses at 16–24 months and 5 years of age.
3. OPV (oral polio vaccine) five doses; zero dose at birth, three primary doses at 6, 10 and 14 weeks and one booster dose at 16–24 months of age.
4. Hepatitis B vaccine four doses; zero dose within 24 hours of birth and three doses at 6, 10 and 14 weeks of age.
5. Measles two doses; the first dose at 9–12 months of age and the second dose at 16–24 months of age.
6. TT (tetanus toxoid) two doses at 10 and 16 years of age,
7. TT – For pregnant women, two doses or one dose if previously vaccinated within 3 years.
8. In addition, Japanese encephalitis (JE) vaccine was introduced in 112 endemic districts in the campaign mode in a phased manner from 2006 to 2010 and has now been incorporated under the Routine Immunization Programme in endemic areas.

Mission Indradhanush

Mission Indradhanush was launched on 25 December 2014 with an aim to cover all those children who are partially vaccinated or unvaccinated. Mission Indradhanush is a nationwide initiative with a special focus on 201 high-focus districts. These districts account for nearly 50% of the total partially vaccinated or unvaccinated children in the country. Mission Indradhanush provides protection against seven life-threatening diseases mentioned under UIP. In addition, vaccination against JE and Hib is included in selected districts of the country. Vaccination against tetanus will be continued to the pregnant women.

Mission Indradhanush, depicting seven colours of the rainbow, aims to cover all those children who are not vaccinated or partially vaccinated by 2020. The Mission Indradhanush initiative is a call for action by the Government of India to intensify efforts to expedite the full immunization coverage in the country.

Measles Supplementary Immunization Activity (SIA)

The Government of India introduced the second dose of measles under the UIP in 2010 through a two-pronged strategy based on the NTAGI recommendation. Twenty-one states where more than 80% coverage had been achieved initiated the second dose of measles. Fourteen states with less than 80% first-dose measles coverage have been targeted for all children between 9 months and 10 years of age for measles vaccination and a second dose of measles vaccination after 6 months. Measles vaccination campaigns are started in a phased manner in all 14 districts.

The Union Ministry of Health and Family Welfare launched a second phase of measles–rubella (MR) vaccination campaign to reduce morbidity. For those who have already received such vaccination, the campaign dose will provide additional booster dose. The Health Ministry has initiated MR vaccination campaign in the age group of 9 months to 15 years in a phased manner.

Polio Eradication and Pulse Polio Immunization

This is a remarkable achievement, particularly considering the fact that in 2009 India accounted for nearly half of the total number of polio cases globally and there were an estimated 2 lakh cases of polio every year in the country in the year 1978. In 1995, the Government of India launched the Pulse Polio immunization programme along with UIP, following global polio eradication initiative of the World Health Organization (WHO) in the year 1988. This programme aimed at making India free of poliomyelitis. With this programme, the last reported cases were in West Bengal and Gujarat on 13 January 2011. On 27 March 2014, WHO declared India a polio-free country. For the last 3 years, there was not a single case reported in India. The Pulse Polio dates in 2017 were 29 January, 2 April, 2 July and 17 September on Sundays.

National Immunization Schedule

Age	Vaccines
Soon after birth, before discharge from the hospital	BCG, OPV (zero dose)
1½ months to 6 weeks	DPT1, OPV1
2½ months or 10 weeks	DPT2, OPV2
3½ months or 14 weeks	DPT3, OPV3
9 months	Measles
1½ year or 18 months	DPT (booster), OPV (booster)
5 years	DT
10 and 16 years	One dose of TT each

General Contraindications to Vaccinations

- Prior allergic reactions to the same or related vaccine.
- Live vaccines, i.e. OPV, BCG and measles, are not to be administered in the following situations: in immunosuppressive therapy, immunodeficiency disorders, leukaemia, lymphoma or generalized malignancy.
- Acute illness with fever above 38°C. Postpone until recovery has occurred.
- Special risk groups in whom the risk of complications from infectious diseases is high include those with chronic lung and congenital heart diseases, Down syndrome, HIV infection, low birth weight (LBW), and asplenia or hyposplenism.

Conditions Not to Be Taken as Contraindication to Vaccinations

Mild or moderately ill children should be immunized to increase individual and community protection. Malnutrition, low-grade fever, mild acute respiratory infection (ARI), or diarrhoea and other minor illnesses are NOT contraindications for vaccination. The general rule is immunizing all children who are not sick enough to be hospitalized.

Live vaccines pose a risk for certain individuals whose immunity is impaired. Examples for such conditions are children undergoing chemotherapy for malignant disease, children treated with immunosuppressants or high-dose systemic steroids, children with impaired cell-mediated immunity (severe combined immunodeficiency syndrome) and children who are HIV-positive.

Specific Contraindications

Measles vaccine is contraindicated if there is a previous anaphylactic reaction to neomycin.
MMR vaccine is safe for children with egg allergies.
Pertussis vaccine is contraindicated in children with convulsions.

Specific Contraindications To EPI Vaccines

Vaccines	Specific Contraindications
BCG	Clinical symptoms of HIV infection.
DPT	Any history of seizures, other than febrile convulsions.
OPV	Nil. If a child has diarrhoea, the OPV dose should be given but not recorded in the regular schedule. The mother must be told to bring the child back as soon as the episode of diarrhoea is over and another dose must be given and duly recorded.
Measles and MMR	Nil. But a female of reproductive age should not become pregnant for 3 months after vaccination.
TT	Nil.
DT	Nil.
Hepatitis B	Nil.

Reactions to EPI Vaccines. Reactions after vaccination are in general mild and of short duration. These may be:
- Mild fever.
- Local pain and swelling at the site of injection.
- Malaise, irritability.
- Transient rash (after measles vaccination).
- A lump or papule appears on the third week after BCG vaccination. It is generally not painful but is tender to touch. The papule increases in size up to 6–10 mm in diameter by the sixth week. The nodule softens with the formation of pus. No treatment is necessary. At the end of 10–12 weeks, only a small scar is visible.
- Regional lymph node enlargement and suppuration observed 2–8 weeks after BCG vaccination is usually a result of the vaccine being injected subcutaneously instead of intradermally.
- In very rare cases, a fever of more than 105°F, convulsions or collapse after DPT vaccination has been observed. In such cases, further doses of DPT should not

be given. DPT vaccination should as far as possible be limited to children under 2 years of age and DT vaccine to children under 7 years of age, as the severity of reactions may increase in the older age groups.

The parents should be informed about the expected side effects, especially when more than one vaccine has been given at the same time, so that they do not worry. If there is any anxiety, they should be encouraged to return to the hospital for consultation.

There are certain myths and false belief related to contraindications of vaccine. They are not contraindications to vaccination. Common such beliefs are as follows:
- Family history of allergic reactions to immunization
- Prematurity (infants <28 weeks of age should have first immunization at the hospital)
- Stable neurological conditions
- Asthma, eczema, hay fever
- Over the age recommended in the standard schedule
- Minor febrile illness

Maintenance and Storage of Vaccines

Remember, the vaccines are kept in a refrigerator at a temperature of 2–8°C. To ensure potency of vaccines, cold chain should be maintained.

Cold chain is the system used for storing vaccines in good condition. It is otherwise called a vaccine supply chain or immunization supply chain. It is a series of links that are designed to keep vaccines within WHO-recommended temperature ranges from the point of manufacture to the point of immunization.

The cold chain is the system which ensures that vaccines remain potent from the moment of manufacture to the moment of immunization. If cold chain is not maintained, vaccines deteriorate quickly when exposed to heat or light. If a child is immunized with a vaccine which has deteriorated, then it is as if that child had not been immunized at all except that the child received additional pain as a result of shots. The cold chain has two components that the nurse must remember. They are the equipment and the procedure. The equipment controls and monitors the temperature of the vaccines. The procedure includes all the actions carried out to ensure that this equipment is correctly installed and maintained. The cold chain must reach from the manufacture to the mother and the child at the periphery where the vaccines are delivered to the child. To maintain cold chain, all EPI vaccines must be stored at correct temperature. They must be kept in darkness. This requirement is met if the vaccines are stored in the refrigeration equipment. It should be exposed only at the immunization session by static units or outreach teams or booths. The temperature required to keep the potency of vaccines is as low as possible, with a temperature range from –20°C to –30°C. OPV and measles vaccines are kept at this temperature at the central laboratory. The immunization unit-level OPV and measles vaccines are stored in the refrigerator at 2–8°C. Vaccines usually kept at this temperature are DPT, TT, BCG, DT and HBV vaccines.

There must be constant supply of electricity to maintain the temperature. If there is a chance to power failure, an absorption system of refrigeration can be used where a combined gas and electricity units are utilized. A standby system of generator or a cold box to store the vaccines is used when electricity failure occurs. Correct positioning of equipment must be maintained so as to ensure cold chain. All refrigerators must be kept in the coolest possible area of the institute. They must never be placed in the direct sunlight. Compression equipment must be at least 6–15 inches away from the wall. It should be placed at the level of the floor. Absorption equipment must also be kept in level and away from draughts and walls.

Correct adjustment of temperature on initial installation of the refrigerator is essential to maintain cold chain. This can be achieved by adjusting the thermostat to the mid position first. Then load the refrigerator with dummy items (e.g. bottles of water). Place a thermometer in the middle of the unit. For the compression equipment, check the temperature after 4 hours; if the temperature is correct, check the temperature again after a further 4 hours and then, if the temperature is still correct, place the vaccines. If the temperature is too high, increase the thermostat, wait for 2 hours and check again. If the temperature is correct, check the temperature after further 4 hours and then place the vaccines. If the temperature is again too high, repeat this sequence until the correct temperature has been obtained and maintained for at least 4 hours. Correct arrangement of the refrigerator must be maintained internally. Ice packs are used when storing vaccines in the ice box, and their correct arrangement helps stabilize the temperature of the refrigerator.

The thermometer kept on the vaccine should show the exact temperature of the vaccine and must therefore be placed on top of the vaccine.

Deep freezers can be used for preparation of ice packs and ice and for storage of polio and measles vaccines at regional centres. **DPT, TT, DT and HBV vaccines should not be kept in deep freezers**.

Vaccine carriers are used for carrying vaccines and storing vaccines during immunization sessions.

Cold box can be for used for collecting large quantities of vaccines for health centres, and transporting vaccines from regional centres and keeping vaccines for several days in need (maximum of 6 days or 150 hours) when electricity fails.

Ice packs are used for lining the walls of cold boxes and vaccine carriers to keep them cold and in the refrigerator to help stabilize temperature at the required level. They are flat plastic bottles filled with water or gel. Ice packs should stand with their edges in contact with the evaporator and not flat on one another in the freezer compartment of the refrigerator.

Cold chain failure: If there is cold chain failure, the affected vaccines should not be used in any case. There is no shame or blame in reporting cold chain failure, although the person-in-charge should do his/her best to avoid such a situation. **A vaccine that does not have potency is better not to be given, as it is only a pain-creating procedure without any benefits.**

Frozen DPT, TT or HBV vaccines should not be used as well. **Shake test** is a reliable method to test the vaccine. Compare the vaccine that you suspect has been frozen and thawed with the vaccine from the same manufacturer that you are sure was never frozen. Shake the containers of the vaccine carefully. Leave the vaccines to stand side by side for 15–30 minutes for the sediment to settle. Inspect the content carefully. The vaccine that is never frozen will be smooth and cloudy immediately after shaking, but the vaccine that is frozen and thawed will not be smooth and there will be particles in it. The vaccine never frozen starts to clear and there will be no sediment in it. But the vaccine that is frozen will be almost clear in the upper part, with thick sediments at the bottom.

Special Points to Remember during Immunization Session

- **Information to the mothers** – Tell the mother which vaccine is given and which are the diseases that can be prevented by that particular immunization. Explain the postimmunization reactions. Give the mother the date of next immunization.
- Maintain cold chain during the immunization session.
- Open a fresh vial of vaccine for even one child, as this is still cheaper than getting a disease to the child.
- Use spirit or alcohol to clean the injection site, as it will not affect the potency of the vaccine as believed.
- Avoid contaminating the vaccine. Use the same needle and syringe to draw up and give the vaccine.
- Discard all partially used vials of vaccines every day. **Measles and BCG vaccines should be discarded at the end of the vaccination session or a maximum of 8 hours.** In developed countries such as USA, it is discarded after 4 hours after opening and reconstituting the vaccine. All other vaccines are discarded at the end of the day.
- Disposal of sharps and used vials as per universal precautions.
- Golden rules for administration are to look directly into the mother's eyes. Smile at the mother and the child as the international language. Congratulate the mother for bringing the child for immunization.
- Parental permission is needed for vaccination.
- There is no change in the schedule of immunization to children with mental retardation and other condition such as cerebral palsy. But children with seizures should not be given pertussis vaccine until the condition gets stabilized.
- Premature babies are immunized as per the chronologic age. But OPV should be deferred until discharge to minimize the possibility of exposing other infants to a live vaccine that might be spread by stools.
- When giving intramuscular vaccines, use anterior–lateral aspect of thigh in infants. In children, the deltoid muscle can be used if they have sufficient muscle bulk.
- Live vaccines are contraindicated in children with congenital disorders of immune function or immunodeficiency disorders and children undergoing immunosuppressant therapy.
- Pregnant women also should not receive live vaccines until there is a special indication necessitating a high risk of exposure. The safest vaccines during pregnancy are tetanus toxoid and diphtheria.
- Before giving pertussis vaccine to a child, ascertain the following: Has the child had a current febrile illness? Has the child had previous serious reactions to the vaccines? Has the child ever suffered from fits, delayed development or any other serious illnesses? If so, withheld pertussis vaccine administration.

- Breastfeeding is not contraindicated after OPV administration, as breastfeeding does not affect the success of immunization. No interruption of breastfeeding schedule is necessary. Mild viral gastroenteritis is not a contraindication to OPV administration, but a severe gastroenteritis is a contraindication to OPV administration.
- There are few merits of OPV above injectable polio vaccine (IPV). OPV is administered orally and does not need shots and is easy to administer. It confers immunity to the population at large because it spreads from person to person and effective in eliminating polio. Hence, it is used for Pulse Polio immunization for eradication of polio. But it causes disease in immunocompromised individuals. It increases the risk by increasing the number of HIV-infected people. IPV is a killed vaccine and is preferred in immunocompromised individuals. It requires booster doses, too. Now, IPV is used in pentavaccines.
- All live vaccines are contraindicated in children with immunosuppression.
- MMR vaccination in a prepubescent female avoids the risk of infection during pregnancy. After administration of rubella vaccine, a female of reproductive age should not become pregnant for 3 months. Rubella syndrome (handicaps of vision, hearing, brain function and congenital heart disease) can be prevented by rubella vaccination.
- Children with sickle cell anaemia, aplastic anaemia, thalassaemia, nephritic syndrome and Hodgkin lymphoma undergoing chemotherapy are the recommended candidates for *H. influenzae*, chicken pox, pneumococcal and meningococcal vaccines.
- There are two types of hepatitis vaccine. All individuals who are at risk of exposure to hepatitis B need to be immunized. Persons with health care-related jobs who are frequently exposed to blood and blood products should be immunized. One millilitre of vaccine should be given intramuscularly initially and repeated at 1 and 6 months. Neonates should receive 0.5 mL of vaccine.
- Remember, no chance for immunizing a child should be wasted, as it counts a lot for the country.

One must maintain reliable vaccine cold chain at all levels. Following procedure must be maintained for this:
- Store vaccines and diluents within the required temperature range at all sites.
- Pack and transport vaccines to and from outreach sites according to recommended procedures.
- Keep vaccines and diluents within recommended cold chain conditions during immunization sessions.

Temperature Requirements for Vaccines

Vaccines are sensitive biological products. Some of the vaccines are sensitive to freezing, yet others are sensitive to heat and others to light. Vaccine potency (ability to adequately protect the vaccinated patient) can diminish when the vaccine is exposed to inappropriate temperatures. If vaccine potency is lost, it cannot be regained. To maintain potency and quality, the vaccine must be protected from extreme temperatures. Vaccine quality and potency are maintained with cold chain that meets specific temperature requirements.

The vaccines are grouped into six categories. Within each of these six categories, the vaccines are arranged in alphabetical order, not in the order of sensitivity to heat, within the group. The most heat-sensitive vaccines are in group A and the least heat-sensitive vaccines are in group F.

Vaccine Heat Sensitivity

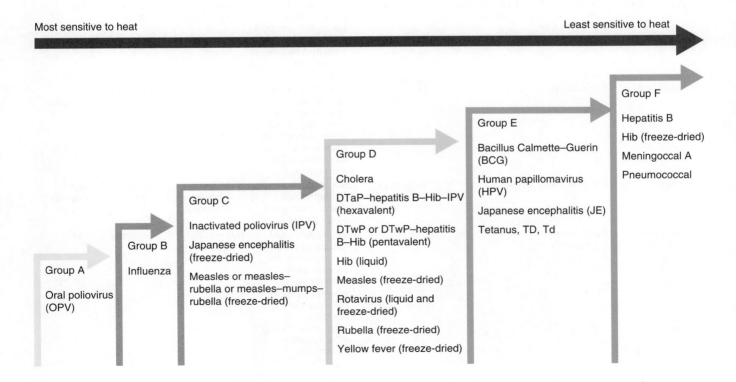

Freeze-Sensitive Vaccines

DO NOT FREEZE THESE VACCINES!!!
- Cholera
- DTaP–hepatitis B–Hib–IPV (hexavalent)
- DTwP or DTwP–hepatitis B–Hib (pentavalent)
- Hepatitis B (Hep B)
- Hib (liquid)
- Human papillomavirus (HPV)
- Inactivated poliovirus (IPV)
- Influenza
- Pneumococcal
- Rotavirus (liquid and freeze-dried)
- Tetanus, DT, Td

Sensitivity to Light

Some vaccines are very sensitive to light and lose potency when exposed to it. These types of vaccines should be protected against sunlight and heat. BCG, MR, MMR are light- and heat-sensitive vaccines. They are supplied in dark glass vials and should be kept in their secondary packaging for as long as possible to ensure light protection during storage and transport.

COMMON COMMUNICABLE DISEASES

Common Communicable Diseases for which Immunization is Available as a Routine

Diseases	Causative Agent	Mode of Transmission	Incubation Period	Major Signs and Symptoms	Complications	Specific Treatment	Immunity
Neonatal tetanus	*Clostridium tetani*	Contaminated umbilical cord	3–14 days	A week later, inability to suck and fits worsened by noise or movement; sucks well at birth.		Available	No
Tetanus	*C. tetani*	Broken skin, discharging ear, etc.	10–15 days	Locked jaw, unable to open the mouth fully. Painful contractions of muscles of the neck and trunk, bending the body like a bow.		Available	No
Diphtheria	*Corynebacterium diphtheriae*	Air	2–10 days	Fever, swollen neck, membrane in the throat, difficulty breathing.	Toxins can affect heart muscle and nerves.	Available	No
Poliomyelitis	Poliovirus I, II, III	Food, water and air	5–14 days	Weakness in the arms or legs, paralysis flaccid, asymmetrical pain and tactile sensations normal.	Residual paralysis	Not available	No
Tuberculosis	*Mycobacterium tuberculosis*	Air	Not known	Fever, listlessness, loss of weight, loss of appetite, coughing, headache, stiffness of neck and convulsions when TB meningitis.		Available	Not known
Measles	Measles virus	Air	9–10 days	Fever, catarrhal, conjunctivitis, rash on the third to fourth days.	Malnutrition secondary infections	Not available	Not available
Whooping cough	*Bordetella pertussis*	Air	5–8 days	Fever, cough, cold, coughing paroxysms during the second week, bulging eyes, haemorrhage in the eyes during coughing spasms, vomiting after coughing spasms.	Malnutrition secondary infections	Available	Yes

Common Communicable Diseases for which Immunization is Available as a Routine—cont'd

Diseases	Causative Agent	Mode of Transmission	Incubation Period	Major Signs and Symptoms	Complications	Specific Treatment	Immunity
Hepatitis B	Hepatitis B virus	Blood, contaminated needles and with sexual activity	45–160 days	Onset insidious, anorexia, nausea, vomiting, jaundice hepatomegaly.	Cirrhosis liver/hepatocellular carcinoma	Not available	Yes

INTEGRATED MANAGEMENT OF NEONATAL AND CHILDHOOD ILLNESS

The Government of India as a part of strengthening child health activities in the country appointed a core committee to decide on the Indian version of the Integrated Management of Childhood Illness (IMCI). Integrated Management of Neonatal and Childhood Illness, adapted from the global IMCI, to enhance the focus on newborns below 7 days of age and on training of community health workers within the National Reproductive and Child Health Programme to address high infant mortality. A Core Group was constituted which included representatives from Indian Academy of Pediatrics (IAP), National Neonatology Forum of India (NNF), National Anti-Malaria Program (NAMP), Department of Women and Child Development (DWCD), Child in Need Institute (CINI), WHO, UNICEF, eminent paediatricians and neonatologists, and the representatives from Ministry of Health and Family Welfare, Government of India. The Adaptation Group developed the Indian version of IMCI guidelines and renamed it as the 'Integrated Management of Neonatal and Childhood Illness'. The original version of IMNCI is only the Integrated Management of Childhood Illness. In this, the early neonatal period (birth to first 7 days of life) was not included.

The major highlights of Indian version are as follows:
- Incorporation of neonatal care as it now constitutes two-thirds of infant mortality.
- Incorporating national guidelines on malaria, anaemia, vitamin A supplementation, and immunization schedule and rescheduling training.

The government has first initiated implementation of the IMNCI strategy in four districts each in nine selected states of Odisha, Rajasthan, Madhya Pradesh, Haryana, Delhi, Gujarat, Uttarakhand, Tamil Nadu and Rajasthan.

IMNCI offers a comprehensive package for the management of the most common causes of childhood illnesses, namely sepsis, measles, malaria, diarrhoea, pneumonia and malnutrition. The following programmes are integrated into this as a routine.

Breastfeeding, iron and folic acid supplementation, and vitamin A supplementation strategy

IMNCI and Its Significance to Child Health and Survival

Every year more than 10 million children die in developing countries before they reach their fifth birthday. Seven in 10 of these deaths are a result of ARIs (mostly pneumonia), diarrhoea, measles, malaria or malnutrition and often to a combination of these illnesses.

According to the National Family Health Survey, in India, common illnesses in children under 3 years of age include fever (27%), ARIs (17%), diarrhoea (13%) and malnutrition (43%) and often occur in combination. Neonatal mortality contributes to more than 64% of infant deaths, and most of these deaths occur during the first week of life. Infant mortality rate (IMR) continues to be high at 68 per 1000 live births and under-five mortality rate at 95 per 1000 live births per year. These are sensitive indicators of the health services provided in a country.

Need for IMNCI

Many of the child welfare programmes such as immunizations for communicable diseases and oral rehydration therapy for diarrhoea are already found to be effective in promoting health and reducing IMR and neonatal mortality rate (NNR). Even the modest breastfeeding programme initiated with BFHI has proven to reduce neonatal and infant mortality. So an integrated approach was planned to manage sick children to achieve better outcomes.

The causes of neonatal mortality can be tackled because much of them are preventable. The major causes of neonatal mortality in India belong to late fetal (28 weeks up to delivery), early neonatal (0–7 days of birth) and late neonatal deaths (8–28 days). The causes of these deaths are as follows:

Late fetal deaths (28 weeks up to delivery)
- Fresh still birth
- Intrapartum birth
- Asphyxia
- Preterm birth
- Birth defects
- Macerated still birth
- Infection, especially sexually transmitted infections
- Hypertension/preeclampsia
- Placental abruption
- Birth defects
- Maternal diabetes
- Post-term pregnancy (more than 42 weeks' gestation)

Early neonatal deaths (0–7 days)
- Birth asphyxia/birth injuries
- Infection
  - Sepsis
  - Meningitis
  - Tetanus
  - Acute lower respiratory tract infection
  - Diarrhoea
  - Complications of preterm birth

- Respiratory distress
- Jaundice
- Increased risk of sepsis
- Birth defects

Late neonatal deaths (8–28 days)

- Infection
- Sepsis
- Meningitis
- Tetanus
- Acute lower respiratory tract infection
- Diarrhoea
- Early feeding failures (more common among preterm and LBW babies)
- Infanticide/neglect

A majority of these causes can be prevented if the health care workers are trained to provide affordable health facilities at the grassroots level for people who are below poverty line. This is one of the major reasons why India had included neonatal services too in IMCI. The first 7 days after birth was not included in the original IMNCI. (Two countries that had formulated their version of IMNCI are India and Ethiopia.)

IMNCI had implemented to go beyond tackling single diseases in order to address the overall health and well-being of the child. During the mid-1990s, WHO, in collaboration with UNICEF and many other agencies, institutions and individuals, developed a strategy known as the Integrated Management of Childhood Illness (IMCI). Although the major reason for developing the IMCI strategy was to provide curative care, it also addressed aspects of nutrition, immunization and other important elements of disease prevention and health promotion, giving a holistic approach to the care of children. The objectives of the strategy were to reduce death and the frequency and severity of illness and disability and to contribute to improved growth and development. In India, the strategy was expanded to include neonates, as much of the infant mortality was due to perinatal (birth to 7 days) and neonatal deaths and renamed as 'Integrated Management of Neonatal and Childhood Illness'. The IMNCI clinical guidelines target children younger than 5 years. IMNCI guidelines are evidence-based, syndromic approach to case management that includes rational, effective and affordable use of drugs and diagnostic tools.

Components of the Integrated Approach

The IMNCI strategy includes both preventive and curative care. The aim of IMNCI is to improve practices in health facilities, in the health system and at home. IMNCI focuses on management of the most common neonatal and childhood problems that cause death in children.

IMNCI protocol includes three main components:

- Improvements in the case management skills of health workers with locally adapted guidelines.
- Improvements in the overall health system required for effective management of neonatal and childhood illnesses.
- Improvements in family and community health care practices.

Principles of Integrated Care

IMNCI guidelines give direction for care of two groups of children:

- Young infants up to 2 months of age
- Children aged 2 months to 5 years

According to IMNCI guidelines, all sick infants up to 2 months of age must be evaluated for possible bacterial infection and jaundice. They must also be evaluated routinely for diarrhoea. All sick infants and children 2 months to 5 years of age need to be evaluated for nutritional and immunization status, feeding problems and other potential problems. In IMNCI, the child's sickness is classified using specific actions and not diagnosis. The classification is based on whether the child needs urgent referral or a higher level of care; the child who needs specific treatment or the child can be cared at home. The child who can be cared for at home and whose mother may be given advice and send home is colour coded as green. The child who needs a specific treatment is colour coded as yellow, and the child who needs a referral is coded as pink.

If the colour code is pink, the health worker has to give the needed prereferral treatment at the health facility and refer the child to a centre where advanced care is available. If the colour code is yellow, the child or infant needs to be given a specific treatment in the health facility that includes treatment of local infections by oral drugs and advise to the caretaker for follow-up. If the colour is green, home management is advised. These infants and children may be given oral drugs to treat local infections, advised to continue breastfeeding if the child is an infant and to keep the infant warm and to return immediately if there are any untoward symptoms.

Treatment of possible infections in young infants up to 2 months of age includes possible bacterial infections/jaundice, diarrhoea, feeding problems, immunization status and other problems. All sick infants will be evaluated first for signs and symptoms of possible infections and jaundice, as they may become serious within no time and die. The major signs to be assessed are convulsions, fast breathing, chest retractions and nasal flaring, grunting, bulging fontanels, discharge from ear, umbilical infections, hyper- or hypothermia, lethargy and unconsciousness.

Jaundice may be looked for at soles and palms, especially within first 24 hours.

Dehydration and diarrhoea may be assessed and treated according to the schedule. Duration of diarrhoea, severity of dehydration, general condition, lethargy, sunken eyes and elasticity of skin using pinch test may be done.

Feeding problem and malnutrition may be assessed by finding out feeding difficulties present, whether breastfed or any other types of feeding, and by checking weight for age.

Immunization status needs to be checked and verified. An infant up to 2 months of age should receive BCG and OPV0 doses and at 6 weeks DPT1, OPV1 and HEP-B1.

Treatment of Infants up to 2 Months (Prereferral). For the first dose of intramuscular or oral antibiotics, keep the infant warm during transfer and prevent hypoglycaemia with breastfeeds or ORS. If the baby has convulsions, the preferred drug is diazepam 0.2 mg/kg i.v. or rectal. For infections, the first dose is intramuscular antibiotics. The usual choice is gentamycin or ampicillin.

IMNCI Guideline for Children Aged 2 Months to 5 Years. History needs to be taken. Check for general danger signs such as lethargy, convulsions, vomiting and inability to drink or feed. The other main symptoms to be checked are cough or difficulty in breathing, diarrhoea, fever and ear problems. They should be assessed for symptoms of malaria if present with fever. Immunization status also needs to be assessed according to age. For infections, antibiotics must be administered according to the schedule and diarrhoea may be treated according to WHO recommendations. Severe malnutrition also needs to be assessed and treated with nutritional supplements, especially vitamin D. Persistent diarrhoea and dysentery also may be treated as per the IMNCI protocol.

IMNCI guidelines do not cover trauma or injuries. This process uses a limited number of drugs and encourages active participation of caretakers/mothers.

MILLENNIUM DEVELOPMENT GOALS

India being a signatory to WHO's MDGs, the 10th Five-Year Plan of the country made the following commitments:

Poverty

By 2007: Poverty ratio reduced by 5%.
By 2012: Poverty ratio reduced by 15%.

Education

By 2003: All children in school.
By 2007: All children to complete 5 years of schooling.

Literacy

By 2007: At least 50% reduction in gender gap in literacy and 75% increase in birth literacy rates.
By 2010: There would be 80% institutional deliveries and 100% deliveries would be attended by trained birth attendants; 100% registration of births also expected.

Infant mortality

By 2007: Reduction in IMR to 45 per 1000 live births.
By 2012: Reduction in IMR to 28 per 1000 live births.

Water

By 2007: All villages to have sustained access to potable drinking water. All major polluted rivers cleaned.
By 2007: 80% coverage of high-risk groups through targeted interventions.
90% coverage of schools and colleges through educational programmes.
80% awareness among the general population in rural areas on HIV/AIDS, its transmission and cause

Millennium Development Goals and Targets

Goal 1 – Eradicate extreme poverty and hunger	**Target 1** – Halve, between 1990 and 2015, the proportion of people whose income is less than US $1 a day. **Target 2** – Halve, between 1990 and 2015, the proportion of people who suffer from hunger.
Goal 2 – Achieve universal primary education	**Target 3** – Ensure that, by 2015, children everywhere, boys and girls alike, will be able to complete a full course of primary schooling.
Goal 3 – Promote gender equality and empower women	**Target 4** – Eliminate gender disparity in primary and secondary education, preferably by 2005, and in all levels of education no later than 2015.
Goal 4 – Reduce child mortality	**Target 5** – Reduce by two-thirds, between 1990 and 2015, the under-five mortality rate.
Goal 5 –Improve maternal health	**Target 6** – Reduce by three-fourths, between 1990 and 2015, the maternal mortality ratio.
Goal 6 – Combat HIV/AIDS, malaria and other diseases	**Target 7** – Have halted by 2015 and begun to reverse the spread of HIV/AIDS. **Target 8** – Have halted by 2015 and begun to reverse the incidence of malaria and other major diseases.
Goal 7 –Ensure environmental sustainability	**Target 9** – Integrate the principles of sustainable development into country policies and programmes and reverse the loss of environmental resources. **Target 10** – Halve, by 2015, the proportion of people without sustainable access to safe drinking water and basic sanitation. **Target 11** – Have achieved by 2020 a significant improvement in the lives of at least 100 million slum dwellers.
Goal 8 – Develop a global partnership for development	**Target 12** – Develop further an open, rule-based, predictable, nondiscriminatory trading and financial partnership for the development system (includes a commitment to good governance, development and poverty reduction, both nationally and internationally). **Target 13** – Address the special needs of the Least Developed Countries ([LDCs] includes tariff and quota-free access for LDC exports, enhanced programme of debt relief for heavily indebted poor countries [HIPCs] and cancellation of official bilateral debt, and more generous official development assistance for countries committed to poverty reduction). **Target 14** – Address the special needs of landlocked developing countries and small island developing states (through the Programme of Action for the Sustainable Development of Small Island Developing States and 22nd General Assembly provisions). **Target 15** – Deal comprehensively with the debt problems of developing countries through national and international measures in order to make debt sustainable in the long term.

Continued

Some of the indicators listed below are monitored separately for the LDCs, Africa, landlocked developed countries and small island developing states.

Target 16 – In cooperation with developing countries, develop and implement strategies for decent and productive work for youth.

Target 17 – In cooperation with pharmaceutical companies, provide access to affordable essential drugs in developing countries.

Target 18 – In cooperation with the private sector, make available the benefits of new technologies, especially information and communications technologies.

The Planning Commission of India evolved the National Development Goals (NDGs) as part of its 10th Five-Year Plan targets. These were essentially based on eight MDGs. The development commitments highlighted in the National Common Minimum Programme (NCMP) of the then central government (UPA) were also concurrent with NDGs and MDGs. Overall, these guidelines gave rise to eight goals, 18 targets and 48 indicators of MDGs. The civil society is committed to a reality check to implement MDGs with the so-called campaign 'Wada Na Todo Abhiyan' (Keep the Promise).

SUSTAINABLE DEVELOPMENT GOALS AND CHILDREN

The **MDGs** were the world's time-bound and quantified targets for addressing extreme poverty in its many dimensions – income, poverty, hunger, disease, lack of adequate shelter and exclusion – while promoting gender equality, education and environmental sustainability. The MDGs concentrated only on developing countries, whereas the SDGs are global and no distinction is made between developed and developing countries and also between rural and urban areas. There is special focus on urban areas, too. The SDGs concentrate on overall development and if the SDGs could be achieved, the major threat of poverty, water scarcity and illiteracy can be removed from the face of the earth.

The SDGs build on the MDGs, eight antipoverty targets that the world committed to achieving by 2015. They were eradicate extreme poverty and hunger; achieve universal primary education; promote gender equality; reduce child mortality; improve maternal health; combat HIV/AIDS, malaria and other diseases; ensure environmental sustainability; and develop a global partnership for development. All these goals had a great impact on child health.

These MDGs aimed at an array of issues that included slashing poverty, hunger, disease, gender inequality and access to water and sanitation. The MDGs have brought enormous change in the world situation, specifically on child health, morbidity and mortality. But poverty and inequality still exist. So the SDGs and the broader SDG agenda go much more than the MDGs to address the root causes of poverty and universal need for development that works for people. On September 2015 at the Sustainable Development Summit at Rio, the member states of UN adopted the 2030 Agenda for Sustainable Development that included 17 goals with 169 targets between them to achieve by 2030. On 1 January 2016, the 17 SDGs of the **2030 Agenda for Sustainable Development** came into force. The **SDGs** are a new, universal set of goals, targets and indicators that UN member states will be expected to use to frame their agenda and political policies over the next 15 years. The foundational principle of UN Agenda 2030 is '**leave no one behind**'. It talks about comprehensive plans for eliminating extreme poverty, reducing inequality and, above all, protecting the world planet. These goals are as follows:

S.No.	Goals	Remarks
1	No poverty	End poverty in all its forms everywhere
2	Zero hunger	End hunger, achieve food security, ensure improved nutrition and promote sustainable agriculture
3	Good health and well-being	Ensure healthy lives and promote well-being for all at all ages
4	Quality education	Ensure inclusive and equitable quality education and promote lifelong learning opportunities for all
5	Gender equality	Achieve gender equality and empower all women and girls
6	Clean water and sanitation	Ensure availability and sustainable management of water and sanitation for all
7	Affordable and clean energy	Ensure access to affordable, reliable, sustainable and modern energy for all
8	Decent work and economic growth	Promote sustained, inclusive and sustainable economic growth, full and productive employment and decent work for all
9	Industry, innovation and infrastructure	Promote sustained inclusive and sustainable economic growth, full and productive employment and decent work for all
10	Reduced inequalities	Reduce income inequality within and among countries. Build resilient infrastructure, promote inclusive and sustainable industrialization and foster innovation
11	Sustainable cities and communities	Make cities and human settlements inclusive, safe, resilient and sustainable
12	Responsible consumption and production	Ensure sustainable consumption and production patterns

S.No.	Goals	Remarks
13	Climate action	Take urgent action to combat climate change and its impacts by regulating emissions and promoting developments in renewable energy
14	Life below water	Conserve and sustainably use the oceans, seas and marine resources for sustainable development
15	Life on land	Protect, restore and promote sustainable use of terrestrial ecosystems, sustainably manage forests, combat desertification, halt and reverse land degradation and halt biodiversity loss
16	Peace, justice and strong institutions	Promote peaceful and inclusive societies for sustainable development, provide access to justice for all and build effective, accountable and inclusive institutions at all levels
17	Partnerships for the goals	Strengthen the means of implementation and revitalize the global partnership for sustainable development

Of the 17 goals accepted to achieve, there are three extraordinary goals: to **end extreme poverty, fight inequality and for justice, and fix climate change. 'Sustainable development** is the **development** that meets the needs of the present without compromising the ability of future generations to meet their own needs' (Brundtland Report, 1987). Sustainable development and child health are closely related.

Great global health success has been witnessed by increasing the immunization of children to prevent communicable diseases. Ensuring vaccination to millions of world children is not an easy task and has been achieved through a systematic protocol for delivery, systematic counting at multiple levels, various behavioural change communication strategies to educate public and through proper training of health workers. The SDGs call for reduction in maternal and child health morbidity and mortality through universal access to sexual and reproductive health services by 2030.

Facts and figures related to child health are given later concerning goal 3 of SDGs. These facts are very important as far as child health is concerned and give importance to including child health improvement activities in all national and international programmes. Though the MDGs have brought drastic changes in improving child health, it is essential to continue child health activities to mould a healthy population, as children are the next productive citizens of the land.

Child Health Facts and Figures

- 17,000 fewer children die each day than those in 1990, but more than 6 million children still die before their fifth birthday each year.
- Since 2000, measles vaccines have averted nearly 15.6 million deaths.
- Despite determined global progress, an increasing proportion of child deaths are in sub-Saharan Africa and Southern Asia. Four out of every five deaths of children under 5 years of age occur in these regions.
- Children born into poverty are almost twice as likely to die before the age of 5 years as those from wealthier families.
- Children of educated mothers – even mothers with only primary schooling – are more likely to survive than children of mothers with no education.

Maternal Health

- Maternal mortality has fallen by almost 50% since 1990.
- In Eastern Asia, Northern Africa and Southern Asia, maternal mortality has declined by around two-thirds.
- But maternal mortality ratio – the proportion of mothers who do not survive childbirth compared with those who do – in developing regions is still 14 times higher than that in the developed regions.
- More women are receiving antenatal care. In developing regions, antenatal care increased from 65% in 1990 to 83% in 2012.
- Only half of the women in developing regions receive the recommended amount of health care they need.
- Fewer teens are having children in most developing regions, but the progress has slowed. The large increase in contraceptive use in the 1990s was not matched in the 2000s.
- The need for family planning is slowly being met for more women, but demand is increasing at a rapid pace.

HIV/AIDS, Malaria and Other Diseases

- At the end of 2014, there were 13.6 million people accessing antiretroviral therapy.
- New HIV infections in 2013 were estimated at 2.1 million, which were 38% lower than those in 2001.
- At the end of 2013, there were an estimated 35 million people living with HIV infection.
- At the end of 2013, 240,000 children were newly infected with HIV.
- New HIV infections among children have declined by 58% since 2001.
- Globally, adolescent girls and young women face gender-based inequalities, exclusion, discrimination and violence, which put them at an increased risk of acquiring HIV infection.
- HIV infection is the leading cause of death among women of reproductive age worldwide.
- TB-related deaths in people living with HIV have fallen by 36% since 2004.
- There were 250,000 new cases of HIV infections among adolescents in 2013, two-thirds of which were among adolescent girls.
- AIDS is now the leading cause of death among adolescents (aged 10–19 years) in Africa and the second most common cause of death among adolescents globally.

- In many settings, adolescent girls' right to privacy and bodily autonomy are not respected, as many report that their first sexual experience was forced.
- As of 2013, 2.1 million adolescents were living with HIV infection.
- More than 6.2 million malaria deaths have been averted between 2000 and 2015, primarily among children under 5 years of age in sub-Saharan Africa. The global malaria incidence rate has fallen by an estimated 37% and the mortality rates by 58%.
- Between 2000 and 2013, TB prevention, diagnosis and treatment interventions saved an estimated 37 million lives. The TB mortality rate fell by 45% and the prevalence rate by 41% between 1990 and 2013.

These are important facts and figures, as healthy women and children are at the centre of the SDGs to transform the world into a healthy one. Goal 3 includes a broad range of targets relating to reproductive, maternal, newborn, child and adolescent health (RMNCAH).

Children at the Centre of SDGs

The children of today and tomorrow are central to sustainable development and the future of our planet and all its inhabitants. Children and young people are both shapers of and shaped by the world around them. When a child is not healthy, has compromised brain functionality as a result of chronic poor nutrition, does not receive a quality education and does not feel safe in his/her home, school or community, that child will not be able to fulfil his/her potential and responsibilities as a parent, an employee or entrepreneur, a consumer or a citizen. A society that denies the individual child rights will not promote full development and potential of children as adults.

In many cases, the answer is 'no' and that not only denies the individual child his/her rights *but also* deprives the entire human family of the intellectual, social and moral benefits that derive from the fulfilment of these rights. It is essential to invest in individual child rights to keep the child's well-being; otherwise, sustainable development will never occur. So the policy makers and administrators of the states need to consider the child rights (Convention of Rights of Children, 1977, CRC) and follow UNICEF's 10 key messages in their planning and implementation of child protection activities for developing a sustainable society. In UNICEF's 10 key messages, the first section sets the context and describes how and why children are central to the concept, principles and future progress on the SDGs. The second section talks about three key messages that are important for policy makers in the Post-2015 Development Agenda on centrality of children and young people to the SDGs.

These are as follows:
1. *Sustainable development starts with safe, healthy and well-educated children;*
2. *Safe and sustainable societies are, in turn, essential for children; and*
3. *Children's voices, choices and participation are critical for the sustainable future we want.*

The third and final section **'makes the case'** to support these key messages by providing powerful supporting evidence and recommendations on how to integrate consideration of children's rights and well-being into the Post-2015 Development Agenda. The actions required are aggregate reductions in household poverty, more children in school than ever before, more rapid reductions in child death rates and rising access to clean drinking water. Almost all countries of the world are concentrating on these issues in their policy making and implementation of national programmes. However, in many parts of the world, there still exist poverty, civil wars and increasing gaps between the rich and the poor; widespread toxic pollution and unplanned urbanization, far-reaching social impacts of violence and conflict, excessive stress on vital ecosystems and refugee problems are badly affecting the child health activities and harming further development. It is essential to create a world fit for children to grow and develop as good human beings by understanding the value of life in the planet. The adults of today should provide a safe, liveable world to children.

Children represent approximately one-third of the world's population and have the right to survive, live and grow up in a decent environment, which permits them to attend school, enjoy good health and nutrition, and live and grow in a safe and secure environment. Sustainable development is inherent in the provision of child rights. It is our collective responsibilities to ensure a safer, cleaner, healthier and more inclusive world for both today's children and for their children.

BABY-FRIENDLY HOSPITAL INITIATIVE

WHO in collaboration with UNICEF introduced 'Baby-Friendly Hospital Initiative' in the year 1991 to encourage breastfeeding practices. The global BFHI is based on 10 steps for a hospital to fulfil to get certification as a baby-friendly hospital. In India, more than 1300 hospitals are certified as baby friendly. Exclusive breastfeeding has been accepted as the most vital intervention to reduce infant mortality and to ensure optimal growth and development of children. BFHI was initiated to reduce infant mortality. In developing countries, it is very important, as infants who are not breastfed are six to 10 times more at risk of mortality even in the first month of life.

In India, BFHI is supported by associations of various health care professionals, especially the medical and nursing fraternity. The Indian Nursing Council had included BFHI in its curriculum on child health nursing.

The BFHI programme emphasizes the irreplaceability of breast milk, the emotional bond between the mother and the child, and psychomotor and social developmental outcomes. BFHI aims protection, promotion and support of breastfeeding in maternity facilities all around the world. It also incentivizes the adoption of policies and care practices for the successful start to exclusive breastfeeding. It promotes adherence to the

International Code of Marketing of Breast Milk Substitutes (BMS).

BFHI can provide the detail and infrastructure of support to ensure that breastfeeding support is appropriately managed.

Ten Steps to Successful Breastfeeding

Every facility providing maternity services and care for newborn infants should:

1. Have a written breastfeeding policy that is routinely communicated to all health care staff;
2. Train all health care staff in skills necessary to implement this policy;
3. Inform all pregnant women about the benefits and management of breastfeeding;
4. Help mothers initiate breastfeeding within half an hour of birth;
5. Show mothers how to breastfeed and how to maintain lactation even if they should be separated from their infants;
6. Give newborn infants no food or drink other than breast milk unless *medically* indicated;
7. Practice rooming in – Allow mothers and infants to remain together 24 hours a day;
8. Encourage breastfeeding on demand;
9. Give no artificial teats or pacifiers (also called dummies or soothers) to breastfeeding infants; and
10. Foster the establishment of breastfeeding support groups and refer them to mothers.

WHO and UNICEF in 2015 established a steering committee (Guideline Development Group) to revise the BFHI guidance. Two simultaneous processes are underway. The first group is working to revise guidelines on patient care, commonly referred as the Ten Steps to Successful Breastfeeding. The work was expected to conclude by mid-2017. WHO and UNICEF also developed an External Review Group (ERG) to monitor implementation of BFHI in countries operating BFHI programmes. The ERG has met since December 2015 to collect information from case studies, key informant interviews, WHO's global policy survey and review of key documents and to craft updated Operational Guidance. In 2017, the work of these two committees would be merged together into a single guidance document for implementation of BFHI. BFHI clearly delineates the role of maternity facilities in protecting, promoting and supporting breastfeeding. Because preterm and LBW babies constitute a substantial number of deliveries, these groups are seriously thinking on this matter in the maternity facilities. The new guidance will include these population. It will focus on the care of infant feeding, as well as on the care aspects of breastfeeding, not mother-friendly aspects of care, as did the 2009 guidance.

The BFHI congress 2016 summarized seven key directions from the new guidance:

1. The Ten Steps to Successful Breastfeeding are the responsibility of every maternity facility and should not be limited to facilities that voluntarily want to do something extra.
2. Countries need to establish national standards of care based on the Ten Steps that apply to all facilities.
3. BFHI must include private facilities, not just public ones.
4. BFHI needs to be integrated with other health care improvement and quality assurance initiatives in order to be sustainable over time.
5. Although designation as a baby-friendly hospital is one way to incentivize facilities to make needed changes, other incentives for participation are encouraged.
6. Regular internal monitoring within facilities of both practices and outcomes is a crucial element of BFHI.
7. Maternity facilities need external assessment for quality assurance, but the process needs to be streamlined enough to be manageable within existing resources.

The International Code of Marketing of Breast Milk Substitutes within BFHI is a critical component of the protection of breastfeeding. It contains several restrictions on marketing that pertain to health care systems and to health workers, including:

- No advertising of BMS;
- No donations of BMS to hospitals;
- No free samples;
- No promotion in health services;
- No company personnel to advise mothers;
- No gifts or personal samples to health workers; and
- No use of space by companies when educating mothers.

STUDY QUESTIONS

- Describe the immunization schedule as per UIP.
- What is a cold chain? How will you maintain a cold chain at a primary health centre?
- What is Mission Indradhanush?
- Explain the evolution of UIP.
- What are the vaccine-specific contraindications for UIP vaccines? How will you motivate parents to have immunizations for their children?
- What are live vaccines? Give examples of them. How will you administer live vaccines?
- What are killed vaccines? Give examples.
- How will you differentiate a serum and a toxin that are used for vaccinations?
- Differentiate between active immunization and passive immunization.
- Describe the functioning of under-five clinics.
- What is IMNCI?
- Why India adopted IMNCI rather than IMCI?
- What is the difference between IMCI and IMNCI?
- Describe the functioning of IMNCI.
- What are Millennium Development Goals?
- How will you differentiate between Millennium Development Goals and Sustainable Development Goals?
- Describe the importance of BFHI.

BIBLIOGRAPHY

1. Chopra, M., Patel, S., Cloete, K., Sanders, D., & Petrson, S. (Apr. 2005). Effect of an IMCI intervention on quality of care across four districts in Cape Town, South Africa. *Arch Dis Child*, Vol. 90. Issue 4. pp. 397–401.

2. Press Information Bureau of India. Mission Indradhanush. March 23, 2015.

3. Duclos P, Bentsi-Enchill AD, Pfeifer D. 'Vaccine safety and adverse events: lessons learnt,' In: Kaufmann SHE and Lamert PH. The Grand Challenge for the Future, Basel, Switzerland: 2005: 209–229.

4. Gera T, Shah D, Garner P, Richardson M, Sachdev HS. Integrated management of childhood illness (IMCI) strategy for children under five. Cochrane Database Syst Rev. 2016 Jun 22;(6):CD010123. doi: 10.1002/14651858.CD010123.pub2.

5. Gold R. Your Child's Best Shot: A parent's guide to vaccination. 3rd edition, Canadian Paediatric Society, Canada, 2006.

6. Milstien, JB. 'Regulation of vaccines: strengthening the science base,' Journal Public Health Policy, 2004: 25(2):173–189.

7. Patwari AK, Raina N. Integrated Management of Childhood Illness (IMCI): a robust strategy. Indian J Pediatr. 2002 Jan;69(1):41-8.

8. Plotkin SL, Plotkin SA. 'A short history of vaccination,' In: Plotkin S, Orenstein W, Offit PA. Vaccines, 5th edition, Philadelphia: Saunders, 2008.

9. Wilson, CB, Marcuse, EK. 'Vaccine safety – vaccine benefits: science and the public's perception,' Nature Reviews Immunology, 2001: 1:160–165.

10. CDC. Why immunize? http://www.cdc.gov/vaccines/vac-gen/why.htm. Accessed July 1, 2015.

11. CDC. Vaccines & Immunizations. Basics and Common Questions: Some common misconceptions. http://www.cdc.gov/vaccines/vac-gen/6mishome.htm. Accessed July 1, 2015.

12. CDC. Vaccines & Immunizations. Vaccines and Preventable Diseases. Meningococcal: who needs to be vaccinated? http://www.cdc.gov/vaccines/vpd-vac/mening/who-vaccinate.htm. Accessed July 1, 2015.

13. Integrated Management of Childhood Illness (IMCI), WHO. website: Available at: http://www.who.int/maternal_child_adolescent/topics/child/imci/en/ accessed on 5th August 2017.

14. Ministry of Health & Family Welfare Government of India New Delhi 2009; INTEGRATED MANAGEMENT OF NEONATAL AND CHILDHOOD ILLNESS (IMNCI) Modules 1 to 9.

15. Ministry of Health & Family Welfare Government of India New Delhi 2009; Facility Based (F-IMNCI) Participants Manual for lecture on IMNCI: http://www.ihatepsm.com/resource/integrated-management-neonatal-and-chil.

16. Resolution WHA39.28. Infant and Young Child Feeding; Thirty-ninth World Health Assembly; Resolutions and records. Final; Geneva. 5–16 May 1986; Geneva: World Health Organization; 1986. pp. 122–135. (WHA39/1986/REC/1), Annex 6.

17. Technical updates of the guidelines on Integrated Management of Childhood Illness (IMCI) Evidence and recommendations for further adaptations. Geneva: World Health Organization; 2005.

18. WHO Second Working Group Meeting on Developing WHO Guidelines on safe production of polio vaccines, WHO HQ Salle D, 19-20 September 2017.

19. WHO Workshop on Implementation of Good Manufacturing Practices for Biological Products, Bangkok, Thailand 15-17 November 2017.

20. World Health Organization (WHO). United Nations Children's Fund (UNICEF), World Bank. State of the world's vaccines and immunization, 3rd ed, Geneva: WHO, 2009.

21. World Health Organization (WHO). 'Introduction of inactivated poliovirus vaccine into oral poliovirus vaccine-using countries', Weekly Epidemiological Record, Geneva: 2003:78(28):241–252.

22. World Health Organization (WHO). 'Pertussis vaccine: WHO position paper', Weekly Epidemiological Record, Geneva: 2005: 80(4):29–40.

23. World Health Organization (WHO). 'Measles vaccines: WHO position paper', Weekly Epidemiological Record, Geneva: 2009:84(35):349–360.

24. World Health Organization (WHO). 'Module 3: The cold chain'. In: Immunization in Practice, Geneva: WHO/IVB/04/06, 2004.

25. World Health Organization (WHO). 'Module 4: Ensuring safe injections'. In: Immunization in Practice, Geneva: WHO/IVB/04/06, 2004.

26. World Health Organization (WHO). 'Module 6: Holding an immunization session'. In: Immunization in Practice, Geneva: WHO/IVB/04/06, 2004.

27. World Health Organization and UNICEF. (2009) WHO Press, World Health Organization, 20 Avenue Appia, 1211 Geneva 27, Switzerland .

28. World Health Organization. Baby-friendly Hospital Initiative. Accessed 4 August 2011.

29. New Delhi: The Government of India, Ministry of Health and Family Welfare; 1996. Annual report of MoHFW 1995-96.

30. Pasteur Institute of India, Coonoor, Nilgiris. [accessed on May 30, 2012]. Available from: http://www.pasteurinstituteindia.com.

31. New Delhi: Ministry of Health and Family Welfare; 2005. Government of India. *Multi Year Strategic Plan for Universal Immunization Program in India (2005-2010).*

32. New Delhi: Ministry of Health and Family Welfare, Government of India; 2005. Government of India. *Report of National Universal Immunization Program review 2004.*

33. Govt's vaccination programme failed due to non-participation of private sectors, Neetu Chandra Sharma, 10 March 2016, India Today.

34. Verma, I. C., & Kumar, S. (Dec.1968). Causes of morbidity in children attending a primary health centre. *The Indian Journal of Paediatric.* Vol. 35. Issue 12 pp. 543–549.

35. Gladstone, B. P, Muliyil, J. P, Jaffar, S., Wheeler J. G., Fevre, A. Le., Iturriza-Gomara, M., et al. (2008). Infant morbidity in an Indian slum birth cohort. *Arch Dis Child*, 93:479–484.

36. Anathakrishan, S., Pani, S. P., & Nalini, P. (2001). A comprehensive Study of Morbidity in School Age Children. *Indian Pediatrics*, Vol. 38. pp.1009–1017.

CHILD HEALTH ASSESSMENT

LEARNING OBJECTIVES

At the end of the chapter, the learner will be able to:

- Describe the general guidelines and technique for performing child health assessment.
- Explain the age-specific approach to paediatric assessment.
- Identify the components of the medical history and questions necessary to clinical assessment data.

Irrespective of place of assessment, the child health assessment is usually done to determine how sick the child is and what kind of intervention he/she needs. Evaluating children is a challenge to health care providers, as they are different from adults – anatomically, physiologically and psychologically. The causes for seeking medical help also differ from that of adults.

Essentially, there are three parts to a paediatric assessment, each of which can be completed in minutes:
- Across-the-room assessment
- Physical assessment (head-to-toe assessment)
- The patient's medical history

'ACROSS-THE-ROOM' ASSESSMENT

This starts as the examiner asks the parent or whoever is with the child about the complaint or injury for which the child needs medical help. This assessment can be done by:
- Not touching the child – Merely looking at the child is enough to tell you how sick the child is and how serious the child is injured in the case of an accident.
- Notice the child's general appearance – Is he/she playful and energetic or lethargic and unresponsive? Is he/she clean? Do you see any rashes or bruises? Inspect the face, head, neck and hands. This will help you identify the severity of illness, behaviours and social response, and level of hygiene.
- Obtaining the child's cooperation is the first thing to do. There are some cues for the same.
- Make friends with the child.
- Be gentle and confident.
- Smile at the child in a nonthreatening manner.
- Use tactics such as short mock examination, e.g. auscultate a doll or teddy bear before staring examination of the child.
- Explain to the child, what you are going to do in a language that the child can understand.
- Examine first a nonthreatening area, such as holding and cuddling the baby's hand and examine the hands, fingers and nails.
- Examine the private area and the unpleasant procedure until last.
- Babies in the first few months of age can be examined in the mother's lap or in an examination couch.
- A toddler is best initially evaluated on mother's/parent's shoulders or mother's lap.
- Parents' reassurance is essential.
- Preschoolers can be examined while they are playing.
- For older children and adolescents, privacy needs to be provided; the girls are best evaluated in the presence of their mothers, if possible.

Age-Related Features and Approach for Assessment

Age and Characteristics	Approach to Assessment
Infants	
Children up to 1-year-old derive pleasure from tactile stimulation and have increasing curiosity about their environment. After the age of 6 months, common fears include strangers and separation from parents.	Evaluate the infant while he/she is on the lap. Use a quiet smoothening voice. The infant will respond to your tone more than your words.

Continued

Age-Related Features and Approach for Assessment—cont'd

Age and Characteristics	Approach to Assessment
Toddlers 1- and 2-year-olds enjoy exploring the environment and have some control over body functions and activity. Common fears include separation, loss of control, pain and changes to rituals.	Approach the child slowly and calmly. Allow the caregiver to remain with the child and let the child handle simple equipment or hold a familiar security object. Expose only one area of the child's body at a time. Prepare the child emotionally immediately before a procedure, using simple, concrete terms.
Preschoolers Children 3–5 years of age have achieved greater independence, but they need their parents or caregivers when they are under stress. They usually take illness as a punishment to wrongdoing or bad behaviour. Common fears include mutilation, loss of control, death, darkness and ghosts.	Ask the child to point to the area of pain or hurt. Provide privacy during the examination and let him/her handle simple equipment. Offer reasonable choices whenever possible, though limit setting is essential. Use simple explanations. Apply dressings and bandages to even minute injuries to provide security and comfort, as these children will have a feeling that their body will ooze out through the cuts.
School children These children view their sickness in terms of effects that it produces on their activities, and the possible consequences of illness. Common fears of these children include separation from friends, loss of control and physical disability.	Ask the caregiver and the child to describe their sickness. Allow caregiver to remain with the child during physical examination. Encourage questions. Give adequate explanation for every activity. Provide adequate privacy.
Adolescents These individuals are 11–18 years of age. They have risk-taking behaviours and are prone to accidents. They have feeling that they are immune to harm. They are conscious about their body image and believe in imaginary audience. They like acceptance of the peers; their common fears include body image disturbances, dependency and loss of control.	Allow the adolescent to choose whether he/she needs the presence of caregivers or not during examination and interview. Provide privacy. Avoid confronting languages. Provide feedback about adolescent's health status and explain properly all the procedures. Encourage questioning.

IMPORTANT DIFFERENCES BETWEEN CHILDREN AND ADULTS

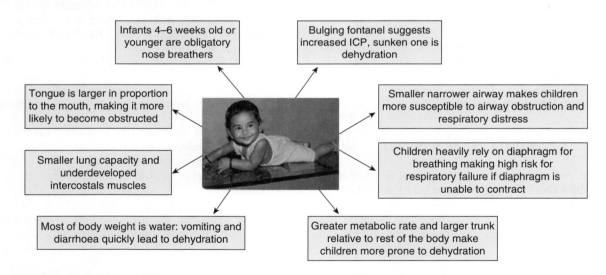

Infants 4–6 weeks old or younger are obligatory nose breathers

Bulging fontanel suggests increased ICP, sunken one is dehydration

Tongue is larger in proportion to the mouth, making it more likely to become obstructed

Smaller narrower airway makes children more susceptible to airway obstruction and respiratory distress

Smaller lung capacity and underdeveloped intercostals muscles

Children heavily rely on diaphragm for breathing making high risk for respiratory failure if diaphragm is unable to contract

Most of body weight is water: vomiting and diarrhoea quickly lead to dehydration

Greater metabolic rate and larger trunk relative to rest of the body make children more prone to dehydration

PHYSICAL ASSESSMENT

Routine physical assessment is little different from an assessment during an emergency. In an emergency, a quick assessment is warranted to get quick overview of the child's condition. In a quick assessment, the examiner assess the ABCDs (refer the assessment of a child during emergency).

While undressing a child, be sensitive to his/her modesty. Expose only needed part, and redress after examining each part of the body. Better get the help of the parent for undressing the child for assessment.

Remember the three WARMS:
- Warm smile
- Warm hands
- Warm stethoscope

Measurements

Because abnormal growth is the first sign of illness in children, it is always advisable to measure and plot a growth chart. It is helpful in comparison of growth as well. But often this is not possible in our set-up, as most of our children will not have properly maintained child health record. Even then it is essential for the nurse to measure weight, height and other circumferences because these measurements are used as landmarks for medicine calculation and fluid and nutrition requirements. So measure weight and length in infants and height in other children.

- Head circumference in children up to 2 years of age
- Chest circumference
- Midarm circumference in preschool children
- Temperature, respiration, blood pressure and heart rate; peak expiratory flow rate if provision for the same is available

General Appearance

Inspect the face, head, neck and the hands. This inspection will help find out chromosomal or dysmorphic syndromes. In infants, palpate the fontanels and sutures.

Respiratory System

- Look for cyanosis – peripheral and central. This is best observed on the tongue.
- Clubbing of the fingers and toes – It is usually associated with chronic suppurative lung disease or cyanotic heart disease.
- Tachycardia – Check the rate of respiration. It is age dependent (refer to the chapter on difference between child nursing and adult nursing).
- Dyspnoea – Look for:
  - Laboured breathing
  - Nasal flaring (flaring of alae nasi)
  - Expiratory grunting
  - Retractions (recession) of the chest wall suprasternal, intercostal, subcostal and infrasternal muscles
  - Use of accessory muscles
  - Difficulty in speaking and feeding
- Chest shape:
  - Barrel shape – Asthma
  - Hollow chest – Pectus excavatum
  - Pigeon chest – Pectus carinatum
  - Harrison's sulcus (as a result of diaphragmatic tug developing from poorly controlled asthma)
  - Symmetry of chest movement

Palpation

- Chest expansion can be noted in school children and measured using a tape.
- Check the tracheal position.
- Locate the apex beat to detect mediastinal shift.
- Percussion has not much value in infants. Localized dullness indicates collapse, consolidation or presence of fluid.

Auscultate for Breath Sounds

- Note quality and symmetry of breath sounds.
- Hoarse voice indicates abnormality of the vocal cord.
- Stridor – Harsh, low-pitched, mainly inspiratory sound as a result of upper airway obstruction.

   Remember: Normal breath sounds are vesicular; bronchial breathing is high pitched. Lengths of inspiration and expiration are equal in normal situations.

- Wheeze – High-pitched expiratory sound from distal airway obstruction
- Crackles – Discontinuous moist sounds from the opening of bronchioles

Cardiovascular System

- Look for cyanosis and clubbing.
- Check pulse.
- Check rate.
- Check rhythm – Sinus arrhythmia.
- Check volume – Small in circulatory insufficiency and aortic stenosis, increased in high-output states (stress, anaemia) and collapsing in patent ductus arteriosus and aortic regurgitation.
- Inspection – Look for respiratory distress.
- Precordial bulge is caused by cardiac enlargement.
- Ventricular impulse – Visible if thin, hyperdynamic circulation or left ventricular hypertrophy.
- Operative scars – Mostly sternotomy or left lateral thoracotomy.

Palpation. (thrill = palpable murmur)
- Apex – (fourth to fifth intercostal space, midclavicular line) not palpable in some healthy infants, plump children or dextrocardia.
- Heave – Left ventricular hypertrophy.
- Right ventricular heave at the lower left sternal edge – Right ventricular hypertrophy.

Percussion. Cardiac border percussion is rarely helpful in children.

Auscultation. Listen for heart sounds and murmurs.
- Heart sounds – Splitting of the second heart sound in atrial septal defects.
- Third heart sound in the mitral area is normal in young children.
- Murmurs – timing, duration, loudness – Grading of loudness is to be done:
  - 1–2: soft, difficult to hear
  - 3: easily audible, no thrill
  - 4–6: loud with thrill
- Site of maximal intensity mitral/pulmonary/aortic and tricuspid areas.

Radiation

- To the neck in aortic stenosis.
- To the back in coarctation of aorta or pulmonary stenosis.

Femoral Pulses
- Decreased volume or may be impalpable in infants.
- Brachiofemoral delay in older children in coarctation of aorta.

Blood Pressure
- Use the largest cuff which fits comfortably, covering at least two-thirds of the upper arm.
- Systolic pressure is the easiest to determine in young children and clinically the most useful in comparison with diastolic pressure.

> **Remember: Hepatomegaly is an important sign of heart failure in infants. An infant's liver is normally palpable 1–2 cm below the costal margin.**

Abdomen

Inspection
Shape – It is protuberant in toddlers and young children. Causes of generalized abdominal distension can be:
- Fat
- Fluid (ascites from nephritic syndrome)
- Faeces (constipation)
- Flatus (malabsorption, intestinal obstruction)
- Fetus (after puberty), though uncommon and usually a result of child abuse

Spleen and liver enlargement can also lead to abdominal distension.

Causes of localized abdominal distension are as follows:
- Upper abdominal – Gastric dilatation from pyloric stenosis and hepatosplenomegaly.
- Lower abdominal distension – Distended bladder, abdominal masses (Wilms tumour or rhabdomyosarcoma).
- Other signs are dilated veins, abdominal striae, operative scars and visible peristalsis (pyloric stenosis).
- Buttocks are rounded (normal) or wasted as in coeliac disease or malnutrition.

Palpation. Palpate in a systematic fashion – liver/spleen, kidneys, bladder through four abdominal quadrants.

Identify areas of tenderness:
- Location – Localized in appendicitis (McBurney's point), hepatitis and pyelonephritis.
- Generalized in peritonitis and mesenteric adenitis.
- Guarding may result from pain.

Palpate liver for hepatosplenomegaly from right iliac fossa. Locate edge with the side of fingers and measure (in cm) extension below the costal margin in the midclavicular line.

Tenderness of liver is usually as a result of hepatitis. Spleen is usually not palpable but could be palpable in those with hereditary spherocytosis/thalassaemia. If palpable, it is at least twice its normal size.

Kidneys

- Normally not palpable after the neonatal period.
- It is palpable for abdominal masses such as Wilms tumour, neuroblastoma – irregular mass.

- It needs to be differentiated from palpable faecal masses – mobile and tender, intussusception – often felt in the right upper quadrant.

Percussion. Dullness at the liver and spleen, shifting dullness in ascites

Auscultation. It is not useful in routine examination. Increased bowel sounds are observed in intestinal obstruction and acute diarrhoea and decreased or absent bowel sounds as in paralytic ileus.

Genitourinary System

Males. Inspect size and shape of the penis. Normal length is 3 cm in neonates. Look for hypospadias, epispadias and ambiguous genitalia.

Find whether the scrotum is well developed or not and whether testes are palpable in the scrotal sac. Look for any scrotal swelling.

Females. Inspect the external genitalia for any abnormality, ectopic bladder, ambiguous genitalia, fistula, etc.

Rectal Examination. Inspect for anal opening in neonates. Routine rectal examination is not essential except in acute abdomen and is usually performed by a paediatric surgeon.

Limbs

- Muscle bulk – Wasting may be secondary to cerebral palsy/muscle disorder/meningomyeloceles or previous poliomyelitis.
- Increased bulk of calf muscle usually seen in Duchenne muscular dystrophy.

Muscle tone. Tone in the limbs is best assessed by observing the following:
- Truncal tone
- Head lag
- Reflexes
- Plantar responses
- Sensation
- Cranial nerve

Bone and Joints

Assess for pain, unwillingness to move limb, limp, joint swelling and muscle wasting.

Palpate for heat, tenderness, fluctuating movements, both active and passive.

Scoliosis – Inspect the spine, especially in adolescents.

Neck

Inspect thyroid for swelling, usually uncommon in children.

Palpate the front of the neck for swelling, nodule or thrill and auscultate if enlarged. Look for signs of hypo- or hyperthyroidism.

Lymph nodes – Examine systematically for occipital, cervical, axillary, and inguinal lymph nodes. Note the size, number and consistency.

- Small, discrete, pea-sized, mobile nodes in the neck, groin and axilla – common in healthy children.
- Small multiple nodes on the neck – Common after upper respiratory tract infection of viral or bacterial origin.
- Multiple lymph nodes of variable size in children with extensive atopic eczema.
- A large nontender, sometimes fluctuating, node usually in the neck is a sign of infected node or abscess.
- Variable size and shape of lymph nodes are seen in viral infections such as infectious mononucleosis and tuberculosis. Rare causes are malignant diseases, such as Kawasaki disease, cat scratch, etc.

Eyes

Inspect pupils, iris and sclera for Bitot spot, infections and growths.

- Movements full and symmetrical? Are there any squint, nystagmus, position or epicanthal folds?
- Perform ophthalmoscopy to check for red reflexes for a distance of 20–30 cm. Absence of red reflexes occurs in corneal clouding, cataract and retinoblastoma.
- **Fundoscopy** is difficult and requires experience and cooperation.
- In older children with headaches, diabetes mellitus or hypertension, optic fundi should be examined.

Ear and Throat

They should be inspected last, as they are usually unpleasant. Proper age-appropriate explanation should be given before starting examination.

Throat: Look at the tonsils, uvula, pharynx and posterior palate swiftly. Older children cooperate during examination. Look for redness, swelling, pus or palatal petechiae. Check for dental hygiene.

Ear: Examine ear canals and drums gently; try not to hurt the child. Look for anatomical landmarks on the ear drum and for swelling, redness, perforation, dullness and fluid.

Skin

Look for rashes that are common in children, not usually serious. But a purpuric or petechial rash along with fever is serious, as it suggests bacterial or viral infections or haematological dysfunction. Inspect for bruises that indicate child abuse (e.g. belt marks, cigarette burns or other injuries). Look for signs of sexual abuse that include bruising or tears around vagina or anus or sexually precocious behaviour.

Look for skin turgor, which is important to find out the level of hydration.

Back: Inspect for injuries, including the back of the head.

NEUROLOGICAL OR DEVELOPMENTAL ASSESSMENT

It must be adapted according to the child's age and a history of developmental milestones should be collected from parents. Infants' evaluation is primarily by conducted by observation. Observe while picking them up for muscle tone, and check head lag on pulling to the sitting position. In older children, watch them play, as well as their writing, manipulative and walking skills.

Observe patterns of movement; normal walking is with a heel-to-toe gait. A toe-to-heel gait is suggestive of pyramidal trait dysfunction.

Developmental Assessment

Developmental skills can be assessed by watching the child's play and is nice to do before physical assessment to obtain maximum cooperation.

Patterns of Movement

Observe walking and running.

- Normal walking is with a heel-to-toe gait.
- A toe-to-heel pattern of walking is suggestive of abnormality of the pyramidal tract. An abnormal gait needs further assessment.
- A broad based gait may be a result of an immature gait or secondary to a cerebellar disease/disorder.
- Observe standing from a lying down position to a supine position. Children up to 3 years of age will turn to the prone position in order to stand because of poor muscle fixation.

Assess Coordination

- Ask the child to build one brick upon another.
- Ask the child to hold his/her arms out stretched straight, close his/her eyes and observe for drift or tremor.
- Perform finger-to-nose testing.
- Check for rapid alternating movements of hands and fingers.
- Touch tip of each finger in turn with the thumb.
- Ask the child to walk heel-to-toe, jump and hop.

Medical History

Obtain a patient's history along with head-to-toe assessment. It should include the following:

- Birth history in the case of a neonate.
- Past medical history, allergies, immunization, medications and diet history.
- Focused medical history denoting the reason for present admission.
  AMPLE
  A – Allergies
  M – Medications
  P – Past medical history
  L – Last meal
  E – Events leading to current injury

- Parents' socioeconomic background and educational status to identify their level of understanding and living status.

All pertinent investigations may be accompanied as per the child's condition, which are detailed along with dysfunctions of each system.

STUDY QUESTIONS

1. What are the important differences between children and adults?
2. Explain the age-related features and approach for child health assessment?

CHAPTER 6

FACTORS AFFECTING CHILD HEALTH

CHAPTER OUTLINE

- Factors Affecting Child Health
- Childhood Illnesses
- Factors Contributing to Illness in Children
- Childhood Problems of Significance
- Special Attributes of Indian Children
- Situation in Kerala

LEARNING OBJECTIVES

At the end of the chapter, the learner will be able to:

- Describe the factors affecting child health.
- Understand the factors contributing to illness in children.
- Enumerate the common childhood illnesses.

There are many factors that affect the health of children. These factors are broadly classified into seven major heads.

1. **Factors inherent to the child**
   a. *Weight and age at birth:* Babies born with low birth weight or are small for date or gestational age have many risk problems as compared with babies born with normal birth weight (refer to high-risk neonates). The problems of preterm babies are different from those of small for gestational age neonates.
   b. *Condition at birth:* Babies born to mothers with high-risk pregnancy (refer to the causes of high-risk neonates) face many problems as compared with term babies.
   c. *Associated congenital abnormalities:* Presence of associated congenital abnormalities adds risk to the survival and health status of children.
   d. *Child's age:* Under-five children have many threats to overcome as compared with children of other age group. They have higher chances of contacting communicable diseases. School children are more prone to accidents and so are the adolescents.
   e. *Sex:* In India, male children are given preferences as a result of our cultural habits. They are brought up with more care. However, our female children have a better survival rate than the male children. Overall morbidity and mortality among male children are more than those in female children.
   f. *Genetic factors:* Genetic inheritance of certain diseases decides the health of children. Genetic diseases are transmitted to the offspring from parents that affect the health of children.
   g. *Temperament:* Some children have vigorous temperament, making them more prone to accidents, so also their attitude towards caregivers. Children with bad temperament are cared for with difficulty and may not get adequate care from caregivers. This makes them prone to ill health.

2. **Family factors**
   Young children are the organic part of the family. Whatever happens to them affects the entire family. A family's physical and social environment is important to maintain child health. There is a saying that 'child heath equals family health'.
   a. *Family structure:* Not only small family norm has improved the standard of living but it has also increased their expectations from their children, which puts more pressure on children. For example, the entrance examination for professional courses and its effects on children is leading to an increased number of suicides by adolescents. In a small family, both parents may be working; there are greater demands for childcare centres or home nursing facilities. In addition, parents have to look for better child minding facilities. Often children may not get adequate and appropriate care from the caregivers. Large families also have their effect on child health. For example, transmission of communicable diseases such as respiratory tract infections and diarrhoea from adult family members to children is common.
   b. *Single-parent families* have many disadvantages as far as child health is concerned. These families have a high rate of unemployment, poor housing and financial hardships as compared with families with double biological parents. If the single parent goes to work, there may not be anyone to look after children at home. Studies have reported an increased incidence of behavioural problems in these children. This is not a major problem in India, as like other developed

and developing countries, we only have few single-parent families towing to our cultural habits. If we have some single-parent families, it may be owing to death of a spouse or in a few cases owing to marital discord. The relatives of the family usually help. Abandoned and orphaned children may have to resort to childcare centres or live as destitute children. These children also have to face many hardships.

c. *Parenting styles:* Child's development is affected by the parenting style. Parents who neglect or abuse their children may damage their children's emotional development. Warm and receptive parenting by imposing reasonable and constant discipline promotes healthy development in children. Temperament of children and parenting styles have direct relationships. A child with a very determined temperament will be in constant conflict with an authoritarian parent. These result in tantrums and other behavioural problems in children.

d. *Siblings:* Behaviours and attitudes of siblings have a marked influence on family dynamics. Sibling rivalry and feelings of insecurity may affect the physical health and development of children.

e. *Child-rearing practices:* Certain harmful child-rearing practices endanger the life of children. For example, application of cow dung and other powders on the umbilical stump of newborns, withholding food and fluid to children with diarrhoea, hostile attitude of parents towards immunizations, use of physical punishment by parents and adults to discipline children, etc.

f. *Maternal health* is a major determinant of child health. Only a healthy mother can bring a healthy baby. The common maternal risk factors that affect child health are maternal malnutrition, maternal age under 18 years or over 35 years, mothers with more than four deliveries and mothers with no basic pregnancy care.

3. **Socioeconomic and educational status of parents**
Physical and intellectual development of children varies with the socioeconomic level of family. Underprivileged children of the same age are smaller, of lower weight and less advanced in psychomotor and intellectual performance. Poverty, illiteracy and sickness create a vicious cycle, which repeats from one generation to the next and is often difficult to escape.

a. *Family income* is an indicator that decides the rearing capacity of parents. If the family income is less than the average national income, then the family has the below poverty line status and children of such family suffer from poverty. Poverty determines the health and well-being of children. Children belonging to a poor socioeconomic class have threat of low birth weight, household injuries, frequent infections, diarrhoea, asthma and malnutrition. They experience frequent hospital admissions and have many behavioural problems. Infant and childhood morbidity and mortality are more common among these children. Lack of good enough parenting, inadequate housing, poor nutrition and low-level literacy are their major problems. Parental literacy and educational status also have a greater impact on child health. Parents who are educated use good parenting styles and are aware of health promotion activities. Mother's education has more impact, as mothers are the primary caregivers to children.

b. *Social custom and habits:* In India, we have many customs that are harmful to children. Late weaning or introduction of complementary feeds with commercially available tin foods causes many health hazards to children. The practice of 'Annaprasa' is performed in temples usually after 6 months of age. If the parents could not do this in time owing to various reasons, they may postpone the same for months, further delaying introduction of rice as a staple food that yields energy. The most appropriate weaning food is rice, and this is withheld until the parents could take the baby to the temple for the customary ceremony. This promotes utilization of other foods which may not be good like rice or promote late weaning, leading to protein–energy malnutrition (PEM), namely marasmus.

4. **Lifestyle issues**
In some cultures in India, child marriage is still prevalent, though prohibited through legislation. Early marriage leads to teenage pregnancy, and its complications cause human wastage.

5. **Environment**
Environment plays a great role in childhood morbidity and mortality. Epidemiological conditions, contact with earth, supply of safe water, inadequate disposal of human excreta and other waste materials, living in slums, abundance of insects, ecological conditions, prevalence of infections, endemic as well as epidemics, pollution, etc. in the environment affect the health of children, as they are more vulnerable to such hazards. The environment consists of both internal environment and external environment. The internal environment constitutes siblings, parents and relatives. Family hygiene and environmental stimulation that the child receives from its relatives contribute to intellectual development of children.

Role of Environment in Child Development

Physical Needs	Psychological Needs
Warmth, clothing and shelter	Personal identity, self-respect, independence
Functioning senses	Affection and care
Food	
Activity with rest	
Security	
Good health	
Play	
Opportunity to learn	
Role models	

External environment includes child's neighbourhood and community that have a profound influence on child's health. Cohesive community and amicable neighbourhood have a positive influence on children. Clan, caste and class differences existing in our country have led to tension and other social adversities such as violence, leaving many children homeless and mutilated. Children and women are the real victims of these calamities. Tension prevailing in the social arena has bad effects on health of these children, which leads to insecurity. This causes emotional and behavioural problems in children. Presence of radioactive materials in the environment is harmful as well, as it produces congenital anomalies and certain malignancies.

6. **Health services available**

The health promotion facilities available to public have a great impact on the health of children. The preventive medicine facility available decides the prevalence of communicable diseases and morbidity and mortality related to such problems. If the primary care facilities provided are good, then the index of child health will be better. The national health facilities provided by the country should concentrate on the prevention and health promotion activities to safeguard the health of its children.

7. **National and international environment**

Conducive national and international environment is essential for proper growth and development of children. Tension prevailing in a country related to civil war or political instability affects the health services such as other basic conditions of food and education. Children in these countries live under tension and threat and may have to live without food and water, sleep under tents or on road/pathways, run away from home for security or for shelter to sustain life. These affect the health of children and their right to live.

International stability is also important. The Gulf War has produced a financial setback in many countries, including India. Kerala suffered most because of remigration of '*pravasees*'.

Frequently, the natural calamities also make many people homeless and create problems of living conditions. The great example of this is the recent tsunami that affected the costal parts of Kerala and Tamil Nadu. Frequently occurring earthquakes and floods in different states of India are examples of natural calamities that alter basic living conditions. These directly affect the health of this vulnerable population.

CHILDHOOD ILLNESSES

Paediatric population is at risk of developing certain diseases specific to their age. The two major causes of paediatric illness are malnutrition and infections. Susceptibility to specific infectious agents is a direct consequence of the maturity of the immune system, exposure to potential infectious agents and the presence of underlying diseases. The host response varies with age. Hence, neonates are at risk for developing different types of infections compared with school-aged children or adolescents.

Malnutrition

It is common among infants and children of lower- and middle-class families. About 190 million children under 5 years of age are malnourished as per estimate of the developing countries. Only 1%–2% have visible signs of malnutrition. Studies conducted on infants belonging to 25 developing countries show that the prevalence of malnutrition is about 25% on weight for age basis. In India, 90% of preschool children have growth retardation related to malnutrition. About 250,000 children suffer from vitamin A deficiency, leading to nutritional blindness, every year in India. Eight million people in the developing world are living in areas endemic to iodine deficiency, leading to cretinism and mental impairment. The National Nutrition Monitoring Bureau had conducted a study in 10 states of India and found that about 8.4% of preschool children suffer from severe malnutrition and 3.4% of children suffer from moderate malnutrition. As far as the agent factors are concerned, energy deficiency along with protein deficiency ranks first. Other nutrient deficiencies lead to specific conditions such as night blindness, beriberi, pellagra, anaemia, rickets, cretinism, etc.

Factors Leading to Malnutrition

a. *Age and sex:* Basal metabolic rate (BMR) and physiological expenditure of energy vary with age and sex. Protein requirement is high in children, and 90% of the brain growth occurs by the age of 2 years. Hence, kwashiorkor is seen in young children compared with their older counterparts, especially preschool children.

b. *Habits, customs and food fads:* Late weaning, feeding children with cooked and strained rice alone, custom of discarding colostrums, increased use of processed foods, fast foods that contain harmful preservatives, etc.

c. *Physiological and pathological stress:* Undernutrition may be secondary to interference with digestion, absorption and utilization of food. Children with various congenital abnormalities of the gastrointestinal tract, cardiovascular system and metabolic problems suffer from malnutrition.

d. *Environmental factors:* Physical, socioeconomic or biological environments are important factors that predispose a person to malnutrition. Among these, socioeconomic factors have a major contribution. A majority of people living in developing countries have low purchasing capacity. A large part of our population obtains food by purchase or barter. Those who are living below the poverty line suffer from scarcity of food and malnutrition owing to less purchasing power.

Infections – The Second Major Cause of Childhood Illnesses

The two major infections in children are acute respiratory infections (ARIs) and diarrhoea. ARIs are the leading cause of morbidity and mortality in children. The World Health Assembly resolved in 1976 to give priority to this area. The ARI control programme was launched in India in the 1980s. About 750,000 children below 5 years of age die of ARI complications in India every year, i.e. 2000 deaths per day or 85 deaths per hour. The risk of Indian children dying from ARI complications is 30–75 times more than that in developed countries. ARIs account for 14.3% of deaths in infants and 15.9% of deaths in 1–5 years old. A child experiences five to eight episodes of ARIs per year in urban areas and two to three episodes in rural areas. ARIs are the current leading cause of deaths in children, and pneumonia ranks first. Of 2000 million episodes of ARIs of which 1 of 50 cases are of pneumonia, 10%–20% result in deaths. ARIs comprise 25%–30% of hospital consultations and 20%–40% of total hospital admissions in children. ARIs include influenza, sinusitis, acute otitis media, nasopharyngitis, tonsillitis, epiglottis, laryngitis, tracheitis, bronchitis, bronchiolitis and pneumonia. Preventable ARIs are measles, diphtheria, pertussis and childhood tuberculosis.

The contributing factors are grouped as host factors and environmental factors. The host factors include low birth weight, malnutrition, lack of immunization and antecedent viral infections. The environmental factors include air pollution, passive smoking, pollution from biomass fuels and overcrowding.

Infestations

These are a common health problem in children. Intestinal parasites such as *Ascaris*, hookworm, *Giardia* and amoeba are common because of poor environmental hygiene and paucity of potable drinking water.

Accidents and Poisoning

Accidents and poisoning also take a heavy toll on children's life. More children in developing countries die as a result of burns and trauma related to unsafe home environment and traffic accidents. The International Union for Child Welfare has estimated that there are 1.5 million such children in India alone.

The common accidents and poisoning in developing countries include falls, burns, poisoning with organophosphorus, chocking, drowning and automobile accidents that cause wounds, bleeding, fractures, shock and head injuries (see emergency care).

Behavioural problems are also on the rise in the child population in our country as a result of lifestyle changes.

Factors Contributing to Illness in Children

The major contributing factors of illness in children can be categorized as follows:
- Genetic factors
- Maternal factors
- Childhood problems
- Predisposing factors

Genetic factors are hereditary factors, genetically transmitted problems and mutation effects.

Maternal factors are maternal infections during pregnancy such as TORCH infections, sexually transmitted infections, HIV infection, drugs taken during pregnancy, environment, radiation exposure and nutrition during the gestational period. Adolescents and pregnant women need to be warned about ingestion and handling of uncooked meat or infected cat containing cyst to prevent toxoplasmosis. They must be warned against the possible hazardous effects of toxoplasmosis that cause blindness and deterioration of brain in the developing fetus.

Cytomegalovirus has a 2% chance to produce deleterious effects in the fetus. It is usually transmitted transplacentally. It infects the baby during the birth process and can cause severe brain damage.

Herpes simplex virus also infects the baby during the birth process, and the mortality rate is about 85%. Maternal syphilitic infections affect the baby in utero before 16th week of gestation, resulting in congenital syphilis.

Other maternal factors include maternal medications, sedations, alcoholism and smoking, environmental hazards, exposure to X-rays, hormonal imbalances, pregnancy-induced hypertension (PIH), pregnancy complicating diseases such as diabetes and hypertension, increased maternal age, etc.

Childhood Problems of Significance

- Communicable diseases and infectious diseases, scabies, respiratory tract infections, acute diarrhoea, worm infestations
- Nutritional disorders such as PEM, vitamin deficiencies
- Inborn errors of metabolism
- Congenital and hereditary disorders
- Accidents and poisoning
- Neoplasms of different types
- Miscellaneous ones include use of indigenous medicines, lack of knowledge regarding child-rearing practices and poor socioeconomic status.

Specific Attributes of Indian Children

India is home to the largest number of children (414 million), i.e. 19% of world's children; 26 million more children are born every year. Out of a hundred children born in India,

35 of those births will be registered;
93 will make it to their first birthday;
51 will be fully immunized;
5 will die of malnutrition;
42 will remain underweight, which will affect their performance throughout their lives; 25 will complete primary school.

These data give a clear picture of the plight of Indian children. Though India made progress after independence, one out of every two children under 3 years of age is malnourished. Nearly 1.8 million infants die each year; most of them die from preventable causes. Every 4 minutes, a woman dies during childbirth. The life expectancy at birth has doubled (32 years at 1951 to 64 in 2001). Literacy rates have also increased (27% in 1951 to 76% in 2001).

India is a country of contrasts and great complexity. There are marked disparities among different geographical regions and between social groups, among different income levels and between the sexes. Malnutrition affects more than half of all rural children. Obesity is a problem among affluent children.

India has some state-of-the-art hospitals that offer some of the best medical care in the world. However, there are communities where a health worker has not been seen for years.

Indian Institutes of Technology provide world-class education to thousands; however, 190 million Indian women remain illiterate. For example, female literacy rates in Maharashtra range from 83% in the district of Mumbai to 46% in Nandurbag.

The number of girls per 1000 boys in the 0–6 years age group fell sharply from 945 in 1991 to 927 in 2001. Some of the worst decline is seen in the more prosperous states such as Gujarat, Haryana, Punjab, Himachal Pradesh and Kerala. Easy access to prenatal diagnostic tests helps determine sex and selective abortion of female fetuses.

Rural–urban geography of gender disadvantage is more acutely reflected in school education data. In total, 80% of girls aged 6–14 years attend school in urban areas as opposed to 70% in rural areas. Malnutrition is common across the whole of India; highest is seen in 'BIMARU' states of India and lowest in Kerala. Factors contributing to this are parent's level of knowledge about infant feeding, hygiene, care of sick child, health service delivery, gender, socioeconomic issues, etc.

SITUATION IN KERALA

Kerala stands first in literacy and health among other Indian states. However, when considering the state of children, Keralites need to have introspection whether their children are given due attention or not. Infant and childhood mortality is low compared with other states and is at par with developed countries of the world. The birth rate of children in Kerala is on the whole declining.

The cause for this is attributed to lifestyle changes and family planning. The total number of children is about 31% of the total population. The statistics show that under-five children are only 6%, children between 5 and 10 years of age are only 7% and children between 10 and 14 years are 8%. Children between 15 and 19 of age are 9% of the total population. This statistics shows similarity with the statistics available from the USA. The number of children who were enrolled in school from 2002 to 2006 is also less than that of the previous years.

The statistics also show that children who are kept in orphanages run by both the state government and voluntary agencies are equally maltreated, except very few children. This was brought out by the legislative assembly report (773/2003). There are about 800 children in seven juvenile homes in Kerala. Many children have been placed for adoption.

STUDY QUESTIONS

1. What are the factors affecting child health?
2. Describe the factors contributing to illness in childhood.
3. Enumerate the common childhood illnesses.

BIBLIOGRAPHY

1. Ahmann. E. (1994). Family Centered Care: Shifting Orientation. Paediatric Nursing, 20(2), pp. 113-117.
2. Band, W. A. (1991). Creating Value for Customers: Designing and Implementing a Corporate Strategy. Executive Vol.5. No.3. pp.99–101.
3. Cone, T.E. Jr. (1979). History of American Pediatrics. Boston: Little Brown.
4. Cone T.E. Jr. (1985). History of the care and feeding of the premature infant. Boston: Little Brown.
5. Heller, R., McKlindon, D. (1996). Families as Faculty: Parents Educating Care givers About Family Centered Care. Paediatric Nursing, 22(5), pp. 428-431.
6. Manoj, K.M. "Kudumbum thedi kunjungal: kunjine thedi kudumbagal" Mathrubhumi Daily-31/10/06; 1/11/06; 2/11/06; 3/11/06; 4/11/06.
7. Pearson, H.A. (1988). The Centennial History of the American Pediatrics Society. New Haven: American Paediatric Society.
8. Spiro, H., Curnen, M.G.M., Peschel, E., St. James, D. (1993). Empathy and The Practice of Medicine. New Haven, CT: Yale University.
9. Wong, D.L, Hockenberry, M.J. (2003). Wong's Nursing Care of Infants and Children. 7th Edn. St. Louis: Mosby.

ACCIDENTS IN CHILDREN

LEARNING OBJECTIVES

At the end of the chapter, the learner will be able to:
- Describe the common accidents in children.
- Explain the strategies which help the parents to prevent accidents in children.
- Describe the general safety precautions that need to be taken by the parents to prevent accidents.

TABLE 7-1   Age-wise Accidents

Age	Common Accidents
Infants	Burns
	Choking
	Extremity fractures
	Head injuries
	Motor vehicle accidents
	Near drowning
	Toxic ingestions
Toddlers	Burns
	Choking
	Extremity fractures
	Head injuries
	Motor vehicle accidents
	Near drowning
	Toxic ingestions
	Bicycle injuries
Preschoolers	Burns
	Extremity fractures
	Falls
	Motor vehicle accidents
	Toxic ingestions
	Bicycle injuries
School-aged children	Extremity fractures
	Motor vehicle accidents
	Sports injuries
Adolescents	Extremity fractures
	Motor vehicle accidents
	Sports injuries
	Near drowning (more common among adolescent boys)

Accidents are the common unintentional injuries that take a heavy toll on human life and cripple many lives. Childhood accidents at home and outside are common but preventable. Parents need to know what accidents are common and how to avoid them. The age is the most important factor that affects children with accidents. It is described in the Table 7.1.

The following section of the text describes the common accidents in children as per age and the preventive measures to be taken in order to prevent them.

ROAD TRAFFIC ACCIDENTS

Road traffic accidents (RTAs) are the most common type of accidents that lead to death of children in our state. These can occur as a pedestrian or as a passenger. But most of the time, RTAs occur to children as pedestrians. Boys between the ages of 5 and 12 years mostly experience this type of accidents. Children of this age group are school going and will not be able to estimate the speed of vehicles or dangers of traffic while crossing roads. Though the school curriculum emphasizes the need of road safety, the practical aspects of road safety are not followed properly. Hence, children must be taught the practical aspects of road safety through demonstration classes.

Child Passengers

During crashes, unrestrained children become missiles and get injured or they may not be able to escape like that of adults. Safety belts in cars have proved to be effective as safe restraints to child passengers that prevent death of children as a result of being thrown away from vehicles during accidents.

Bicycle Accidents

Children sustain bicycle accidents frequently. These are one of the most important causes of head injuries in children. Motorbike accidents are also common among children as passengers. In Kerala, this is a common form of accidents that take lives of many children.

Falls of Other Forms

Either falling from a height or falling down in house and premises can result in head injuries or internal and external injuries. Children can suffer from abdominal and chest injuries associated with severe trauma.

Prevention

- Do not allow children to sit in the car without wearing a seat belt. Ensure that their seat belts are fastened.
- Do not put babies or young children in the car without a child seat or restraint. Ensure that special child seats are used for babies and young children.
- Do not give children the opportunity to open the car doors. Put safety lock in car doors.
- Do not put children in the front seat of the car; they are more likely to get hurt. Make sure that they sit in the back seat with the seat belt fastened.
- Do not let children play near cars that are reversing or being parked, as they might get hit or run over.
- Do not leave keys in the ignition while children are in the car. They might start the car by accident. Ensure that you always take keys with you and keep the parking on.
- Provide seats for people carrying or accompanying children in public transports. Never allow ladies to carry children and keep standing in a running public transport.
- Falls can be prevented by supervising children railing around stairs and teaching children about the dangers of height.
- Do not leave children unattended on an upper storey, on balcony or any high place. Install sturdy gates for the stairways. Keep the balcony door closed at all times. Put the baby in a cot with side rails up, and use straps when the baby is placed in a high chair.
- Do not place the baby on a sofa. He/she could fall down if he/she is very active. Place the baby in a cot bed if you have to leave him/her alone. Make sure that the hinges are strong, the wood rim is not chopped and paint is lead free.
- Do not leave the baby alone in a movable play pan or walker when you are not within a watching distance. Make sure your baby's walker is stable and sturdy so that it will not collapse or overturn.
- Do not let young children sleep on the upper deck of a bunk bed which has no railing on it. Fix railings on the upper deck before you let your child sleep in it. Make sure that the bed and the ladder have a solid construction.
- Do not place furniture near an open window. Children may climb on it and fall down accidentally. Fix grills on all windows, especially those on an upper storey.
- Do not leave spilled liquids or patches of water on the floor, and never polish under the rugs. Children may slip on it. Wipe off liquids spilled on the floor immediately.

BURNS AND SCALDS

These are the second most common cause of death from accidents. Most of these deaths are caused by carelessness of parents or caretakers. In rural Kerala, the most common cause of burns is the unsafe use of kerosene lamps. Burns from fireplaces are also common. Scalds from boiling water and hot drinks are common among children, especially in toddlers. The common victims of burns with kerosene lamps are school-aged children, who use kerosene lamps for studying.

Prevention

Burns and scalds can be prevented by ensuring a safe cooking place, making hot things not accessible and teaching children the dangers of fire, hot liquids, etc.
- Do not allow children to burn firecrackers unsupervised or allow children access to matches or lighters.
- Do not allow children play near the cooking stove or fireplace.
- Do not put a tablecloth on the dining table if you have small children around. They could playfully pull the table cloth, causing everything on the table to fall on them. Use table mats instead of a tablecloth.
- Do not place containers of hot liquid near the edge of the table or on stove with handles jutting out or at the ground level. Keep all containers out of reach of children.
- Do not pour hot water into a basin and leave the child alone near it even for a minute. The child may think the bath is ready for him/her. Better fill the basin with cold water first and then add hot water for mixing into a warm bath.

ELECTROCUTION

This is yet another cause of death in children.

Prevention

- Do not expose empty wall sockets which your child could tamper with. It is best not to allow them to play near electrical points. Put safety caps on all unused electric outlets and switch them off when not in use. Cover up electrical points with heavy furniture so as to be kept out of reach of children.
- Do not leave any unused appliances connected to the electrical point. It is extremely dangerous, especially if the switch is still on. Unplug the appliances and keep them in a safe place.
- Do not leave faulty electrical appliances around the house. Children may accidentally get electrocuted. Ensure electrical appliances are safe for use and the electrical system in the house is in a proper order.

DROWNING AND NEAR-DROWNING

Drowning and near-drowning also cause death in children, especially in preschoolers and school-aged children. Children may get drowned in streams, rivers, lakes, swimming pools, as well as in pits where water is stagnated. Drowning can occur in pits where the clay or soil is removed for making bricks and tiles. This is very common in northern Kerala. Infants and toddlers are also not free from the risk of drowning. This usually occurs at home. They get drowned in bathtubs and water-filled vessels.

Prevention

- Do not leave the baby alone in or near a tub of water. He/she could turn face downwards and drown within seconds. Pick up the baby and take him/her along if you have to attend to something urgently; do not leave the baby near to a water-filled vessel or tub.
- Do not leave children alone with uncovered water storage containers such as wells and fish tanks. They could fall into it and get drowned. Cover all water storage containers securely after use.
- Do not let children play near pools, drains, rivers and streams, as they might fall into it and get drowned. Ensure that they are always free of imminent danger. Teach swimming to children.

CHOCKING, SUFFOCATION AND STRANGULATION

Children may choke on vomit, toy parts or aspiration of food and fluids. Children strangle themselves on curtains, cloth cradles, beddings and even necklaces and neckties. Some children try to imitate TV and cinema scenes and get strangulated. Some intentionally do the same.

Airway obstruction from aspirated foreign bodies can be relieved using Heimlich manoeuvre in older children.

Prevention

- Do not put strings holding a pacifier or gold chain or any such things around the neck. They get entangled and strangle the baby. Avoid putting chains or strings of any type around the neck of the baby.
- Do not put plastic sheets on mattress or leave plastic bags within a child's reach. They could result in suffocation. Use a thick rubber mat if you must line the baby's mattress and store plastic bags out of the child's reach.
- Do not leave objects such as hard candies, sweets, nuts, marbles, pins and buttons that could be accidentally swallowed or inhaled within the child's reach. Store such items away in a safe place. Make sure your child's toys do not have small parts that can be easily detached (e.g. eyes of dolls, buttons).
- Do not let bottle-fed baby unattended. This may lead to chocking; always hold the baby while bottle-feeding.

- Do not let children play near the unused fridge, cupboard or washing machine. They may be trapped inside and may suffocate to death. Store away and securely lock such bulky unused items.
- Do not put too many bolsters and pillows around your sleeping infant. It may cause suffocation. Let the baby sleep in comfort in an uncluttered cot.

POISONING

Many children are hospitalized because they have been poisoned by eating or drinking or even inhaling poisonous substances. Some of these children die. To prevent such types of deaths, adults need to be vigilant. Substances such as medicines, petrol and household cleaning materials need to be stored high up so that children cannot reach them.

Prevention

- Do not leave harmful chemicals within easy reach of children. They like to imitate adults; any aerosol can is just like hair sprays that their mother or father use. Lock away all harmful items in a high, safe place that is inaccessible to children.
- Do not use empty soft drink bottles to store poisonous liquids such as kerosene, turpentine oil and pesticide; a child may drink it by mistake. Throw away all empty bottles. Poisons should be retained in their original containers which cannot be easily uncapped by children. Colourful tablets could be mistaken for sweets. Keep medicines in child-proof bottles and containers and under lock-and-key.
- Do not place medicinal items together with foods. They could be accidentally consumed by the children. Keep medicines away in places specially meant for them.
- Do not put potted plants in places within easy reach of young children. Out of curiosity, they may pick and eat the leaves and earth.
- Do not use pest control chemicals carelessly (e.g. mothballs). A child could be poisoned if he/she swallows them. Put such chemicals in places away from children's inquisitive eyes.

CUTS

Cut injuries are also common among children. They may pick carelessly placed knives, razors and blades to experiment. Sharp edges of furniture can also be injurious to children.

Prevention

- Do not use furniture with sharp edges. A child could easily hurt himself/herself if he/she knocks into it accidentally. Use furniture that is sturdy, steady and without sharp edges, so it will not overturn or break easily.
- Do not have glass sliding doors closed when children are around; they may accidentally walk into

them. Avoid use of glass for household fittings and tables.

- Do not keep sharp cutting instruments lying around or where children can get them easily. Make it a point to put away sharp instruments after use.
- Do not have faulty or ill-fitting flooring unattended. Make sure all floorings are properly fitted to avoid children tripping on them.
- Do not give breakable toys or items made of glass or ceramics to children. They could get a bad cut. Give sensible toys that are appropriate to the child's age.
- Do not place table fans within children's reach. Place the fan on a high place to avoid the possibility of children playing with its blades.

GENERAL SAFETY PRECAUTIONS THAT NEED TO BE TAKEN BY THE PARENTS OR CAREGIVERS

Following are some of the age-wise precautions to be taken for preventing accidents in children.

Infants

- Provide rails with small-distance slats for wooden cribs.
- Avoid pins in dresses.
- Avoid small objects, removable screws, etc. in toys.
- Place infants in safe feeding and post-feeding positions.
- Do not leave infants unattended into or near a water container.
- Child car or vehicle safety must be followed.

Toddlers

- Avoid knives, sharp tools, scissors and matches within children's reach.
- Keep stove, top pots or bottle warmers on back gas burners.
- Lock away cleaning solutions, chemicals, insecticides and medicines. Never say medicines are candy.
- Play area safety must be established.
- Do not leave swimming pools, even baby style, unattended.
- Use 'NO' and 'DO NOT' with discretion.
- Follow child car safety precautions.
- Keep an eye on inquisitive walkers and climbers.

Preschoolers

- Teach them to expect falls.
- Stress importance of sidewalks, play versus playing on the street.
- Provide swimming lessons.
- Prevent children from running while carrying sharp utensils.
- Teach children not to accept rides or gift from strangers.
- Teach children to use regular safety belts in cars.

School-aged Children

- Teach safe use of play and sports equipment.
- Teach traffic and bicycle safety rules.
- Teach use of seat belts in vehicles.
- Teach children to follow animal safety.
- Provide swimming and first aid instructions.
- Reinforce the need of caution with strangers.

Adolescents

- Provide constructive diversionary activities.
- Promote development of inner discipline.
- Provide appropriate safety teaching (e.g. use of helmets) and instruction for avoiding sports accidents.
- Teach the danger of alcohol and drug abuse.
- Teach first aid and cardiopulmonary resuscitation (CPR).
- Reinforce the need for caution against strangers and need for safety precautions during driving.

STUDY QUESTIONS

1. What are the common accidents encountered in children and how can you prevent them?
2. Conduct a health talk on prevention of accidents in toddlers to a group of mothers of toddlers?

BIBLIOGRAPHY

1. Atkuri, R. (May 2006). Millennium Development Goals. Health Action, 2(3), pp. 4–8.
2. Bass, J.L., et al. (Feb 1985). Educating Parents About Injury Prevention. Pediatric Clinics of North America, 32, p. 233.
3. Bonadio, M. (1993). Defining Fever and Other Aspects of Body Temperature in Infants and Children. Paediatric Annals, 22(8), p. 467.
4. Cantor, R. and Learning, J. (Feb 1998). Evaluation and Management of Pediatric Major Trauma. Emergency Medicine Clinics of North America, 16(1), pp. 229–256.
5. Cortiella, J. and Marvin, J. (June 1997). Management of Pediatric Burn Patient. Nursing Clinics of North America, 32(2), pp. 311–329.
6. Expert Committee on School Health. (1951). WHO Technical Report Series No. 30.
7. Fernado, A. (1990). High-risk Pregnancy and Delivery. New Delhi: Jaypee Brothers.
8. Garot, P.A. (April 1986). Therapeutic Play: Work of Both Child and the Nurse. Journal Pediatric Nursing, 1, p. 111.
9. Gill, D., O'Brien, N. (1998). Paediatric Clinical Examination. 3rd Edn. Churchill Livingstone: Edinburgh.
10. Gopalan, C. (1992). Growth Charts in Primary Child Health Care: Time for Assessment. Indian Journal of Maternal and Child Health, 3(4), pp. 98–103.
11. Gopalan, K.C. (28 Aug 2005). Evils of Child Marriage. The Hindu.
12. Gopalan, C., Chatterjee, M. (1985). Use of Growth Charts for Promoting Child Nutrition. Special Publication Series 2. Nutrition Foundation of India.
13. Growth and Physical Development of Indian Infants and Children. (1989). ICMR Technical Report Series No. 18.
14. Growth Chart for International Use in Maternal and Child Health Care. (1986).
15. Haszinski, M.F. (1992). Nursing Care of the Critically Ill Child. St. Louis: Mosby.
16. Herzog, L. and Coyne, L. (1993). What is Fever? Normal Temperature in Infants Less Than Three Months Old. Clinical Paediatrics, 32(3), p. 142.

17. Higgins, B. (24 July 1980). Building Play Skills. Nursing Times, 76, p. 1317.
18. Kelley, S.J. (1994). Paediatric Emergency Nursing. 2nd Edn. Norwlk, CT: Appleton & Lange.
19. Krishna Menon, M.K., Palaniyappan, B., Mudaliar and Menon. (1990). Clinical Obstetrics, Madras: Orient Longman.
20. Latheef, N.A. Vettilakolli Tribals in Penury. (29 Aug 2005). The Hindu.
21. Naushad. Immunization Programme. (23 Aug 2005). The Hindu.
22. Profile of the Child in India: Policies and Programmes. (1997). Govt. of India.
23. Park, K. (2007). Park's Text Book of Preventive and Social Medicine. 19th Edn. M/s Banarsidas Bhanot, Jabalpur.
24. Rajaram, P. (1992). Child Survival: Maternal Factors. Indian Journal of Maternal and Child Health, 1(2), pp. 39–45.
25. Reproductive and Child Health Programme: Scheme for Implementation. (1997). Govt. of India.
26. Risk Approach for Maternal and Childcare. WHO Offset Publication No. 39, 1978005.
27. Schuman, W. (Sept 1984). The Importance of Play. Parents, 59, p. 56.
28. Sharma K. (18 Sept 2005). The Sensex, Sania and Starvation. The Hindu.
29. Staff Reporter. Only Slender Shoulders to Lean. (24 Aug 2005). The Hindu.
30. Thomas, D.O. (April 1996). Assessing Children—It's Different. RN, pp. 38–42.
31. Wilson, M., Baker, S.P., Teret, S., et al. (1991). Saving Children: Guide to Injury Prevention. Oxford University Press: New York.

UNIT 3

HEALTHY CHILD

Human growth is a biological phenomenon that makes an individual grow physically and naturally based on different factors. Development is also a process that makes an individual mature physically as well as emotionally. Growth and development is a continuous process, and the individual goes through different stages to reach the final stage of growth and development. Development growth includes the psychological growth and is also influenced by different factors, namely environmental, social and individual factors.

This unit consists of ten chapters.

FACTORS AFFECTING GROWTH AND DEVELOPMENT

LEARNING OBJECTIVES

At the end of the chapter, the learner will be able to:
- Describe the factors affecting growth and development.
- Discuss play as an important aspect of growth and development in children.

The major difference between children and adults is that of growth. It influences every aspect of childcare. For this reason, knowledge of human growth and development is basic to paediatric nursing, including general principles that govern growth, understanding of physical and psychological growth and role of play/recreation in the development of a child.

It should be remembered that the growth and development of a child from conception to adulthood are not simply a result of single factor but also a result of amalgamation of various factors, including child's reactions to his/her interaction with such influences.

INHERITANCE

Inheritance plays an important part in the future growth and development of a child. It is responsible for many disorders. Heredity influences the ultimate constitution of the body. For example, taller parents are likely to have taller children. Transmission of some abnormal genes may result in familial illnesses. Thalassaemia, sickle cell anaemia, Phenylketonuria (PKU), etc. are a few such examples.

Heredity of men and women determine their children's growth. The embryonic life begins with the cytoplasm and nucleus of the fertilized ovum genetically determined by both parents. Rate of growth is more alike among siblings than among other children. Some children are small,

not because of endocrine or nutritional disturbances but because of their genetic constitution.

Genetic predisposition influences the growth and development of children, as it decides the phenotype, characteristics of parents, race, sex, biorhythm and maturation, and genetic disorders. It is a proven fact that DNA directs the growth and differentiation; the structural genes are involved in protein synthesis, the operator genes regulate structural genes and the regulatory genes regulate the operator genes. From this, it is evident that genetic factors affect growth and development. Even though there are other factors that affect growth and development, an individual cannot exceed his/her genetic potential. So the genes inherited from parents decide the gender, physical features, behavioural developments and even the number of fetuses or babies in each pregnancy. Genes also decide height, weight, facial features, hip and breast size, intelligence, eye and hair colour.

INTRAUTERINE LIFE

A number of factors can affect the embryo after conception while it is still growing and developing within the mother. Such factors include placental defects, drugs taken during pregnancy, maternal alcohol intake, smoking and radiation exposure, maternal nutrition, etc. Even the emotional deprivation of the mother during pregnancy can adversely affect the growth and development of the fetus inside her womb.

BIRTH

Although the birth process is an arduous experience for the infant, the effects are normally temporary and do not affect future growth and development. Few exceptions relate to oxygen deprivation and nerve injuries. If brain cells are without enough oxygen for even a few minutes, the cells die and cause a permanent brain damage. If the birth is difficult, there may be permanent brain injury to nerves, causing muscle paralysis and a variety of serious developmental problems. Prenatal factors such as mother's age, father's age, maternal health, maternal nutrition during pregnancy, etc. also affect growth and development. Harmful maternal factors such as maternal nutritional deficiencies; malpositions; metabolic and endocrine disturbances; maternal infections such as toxoplasmosis, rubella, herpes, syphilis, etc.; Rh incompatibility; smoking; alcohol use; and intake of certain drugs. If the neonate is of low birth weight, the growth will be affected. Neonates with seizures may have developmental delay. Postnatal factors that affect growth and development include sex of the child (male children get more care in the Indian culture), hormonal influence, nutrition, infection, trauma and socioeconomic factors. Boys are heavier and taller than girls at birth, and this is maintained till 11 years of age. Prepubertal growth spurt occurs in girls earlier than in boys. Boys grow taller than girls when they reach prepubertal growth spurt.

ENVIRONMENT AND NUTRITION

When infants are born, they bring with them an inherited potential, a physical body and an underdeveloped personality. The environment into which they arrive and the diet they receive profoundly affect their growth and development. So one must remember the dictum 'nature versus nurture'.

Environment is the surroundings of the child namely, air, sunshine, home, family, diseases, emotional climate, religious and social customs etc. All these influence a child's growth and development. Exposure to lead, pesticides, etc. affects the growth and development. Use of pesticides in different parts of India (best example is cashew plantations of Kasargod, Kerala) has proven this effect of environment on child growth and development. Pollution, housing conditions and access to health and welfare measures are also important. Other environmental factors that also affect growth and development are pollution, chemicals and environmental radiation such as that happened after nuclear and atomic bombings at Hiroshima and Nagasaki in Japan. They interfere with early development.

External environment such as school, neighbourhood, religious institutions and social clubs also affect growth and development. Political unrest, civil wars and immigration problems also affect growth and development of children.

Adequate nutrition is essential for a normal physical growth. This includes enough of all necessary dietary nutrients and the quality of the diet, not just enough food to fill an empty stomach. Nutritional deficiency of protein, carbohydrates, minerals, vitamins and essential amino acids, both quantitatively and qualitatively, considerably affects physical and mental development. Even problems resulting from inadequate absorption lead to retarded growth.

Nutritional deficiencies affect the growth and development of fetuses, leading to intrauterine growth retardation.

It can further manifest in childhood undernutrition if they are not adequately fed, leading to stunted growth. Deficiency of microelements such as iodine deficiency, iron deficiency, zinc deficiency and inadequate breastfeeding all can lead to stunted growth.

Significant difference between the growth rates of formula- and breastfed infants was first reported in the DARLING (US) study [10][6], which showed that breastfed infants grew more quickly initially, for the first 3–6 months, and then more slowly over the next 6–9 months. At the end of 12 months, breastfed infants were generally 0.5–0.6 kg lighter than the formula-fed infants.

ENDOCRINE FUNCTION

The endocrine glands play an important role in growth and development. Deficiency of thyroid hormone can lead to 'cretinism' – a condition in which retarded physical and mental growth and development lead to mental retardation. Thyroxin regulates metabolism and aids in body heat production. Pituitary hormone deficiency and overproduction can lead to dwarfism and gigantism, respectively.

Abnormalities in circulating hormones such as growth hormone, insulin-like growth factor, testosterone, oestrogen, thyroid hormone, cortisol and insulin affect birth weight and growth. Best example for this is the large for gestational age babies of diabetic mothers.

SOCIOECONOMIC FACTORS

Poverty relates to diminished growth and affluence to healthy growth. Children from well-to-do families are usually well nourished. Poor children have diminished growth owing to poor nutrition and low socioeconomic status.

SEASONAL FACTORS

It has been observed that maximum weight gain occurs during autumn and maximum height gain during spring, so also are certain diseases. Seasonal variations are observed in the development of respiratory tract infections (winter) and acute diarrhoeal diseases in summer.

CHRONIC DISEASES

Chronic diseases such as congenital heart disease, rheumatic heart disease, asthma, cystic fibrosis, etc. affect growth. Retarded growth is a feature of some of these diseases. Adrenocortical overactivity causes excessive height. Metabolic disorders cause mental retardation. There are various chronic diseases that can lead to failure to thrive in children.

GROWTH POTENTIAL

It is influenced by various genetic and environmental factors. The smaller the child is at birth, the smaller he/she is likely to be in subsequent years, and vice versa. Thus, growth potential is to some extent indicated by the child's size at birth. The child's height potential can be predicted on the basis of his/her parents' heights through complex calculations, which is obtained by calculating midparental height by adding both parents' heights and dividing by 2.

EMOTIONAL FACTORS

Emotional trauma from unstable family, insecurity, sibling rivalry, loss of parents, etc. negatively affects the growth and development of a child. Psychosocial risk factors such as deficient cognitive stimulation, lack of caregiver sensitivity and responsiveness to child are factors that affect the emotional growth of children. Contextual risk factors such as maternal depression, maternal deprivation and exposure to violence also affect children's emotional development and, in turn, affect growth and development. Emotionally deprived children, even if they have received good nutrition, may not show expected weight gain and are pale and unresponsive. Prolonged periods of emotional deprivation will lead to growth retardation and repeated illness, and they can become emotionally ill. A child who is given love and affection grows well as a good citizen with right attitudes. Good relationships with family members, mother, father and siblings, are essential. Undue stress in the family also negatively affects the growth and development of children. There are 10 identified emotional foods for proper growth and development:

1. Love
2. Affection
3. Security
4. Acceptance
5. Self-respect
6. Achievement
7. Recognition
8. Independence
9. Authority
10. Play

CULTURAL FACTORS

Methods of child rearing are dependent on culture. The feeding habits of infants vary in different societies. Some religious customs such as 'Anna Prassa' followed in Kerala will not allow the introduction of rice as a major source of carbohydrate till the child is taken to the temple and fed first time there. If the ceremony is delayed because of any reason, the child is denied rice and rice products. This can lead to protein–energy malnutrition, wasting or growth retardation. It is scientifically proven fact that rice is the best staple food to be used for early feeding by 6 months of age, as rice is devoid of gluten that can produce food allergy. Cultural deprivation is also important. Many working-class families fail to provide their children with skills to be successful in life. They grow culturally deprived, leading to stunted growth.

STUDY QUESTIONS

1. What are the factors affecting growth and development?
2. How environment and nutrition affect the growth and development of a child?
3. What are the endocrine functions that affect growth and development?
4. How emotional factors affect growth and development?

BIBLIOGRAPHY

1. de Onis, M. (2006). Comparison of the World Health Organization (WHO) Child Growth Standards and National Center for Health Statistics? WHO International growth Reference; implications for child health programmes. *Public Health Nutrition, 9*(7), 942–947.
2. Risnes, K.R., et al., Birthweight and mortality in adulthood: a systematic review and meta-analysis. International Journal of Epidemiology, 2011. 40(3): p. 647-661.
3. Stenhouse, E., et al., The accuracy of birth weight. Journal of Clinical Nursing, 2004. 13(6): p. 767-768.
4. Kitchen, W.H., H.P. Robinson, and A.J. Dickinson, Revised intra-uterine growth curves for an Australian hospital population. Journal of Paediatrics and Child Health, 1983. 19(3): p. 157-161.
5. Gluckman, P.D., et al., Losing the war against obesity: the need for a developmental perspective. Science Translational Medicine, 2011. 3(93): p. 93cm19.
6. Dewey, K.G., et al., Growth of breast-fed and formula-fed infants from 0 to 18 months: the DARLING study. Pediatrics, 1992. 89(6): p. 1035-1041.
7. Delemarre-van de Waal, H.A. Environmental factors influencing growth and pubertal development. Environmental Health Perspectives, 1993 Jul; 101(Suppl 2): p. 39–44.
8. Taylor, H. and Beckett, C. (2009). Human Growth and Development, 2nd edition, SAGE Publications Limited.

PLAY IN CHILDREN

LEARNING OBJECTIVES

At the end of the chapter, the learner will be able to:
- Describe the role of play in child development.
- Discuss the functions of play.
- Discuss the types of play in children.
- Describe the therapeutic role of play in the care of hospitalized children.

Play is essential for human beings to reach their full potential. Children love to play. Play gives a real a picture of what is important in their life. For children, it is fun being with their friends. Play takes different forms. It can be quiet, noisy, funny, serious, strenuous, effortless, orderly or messy, or outside or inside, and children play for different reasons. Play is a way of 'doing things'. Play has been defined as any activity freely chosen, intrinsically motivated and personally directed. It stands outside 'ordinary' life and is nonserious but at the same time absorbing the player intensely. It has no particular goal other than itself. Through play children experience their world and the world of others. According to Stuart Brown, a famous psychiatrist, play is '*the basis of all art, games, books, sports, movies, fashion, fun, and wonder – in short, the basis of what we think of as civilization*' (Brown, 2009).

'Play' is a generic word, and it is used for both children and adults. But it is innate in children. All the activities children do when not being told by adults to do is play for children. They do it by their instincts and not under any direction. Then it is real play for children. Adults take responsibility for providing provisions for play to children, as they know it is essential for growth and development of children. So, 'Play is what children and young people do when they follow their own ideas and interests, in their own way and for their own reasons' (DCMS, 2004).

Play is a serious business to children. It is their vehicle for development. Through play, children learn about themselves and the world in which they live. Play serves several specific functions. As children grow and mature, play changes in form or type, to fit into the complex needs of the growing child.

FUNCTIONS OF PLAY

- **Physical and motor development**
  Physical and motor development is the immediate and continuing result of play. Play activities help exercise the muscles and teach motor coordination. The whole body is involved in play, as the child bends and twists, jumps and runs, lifts and handles objects, pushes and pulls. Through play, surplus energy can be worked off. Active play promotes general good health.
  Physical benefits of play are as follows:
  - Reduces obesity
  - Increases positive emotions and increases the efficiency of immune, endocrine, and cardiovascular systems
  - Decreases stress, fatigue, injury and depression
  - Increases range of motion, agility, coordination, balance, flexibility, and fine and gross motor exploration
- **Social development**
  Social development occurs as a result of play with other children. At first, the child is satisfied to be

near others and then begins to play with them. The child learns to share, take turns, communicate, enjoy the friendship of others, compete, be a good sport and relate to individuals and groups through play. In play, the child has an opportunity to practice the art of interacting successfully with others, thus preparing for adult relationships.

Social benefits of play are as follows:
- Increases empathy, compassion and sharing
- Creates options and choices
- Models relationships based on inclusion rather than exclusion
- Improves nonverbal skills
- Increases attention and attachment

- **Emotional development/expression**

 Emotional expression is one of the valuable functions of play. The toddler can relieve anger by hammering pegs through a peg board. The preschooler can act out feelings by imaginative play. The school-aged child and the adolescent may use competitive sports to vent hostility. Play can be flexible according to the child's need. Therefore, play acts as an indispensable item for the maintenance of mental health in children. According to Azar (2000), learning to play successfully with others requires 'emotional intelligence', the ability to understand others' emotions and intentions. Play helps level the playing field and promotes fairness. Justice begins with healthy social play.

 Emotional–behavioural benefits of play are as follows:
- Reduces fear, anxiety, stress and irritability
- Creates joy, intimacy, self-esteem and concern for others
- Improves emotional flexibility and openness
- Increases calmness, resilience and adaptability and ability to deal with surprise and change and to heal emotional pain

- **Intellectual education**

 Intellectual education could be called 'play' if it were not made 'work' by school teachers and others. In young children, all bodily senses are involved in the process of learning through their play. The child feels, sees, tastes, hears and smells the information gained and puts them together to form concepts. This process of gathering information, putting together and coming to conclusions is called education. When all these process are enjoyed, it is called play.

- **Play and the brain:**

 Play increases brain development and growth. It helps in establishing new neural connections, making the player more intelligent. Play is more frequent during the rapid brain growth. It helps children perceive others' emotional state and adapt to ever-changing circumstances.

 Through play children develop the neurological foundations that help them solve problems and help in language development and creativity.

 Neuroscientist Jaak Panksepp found that play stimulates production of a protein, 'brain-derived neurotrophic factor', in the amygdala and the prefrontal cortex, which are responsible for organizing, monitoring and planning for the future.

- **Development of moral values**

 The development of moral values takes place as children interact with other children during play. They begin to learn that good actions help and that bad actions hurt others. At first, their sense of right and wrong is limited to simple situations, such as taking toy from another child or playing roughly. As children grow, they learn about telling the truth and lying. Later on, they learn about gossiping and hurting the feelings of classmates. Through play adolescents learn about paying debts, honesty, loyalty to friends, and sexual relationships and responsibility; thus, moral values evolve as a result of interaction with others and with the code of ethics taught by meaningful persons in the society.

TYPES OF PLAY

As children grow and develop, the types of play characteristics of their age change (Table 9.1). Babies play by themselves with objects that they move about. In infancy, the type of play observed is solitary, as infants play with their own hands and legs or by observing, listening and manipulating toys in and around them. Toddlers still play by themselves but enjoy plying near other children. This is called *parallel play*.

By 3 years of age, they begin to play together in a simple direct way, such as one child being doctor and the other being patient. This called *cooperative play*. Imaginative play has its own value for preschool children. They attribute life to inanimate objects such as chair, table, cot, etc. and play with them as if they have life. In cooperative play, children interact, take turns, share and decide how and what to play. They collaborate, develop and negotiate ideas for their play. **In associative/partnership play,** children begin to play together, developing interactions through doing the same activities or playing with similar equipment or by imitating.

During the school years, games and plays usually involve a group of children in activities such as hide and seek, baseball, board games and Bobo and Coco. 'Make-believe play' serves a special need for 8–10 years old children.

Solitary play has a place at every age, including fishing, making models, painting and just walking alone. Adolescents usually do not consider these activities as play anymore, even though they serve the same purposes as before.

Adolescents tend to think of work and school as separate from recreating. Adults work instead of play. When adolescents play baseball, go for skiing or diving or attend dance, they think of these activities as recreation and so these activities also serve to provide physical, motor, social and moral development, emotional expression and education.

Adolescents may require specialist coaching to excel in sports and games and also to participate in games and

TABLE 9-1 Interests and Activities of Children According to Age

Age	Interest	Activities	Music and Books
Infants (0–1 year)	Objects that attract eyes and ears but go into the mouth	Bright mobiles, bells, rattles, rings, etc.	Enjoy being sung songs
Toddlers (1–3 years)	Play things that allow parallel play and muscle coordination and give attention and security	Sand pail and shovel, peg board and mallet, kiddie car, jumping horse, pull toys cuddly animals, large dolls	Like large print books, to hear the same story over and over and to hear stories about animals
Preschool children (3–5 years)	Toys, equipment that stimulates imaginative, creative and active play	Playhouses, tinker toys, trains, trucks, dolls, finger paint, tricycle	Enjoy stories about fire engines, trains and action, like to read books with pictures, enjoy singing and action songs in groups
Early school-aged children (5–9 years)	Activities that use mental and physical skills, play with other children of the same sex, enjoy surprises	Crafts, metal, beads, leather, spool knitting; games: board games, old maid, rook; puzzles; hide and seek; swimming; riding tricycle and bike; imaginative play with mother's clothes, trains cars, buses, etc.	Still enjoy hearing stories; read for self; enjoy fairy tales, adventures and think-do books; enjoy group songs; sing solo; play musical instrument
Middle school-aged children (9–12 years)	Activities that use mental and physical skills, doing things with gang, enjoying team play, having buddy works for awards, prizes	Active team sports, e.g. baseball, soccer, basket ball; swimming, cycling; boys scout and girls guide crafts; metal, leather, modelling, carving, games: checkers, chess board, cards, ludo board, snake and ladder	Enjoy adventures, stories, biographies, comics, group singing solo and instrument
Early adolescents (12–15 years)	Budding interest in the opposite sex, activities that require skill related to the body and mind, want to earn to spend money	Active sports, every kind of more advanced hobbies, photography, radio, TV, telescope, microscope, complicated models to attract attention; cosmetics for girls; games: chess, cards	Adventure and love stories; technical or specialized books in the interested area; popular music, some group singing; solo instrument
Adolescents (15–18 years)	Recreational activities much like adults, opposite sex attraction, vocational activity search	Active sports, automobiles, boats, motorbikes, swimming, team sports, games; adult-type dances, dating, relaxing	Read or write any type of books, perform or audit popular, classical or folk music

sports competitions at the state, national and international levels. Youth groups, special interest groups, opportunities to develop physical fitness through formal and informal training, etc. will help adolescents develop physically, mentally and emotionally. Teenagers are risk takers, and in the name of sports and games, they may take any level of risk that may harm them, even their life. So, adult supervision is required even during play. Adult supervision is required at all venues and events of teenage sports, games and get together, as alcohol, drugs and negative social alignments could cause threats to their life. Adults need to be available to facilitate accepted behaviours at these places and help them take responsible decision at all times. Play provision suggestions that are healthy and appropriate should be arranged for this turbulent group of youngsters.

Other Types of Play

Creative play: Here children explore and use their body and materials to make and do things and to share their feelings, ideas and thoughts. They create materials and models with recycled materials and play with clay or dough using their imaginative actions. They do action dance and make and sing parody songs that give fun and inner meanings.

Games with rules: In the early stages of development, often children play by their own rules. But as and when time passes and children mature, they go to play with external and internal rules. The most common example for this is *Antakshari* (reciting poems, film songs, etc). Children negotiate the rules.

Language play: In this type of play, children play with sounds and words. It includes unrehearsed and spontaneous manipulation of words using rhythmic and repetitive elements. They enjoy playing with language, its patterns, sounds and meaningless words. They enjoy this as a joke.

Physical play: There are many types of physical play prevailing in every society, and children also use these types of play by practising and refining body movements and control. This provides children with control over their body and better coordination.

Exploratory play: In this type of play, children use both physical skills and their senses to find out what things feel like and what they can be done with them.

Children explore their body parts to identify the differences among friends and opposite sexes.

Manipulative play: Here they practice and refine motor skills. They fix missed parts and identify the appropriate items. This enhances their physical dexterity and eye–hand coordination.

Constructive play: They make houses, buildings, animals, trees, etc. using different types of blocks, natural or manufactured, and cubes. This type of play becomes complex as the child grows.

Pretend, dramatic, make-believe, role- and **fantasy play:** Here children use their imagination and pretend as objects or perform actions (mimicry). This type of play also becomes complex as the child grows. They can even role-play real-life events and do mime and perform mimicry. As thinking capacity changes from concrete to abstract, they even create and write dramas, scripts, and stories and create artificial scenarios.

Early literary and numeracy: This type of play is seen more among school children, and they use bus tickets, cinema tickets and multiplication tables. Interdictive Computer Techniques (ICT), mobiles, laptops, etc. are used precisely by children in this type of play.

Small-world play: Children play miniature representations of real things such as animals, dolls, cars, train, truck, etc.

Sociodramatic play: Here children play with other children and/or adults. This type of play makes children develop friendship, communication skills and skills for negotiation and ability to write.

PLAY AND RIGHTS OF CHILDREN

The United Nations (UN) Convention of Child Rights specifically mentions that no child should be discriminated on any basis and every child has the right to play. The Article 31 of UN Convention on Rights of Child specifically mentions the rights of all children and young people up to 18 years of age. It states that:

1. Parties recognize the right of the child to rest and leisure, to engage in play and recreational activities appropriate to the age of the child and to participate freely in cultural life and the arts.
2. Parties shall respect and promote the right of the child to participate fully in cultural and artistic life and shall encourage the provision of appropriate and equal opportunities for cultural, artistic, recreational and leisure activities.

GENDER AND PLAY

Equal opportunities for play for both boys and girls should be provided. In our culture, boys have more independence and are allowed to play away from home more often. Girls are kept close to home (usually security reasons and culture). Girls are often burdened with home responsibilities and taking care of younger children that limit their play requirements. Boys are given more encouragement in sports, and their achievements in sports and games are celebrated rather than the girls' achievements. This is seen in most of the societies.

Toys and game traditions socialize children in particular gender roles. Some roles limit holistic developments of children of both sexes. The gender issues in play are about ensuring equal opportunity for both genders, as play is important for overall development of the children. One must be careful and should reflect on play patterns that might promote negative stereotypes and behaviours of children of both genders.

Children show gender preferences in their play and interest in certain types of toys. By 8 months of age, this pattern is evident. Boys are more physically active than girls, and this is reflected in their play. Girls prefer to play more quietly and in smaller groups than boys. Boys will run around, make noise and be vigorous than girls.

Girls show visual preference for dolls over a toy truck or car. But boys are more often interested in a toy truck or car. Certain features such as colour, shape and purpose of toys make masculine and feminine preferences by children, showing their gender preferences.

These types of early sex differences could reflect inborn tendencies for girls and boys to prefer different toys. Preference for sex-linked toys usually emerges before the children develop gender identity.

Adults should be vigilant to a right approach about how children are treated during play, not to be discriminated because of any reason (gender, socioeconomic status, race, creed, etc. and also disability), what forms of play are supported and what values are conveyed in the purpose, rules and image of play.

PLAY AND CHILDREN WITH DISABILITIES

Children with disabilities should not be excluded from play. A child health nurse must concentrate on the child rather than on his/her disabilities. Play needs are equal for all children with or without disabilities. Children with disabilities require more attention to play actually in order to improve their development and self-help abilities. They require more opportunities, support and encouragement to improve self-esteem. Nurses need to explore innovative ideas for planning age-appropriate and disability-oriented play materials and types of play for these children. Play can be very well utilized for training on self-help abilities such as brushing teeth, combing hair and meeting hygienic needs.

PLAY AND HEALTH

Play has the potential to improve many aspects of emotional well-being, such as reducing anxiety, depression, aggression and sleep problems. It prevents obesity in children by increasing metabolic rates. That is why play has been used as a routine part of assessment, training and therapy for children. Researchers report that active play helps in managing children with ADHD (attention-deficit/hyperactivity disorders). Physical activity has important benefits for children's physical health and mental well-being if they meet recommended levels of play. The most undeniable feature of play is fun; hence, it improves quality of life of children. Enjoyment is the main reason for playing. Positive emotions contribute significantly to a sense of well-being and health.

PLAY DEPRIVATION

Because play promotes brain growth and development, its deprivation will lead to impaired brain development and flexibility. Play deprivation can cause increased risk for abnormal development, deviant behaviour and loss of self-control in children. It is like sleep deprivation. Play deprivation can affect optimal learning, normal social functioning and improper cognition, and they may not mature properly. According to Peter Gray (2011), the decline in play has causally contributed to the rise in psychopathology of young people. Play functions as the major means by which children (1) develop intrinsic interests and competencies; (2) learn how to make decisions, solve problems, exert self-control and follow rules; (3) learn to regulate their emotions; (4) make friends and learn to get along with others as equals; and (5) experience joy. So restoring children's free play is the best gift an adult can promise for better future of children as adults. Free play is the gift that can be offered to children. Play can be either structured or unstructured. Unstructured play promotes more creativity and increases intellectual development.

As adults, the child health nurse can promote play in children and can be an advocate for children in promoting play inside the hospital, home or outside. He/she can be the supporter of finding space for children's play too, as the free space for play is diminishing or shrinking in the name of development.

Managing Behaviour through Play

Certain paediatric procedures can be carried out easily using play. Few such procedures and nursing interventions are listed as follows:

Procedure	Nursing Interventions
Bathing	Give tub toys such as boats, cups and water syringes without needles. To play fountain experiences. Give the child a doll he/she can give a bath.
Encourage deep breathing	Give the child bubbles, balloons or surgical gloves to blow. Have the child blow through straws to race cotton balls. Older children can play mouth organ if available. Give the child straws to suck up pieces of paper or cotton balls.
Encourage coughing	Keep sneaking toys on child's abdomen, so toy makes a noise when the child coughs.
Encourage mobility	Arrange fantasy trips to an external environment. Decoration of the bed and surroundings with the help of the child. Arrange visits to other children. Use video games for older children.
Ambulation	Give the child something to pull or push. Set reasonable distance goal for the child to reach. Take the child for a visit to other children or place. Have a parade with fancy hats, horns and mask. Give the child a reward for a walk.
Maintain NPO status	Arrange special activities during mealtime, e.g. walk or visit to a special place in the hospital or any setting.
Encourage the child to eat	Make the child sit with other children who are eating. Serve food in a small portion on a small plate. Use a game or story to encourage eating. Involve the child in preparation/arrangement of food.
Restrict fluid intake	Give the child a choice of fluid and also a choice of time to drink.
Encourage the increase of fluid intake	Give a small amount of liquid over a period of time. Use a special decorated cup. Use syringes instead of a straw or cup. Arrange a mock teen party with other children.
Depressed behaviour	Encourage the child to express himself/herself through play. Talk through a doll or stuffed animal with younger children. Determine the child's level of understanding and clarify misconceptions. Do not avoid the child; continue to interact and support. Structure the child's day.
Aggressive behaviour	Channel energy positively; older children may enjoy competitive activities, whereas younger children can release tension through pounding boards, large motor activity or clay projects. Set limits. Praise for jobs well done. Help the child gain a sense of mastery.

Procedure	Nursing Interventions
Passive behaviour	Structure the child's day.
	Give simple choices.
	Encourage self-care.
	Spend more time with the child and attempt to stimulate interest.
Regressed behaviour	Regression is acceptable to a point because it allows the child a brief return to a less mature and demanding time.
	Support independence, mastery of tasks and self-care.
	Give attention to regressive behaviour; do not reprimand or shame regressive behaviour.

PLAY AND TECHNOLOGY

Toys always reflect the latest developments in science and technology. The best examples are the music boxes, cartoon features, electric vehicles, games, robots, etc. Toys are embedded with electronics to adapt to the abilities of the player. Smartphone, tablets or toy computers have different functions that aid children to use technology. There are many types of toys, with LEDs of different colours and sounds inbuilt with toys. These toys are used to teach phonics, speech, vocabulary and prereading skills. But the natural toys that are made at home with natural raw materials are as good as these high-tech toys.

Smart toys have different advantages. They are designed to teach a skill, make learning fun and engage children in physical activity rather than watching TV.

THERAPEUTIC PLAY AND PLAY IN THE HOSPITAL

Therapeutic play is used as a method for detecting more serious problems. It is usually provided by a certified play therapist, child psychologist or mental health expert. Therapeutic play helps in preventing slight or mild problems becoming worse and assists children resolve emotional or psychological issues that prevent them from reaching their goal. Usually, children play by themselves. But therapeutic play is administered by a therapist with an intention to resolve the child's mental health issues. In play therapy, the therapeutic use of play is applied to provide emotional and psychological help to children. Therapeutic play is activity based and play therapy is relationship based.

Play in the hospital is not play therapy or therapeutic play. For hospitalized children, it is essential to arrange play materials for them. Play helps children in all aspects of development. Children who are ill require more age-appropriate and safe toys. In child-friendly hospitals, designated spaces are arranged as play area and safe and age-appropriate play materials for different age group are provided. Children who are not very sick and ambulatory and not suffering from contagious disease can spend time playing without affecting their development. This will reduce the traumatic experience of hospitalization, as play can be therapeutic and help children deal with difficult situations such as emotional stress or medical treatment.

Selection of Toys

A child health nurse is in a unique position to select toys for his/her hospital paediatric set-up either in paediatrician's office or in the admission unit. He/she is also a child advocate and a health educator. So, the child health nurse should follow all safety precautions while selecting toys. Irrespective of the setting, when children are involved, play is their right and they are free to choose what they do lively or relaxed, noisy or quiet, take risks and enjoy freedom. But the adults who are selecting toys for children should be vigilant to protect children from harm. So judicious selection of toys is important. Toys selected should be age appropriate and safe. It should not contain small or easily removable parts so that aspiration of such parts can be avoided. This is important in the case of infants and toddlers. The toys should not have lead paint, soft fur and chemicals.

Adult supervision is required to prevent accidents met by children during play. Play spaces should be accident free, as children like challenging environments for exploring and developing their abilities. Children should not be exposed to unacceptable risks of death or serious injuries from play. So it is a serious responsibility of the child health nurse to look into the safety aspects of play in children.

STUDY QUESTIONS

1. Define play.
2. Why is it important to allow children to play?
3. What are the types of play?
4. What are the important points to be remembered while selecting toys for children?
5. How will you manage abnormal behaviours of children through play?
6. How play assist children develop emotionally, socially and physically?
7. Discuss the advantages of play for children.
8. Discuss the categories of play for children.
9. How gender affect play in children?
10. What are the age-appropriate ways for planning play in children?
11. As a nurse, how will you provide play opportunities for children in your hospital?
12. How will you differentiate therapeutic play from play therapy?

BIBLIOGRAPHY

1. Alexandria, G. M & Melissa H., and Hines, Melissa. (2002). Sex differences in response to children's toys in nonhuman primates (*Cercopithecus aethiops sabaeus*). Evolution and Human Behaviour, 23, 467-479.
2. Alexander, Gerianne, Wilcox, Teresa, and Woods, Rebecca. (2009). Sex differences in infants' visual interest in toys. Archives of Sexual Behaviour, 38, 427-433.
3. Ashiabi, G. S. (2007). Play in the preschool classroom: Its socio-emotional significance and the teacher's role in play. Early Childhood Education Journal, 35, 199-207.
4. Azar, Beth. (Mar, 2002). It's more than fun and games. Monitor on Psychology.
5. Benenson, Joyce F., Tennyson, Robert, and Wrangham, Richard W. (2011). Male more than female infants imitate propulsive motion. Cognition, 121, 262-267.
6. Bergen, Doris. (2004). Preschool children's play with 'talking' and 'nontalking' Rescue Heroes: Effects of technology-enhanced figures on the types and themes of play. In J. Goldstein, D. Buckingham, and G. Brougére (Eds.). Toys, Games, and Media. Mahwah, NJ: Lawrence Erlbaum Associates.
7. Bradley, R. H. (1985). Play materials and intellectual development. In C. C. Brown and A. W. Gottfried (Eds.), Play Interactions. Skillman, NJ: Johnson and Johnson.
8. Brezinka, Veronika, and Hovestadt, Ludger. (2007). Serious games can support psychotherapy of children and adolescents. Lecture Notes in Computer Science, 4799, 357-364.
9. DCMS. (2004) Getting Serious About Play – A review of children's play. London: Department for Culture, Media and Sport.
10. Gray, Peter. (2011). The special value of children's age-mixed play. American Journal of Play, 3, 500-522.
11. Gray, Peter. (2011). The Decline of Play and the Rise of Psychopathology in Children and Adolescents. American Journal of Play, 3, 443-463.
12. Panksepp, Jaak. (2007). Can play diminish ADHD and facilitate the construction of the social brain? Journal of the Canadian Academy of Child and Adolescent Psychiatry, 16, 57–66.
13. Pellis, S., and Pellis, V. (2010). The playful brain. Oneworld.
14. Stevens, Karen. (2009). Imaginative play during childhood: Required for reaching full potential. Exchange: The Early Childhood Leaders' Magazine, no. 186, 53-56.
15. Jadva, Vasanti, Hines, Melissa, and Golombok, Susan. (2010). Infants' preferences for toys, colours, and shapes: Sex differences and similarities. Archives of Sexual Behaviour, 39, 1261-1273.
16. Howard-Jones, P. A., and others. (2002). The effect of play on the creativity of young children during subsequent activity. Early Child Development and Care, 172, 323-328.
17. Pellis, S., and Pellis, V. (2010). The playful brain. Oneworld.
18. Panksepp, Jaak. (2007). Can play diminish ADHD and facilitate the construction of the social brain? Journal of the Canadian Academy of Child and Adolescent Psychiatry, 16, 57–66.

PRINCIPLES OF GROWTH AND DEVELOPMENT

LEARNING OBJECTIVES

At the end of the chapter, the learner will be able to:
- Identify the general principles of growth and development.
- Differentiate between growth, development and maturation.
- Describe the stages of growth and development.
- Explain the pattern of growth and development.
- Identify the various parameters of growth measurement.
- Assess growth and development.
- Describe various growth and development assessment tools.

GENERAL PRINCIPLES OF GROWTH AND DEVELOPMENT

Growth

Normal growth from birth to adulthood is characterized by certain general observations that have been found to be true for all healthy children.

Continuous Growth

Growth occurs continuously from conception onwards, but it is not even or regular. There are spurts when growth is largely accelerated, followed by rest periods when it is slowed. Growth is higher during infancy and early childhood and then there is rapid growth spurt during early puberty that tapers off in the late adolescence. Growth never really stops until the maximum size is attained.

Variable Rates

Growth rates vary from child to child, from time to time and from body structure to body structure. There are periods of growth in all children when they have their own ultimate size. For example, in infancy, most rapid growth is observed. During prepubescent, a slow rate is seen; during puberty, another growth spurt is observed, and after puberty, a decline in the growth rate occurs till death.

Orderly Sequence

Normal growth follows an orderly sequence. The increase in size of children proceeds without interruption. Even if they may seem to grow rapidly, they never skip a stage. They do simple things and then more complex ones. For example, they first learn to roll over, then to get onto their hands, afterwards to creep, subsequently to stand and finally to walk.

Total Process

Growth is a total process involving the entire child. All parts of a child grow simultaneously. The mind and emotions do not grow in one day and physical body the next day. The child develops as a whole being – physically, mentally, emotionally and socially.

The word 'growth' refers to the increasing size of the physical structure of a body. It is measured by 'inches and pounds' or 'centimetres and kilograms'. Altogether, growth is a quantitative change. The ultimate size that an individual acquires when growth stops is called the extent of growth. The rate of growth is the amount of growth measured within a given time. There are distinct periods of growth, and each child goes through well-defined periods of growth. A series of growth periods in a given child is called a growth pattern. All the body tissues and systems follow a general pattern described by these periods of growth, with three exceptions:

1. The nervous system grows most rapidly during infancy and reaches to a maximum size by puberty.

2. The reproductive system grows very slowly until pubertal spurt that accompanies sexual maturity.

3. Lymphoid tissue grows at a greatly accelerated pace until the child is 12 years of age when it gradually shrinks to adult proportions.

Development

Development refers to a gradual growth and change from a lower stage to a more advanced state of complexity. It is the increasing capacity of children to use their bodies. Growth and development are interrelated. They go hand in hand; growth having to do with the physical structure of the body and development with its function. The extent of development is the ultimate degree of achievement and depends on genetic inheritance, adequate nutrition, normal hormonal activity and a favourable emotional environment. It involves expansion of child's capacities through growth, maturation and progressive gains in functional ability.

Maturation is the total process by which a child grows and develops according to individual inherited patterns of physical, mental and emotional potential. Maturity means full or complete growth. Physical maturity is normally complete by 20–25 years of age. It is generally expected that a certain level of emotional maturity will have been attained by the age of about 25 years.

STAGES OF GROWTH AND DEVELOPMENT

Child growth and development are commonly classified into seven stages based on a consideration of the physical, emotional, intellectual and social maturity of the child.

- Prenatal   Conception to birth
- Neonatal   Birth to 1 month
                       (precisely 28 days)
- Infancy   1 month to 1 year
- Toddlerhood   1–3 years
- Preschool-aged   3–6 years
- School-aged   6–12 years
- Puberty (adolescence) 12–18 years
  - Prepubescent
  - Pubescent

PATTERNS OF GROWTH AND DEVELOPMENT

Growth and development occur in definite and predictable patterns or trends such as directional, sequential and secular trends.

Directional trends occur in regular directions or gradients, depicting the development and maturation of neuromuscular functions. These trends apply to physical, mental, social and emotional development and include the following:

- Cephalocaudal or head-to-tail development, occurring along the body's long axis, in which control over the head, mouth and eye movements precedes control over the upper body, torso and legs.
- Proximodistal or midline to peripheral development, progressing from the centre of the body to the extremities; here, the child develops arm movements before fine motor finger ability. Proximodistal development is symmetrical; both sides develop in the same direction and at the same rate.
- Mass to specific development, sometimes referred to as differentiation in which a child masters simple operations before complex functions and moves from broad general patterns of behaviour to more refined patterns.
- Sequential trends involving a predictable sequence of growth and development stages. Sequential trends are identified in the development of motor skills such as locomotion (e.g. a child crawls before creeping, creeps before standing and stands before walking) and behaviours such as language and social skills (e.g. a child first play alone and then with others in increasing numbers and in progressively complex activities). The language development shows that the baby starts with vowels, monosyllables, simple sentences, and so on.
- Secular trends refer to worldwide trends in the rate and age of maturation. In general, children are maturing earlier and growing larger at each age as compared with their preceding generation.

GROWTH MONITORING

Growth is a highly individual process, so also the comparison of a child with others and with the child's own past growth is a valuable means of evaluating progress. One common method is to plot the results on a graph paper. This can be called as a growth chart. Different standardized growth charts are available.

Growth is measured in a number of ways, including weight, height, body proportions, bone development and motor development. The nurse is expected to make these measurements, to understand its significance and to empathize what is considered normal for children of all ages.

Weight

Weight is influenced by all the other factors; therefore, an increase in body size is the best indicator of nutrition and growth. A full-term baby weighs an average of 3 kg at birth. This is doubled during next 6 months, tripled by 1 year, quadrupled by 2 years, after which yearly steady increase of about 2.25–2.75 kg per year. However, at the onset of adolescence, boys may add 20 kg and girls about 16 kg to their respective weights. Rapid weight gain occurs in both boys and girls during puberty, corresponding to the gain in height. Girls begin their preadolescent growth spurt at about 10–12 years of age, reaching adult proportions at about 16–18 years of age. Boys follow girls by 2 years, growing to be heavier and taller than girls. During the first 3–4 days after birth, babies lose up to

10% of their birth weight. Birth weight is regained by the 10th postnatal day. The rate of weight gain in the first 3 months is 30 g/day. In the remainder of the first year, infants gain about 15 g/day.

Other formulae used in estimating the weight of a child are as follows:

3–12 months: Age (month) + 9 ÷ 2
1–6 years: Age (year) × 2 + 8
7–12 years: Age (year) × 7 − 5 ÷ 2

Easy Nursing Tips for Weight/Height for Children

Age	Weight (kg)	Age	Height (cm)
At birth	3	At birth	50
5 months	6 (BW × 2)	3 months	60
1 year	9 (BW × 3)	9 months	70
2 years	12 (BW × 4)	1 year	75
3 years	15 (BW × 5)	3 years	90
7 years	21 (BW × 9)	4.5 years	100
10 years	30 (BW × 10)	Up to 10 years	5 (every year)

BW, birth weight.

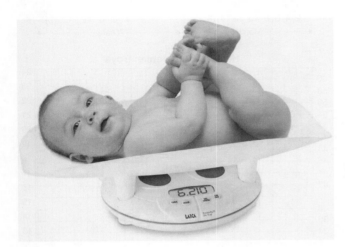

Weighing a newborn in baby weighing scale.

Height

The average length of a newborn is 50 cm (20 inches). The periods of rapid growth are during infancy and puberty. By 1 year of age, there will be 50% increase in birth length. That is, an infant aged 1 year will approximately measure 75 cm. During the second year, there will be an increase of 12.5 cm. In the third year, there will be an increase of 12.5 cm. The height of an adult is about twice what it was in the same individual at 2 years of age. So, we can predict the adult height of a baby of 2 years by the following formula: Height at 2 years × 2 ± 2. Males tend to be somewhat taller than females. After 3 years, until the onset of pubertal growth spurt, children grow at a steady rate of 6 cm/year. After 2 years of age and up to 12 years, the following simple formula may be used to calculate the expected height:

$$\text{Expected height (cm)} = \text{Age (year)} \times 6 + 77$$

General Trends in Weight and Height Gain During Childhood

Age	Weight	Height
Infants Birth to 6 months	Weekly gain: 140–200 g Birth weight doubles by the end of 5–6 months	Monthly gain: 2.5 cm (1 inch)
6–12 months	Weight gain: 85-140 g Birth weight triples by the end of the first year	Monthly gain: 1.25 cm (½ inch) Birth length increases by approximately 50% by the end of the first year
Toddlers	Birth weight quadruples by the age of 1–2 years Yearly gain is 2–3 kg.	Height at the age of 2 years is approximately 50% of the eventual adult height Gain during the second year is about 12 cm Gain during the third year is about 6–8 cm
Preschoolers	Yearly gain of 2–3 kg	Birth height doubles by 4 years Yearly gain of 5–7.5 cm
School-aged	Yearly gain of 2–3 kg	Yearly gain after the age of 7 years is 5 cm Birth length triples by the age of 13 years
Pubertal growth spurt: Females 10–14 years	Weight gain: 7–25 kg, with a mean gain of 17.8 kg	Height gain 5–25 cm 95% of mature height achieved by the skeletal age of 13 years Mean height gain is 20.5 cm
Males 11–16 years	Weight gain is 7–30 kg, with a mean gain of 23.7 kg	Height gain is 10–13 cm Approximately 95% of the mature height achieved by the skeletal age of 15 years Mean gain is 27.5 kg

Upper Segment/Lower Segment Ratio

The upper segment (US) is measured from the vertex to the symphysis pubis. The lower segment (LS) is measured from the heel to the symphysis pubis. The ratio of US/LS at different ages is given as follows:

US/LS Ratio

Age	US/LS
Birth	1.7
6 months	1.62
1 year	1.54
2 years	1.4
3 years	1.33
4 years	1.25
5 years	1.17
10 years	1

The US/LS ratio remains high in children with hypothyroidism and short-limbed dwarfism such as achondroplasia. The ratio is lower than expected in some rare disorders such as Marfan syndrome.

Mean stem–stature index =

$$\frac{\text{Stem length (crow to rump or sitting height)}}{\text{Recumbent length or standing height}} \times 100$$

Age	Percentage
At birth	67
6 months	66
1 year	64
2 years	61
3 years	58
5 years	55
10 years	52

Head Circumference

Head circumference at birth is between 33 and 35 cm. The rate of increase is 2 cm/month in the first 3 months, 1 cm/month from 3 to 6 months and 0.5 cm/month from 6 to 12 months. Head circumference reaches 45–47 cm by 1 year of age.

The mean head circumferences at various ages are as follows:

Head Circumferences at Various Ages

Age	HC (cm)	Age	HC (cm)	Age	HC (cm)
Birth	33	6 months	43	1 year	46
1 month	36	7 months	43.5	2 years	49
2 months	38	8 months	44	3 years	50
3 months	40	9 months	44.5	5 years	50.8
4 months	41	1 months	45	8 years	52.5
5 months	42	11 months	45.5	12 years	53.5

HC, head circumference.

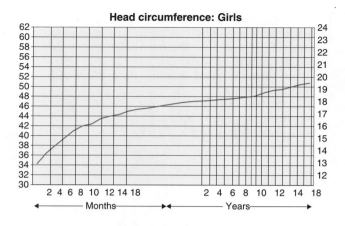

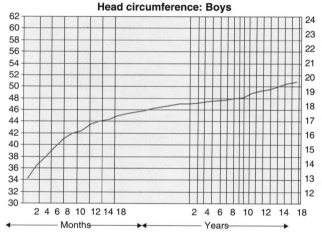

Microcephaly is diagnosed when the head circumference is less than −3 SD of the mean (i.e. ~3 cm less than expected) for age. A faster than expected increase in the head circumference when measured serially is suggestive of hydrocephalus. The head circumference exceeds the chest circumference at birth. Both approximate around 10 months of age in well-nourished children and equal in almost all children by 1 year of age. It can be roughly estimated in an infant using the following formula: Length (cm) + 9.5 ÷ 2. Later, the chest circumference exceeds the head circumference.

Chest Circumference at Various Ages

At birth	32 cm (>35 cm of the head)
1 year	45 cm (chest = head)

At the remaining periods, chest circumference will be more than the head circumference.

The Fontanels

The anterior fontanel closes between 9 and 18 months of age. The posterior fontanel is usually closed at birth or within 2–6 months. Delayed closure of fontanels is seen in hydrocephalus, hypothyroidism, rickets, severe protein–energy malnutrition (PEM) and certain bone disorders.

Dental Development

The time and sequence of eruption of teeth and shedding of deciduous teeth are as follows:

Time of Eruption and Shedding of Deciduous Teeth

Name of Teeth	Eruption Age (Month)		Shedding Age (Year)	
	Lower	Upper	Lower	Upper
Central incisors	6	7½	6	7½
Lateral incisors	7	9	7	8
Cuspids	16	18	9½	11½
First molar	13	14	10	10½
Second molar	20	24	11	10½

Incisors = 2 months. Range = 6 months. Molar = 4 months. A rough formula to remember: Age (month) = Number of deciduous teeth

Time of Eruption of Permanent Teeth

Name of Teeth	Age (Year)	
	Lower	Upper
Central incisors	6–7	7–8
Lateral incisors	7–8	8–9
Cuspids	9–11	11–12
First premolar	10–12	10–11
Second premolar	11–13	10–12
First molar	6–7	6–7
Second molar	12–13	12–13
Third molar	17–22	17–22

Bone Age

The ossification centres of the upper tibial and lower femoral epiphyses are visible at birth in a normal full-term infant. This may also be used prenatally to decide on maturity of the fetus when termination of the pregnancy becomes essential. During the later part of infancy and preschool years, X-ray of the wrist shows ossification centres for capitate and hamate by 6 years of age. The lower end of the radius appears in the early months of the second year. One more carpal bone triquetral appears in the beginning of the third year and the lunate appears in the fourth year. A rough guide to follow in the first 5 years can be as follows: Age (year) = Number of ossification centres seen at the wrist – 1.

In older children, X-rays of the anteroposterior and lateral views of the elbow are obtained. The mean age at the appearance of ossification centres at the elbow is as follows:

Ossification Centres	Boys	Girls
Capitulum	4M	3M
Radial head	5Y 3M	3Y 10M
Medial epicondyle	6Y 3M	3Y 5M
Olecranon of the ulna	9Y 8M	8Y
Lateral epicondyle	11Y 3M	9Y 3M

M, month; Y, year.

Bone age is markedly delayed in severe PEM, rickets, hypothyroidism and Cushing syndrome. It is also delayed in children with a constitutional short stature. Bone age is the average osseous development of children of a given chronological age as determined by X-ray examination. By comparing an individual child's bone development with standard bone age studies, the skeletal growth can be evaluated.

Body Proportions

One of the most obvious ways in which a child is not a miniature adult is the body proportions. At birth, the head is one-fourth of the total body length. The arms and legs are relatively short, and the chest and the abdomen are more or less barrel shaped. As the growth precedes, the midpoint of the total height moves from the umbilicus to the pubis bone, the chest flattens and extremities grow longer. During puberty, adult proportions are attained and the characteristic male/female contours develop.

Growth Monitoring

Assessment of growth may be done by longitudinal and cross-sectional studies. The common parameters used for growth monitoring include weight, height, head circumference, chest circumference, US/LS ratio and mean stem–stature index. These characteristics are measured and compared with reference standards. The following are the three methods used for comparisons:

- Use of mean/median values. A variation of 2 SD from either side of the mean is considered as within normal limits.
- Use of percentile or centiles. This is much easier than the use of mean or median. It refers to the percentage of individuals falling below the third percentile and a farther 3% of children are above the 97th percentile. The percentage of individuals falling between the 97th and third percentiles is considered normal.
- Use of independent indices as weight for height and weight for age.

Common Reference Values

- **Harvard (Boston) standards:** These are based on observations made on children in Boston from 1930 to 1956 by longitudinal studies.
- **World Health Organization (WHO) reference value:** This is based on independent indices for weight and height. The values are obtained on the basis of a cross-sectional study conducted by the US National Center for Health and Statistics. This value is used only for children up to 5 years of age.
- **Indian standards:** Indian Council of Medical Research (ICMR) conducted a nationwide cross-sectional study during the year 1956–1965. This tool is widely used in India as the reference value to assess growth.

NB: Reference value should not be used as the standard value, as reference values are usually different from those of a racially different population.

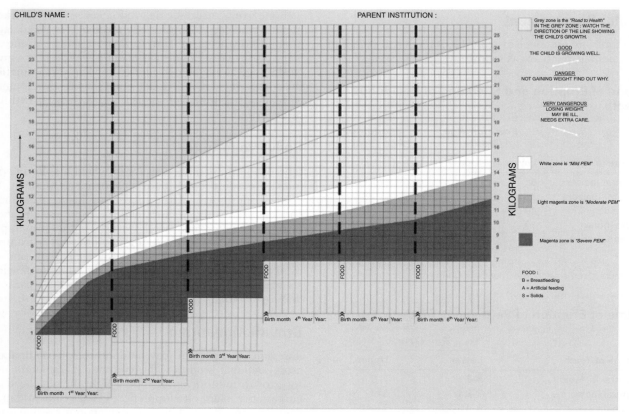

Growth chart.

Monitoring of Child's Growth and Development

Completion of	Motor Development		Language		Cognitive		Social Psychological			Action Taken
3 months	Able to hold the head	Yes No	Coos and squeals	Yes No	Puts finger in the mouth	Yes No	Smiles to his/her mother More		Yes No	REFERRED NIL FOLLOW-UP
	Raises chin above the table	Yes No								
6 months	Sits with or without support	Yes No	Produces vowel sounds, babbles	Yes No	Forgets the rattle if hidden	Yes No	Recognizes the mother		Yes No	REFERRED NIL FOLLOW-UP
15 months	Walks alone	Yes No	Says Mama, Papa Vocabulary of 3–20 words	Yes No	Traces the hidden object (object permanence)	Yes No	Assists and cooperates in dressing		Yes No	REFERRED NIL FFOLLOW-UP
3 years	Runs, rides tricycle, goes up and down stairs, walks tiptoe	Yes No	Three-word sentences;	Yes No	Can identify and name objects (symbolic play); copies + and 0	Yes No	Feeds self well;		Yes No	REFERRED NIL FOLLOW-UP
			tells name and sex	Yes No			puts on sandals	Yes No	Yes No	
6 years	Hops on one foot	Yes No	Can name all colours	Yes No	Identifies long and short copies	Yes No	Plays cooperatively with peers; sex role behaviour		Yes No	REFERRED NIL FOLLOW-UP
	Throws a ball	Yes No	Value of coin	Yes No				Yes No	Yes No	
8–10 years	Can balance on board	Yes No	Can name 10 animals in 1 minute	Yes No	Abstract reasoning	Yes No	Can use knife Combs hair		Yes No Yes No	REFERRED NIL FOLLOW-UP

Assessing Growth

Weight for Age

Measurement of weight and the rate of gain in weight are the best single parameter for assessing physical growth. A single weight record indicates the child's size at that moment. Serial weighing is useful to interpret progress of growth when the age of the child is known. For this reason, several recordings of growth are advocated with the use of a growth chart. Each baby should have its own growth chart. Maintenance of growth chart alerts for malnutrition.

Growth chart or 'road to health' chart designed by David Morley has been modified by the WHO. The charts provide a visible display of growth and development of young children over a period of time. So, changes can be interpreted easily in weight. For age chart, height is not taken into consideration, as weight is considered the most sensible indicator of growth. From this chart, deviation from normal can be detected easily by comparison with reference curves that show the limitation of normal growth.

The WHO growth chart can be adapted to local needs. In this chart, space is given for recording and presenting information such as identification data, date of birth, birth weight, age, history of health, number of sibling, immunizations, introduction of supplementary foods, episodes of sickness and special reason for special care.

Growth Charts Used in India

There are about 50 types of chart used in India. The growth chart recommended by the government of India is shown in the figure (Growth Chart on p. 108). This chart shows four degrees of malnutrition. According to this, the child's weights between 80% and 70% lines indicate first-degree malnutrition. Between 70% and 60% is second-degree malnutrition, below 60% is third-degree malnutrition and below 50% is considered as severe or fourth-degree malnutrition.

Uses of Growth Chart

- Growth monitoring
- Diagnostic tool (high-risk children identification)
- Planning and policy making
- Educational tool
- Tool for action and decision making
- Evaluation

Development

Development occurs with the interaction of two major components such as heredity and environment which have an impact on the developing brain. Heredity determines the potential of the child. Environment influences the extent to which the child achieves the potential. The environment should meet the physical and psychological needs to attain optimal development. Physical and psychological needs are age dependent. For example, an infant is totally dependent on parents for his/her physical and psychological needs. A preschooler usually meets some of his/her physical needs and copes with many social relationships. An adolescent can meet all of his/her physical needs but experiences many complex emotional needs. The nurse needs to decide whether the individual child is within the range of normality for his/her age of development to provide age-appropriate care to children. Setting limit on age is advised to find out delayed development.

The other factors affecting child development include the following:

- Physical factors – Prenatal and postnatal physical insults affect growth and development.
- Nutritional factors – They influence growth and development. Chronic malnutrition causes stunting of physical growth. Prenatal and early postnatal malnutrition affects brain growth and hence development.
- Emotional factors – Factors such as position of the child in the family, the child rearing practices, etc. affect the development.
- Sociocultural factors – This either limits or expands the range of skills the child acquires. Definitely, there are interactions between many of these factors that contribute to proper development of a child.

Developmental Assessment

Developmental assessment constitutes a large part of the neurologic examination. It tests higher cortical functions such as memory, intelligence and language; vision; hearing; and gross and fine motor skills. The standard clinical portion of the examination provides further information on special sensory, motor and reflex functions. The examination of 'soft signs' that mainly consist of abnormalities on tasks, motor skills and maintenance of posture is pathologic only in relationship to age. These signs are normally present in young age which disappear with age. If they persist in older children, they are associated with developmental delays or problems related to neurodevelopmental maturation. This is demonstrated by the presence of Moro reflex in early infancy and disappearance of the same as the child grows.

Functional Areas for Developmental Assessment

Many approaches can be used to assess development. Usually, health workers make use of the approaches exercised by Gessell and co-workers. This provides a very simple framework for assessing development in children. This approach provides simple equipment, standardization of results and the existence of a screening test.

Development is divided into four functional areas, although points of overlap and interdependence obviously exist.

- Gross motor
- Fine motor and adaptive skills
- Speech, language and hearing
- Personal social (emotional and behaviour)
    Gross motor development: Gross motor development refers to skills involving stabilization of the head,

trunk and limbs; postural control; and acts requiring the use of large, proximal muscle groups. In gross motor development, the immobile newborn rapidly progresses to one who is able to adapt an upright posture and then walk and explore his/her environment. For achieving this capability, the child undergoes sequences of activities such as the following:

- Acquisition of tone and head control
- Disappearance of primitive reflexes
- Sitting
- Locomotor pattern
- Running, hopping, jumping and pedalling

Acquisition of tone and head control: With the increase in muscle tone, the infant achieves head control, then sits and finally stands. In the newborn period, the baby will lay in a supine position with limbs flexed and kicks his/her arms and legs. Head control is poor, evidenced by marked head lag when pulled up by his/her arms. By 6 weeks of age, the baby can lift his/her head and move it to both sides. By 3–4 months of age, he/she can hold his/her head upright when held in a sitting position.

Primitive reflexes: The newborn infant is born with some primitive spinal or brainstem reflexes (e.g. Moro reflex, grasp reflex, stepping reflex and atonic neck reflex). These reflexes disappear by 4–6 months of age to allow progression of motor development.

Sitting: By 6 months of age, an infant sits with support. He/she uses the protection response such as parachute reflex (forward propping – putting out his/her arm to the side or forward to protect himself/herself from falling).

Locomotor pattern: The newborn infant shows locomotion by crawling on all fours or by commando crawl with abdomen on the floor or by creeping. But some infants bottom shuffle. Initially, the child stands with support after crawling, then walks with support holding on furniture and finally walks unsupported by 12–14 months of age.

Running, hopping, jumping and pedalling: The walking baby subsequently learns to kick a ball, hop on one leg (20 months), go up and down stairs, jump and pedal a tricycle or bicycle.

This is the most obvious area of development initially. As the child grows older, higher degrees of coordination are required for gross motor tasks.

Gross Motor Milestone	Age
Raises head to 45°	6–8 weeks
Rolls over	3 months
Sits alone with the rounded back	6 months
Sits alone with the straight back	8 months
Crawling	8–9 months
Stands alone	1 year
Walks up steps	1.5 years
Pedals tricycle	2 years
Balances on one foot	3 years

Fine motor and adaptive skills: Fine motor and adaptive skills are considered together because they are highly interdependent, although not identical. In general, fine motor skills involving high degrees of coordination of predominantly distal muscles and the ability to isolate movements and parts of movements are a necessary substrate for performing adaptive tasks. The infant needs to acquire visual attention and pincer grip to develop the dexterity required to perform complex tasks such as feeding, dressing and writing. In fact, some children with neurologic deficits that impair fine motor skills learn nonstandard methods of completing the same tasks.

Fine Motor Adaptive Milestones	Age
Follows face in midline	Newborn
Follows moving objects	6 weeks
Grasps a rattle	3 months
Reaches out for toys	4 months
Passes cube hand-to-hand	6 months
Neat pincer grasp	1 year
Builds tower of four cubes	1½ years
Builds tower of six cubes	2 years
Imitates vertical line	2 years
Builds tower of eight cubes	2½ years
Copies circle	3 years
Draws +	4 years
Draws squares	4½ years

Language development: Language probably correlates more accurately with certain cognitive skills than does any other area of development. Language is more sensitive to environmental factors than are the other functional skills.

Language Milestones	Age
Startles to loud noises	Newborn
Squeals and vocalizes alone/when spoken to coos and laughs	3 months
Turns to voice	6 months
Says 'mama' or 'dada'	1 year
Combines two words	1.5 years
Use plurals	2 years
Gives entire name and talks constantly	3 years

Personal social skills: Personal social skills involve learning in a social setting and are therefore sensitive to environmental factors. Knowledge of intrafamilial and cultural patterns is essential before reaching conclusion.

Personal Social Milestones	Age
Smiles spontaneously	3 months
Feeds self crackers	6 months
Drinks from a cup	1 year
Helps in simple tasks	1.5 years
Plays interactive games	2 years
Buttons clothes	3 years

Screening Tests

By definition, a screening test is not a diagnostic instrument. It consists of a sample of developmental items drawn from a number of sources and selected to determine which children will have a high yield of abnormalities when given a standard test and which children will have a low yield. A well-constructed screening test attempts to strike a balance between errors of omission and commission. A screening test should neither be used to make a developmental diagnosis nor be used to assess developmental progress. It is useful to select only from a pool of patients who should be referred for administration of an accepted standardized developmental examination.

Denver Developmental Screening Test (DDST): The DDST is quite a useful standardized screening test. The equipment needed is simple and administration is rapid and relatively easy. But if it is not used properly, its reliability is compromised.

Bayley Scale of Infant Development (BSID): This scale is used to assess motor, mental and infant behaviours for children up to 30 months of age and can be completed with 30–60 minutes.

Gessell Developmental Schedule: This measures the four functional areas of development in children up to the age of 5 years within 30–40 minutes.

Baroda Developmental Screening Test: It is prepared on the basis of Baroda norms that are standardized to Indian scenario. It evaluates motor and mental development and infant behaviour.

Trivandrum Developmental Screening Chart (TDSC): It is prepared on the basis of 17 selected items from the BSID and Baroda norms and was developed at Sree Avittom Thirunal Hospital, Trivandrum, for children up to 24 months of age. This is a simple tool and can be administered by anyone with very little training. It takes only 5–7 minutes to administer.

Developmental assessment is an essential part of paediatric care for various reasons. The paediatric nurse who does the assessment should have a thorough knowledge of the normal, variations and the reason for such variations. All interpretations should be based not only on through physical assessment but also on a detailed history. The physical assessment should include head circumference in relation to weight, and the assessment of vision and hearing and other factors which affect development. The nurse who does the developmental assessment should understand its great value, its predictive importance and its limitations too. Hasty and unwise comment made by a professional may lead to parental anxiety and mental trauma. So, the nurse must be vigilant not to make unwise comments to parents. The emotional aspect of the parents must be considered while explaining developmental problems to parents about their child.

Laboratory Procedures

Special laboratory examinations are also essential to detect developmental abnormalities. Some of them are discussed as follows:

Biochemical screening tests: The list of inborn errors of metabolism associated with developmental abnormalities is long. The most common problems associated are inborn errors of metabolism of amino acids, carbohydrates, short-chain fatty acids and ammonia metabolism. Broadly, three evaluations are important: urinary metabolic screening tests, screening chromatography and clinical laboratory studies.

Urinary screening tests: It include a series of test-tube studies for aromatic hydroxyl groups, total reducing substances and glucose, cystine and homocystine, and acid mucopolysaccharides.

Screening chromatography: Two-dimensional paper chromatography on blood or urine is performed to separate amino acids and other compounds.

Clinical laboratory studies: If there is a suspicion of problems involving metabolism of ammonia or short-chain fatty acids, serum ammonia, pH, electrolytes, urea nitrogen and complete blood cell count are performed.

When abnormality during screening is documented, quantitative studies are conducted. The best yield of positive results from metabolic studies is obtained when there is clinical suspicion of specific disorder such as Phenylketonuria (PKU) or familial occurrence of a developmental disorder or a history of loss of previously acquired milestone or any central nervous system (CNS) findings indicative of developmental delay.

Immunological studies: Presence of elevated immunoglobulin level in the neonate is a nonspecific screening procedure for intrauterine infection. The most frequently used immunologic studies are the TROCH (toxoplasmosis, rubella, cytomegalovirus, herpes simplex) titres. These titres must be compared with maternal levels because they test immunoglobulin G (IgG) antibodies that cross the placental barrier. Such tests are indicated when intrauterine infections are suspected.

Radiological examination: X-ray is not so significant to identify the developmental anomaly, but computed tomographic scans are indicated when strong suspicion of anatomic malformation is present.

Electrophysiological studies such as electroencephalogram may be indicated in those cases where suspicion of CNS abnormality exists.

STUDY QUESTIONS

1. Explain the general principles of growth and development.
2. What are the trends and patterns of growth and development?
3. What are the uses of growth chart?
4. What is the common assessment parameters used in measuring growth?
5. What are development assessment tools?
6. What are the uses of development assessment tools?
7. Explain Denver Developmental Screening Test.
8. Explain the parameters used in the Baroda Developmental Screening Test and the Trivandrum Developmental Screening Chart.

BIBLIOGRAPHY

1. Bhandari N, Bahl R, Taneja S, de Onis M, Bhan MK. (2002). Growth performance of affluent Indian children is similar to that in developed countries. Bulletin of the World Health Organization, 80:189–195.
2. Edalmarys Santos & Chad A. Noggle. (2011). Cephalocaudal Principle Encyclopedia of Child Behavior and Development. Springer US, pp 321-321.
3. de Onis M, Yip R. (1996). The WHO growth chart: historical considerations and current scientific issues. Bibliotheca Nutritio et Dieta, 53:74–89.
4. JN Sharma (ed). Principles and Practice of Pediatrics. Peepee Publishers and Distributors, Delhi; First Edition: 2014; ISBN: 978-81-8445-135-1.
5. Mukerjee, D and MKC Nair. (2008). Growth And Development. Jaypee publication, New Delhi.
6. Marilyn Hockenberry David Wilson Cheryl Rodgers. (2010). Wong's Essentials of Pediatric Nursing. 10th Edn Mosby Elsevier publication. Philadelphia.
7. MKC Nair (Ed). (2016). IAP Textbook of Pediatrics. 6th Edn. Jaypee publications, New Delhi.
8. WHO. (2006). WHO Child Growth Standards WHO Child Growth Standards 1 year 2 years 3 years 4 years 5 years Length/height-for-age, weight-for-age, weight-for-length, weight-for-height and body mass index-for-age Methods and development. Department of Nutrition for Health and Development. ISBN 92 4 154693 X (NLM classification: WS 103).
9. WHO Multicentre Growth Reference Study Group. (2006b). Breastfeeding in the WHO Multicentre Growth Reference Study. Acta Paediatrica, Suppl 450:16–27.

CHAPTER 11

GROWTH AND DEVELOPMENT – THE INFANT (NEONATE THROUGH 12 MONTHS)

CHAPTER OUTLINE

- Major Development Theories
- Physical Characteristics at Birth
- Play and Age

- Health Maintenance and Anticipatory Guidance
- Accident Prevention and Safety Precautions

LEARNING OBJECTIVES

At the end of the chapter, the learner will be able to:

- Describe the major developmental theories related to infancy.
- Identify the developmental timetable.
- Explain age-appropriate play of children.
- Describe the different health maintenance activities and anticipatory guidance for feeding, play and accident prevention.

The best indication of good health in an infant is steady increasing height, weight, head circumference and chest circumference. Growth and development are monitored by plotting measurement on standard growth charts.

MAJOR DEVELOPMENTAL THEORIES – CHARACTERISTICS

Maslow's Hierarchy of Needs

- Physiological needs for survival
- Safety and security
- Love and belonging

Freud's Psychosexual Theory of Development

Oral stage
- Oral gratification and sucking needs: If successful, feelings of security result and if unsuccessful, an oral-dependent character results.
- Egocentrism is complete.

Erikson's Theory of Psychosocial Development

Trust versus mistrust
- Oral sensory
- Quality of parental–infant relationship important
- Mother: The significant person establishing the core task of trust
- At birth: Views faces and establishes eye contact
- 1–2 months: Smiles responsively
- 2–3 months: Smiles spontaneously
- 6 months: Exhibits stranger anxiety and shows attachment to favourite objects (e.g. teddy bear, dolls or blanket)
- 12 months: Demonstrates emotions of fear, anger and affection and can indicate desires without crying

Piaget's Theory of Cognitive Development

- Substage 1 (0–1 month): Practice of reflexes and reflex-like actions
- Substage 2 (1–4 months): Purposeful reproduction of reflex actions
- Substage 3 (4–8 months): Object-oriented and imitative actions; accidental actions repeated
- Substage 4 (8–12 months): Coordination, intentional goal direction and achievement; other features include experimentation and achievement of object – permanence (searches for a dropped object or person playing hide and seek); infants at this age imitate and model behaviour.

Kohlberg's Theory of Moral Development

Stage I: Preconventional level
- Beginning of punishment related to deprivation or injury but makes no cognitive connection. No moral concepts or rules exist at this age.

Development Table as per Time

| | | Neurological and Motor Development[a] | |
Sound and Language	Vision	Gross Motor	Fine Motor
Newborns prefer high-pitched voices All infants coo and babble, especially at 6 months of age, including deaf infants Newborns are startled at loud noises 2–3 months: Laughs and squeals 4 months: Produces belly laughs 4–5 months: Turns to voice (quiet listening) 8–10 months: Uses words such as 'dada' and 'mamma' (nonspecific), responds to own name at about 10 months of age (receptive language skills develop first), localizes sound above or below 7–11 months: Imitates speech and sounds and understands name and 'yes' or 'no' 10 months: Understands bye and claps hands 1 year: Has one word in spoken vocabulary; comprehends give and stops when told 'no'; has receptive vocabulary of several dozen words 3–12 months: Behaviour is learned rather than being reflexive, recognizes certain sounds and ignores others, attends to quiet sounds more than louder ones	Birth: Fixates on human face and demonstrates preference 2 months: Follows to the midline; produces tears 6 months: Inspects hands, can fixate on objects 3 feet away Strabismus if present, no longer within normal limits 8 months: Has permanent eye colour 10 months: Tilts head backwards to see upwards 12 months: Shows smooth visual pursuit of objects with 20/100 vision	Birth: Turns head when in a prone position but cannot support the head; adjusts the posture when held at the shoulder and may squirm to the corner or edge of the crib when in a prone position; arm and leg movements reflexive 6 weeks–2 months: Holds head up to 45°–90° when in a prone position 3 months: Rolls over from side to side 4 months: May bear weight on legs when assisted to stand, head lag disappears when pulled to a sitting position 5 months: Pulls to a sitting position, rolls from back to the stomach, sits alone momentarily, shows unilateral reaching 6 months: Sits without support, may creep an inch forward or backward, moves from place to place by rolling over 7 months: Stands holding on; early stepping movements, begins to crawl or hitch 8 months: Pulls to a standing position, raises self to a sitting position 9 months: Walks with help; crawls or hitches when permitted; sits down 10 months: Continues walking skill development with help, stands alone and may climb up and down the stairs 11 months: May walk alone, begins to stoop and recover 12 months: Walks alone	Birth to 2 months: Follows to and slightly past the midline 2–3 months: Keeps hands open predominantly; reflex grasp replaced by voluntary grasps of objects such as a rattle in the open hand; may bring hands together at the midline 3–4 months: Uses ulnar–palmar prehension with a cube; reaches for objects 5 months: Attempts to catch dangling objects; begins the use of fingers and thumb in a pincer grasp; retains two cubes, recovers rattle, reaches and grasps objects 6-7 months: Can grasp at will; holds and manipulates objects; transfers from hand to hand; scoops pellet; demonstrates inferior pincer grasps 8–9 months: Combines spoons or cubes at the midline; retains two of three cubes offered; achieves a neat pincer grasp of a pellet, feeds self with finger foods 10–11 months: Plays pat-a-cake, a midline skill, puts several objects in a container; holds a crayon adaptively; bangs two cubes together; looks for hidden objects; achieves a neat pincer grasp of tiny objects

[a]Development is cephalocaudal and proximodistal in nature and direction (arm and hand skills develop prior to leg and feet skills.)

PHYSICAL CHARACTERISTICS

- Loss of 10% of birth weights in the first 3–4 days of life is observed.
- 70%–73% of body weight is water in the newborn.
- 2–3 months to 6 months: Posterior fontanel (soft spots) closes.
- Obligate nose breathers until 5 months of age.
- 5–6 months: Birth weight doubles owing to a gain of 125–175 g per week.
- 6 months: Teething begins with lower central incisors.
- 8 months: Regular bowel and bladder patterns are established.
- 1 year: Average weight is 9 kg (triples birth weight).
- Head circumference and chest circumference become equal by 1 year of age.
- Crown to rump length ratio (upper segment/lower segment [US/LS] ratio) growth is of 1.3–1.9 cm per month.
- Increase of 50% birth length by the age of 12 months to measure 75 cm at 1 year.
- The head to body ratio shows that the head is much larger than that of an adult and is one-third of the body length.
- At birth, normal head circumference is about 35 cm.
- Normal chest circumference is 33 cm.
- Head circumference and chest circumference equalize by 1 year of age.
- Normal chest circumference changes include:
  - Smaller than head circumference at birth.
  - Equal to chest circumference at 12 months of age.

After 2 years of age, chest circumference increases substantially more than head circumference. Normal head circumference changes include:

- Increase of 1.3 cm per month between 1 and 6 months of age.
- Increase of 0.64 cm per month between 7 and 12 months of age.

Cranial suture changes:

- Posterior fontanel measures 1 cm × 1 cm at birth and normally closes by 2–6 months of age.
- Anterior fontanel measures 3.5 cm × 3.5 cm at birth, is diamond shaped and closes by 18 months of age.

Other characteristics include the following:

- Hair gradually takes on the genetically determined colour.
- The blocked sebaceous glands (milia) on the nose will disappear without interference.
- Lip blisters will disappear without interference.
- Sucking pads have an obvious use in feeding.
- Skin pigmentation may be a result of birth trauma or of soreness.
- Persistent marks such as strawberry naevus should be noted but left alone unless causing distress or harm.
- Blue spots (Mongolian spots) are mainly seen on some of the babies and do not require treatment. These tend to fade by the first year of life.

PLAY AND AGE-APPROPRIATE PLAY INTERVENTIONS

- Sensory motor developmental ability controls movements and increases ability.
- Type of play is solitary, exploratory and manipulative.
- Enjoys squeak toys, crumpled paper, mirror and water play, busy boxes, rattles and noisy toys.
- 5–7 months: Resists toy pull, picks up tiny objects, plays hide and seek and works for toys kept out of reach.
- 8–9 months: Enjoys mirror image.
- 10–12 months: Plays ball with examination; baby achievers, object permanence and search for hidden objects.

HEALTH MAINTENANCE AND ANTICIPATORY GUIDANCE

Immunization

BCG, OPV, DPT, HBV vaccines and vitamin A are the immunizations needed during infancy. For schedule, refer the section on 'Immunization'.

Nutrition

Breastfeeding is the ideal choice for the baby, especially for the first 6 months. The stomach is approximately 4 ounce in size and empties every 3–4 hours. Digestive system is immature and hence breast milk is the ideal food.

Requirement = 50 cal/lb per day or 110 kcal/kg per day. Breastfeeding gives 20 cal per oz.

So, a 10-lb baby requires 10 × 20 cal per day = 500 cal per day. A 3-kg baby needs 3 × 110 = 330 cal per day. So, 500 cal/20 cal per oz = 25 oz or 750 mL of breast milk per day. An average Indian woman produces 600–750 mL of breast milk per day.

Demand feeding is preferred over scheduled feeding. Gradually, the need increases. The feeding requirement can be summarized as follows: at the age of 1 month, 4 oz six times a day; 2 months, 4–6 oz for six feeds; at 5 months, 6 oz five times with solid food introduction (for details, refer the chapter on 'Nutritional Requirement').

Complementary Feeding

Introduction of solid foods along with breastfeeding is complementary feeding. First preferred solid food is cereal, and most preferred cereal is rice (for details, refer the chapter on 'Nutritional Requirement').

Dental Care

Prevention of dental caries by proper care, especially not allowing the baby to sleep with feeding bottles, is advised. Studies have shown that breastfed babies have fewer dental problems such as dental caries and misalignment of teeth. It also enhances strong jaw development.

Sleep

In the early neonatal period, babies sleep most of the time. They are awake only for short periods and seldom awake without fussing. They sleep through household noises, oblivious to the surrounding stimuli; thus, a quite environment is not necessary.

ACCIDENT PREVENTION AND SAFETY PRECAUTIONS

- Allow no unsupervised tub bath, and maintain a baby-proof environment by removing hazardous material within the reach of the baby.
- Review normal developmental behaviours for the age and provide anticipatory guidance around the next developmental age (for further details about accident prevention, refer the chapter on 'Accident Prevention').

STUDY QUESTIONS

1. What are the major developmental theories pertaining to growth and development?
2. Describe the psychosocial development and significant others in each stage of development of infants, toddlers, preschoolers, children, school-aged children and adolescents.

Growth and Development – The Toddler (1–3 Years)

LEARNING OBJECTIVES

At the end of the chapter, the learner will be able to:

- Describe the major developmental theories related to the toddlerhood.
- Identify the developmental timetable during different stages.
- Explain age-appropriate play of children.
- Describe the different health maintenance activities and anticipatory guidance for feeding, play and accident prevention for various age groups.

Definition – A young child, especially one who is learning or has recently learned to walk (Cambridge International Dictionary of English).

MAJOR DEVELOPMENTAL THEORIES – CHARACTERISTICS

Maslow's Hierarchy of Needs

- Physiologic
- Safety and security
- Love and belonging
- Self-esteem

Freud's Psychosexual Theory of Development

Anal stage
- Sensual pleasure shifts to anal urethral areas. Toilet training is seen as an area of discipline and authority. If unsuccessful, personality may become possessive or the child may refuse to release possessions, including waste materials.

Erikson's Theory of Psychosocial Development

Autonomy versus shame and doubt

Doubts sense of self-control, and personal behaviour may be self-determined; overprotection and excessive criticism may be related to negative feelings. Need to permit the child to move at own pace. The child will be ritualistic. Ambivalence, walking, toilet training, temper tantrum and negative 'oppositional' behaviour.

Dawdling and magical thinking (wishes makes it so) are common. Inconsistent limit setting disrupts and upsets behaviour patterns.

Piaget's Theory of Cognitive Development

Sensory motor (0–2 years)
- This toddler period encompasses parts of two stages of cognitive development: preoperational and pre-conceptional (2–7 years)
- Substage V (12–18 months): Production of vowel behaviours and curiosity
- Substage VI (18–24 months): Concept of object permanence fully achieved
- Has symbolic plane (expresses intention or feeling that has no practical value)
- Limited concept of time (no tomorrow)
- Very egocentric, animistic (talk to toys, attributes life to inanimate objects, e.g. talking to chair, table, as if they are human beings)
- Imaginary playmates
- Parallel play prevails
- Premature sense of cause and effects
- Goal-directed behaviour initiated

Kohlberg's Theory of Moral Development

Stage II: Preconventional level
- Detects concepts of fairness and sharing
- Instrumental – Relationistic orientation

- Satisfaction of own needs
- Conventional level beginning, good girl/nice boy
- Approval-seeking behaviour coupled with desire to please

Developmental Table as per Age

		Neurologic and Motor Development	
Sound and Language	Vision	Gross Motor	Fine Motor
Beginning of spoken language May occur at the same time as walking Concentration of one or other may occur 300 words and two-word sentences by 2 years 900 words and three-word sentences by the third year 12–18 months: Recognizes naming words, uses gestures to make needs known 18–24 months: Follows directions, points to nose, hair, eyes, etc on command Comprehends gives me by gestures 2–2½ years: Uses colour, understands action-oriented verbs and commands, understands size gradations, designates me, I, mine, etc and uses plurals 3 years: Gives first and last names; progressive comprehension of speech response to musical sounds	18 months: Displays interest in pictures. 2 years: Identifies forms (Snellen testing: 20/40 vision) 3 years: Has 20/30 vision	12–18 months: Walks well, throws ball, stoops and recovers, walks up stairs with help, begins to run, walks sideways and backwards 10 feet; stands on one foot with help 18–24 months: Kicks ball forward, throws overhead, walks down stairs with help, one step at a time 2–3 years: Jumps and runs well, jumps from the bottom step jumps in place, balances on one foot for 1 second, pedals tricycle, walks on a straight line; tiptoes 29–72 months: Broad jumps (distance) 4–14 inches	12–18 months: Scribbles spontaneously, builds tower of two and then four, may untie shoes, uses opposite thumb well (prehension), shows preference for hands 18–24 months: May remove articles of clothing, holds pencil well enough for scribbling; builds tower of four cubes, imitates vertical line within 30° 24–36 months: Builds tower of six to eight cubes, can use paint brush, imitates scribbles, copies a circle, begins to wash and dry hands, and dress with supervision

PHYSICAL CHARACTERISTICS

- Height and weight increase in a step-like fashion, reflecting the growth spurts and lags characteristics of the toddlerhood.
- Protruding abdomen results from underdeveloped abdominal muscles.
- Typical bowleggedness results, as the leg must bear the weight of the large trunk.
- Weight changes include:
  - Slower gain than that in infancy, about 1.8–2.7 kg per year
  - Average weight 12 kg by 2 years of age
  - Birth weight $\times$ 4 = Weight at 2 years
- Height and weight changes are seen.
- Height increases 7–8 cm per year and reaches an average height of 80–87 cm at the age of 2 years.
- This is half of the expected adult height.
- Adult height = Height at $2 \times 2 \pm 2$.
- Head circumference increases about 2.5 cm between 1 and 2 years of age.
- Thereafter, it increases 1.3 cm per year until 5 years of age.
- The anterior fontanelle closes by 18 months of age.
- Need for food relative to size is not as much as like that in infancy.

PLAY AND AGE-APPROPRIATE PLAY INTERVENTIONS

Play is parallel. Plays alongside, not with others; starts imitating adult roles including household.

- 18 months: Starts to do simple task at home.
- 21–36 months: Starts to play interactive games.

Play materials that are preferred for this age group include water (supervised tub play), sand, clay, crayons, puzzle boxes, wheeled vehicles, reading storybooks by adults.

Fantasy make-believe play starts at this age, as well as action games, hide and seek (well-known Kerala play 'sat').

HEALTH MAINTENANCE AND ANTICIPATORY GUIDANCE

Immunization

DPT, OPV booster, MMR and HBV are the vaccines needed in this age group. Immunization must be given as per schedule.

Dental Care

- First dental check-up should take place at 2½ years of age.

- Anticipatory guidance regarding safety and accident prevention protects from falls; locking inside rooms; drowning; aspiration of toy parts, peanuts, manjadi seeds, tamarind seeds, etc.
- Avoid sharp objects – Keep away knives, blades and such harmful articles out of reach of children.
- Ensure prevention of toxic substances such as insecticides and pesticides.
- Keep cabinets closed, as there is chance for toddlers to get locked inside.
- Burns and scalds are also common and need to keep vigil to prevent burns and scalds. Keep away matchboxes, lighters and kerosene lamps out of reach of toddlers.

Nutrition

Encourage eating from the table along with others. Provide drinks in cups. Spilling is common. Try to include table manners in a nonthreatening way.

Sleep

Night awakening may be seen and the child can be reassured to sleep in the presence of parents.

Toilet Training

Children should be oriented and deferred until at least 18 months of age. Signs of readiness include the following:
- A desire to please parents
- A pleasure in imitating the parents
- A desire to develop autonomy and master primitive skills
- Adequate motor development

Common problems and concerns are as follows:
- Temper tantrums
- Night crying
- Stranger anxiety
- Poor appetite
- Teething

STUDY QUESTIONS

1. What are the major developmental theories pertaining to growth and development?
2. What is anticipatory guidance?
3. What is the importance of anticipatory guidance in preventing accidents in toddlers?

CHAPTER 13

GROWTH AND DEVELOPMENT – THE PRESCHOOL CHILD (3–6 YEARS)

LEARNING OBJECTIVES

At the end of the chapter, the learner will be able to:

- Describe the major developmental theories related to preschool age.
- Identify the developmental timetable during different stages.
- Explain age-appropriate play of children.
- Describe the different health maintenance activities and anticipatory guidance for feeding, play and accident prevention.

Definition – A child who has not yet gone to school and not yet started school activities.

MAJOR DEVELOPMENTAL THEORIES – CHARACTERISTICS

Maslow's Hierarchy of Needs

- Physiologic
- Safety and security
- Love and affection and belonging
- Self-esteem
- Cognitive needs

Freud's Psychosexual Theory of Development

Phallic stage.
- Much genital manipulation and exploration (particularly with other children)
- Shows intense alteration and love for the parent of opposite sex (Oedipal complex in males and Electra conflict in females)
- Rivalry with the parent of opposite sex
- Castration anxiety, mutilation fears, intrusive procedures threaten body image and integrity
- Primitive sense of body image begins
- Separates easily from the mother

Erikson's Theory of Psychosocial Development

Initiative versus guilt.
- This stage is characterized by locomotor and genital preferences.
- *Magical thinking:* The child engages in much make-believe play activity, which if stifled is related to guilt.
- When permitted freedom, creativity is enhanced.
- The child imagines many types of fears such as having head chopped off or being sucked down the drain owing to magical thinking.
- Fears become real and logical in the child's mind and takes things literally.

Piaget's Theory of Cognitive Development

Preoperational (2–7 years).
- Egocentrism and omnipotence (inability to distinguish between own perception and that of someone else)
- Thinking concrete and tangible, becoming intuitive towards the end of this stage
- Transudative reasoning from a particular event to another event
- Animism; anthropomorphism (attribute human traits to animals or inanimate objects)
- Magical thinking (imaginary playmates common)

- Artificialism (all things made up for a purpose)
- Irreversibility (cannot backtrack steps in a thinking pattern)
- Centration (inability to consider several aspects of the situation simultaneously)
- Trial versus error (prelogical thought processes)
- Primitive concepts of space, time and causality

Kohlberg's Theory of Moral Development

Stage III: Conventional stage.
- Desires to please others; seeks approval or attention through behaviours
- Social concerns

Developmental Table as per Time

Sound and Language	Vision	Neurologic and Motor Development	
		Gross Motor	Fine Motor
Uses four- to five-word sentences with an adult sense of syntax (refer language development), has vocabulary of about 2100 words Can name body parts, recognizes colours Talks fluently and listens Cooperates on systematic audiometric tests 3–4 years: Can comprehend terms such as 'cold', 'tired' and 'hungry' (two of three), comprehends preposition 4–5 years: Knows opposite analogies (two of three) 5–6 years: Defines words (six of nine), knows composition of objects (three of four) Clues to hearing deficits: Volume of TV, whether the child responds to you, formal audiometric tests, whether 5-year-old's speech is intelligible	3 years: Has 20/30 vision, copies a circle 4 years: Cooperates with Snellen's testing, copies crosses 5 years: Recognizes colours, copies squares Clues to visual deficits, squints, favours one eye over the other, tilts head, bumps into objects	3 years: Hops on one foot 4 years: Skips, balances on one foot for 5 seconds (two out of three tries), dresses without supervision 5 years: Walks backwards heel to toe (two out of three tries), balances on one foot for 10 seconds (two out of three tries)	3–4 years: Buttons large-sized buttons, picks a longer line (three out of four tries) 4–5 years: Ties shoe laces, draws a man with three to six parts, copies a square 5–6 years: Draws a man with six parts, copies a triangle

PHYSICAL CHARACTERISTICS

- As regard to weight, there will be a gain of 2.3 kg per year.
- At the age of 3 years, the average weight is 14.5 kg.
- At the age of 4 years, the average weight is 16.8 kg.
- At the age of 5 years, the average weight is 18.6 kg.
- A healthy preschooler is slender, graceful and agile with a good posture.
- Height and weight changes are as follows:
  - An increase in height of 6.5–7.8 cm occurs per year.
  - At the age of 3 years, the average height is 96 cm.
  - At the age of 4 years, the average height is 103.7 cm.
  - At the age of 5 years, the average height is 118 cm.

PLAY AND AGE-APPROPRIATE PLAY INTERVENTIONS

- Mainly parallel and associative; plays with other children and engages in common activities
- Have no organization or group goals
- Defines own rules and cooperates with other children
- Plays interactive games
- Content of play includes dramatic/socially affective and imitative
- Play materials: Water, sand, wheeled vehicles, tea and kitchen sets, dress-up clothes, storybooks, dolls, action games, cards, etc.

HEALTH MAINTENANCE AND ANTICIPATORY GUIDANCE

- Immunization: Booster doses of DT, TT and OPV should be completed.
- Nutrition: The child eats little, and it causes concern for parents. Parents need nutritional counselling.
- Safety and injury prevention: Topics for discussion should be road traffic accidents, playground safety, bites from pets, fire and water safety, bicycle injury, etc.
- Toilet training: Maintain a child-oriented approach. Do not embarrass the child.
- Dental care: First dental check-up should be by 2–2½ years of age.
- Immunizations: Booster doses of DT, HBV and other EPI schedules to be completed.
- Play: Usually solitary play and parallel forms emerge. Help preserve child's integrity during play.
- Television: Curtail seeing violence on TV shows.
- School readiness needs to be assessed, and prepare the child for an uneventful school day.

ACCIDENT PREVENTION AND SAFETY PRECAUTIONS

- Safety regarding poisoning, playing in the street, drowning, fire and burns, etc. needs to be reinforced.
- Dental care need to be emphasized to prevent dental caries.

DEVELOPMENTAL ISSUES

- Autonomy: Problematic behaviour may be manifested because of child's continuing negativism.
- Attachment: Problem with separation continues, which shows the importance of attachment. But the child should be trained to adjust with separation with slow and short separation experiences.
- Impulse control: The child must be taught for impulse control, and temperament training may be given.

- Motor skills: They are motor minded and engage in rough and tumble play, leading to injuries. Hence, supervision is essential.
- Cognitive development: Preoperational period and mastery of language are the major cognitive issues. Hence, better language and pronunciation to be practiced by parents.
- Gender identity: Concept gender is fixed and stable definition of sex develops. Concept Oedipal complex and castration complex also are evident during this stage.

STUDY QUESTIONS

1. What are the major developmental theories pertaining to growth and development?
2. Describe the psychosocial development and significant others in each stage of development of a preschool child.
3. What is anticipatory guidance?
4. What are the common health problems of preschool children?

CHAPTER 14

GROWTH AND DEVELOPMENT – THE SCHOOL-AGED CHILD (6–12 YEARS)

CHAPTER OUTLINE

- Major Development Theories
- Physical Characteristics
- Play and Age

- Health Maintenance and Anticipatory Guidance
- Accident Prevention and Safety Precautions

LEARNING OBJECTIVES

At the end of the chapter, the learner will be able to:

- Describe the major developmental theories related to school age.
- Identify the developmental timetable during different stages.
- Explain age-appropriate play of children.
- Describe the different health maintenance activities and anticipatory guidance for feeding, play and accident prevention.

Definition – A child who is enrolled in school.

MAJOR DEVELOPMENTAL THEORIES – CHARACTERISTICS

Maslow's Hierarchy of Needs

- Physiologic
- Safety and security
- Love and belonging
- Self-esteem
- Self-actualization (making maximum use of abilities)
- Cognitive needs: Seeking knowledge and understanding

Freud's Psychosexual Theory of Development

Latent stage.
- Sexual impulses are repressed.
- Parents are no longer viewed as omnipotent.
- Privacy becomes important in the later school-aged child.

Erikson's Theory of Psychosocial Development

Industry versus inferiority.

A sense of industry ensues when the child is encouraged to make, build, construct or sew various projects. The child displays keen sense of concern with how things are made, and a sense of inferiority ensues when projects are not praised or creativity is squelched.

Piaget's Theory of Cognitive Development

Concrete operational (7–11 years).
They develop the following:
- Ability to reason
- Concept of reversibility (can reverse actions or thinking as 10 = 10)
- Clarification of objects (e.g. collections of bangle pieces, stamps, coins)
- Concepts of conservation; comprehend amount, weight, physical movement, volume of substances, etc. (e.g. volume of milk poured from a glass to a cup is the same)
- Concept of relativism: Two or more aspects of a problem may be operated simultaneously
- Can place self in another's situation
- Serialization: Makes the ordinal number lines
- Can group and sort/place in a logical order
- Fundamental skills of reading, writing and grammar develop
- Late school-aged child (11 years) capable of abstraction and deductive reasoning

Kohlberg's Theory of Moral Development

Stage IV: Conventional (adult-like) level of moral development.
- Concerns with authority figures; shows fixed rules in moral decisions

- Concerns with obligation to duty
- A bad act breaks a rule or does harm

- Accidents or misfortunes may be interpreted as punishment.
- Develops conscience and sense of value

Developmental Table as per Age

		Neurologic and Motor Development	
Sound and Language	Vision	Gross Motor	Fine Motor
Augment vocabulary and cognitive skills	20/20 vision at the age of 7 years	6 years: Walks a straight line; has mastered all skills on the Denver developmental screening test	Continually refines and improves previously learned skills

PHYSICAL CHARACTERISTICS

- Girls often grow faster than boys and commonly surpass them in height and weight.
- During preadolescence extending from about the age of 10–13 years, a child commonly experiences rapid and uneven growth as compared with age-mates.
- Height and weight changes include:
- A weight gain of 2–2.9 kg per year between the ages of 6 and 12 years.
- Average weight gain of 40 kg at the age of 12 years.
- Height increases about 5–5.2 cm per year.
- At the age of 6 years, average height is 115 cm and at the age of 12 years, the average height is 151 cm.

PLAY AND AGE-APPROPRIATE PLAY INTERVENTIONS

- Cooperative team play
- Skill play (e.g. jumping rope, skipping or skating)
- Enjoys testing model building, exploration and camping
- Collections and classification of items, e.g. dolls, board games such as chess, snake and ladder.
- Reads for pleasure.
- Enjoys swimming, boating and picnic
- Needs to be distracted from continuous hours of idle TV viewing

HEALTH MAINTENANCE AND ANTICIPATORY GUIDANCE

- Accident prevention related to sports, falls, etc.
- Recognizing behaviours such as socialization problems and learning disabilities

- Sex education
- Nutritional counselling needed
- Discretion in viewing media productions (TV/movies)
- Prevention of communicable diseases related to school
- If undergoing antibiotic therapy, stress the importance of completing its full course
- Somatic complaints and fatigue not uncommon; more frequently seen at 6, 9, 11 and 12 years of age
- Fears are common, especially enhanced at 6, 7, 10 and 11 years of age
- School progress: Asking both parents about school performance and identifying school performance are important
  Common problems and concerns are as follows:
  - Exhibiting acting out behaviour, as they are striving to attain independence.
  - Separation anxiety: If an adolescent could not achieve independence from home and family, school phobia and school avoidance may develop
  - Recurrent pains
  - Poor scholastic achievements

STUDY QUESTIONS

1. What are the major developmental theories pertaining to growth and development?
2. Describe the psychosocial development and significant others in each stage of development of a school-aged child.

CHAPTER 15

GROWTH AND DEVELOPMENT – THE ADOLESCENT (12–18 YEARS)

LEARNING OBJECTIVES

At the end of the chapter, the learner will be able to:

- Describe the major developmental theories related to adolescence.
- Identify phases of growth and puberty.
- Explain problems of growth and development: short stature, tall stature, asymmetry of head, premature sexual development and precocious puberty.

Definition – A young person between childhood and adulthood. Adolescence refers to the passage from childhood to adulthood. Puberty refers to those biological changes that lead to reproductive capacity. Puberty occurs in predictable sequence, but the timing of initiation and velocity of changes are highly variable. Integration of pubertal changes into adolescent's self-concept is crucial to normal adolescence.

Girls

Soon after deposition of adipose tissue and changes in bony pelvis that widens the contour of hips, females experience thelarche (breast budding under the areola) and adrenarche or pubarche, the appearance of fine pubic hair over mons veneris. These changes occur at about 11 years of age (range, 8–13 years). This marks the sexual maturity rating (SMR) or Tanner stage II of pubertal development. Breast development proceeds to SMR V (adult) stage over approximately 4 years. But it can vary as short as 18 months to as long as 9 years, with an average of 2½ years. About 1 year after breast development during SMR stage III, girls have very rapid increase in height at the peak of this growth spurt, which precedes the onset of menstruation in normal individuals. Menarche is late pubertal change or event, occurring usually 6 months after the growth spurt during or just before SMR stage IV of development. Girls grow slowly 1–2 inches after menarche.

Boys

Boys also follow a regular sequence of physical changes but with observable milestones like girls. Nocturnal emission in dreams is considered as the counterpart of menstruation, first appearing at SMR stage III. But they are not regular like menses. Testicular growth on the long axis of testis >2.5 cm indicates transition from SMR stage I to SMR stage II. This begins about at 11½ years of age (range, 9½–13½ years). Penile enlargement commences marking SMR stage III, preceded by adrenarche, followed by development of axillary hair. Completion of testicular growth can occur any time at 13½ and 17 years of age. Penile lengthening and ordering begin normally between 10½ and 14½ years of age. Development of penis reaches SMR stage V between 12½ and 16½ years of age. The growth spurt is initiated from 10½ to 16 years of age and is completed by 13½–17½ years of age, depending on individual. Growth in boys continues at slower pace and can continue into the third decade.

MAJOR DEVELOPMENTAL THEORIES – CHARACTERISTICS

Maslow's Hierarchy of Needs

- Physiologic
- Safety and security
- Love and belonging
- Self-esteem
- Self actualisation
- Cognitive
- Aesthetic needs; desire for beauty

Freud's Psychosexual Theory of Development

Genital stage.
- Personality and defence mechanisms become integrated into a person's character
- Oral, anal and phallic sensuality is incorporated into gentility

Erikson's Theory of Psychosocial Development

Identity versus role confusion.
- *Puberty and adolescence:* Sense of formulating an individual identity begins at the age of 12 years and is characterised by the following:
  - Rapid and marked physical changes
  - Shattering of previous trust in one's own body (rapid growth may result in a lack of physical co-ordination)
  - Preoccupation with appearance – feeing of imaginary audience
  - Integration of personal values with those of society; role confusion may ensue
- Later adolescence and young adulthood:
  - Intimacy versus isolation
  - According to Elkind, pseudo-stupidity appears to ask dumb questions
  - The imaginary audience: Super self-consciousness; believes that everybody is watching and evaluating
  - *Personal fable:* Belief of being special and not subject to natural laws
  - Apparent hypocrisy (believing or pretending to believe or feel something that they do not have)

Piaget's Theory of Cognitive Development

Formal operations (abstractions and hypothetical deductive reasoning possible).
- Having adaptability and flexibility
- Thinking in abstract terms
- Using abstract symbols
- Drawing conclusions from a set of observations
- Developing hypothesis and testing them
- Considering abstract theoretical and philosophical matters
- Problem solving (there may be some confusion of the ideal with the practical)
- Having ability to comprehend purely abstract or symbolic content, as well as ability to solve advanced mathematics and logical problems
- Can comprehend value and belief system in the philosophical, moral and political realms
- Capable of sharing self with another to foster an inanimate relationship
- Inability to form intimate relationships may result in a sense of isolation

Kohlberg's Theory of Moral Development

Stage IV – Conventional (12–16 years): Fixed rules in moral decisions with obligation to do no harm and to do well (many adults never get pass this stage of moral development).

Stage V – Postconventional (16 years and above):
- Social contracts understood and formulated
- Laws recognized as changeable
- Correct actions depend on standards and individuals' rights

Stage VI – Adulthood: Moral reasoning may occur in late adolescence but probably will not; abstract moral principles govern behaviours.
- Morality is easily separated from legality
- Orientation is based on universal, ethical orientation
- Situation ethics can be applied by those in this stage of moral reasoning (many individuals do not comprehend this level of development)

Developmental Table as per Age

Sound and Language	Vision, Neurologic and Motor Development
Has an adult verbal skill, with ever-increasing vocabulary	Regular vision testing important; good posture impeded by rapid growth spurt that accompanies puberty
	Those active in sports tend to have fewer problems with poor posture

Physical Characteristics

- Adolescence encompasses puberty, the period when secondary sex characteristics begin to develop.
- In girls, puberty begins between the ages of 8 and 14 years and is completed within 3 years. In boys, puberty begins between the ages of 9 and 16 years and is completed by the ages of 18–20 years.
- During adolescence, hormonal influences cause important developmental changes that include:
  - Body mass reaches adult size.
  - Sebaceous glands become active.
  - Exocrine sweat glands become fully functional.
  - Apocrine sweat glands develop with hair growth in the axillae, areola of breast, genital and anal regions.
  - Body hair assumes characteristic distribution patterns and textural changes.
  - During puberty, girls experience increases in height, weight, breast development and pelvic girth, with the expansion of uterine tissue; menarche (onset of menstrual periods) typically occurs about 2½ years after the onset of puberty.
  - During puberty, boys experience increases in height, weight, muscle mass and penis and testicle size; facial and body hair growth and voice deepening also occur. Onset of spontaneous nocturnal emission of seminal fluid is an overt sign of puberty, analogous to menarche in girls.
- Height and weight changes include:
  - Girls gain 5–20.5 cm and reach adult height by the age of 16–17 years.

- Boys gain 10.2–3.8 cm and reach adult height by 21 years of age.
- Girls gain an average of 6.8–25 kg over a 3-year period.
- Boys gain 6.8–29.5 kg over a period of 4-year period.
- Full height not attained until the ages of 20–24 years when epiphyseal plates close.
- Nutritional requirement increases. Males may consume 3600 calories and females 2600 calories per day.
- At the end of adolescence, male basal metabolic rate is about 10% greater than that of a female.

Health Maintenance and Anticipatory Guidance

- They need entertainment.
- They prefer group or peer activities such as sports or academic teams.
- Thrill-seeking behaviours should be curtailed.
- Motor vehicle safety, sport injuries, drowning, etc. need to be warned.
- Skin care need to be overemphasized because of increased sebaceous gland secretion and acne vulgaris.
- Consequences of drug and alcohol consumption need to be taught.
- Immunizations – booster TT should be scheduled.
- Sex education and family planning need to be emphasized.
- Nutritional counselling also is indicated.
- Developmental issues – Autonomy is emphasized.
- Parental – adult limit setting continues to be sought and desired by the adolescent and should be given, testing of independence continues and is ascertained. Allowing the child to assume increasing responsibility may lessen family conflict. By early adolescence, the drive for autonomy culminates in the child's challenging of long-standing beliefs.
- Peer interaction may create challenges to family values.
- They are in the concrete operational and formal operational states and are able to have hypothetical and abstract reasoning. So, they have a tendency to question certain beliefs and practices of adults.

GROWTH AND PUBERTY

There are four phases of human growth – fetal, infantile, childhood and pubertal growth spurt phases.

Fetal Phase

Fetal phase is the fastest period of growth that causes about 30% of eventual height.

Size at birth – deciding factors are size of the mother, placental nutrient supply (modulates human placental lactogen and insulin IGF2).

The Infantile Phase

Growth during infancy (i.e. up to 18 months of age) is dependent on adequate nutrition, good health and normal thyroid function. During this phase, there is a rapid but decelerating growth rate which accounts for about 15% of eventual height. Decreased rate of weight gain during this phase is called failure to thrive (FTT).

Childhood Phase

It is slow, steady but of prolonged growth which contributes 40% of the final height. Deciding factors of growth at this phase are:

- Adequate nutrition and good health
- Thyroid hormone
- Vitamin D and steroids affect cartilage cell division and bone formation

Pituitary growth hormone (GH) secretion acting to produce insulin-like growth factor-1 (IGF-1) at the epiphysis is the main determinant of growth at this time.

Pubertal Growth Spurt

It accounts for 15% of the final height. Sex hormones, testosterone and oestradiol, stimulate growth hormone secretion that leads to pubertal growth spurt. But same-sex steroids cause fusion of the epiphyseal growth plates to stop growth. This happens with puberty. If early puberty is achieved, there is reduction in pubertal growth spurt.

PROBLEMS OF GROWTH AND DEVELOPMENT

Short Stature

It is defined as a height below the 2nd (2 standard deviation [SD] below the mean) or 0.4th centile (−2.6 SD). Usually, these children will be normal, though short. But if they are below −2.6 SD, there will be a pathological cause. This growth failure can be identified from the child's height falling across centile lines plotted on a growth chart. This allows growth failure to be identified, even though the child's height in still in the 2nd centile.

Height velocity is a sensitive indicator of growth failure. A height velocity persistently below the 25th centile is abnormal.

Procedure

Take two accurate measurements of height in centimetres per year at least 6 months apart (preferably 1 year apart) and plot the measurements at the midpoint in time on a height/velocity chart. Usually, a tall child with a height on the 98th centile will grow at approximately the 75th velocity centile and a short child with a height at the 2nd centile will grow at approximately the 25th velocity centile. So, the normal growth approximates to the 25th–75th centiles. Height velocity calculations are highly dependent on the accuracy of height measurements. Height centile of a child must be compared with weight centile and the estimate of their genetic target centile and range calculated from the height of their parents.

Causes

- *Familial:* Most short statures are psychologically well adjusted to their size as a usual phenomenon in the family.
- *Intrauterine growth retardation (IUGR) and extreme prematurity:* One-third of the children born with severe intrauterine growth restriction or who were extremely premature remain short.
- *Constitutional delay of growth and puberty:* It is usually familial having occurred in the parent of same sex.
- *Endocrinal:* It includes hypothyroidism, growth hormone deficiency and steroid excess. This is associated with overweight. Weight is on a higher centile than that of the height.
- *Hypothyroidism:* This is usually congenital in infancy or caused by autoimmune thyroiditis during childhood.
- *Growth hormone deficiency:* This is secondary to panhypopituitarism. Common conditions leading to growth hormone deficiency are craniopharyngioma, hypothalamic tumour or cranial irradiation.
- *Corticosteroids:* These are usually iatrogenic and are a potent growth suppressor.
- *Nutritional/chronic illness:* This is a relatively common cause of abnormal growth. These children are usually short and underweight. Their weight will be on the same or lower centile than that of the height. Associated common conditions of short stature are:
  - Coeliac diseases, which usually present in the first 2 years of life
  - Crohn disease
  - Chronic renal failure
  - Cystic fibrosis
  - *Psychological deprivation:* Children subjected to physical and emotional deprivation may be short and underweight and show delayed puberty.
  - Chromosomal disorders and syndromes are associated with short stature. Down syndrome (is usually diagnosed at birth) has short stature as a feature. Turner, Noonan and Russell–Silver syndromes may also show short stature.

Disproportionate Short Stature

Confined by measuring the sitting height – base of the spine to top of the head and subischial leg length – subtraction of the sitting height from the total height. Disproportionate short stature is seen in achondroplasia and other short-limbed dysplasias.

Investigations are done by plotting the present and previous heights and weights on appropriate growth charts together with the clinical features that usually help identify the cause.

Treatment of the endocrine causes is achieved with supplementation of respective hormones.

Tall Stature

Tall stature is inherited from parents. Overeating in childhood leads to obesity, which may promote tall stature.

Tall children may have disadvantages as compared with their counterparts because they appear older than their actual age. Tall children are treated with oestrogen therapy to induce premature fusion of the epiphysis. Surgical destruction of epiphysis in legs is also done as an intervention.

Causes

- Familial
- Obesity
- *Secondary causes:*
  - Hyperthyroidism
  - Excess sex steroids
  - Excess adrenal androgen steroids (e.g. congenital adrenal hyperplasia)
  - True gigantism (excess growth hormone)
- *Syndromes:*
  - Long-legged ones like Marfan syndrome
  - Homocystinuria
  - Klinefelter syndrome
  - Proportional tall stature at birth, such as maternal diabetes
  - Primary hyperinsulinism
  - Beckwith syndrome
  - *Sotos syndrome:* Associated with a large head, characteristic facial features and learning difficulties

Asymmetry of Head

The common asymmetrical heads are microcephaly and macrocephaly. The asymmetrical head may result from an imbalance of the growth rate at the coronal, sagittal and lambdoid sutures, although the head circumference increases normally.

Craniostosis: Premature fusion of a suture may lead to distortion of the head shape. Usually, the sutures of the skull bones do not finally unite until about 12 years of age. This condition is treated surgically to decrease intracranial pressure (ICP) and cosmetic reasons.

Macrocephaly: It is head circumference above the 98th centile. The common causes are as follows:

- Tall stature
- Familial
- Increased ICP
- Hydrocephalus
- Subdural hematoma
- Cerebral tumours
- Neurofibromatosis
- Soto syndrome
- CNS disorders

(see also Hydrocephalus)

Premature Sexual Development

The development of secondary sexual characteristics before the age of 8 years in females and 9 years in males is considered as premature sexual development.

Causes

- Precocious puberty (PP) when it is accompanied by growth spurt
- Premature breast development (thelarche)
- Premature pubic hair development (adrenarche)

Precocious Puberty

The cause of PP is unknown, but in some cases, it may be familial. PP is categorized on the basis of levels of pituitary-derived gonadotropins, follicle-stimulating hormone and luteinizing hormone as (i) gonadotropin dependent (central/true PP) developed from premature activation of pituitary and (ii) gonadotropin independent (false/pseudo-PP) from sex steroids.

STUDY QUESTIONS

1. What are the major developmental theories pertaining to growth and development?
2. Describe the psychosocial development and significant others in each stage of development of adolescents.
3. What is tall stature?
4. Mention common asymmetry of head.
5. What are the common health problems seen in adolescents? How will you manage the same?

BIBLIOGRAPHY

1. Algranati, P.S. (1992). The Pediatric Patient: An Approach to History and Physical Examination. Williams and Wilkins: Baltimore, MD.
2. Algranati, P.S. (1998). Effect of Developmental Status on the Approach to Physical Examination. Pediatric Clinics of North America, 45(1), pp. 1-23.
3. Brazelton, T.B. (1975). Anticipatory Guidance. Pediatric Clinics of North America, 22, pp. 533-544.
4. Telzrow, R.W. (1978). Anticipatory Guidance in Pediatric Practice. Journal of Continuing Education in Pediatrics, 20, pp. 14-27.

THEORIES OF DEVELOPMENT

LEARNING OBJECTIVES

At the end of the chapter, the learner will be able to:

- Describe various theories of child development, namely
- Psychosexual development.
- Psychosocial development.
- Intellectual development.
- Moral development.
- Psychoanalytic theory.

Sigmund Freud (1856–1939) was a son of Jewish merchant and was brought up in Vienna in Austria. He started practicing neurology after completing his medical school in 1886. His specialization was hysteria. His psychoanalytic theory had evolved with his struggle to decide the truthfulness of reported sexual encounters with their fathers by his female patients during their pubertal period.

According to Freud, personality or the psychic energy had three components: **id, ego** and **superego. Id** is based on the instinctual drive that works on pleasure principles. Id seeks immediate gratification and tries to avoid physical or psychic pain. It is based on the primary process of thinking and is illogical and indulges in fantasy. Id's drive for pleasure conflicts with societal norms of moral principles. The **ego** emerges to keep the id out of trouble. It balances the id's drive and keeps up the society's norm-based more rational thinking. Ego engages in the secondary process of thinking. It delays gratification to have it in a more realistic and acceptable way. **Superego** develops by internalization of moral standards. So, it is the moral component of the personality. It emerges around 3–5 years of age. This is the individual way of moral policing of his or her behaviour. If superego becomes more demanding, it leads to guilt in an individual.

Freud described awareness as having three levels: **conscious, preconscious** and **unconscious**. Conscious is the awareness of the present. Preconscious is just below the surface where the individual knows about it but does not think about it at the present. Unconscious is the memories, thoughts and desires that are lying deep below and the individual is not aware of them but they have profound influence on the individual's behaviours. Id rests completely in the unconscious.

Psychoanalytic forces (psychic energy) energize all human behaviours. This psychic energy is divided into three components, viz. id, ego and superego (Freud). The id (the unconscious mind) is the inborn component that is driven by instincts. The id obeys the pleasure principle of immediate gratification of needs, whereas the ego (conscious mind) serves the reality principle. The ego helps in controlling self and finds realistic means for gratifying the instincts, blocking the irrational thinking of the id. The superego (the conscience) is the moral arbitrator and represents the ideal. The superego helps the individual keep away from expressing undesirable instincts.

PSYCHOSEXUAL DEVELOPMENT (FREUD)

Freud's psychosexual theory states that the development of personality is affected by sexual instincts. In his view, the psychosexual means the sensual pleasure, and many simple body functions considered to be nonsexual were viewed by him as erotic. Factors motivating these activities are named as sex instincts. Certain regions of the body assume a prominent psychological significance as a source of new pleasure during childhood. As the age advances, new conflicts gradually shift from one part of the body to another as prominent source of pleasure. So, during each stage of development, the child assumes a particular body part as a source of new pleasure. For example, during infancy, mouth is the source of new pleasure, as it is the oral region. He further states that each stage builds on the previous one, and maturation of sex instinct leaves distinct imprints on the developing psyche. Children who face severe conflicts in one stage are reluctant to move to the next phase, showing certain level of regression.

Freud attempted to provide a systematic explanation of human behaviour. His theory focuses on single motive governing behaviour (satisfying biological needs) to release tensions. He derived his theory from retrospective studies of adults and not from direct observation of children. So, it stays nonuseful to predict future behaviours. According to him, conflicts and **defence mechanisms** are developed with internal battles between id, ego and superego. The internal battle creates conflict in their personality. The drives for sex and aggression are conflicted as the social norms. This internal battle causes anxiety and guilt. Defence mechanisms are unconscious and protect the ego from unpleasant feelings such as anxiety and guilt. Common defence mechanisms are rationalization, repression, projection, displacement, reaction formation, regression and identification.

For Freud, sexual means an innate drive for physical pleasure. He divided the whole life cycle into five phases. Children control over these urges through five psychosexual stages. These stages are **oral, anal, phallic, latency and genital stages**. The failure to progress to these stages is referred as fixation.

Oral Stage (Birth to 1 Year)

Oral stage: It is the first year of life, and the main source of pleasure is the mouth. The activities are sucking, biting, etc. Adult oral fixations are eating and smoking.

The major pleasure-seeking region is the oral area, and the activities to arouse the sensual pleasure are sucking, biting, chewing and vocalizing. Children prefer one of these activities over the other. The preferred method of oral gratification can provide a clue or an indication for the type of personality they develop into. Examples of oral personality development are as follows:
- Pessimism versus optimism
- Determination versus submission
- Admiration versus envy
- Gullibility versus suspiciousness

Anal Stage (1–3 Years)

Anal stage: This is seen in the toddler period, and the pleasure is obtained in controlling the bowel movements. Toilet training, the first effort to control the child's self-serving physical drive by the societal norms, creates conflict between the child and care takers. Adult anal fixation is anxiety about being punished for not performing.

Major pleasure-seeking region is the anal region and child develops some level of control to withhold or expel faecal matter at will. The conditions prevailing in the environment during the period of toilet training will create long-lasting effects on child's personality. Common anal personalities are as follows:
- Stinginess or overgenerousness
- Constriction or expansiveness
- Orderliness or messiness
- Rigid or tardiness

Phallic Stage (3–6 Years)

Phallic stage: This period is between third and fifth years of life. Boys find pleasure in self-stimulation and competing with their fathers in their love towards their mother. Girls blame their mothers for not having a penis and compensate for the deficiency by having attachment with their fathers. 'Oedipus complex' is the term coded for the sexual desires for the parent of the opposite sex along with the hostility towards the parent of the same sex. This conflict coincides with emergence of superego. According to Freud, resolution of this conflict with the parent of the same sex is essential for healthy gender identification.

At this stage, areas of sensual pleasure are the genitals. Children identify the difference between sexes and become curious about dissimilarities. The controversial issues of Oedipal complex, castration complex, Electra complex and penis envy develop.

Common phallic personalities are as follows:
- Brashness or bashfulness
- Stylishness or plainness, gaiety or sadness
- Blind courage or timidity
- Gregariousness or isolationism

Latency Period (6–12 Years)

Children elaborate on previously acquired skills. Channelize the physical energy to knowledge acquisition and vigorous play.

Latency stage: This stage is from the age of 5 years to puberty. Sex urge is suppressed as children develop social relationship beyond the family, especially with peers.

Genital Stage (12 Years and Above)

This stage begins at puberty with maturation of the reproductive system and production of sex hormones. The major sources of tension and sensual pleasure are the genital organs. The energies are directed in formal friendship and preparation for marriage. During puberty (adolescence), sexual urge is directed towards peers of the opposite sex. This stage is marked by discontinuation of development, as it implies that development has clearly demarcated points of change.

The stages of psychosexual development and focus of sexual urges are given in the following table for quick reference:

Stage	Age	Focus of Sexual Urges
Oral	First year of life	The mouth (sucking, biting)
Anal	Toddler	Controlling biological urges (e.g. bowel movements)
Phallic	3–5 years	Genital self-pleasure, the Oedipus complex
Latency	5 years–puberty	Suppressing urges
Genital	Puberty	Peers of the opposite sex

The major aim of psychoanalysis is to make awareness of the unconscious conflicts, motives and defences so that they can be resolved. Free association is the spontaneous expression of an individual's thought and feelings.

PSYCHOSOCIAL DEVELOPMENT

Erik Homburger Erikson (1902–1994) emphasized the importance of social environment in shaping child's sense of self. His theory of psychosocial development is based on interactions of human being with the ever-widening circle of people starting with the mother and ending with humankind in general. He had described eight stages of development characterized by a normative development crisis that is resolved on a continuum between opposing positive and negative outcomes. Personality is formed as a result of the resolution of these crises, making people to have strengths and weaknesses. While Freud believed that human beings keep the balance of unhappy childhood experiences, Erikson believed that human beings rework earlier crisis later in life. Erikson was more hopeful than Freud. According to Erikson, reworking is growth enhancing but if reworking is poorly resolved, then revisiting can be disruptive leading to personality disturbances.

The theory of personality development advanced by Erickson (1963) is built on Freudian theory. It emphasizes on development of a healthy personality. There are predictable age-related stages in the life of human being. During each stage, specific changes are assumed to take place. In his theory of psychosocial development, Erickson used the biological concepts of critical periods or core problem that the individual strives to master during each period of personality development. For the development of successful personality, the child needs to conquer the core conflicts/problems successfully in the predicted period itself. That is, mastery of each conflict is build upon the successful completion of the previous conflict.

Children have certain unique problems at each stage of psychosocial development. Resolution of this problem requires lots of efforts from the child by integrating personal needs and skills with social demands and cultural expectations. These individual efforts used by children to resolve the problem are called crises – the normal stresses which the child confronts during each stage of development.

The core conflicts at each stage of personality development have two components, viz. the favourable and unfavourable aspects of the core problem (positive and negative counterparts). No core conflict is ever mastered completely and remains as a recurrent problem throughout life. No life situation is ever secure. Each new situation presents a conflict in a new form. For example, a child who successfully develops trust at home may confront hospitalization as a threat where he/she has to develop a trust on those who care for him/her.

Erickson staged the life periods into eight stages. The outcome of each stage is ego quality that provides the resource for coping. The key socializing agent is the specific person in the environment during each stage. For example, the mother is the significant person (key socializing agent) during infancy. Although there are certain shortcomings, Erickson's theory provides an excellent framework for explaining children's behaviour in mastering developmental tasks.

Stage 1 – Trust versus Mistrust (Birth to 1 Year)

It is a time of getting and taking in through all senses. It exists only in relation to something or someone; therefore, a consistent, loving care by a mothering person is essential for the development of trust. When trust-promoting experiences are deficient or the basic needs are inconsistently or inadequately met, mistrust develops. In Erikson's view, awareness of physical needs is most important, especially for nourishment. If a child' caretaker anticipates and fulfils these needs consistently, the infant learns to trust others. Once the caretaker meets physical needs, mutuality occurs, though there are periods of anxiety and rejection in the infant's life. Trust versus mistrust as the first crisis concerns the child's confidence in other people. If trust is established in the first year, establishment of the trust in later years is found to be easier. All infants express basic needs, and the caretaker's sensitivity to these needs is most important in establishing the child's trust in others.

A baby develops the ego equality of hope through the process of mutuality with the primary caregiver. Once the primary caregiver gives adequate and consistent care, the baby feels that there is someone for it. This results in deep faith and optimism.

Autonomy versus Shame and Doubt (1–3 Years)

It corresponds to Freud's anal stage, where there is holding on and letting go of the sphincter muscles. During this stage, autonomy is expressed by children's increasing ability to control their bodies by themselves and in response to their environment. By now (second year of life), development of the muscular and nervous systems allows the children to acquire new skills.

They use their newly acquired power to perform activities such as clothing, climbing and manipulating. They also use the mental power of decision-making and learn certain social rules. They move around and examine the environment. The wants of children and adults contradict here; the adults are concerned about health and safety of children. The children need guidance and caretaker's decision about how much freedom to allow. In the crisis of autonomy versus shame and doubt, the critical issue is the child's feeling of independence. In a highly permissive environment, infants encounter difficulties that they cannot yet handle and doubting themselves and not developing a sense of independence. If the control is too severe, children feel worthless and shameful of being incapable. The caretaker should take a stand that respects the child's needs and provides careful and constant attention to prevent hazardous environmental factors.

Children may develop negative feelings of shame and doubt when they are *made to feel unimportant or when others are not encouraging them*. The central process is imitation and the key socializing agent is parents.

Initiative versus Guilt (3–6 Years)

This stage corresponds to Freud's phallic stage. After gaining certain amount of independence, the child would like to try various possibilities. Imaginative play exists in this group of children. Imitation work and role-playing make them attempt difficult tasks. A child's willingness to try new things needs to be facilitated in a constructive manner.

Here, children explore the physical world with all their powers. At this stage, they are no longer guided by the outsiders but by their inner voice – conscience – that develops during this age. Children sometime do activities that are confronting with their parents' goals. If they are made to feel that their activities are not right, it makes them feel guilty. Excessive guilt inhibits initiatives, but children must be taught to keep up initiatives without hampering others' rights. Imitating the roles of family members and attributing life to inanimate objects are prominent during this age. The central process is the identification, and the socializing agent is the family. Parents and family set example by developing manners and social behaviours. Preschool children need to be taught appropriate table manners, as they view their parents as examples for social behaviours.

Industry versus Inferiority (6–12 Years)

Corresponds to Freud's latency period where children are workers and producers. They engage in work and make it to completion and need achievement. They are more cooperative, and if they succeed in their activity, they develop a sense of mastery and self-assurance. Feeling of inadequacy and inferiority develops if too much is expected of them. The central process is education, and the key socializing agents are peers and teachers.

In the crisis of industry versus inferiority, the aim is to develop a feeling of competence rather than inability; it is shaped by interaction of inherited and environmental factors. The key concept is readiness.

Identity versus Role Confusion (12–18 Years)

This stage corresponds with the genital stage of Freud. This is characterized by rapid and marked physical changes. They try to play with current rules and fashions adopted by their peers and struggle to fit in the society by integrating their concepts and values. They make decision regarding occupation. Inability to solve the core conflict results in role confusion. The central processes are peer pressure and role experimentation. The key socializing agent is the peer society. The successful outcome of this stage leads to devotion and fidelity. Hero worship is a common feature of this stage, and a role model is essential for successful outcome.

Intimacy versus Isolation

This occurs during adulthood. A sense of intimacy is established as a sense of identity. Intimacy is the capacity to develop an intimate, loving relationship with friends, partners and other significant persons. If there is no intimacy, there is isolation. The central process is mutuality, and the key socializing agents are spouses, lovers and close friends.

Generativity versus Stagnation

This stage is applicable to young middle adulthood. It is mainly concerned with the creation and care of the next generation. The essential element is to nourish and nurture. It may be directed towards one's own children, children of others or products of creativity. The key socializing agents are spouse, children and cultural norms. The central process is person–environment fit and creativity.

The Ego Integrity versus Despair

This stage takes place during old age. A sense of integrity results from satisfaction with life and acceptance of what has been. Despair arises from remorse for what might have been. The central process is introspection, and the favourable outcome is renunciation and wisdom.

THEORY OF INTERPERSONAL DEVELOPMENT

Interpersonal development theory is put forward by Sullivan in 1953. This theory is also build upon Freudian theory. This theory describes the interpersonal relationships that children engage in and the importance of social approval and disproval in developing self-concept.

Unfavourable interactions result in tension and anxiety. Favourable interactions result in a sense of comfort and security. First interactions are between infants and their mothering figure. The bipolar relations change as the infant grows and extends to other family members by the age of 2 years. This gradually extends to neighbours, peers at school, etc., and the horizon widens. Through repeated interactions with others, children learn a set of accepted behaviours to deal with others and try to reduce the tension-producing encounters.

INTELLECTUAL DEVELOPMENT/MENTAL DEVELOPMENT

Children are born with inherited potentialities for thorough intellectual growth. Development of potential occurs through interaction with the environment. The age-related changes in mental activities are called cognitive development. The term 'cognition' means understanding. It refers to mental development that includes not only intelligence but also such complementary processes as perceiving, recognizing, recalling and interpreting information, as well as all forms of reasoning. Most acceptable theory of cognitive development is put forward by the Swiss psychologist Jean Piaget (Swiss epistemologist) in 1969 through conversations and observations with his three children and a nephew. Thinking of normal children is not a simpler version of the thinking of adults. It is qualitatively different. Thinking is based on different understanding of reality. It slowly changes according to maturation and experience. Piaget proposed three stages of reasoning as intuitive, concrete operational and formal operational. According to Piaget, children proceed through the stages of mental activity in an orderly and sequential manner. Children learn through assimilation and accommodation. By assimilation, children incorporate new knowledge, skills, ideas and insights into cognitive schemes (schema according to Piaget). Understanding of a new experience is based on previous experiences of the child. Certain new experiences or situations do not fit into the cognitive schemes to solve difficult problems. The sequence of cognitive changes is divided into four periods according to the chronological age as sensorimotor period, preoperational thought, concrete operational and formal operations.

Stages of Logical Thinking

There are four major stages:

- Sensory motor phase (birth to 2 years): Here the infant is not concerned with thinking about things but experiencing them. The intelligence is called practical intelligence. The child merely senses things and acts upon them. So, this period is called the sensory motor period.

  Here, the infant progresses from reflex behaviour to simple repetitive activity. Three important events take place during this phase.

- The first event is separation. The infant identifies that there are objects in the environment and the other objects also play a part in the environment besides him/her. This stage coincides with Erickson's concept formation of trust. The baby identifies that there is a mother besides him/her for mutual regulation of frustration.
- The second event is object permanence. Here, the infant realizes that objects that leaves the visual field does not vanish and still exists. This can be revealed by a simple game of hide and seek where the baby will be searching for the hidden object/person. This skill develops approximately by 8–10 months of life.
- The third event is symbol or mental representation. The use of symbols allows the infant to think of an object or situation without actually experiencing it. Recognition of symbols is the beginning of understanding of time and space. This can be viewed when the baby sees the cup and spoon that are usually used for feeding, he/she shows reactions similar to that of feeding. The sensory motor period has six stages.

First Stage – Use of Reflexes (Birth to 1 Month)

At this stage, the baby is totally narcissistic being. Repetitious nature of reflexes helps form patterns. For example, when the baby cries with hunger, the mother provides breast, the baby sucks, feel satisfied and go to sleep. They assimilate this experience. The common reflexive activities during this period are sucking, swallowing, rooting, grasping and crying.

Second Stage – Primary Circular Reactions (1–4 Months)

Here, the baby replaces the reflexive activity with voluntary acts. Sucking becomes more deliberate. For example,

observing the responses produced by the baby when pulling mother's hair while in lap or holding the baby shows the deliberate acts of the baby in response to the mother's response. With repetition of acts and its response, the baby identifies a pattern and then helps in function of orderly sequence of events. This orderly sequence of events directs the development of the concept of space and time. For example, while pulling the hair, the mother releases the baby's hands. The baby identifies that the mother will releases its hands in a particular way when he/she pulls the hair. So, they develop a stimulus response pattern. This is assimilation. Gradually, this changes to accommodation. For example, when the baby cries the mother feeds the baby with her breasts. So, there develops an association of cry and nipple. Once this is established, when the baby hears the voice of the mother, he/she stops crying before receiving the breast as he/she accommodates that once the mother is near, she is going to feed as the recognition of the sequence of the activity.

Third Stage – Secondary Circular Reactions (4–8 Months)

It occurs as a continuation of primary circular reactions. Here, the primary circular reactions are repeated. Grasping and holding now change to shaking, banging and pulling. Shaking is done to hear the sounds. This is not only done for the pleasure of shaking but also done to identify the quality and quantity of an act. For example, more or less shaking produces different volume of sounds. At this stage, the baby develops the concept of casualty, time, deliberate intention and separateness from the environment in a rudimentary form. For example, a wet baby cries. The cry depicts urgency. The new processes of human behaviour that occur at this stage are imitation, play and affect. During second-half of the first year, infants imitate sounds and simple gestures. They take pleasure in performing an act after mastering it and it is their play. All waking hours of infants are immersed in sensory motor play. For the first 6 months, the out of sight is out of mind for them. But when the object continues to be remembered, even if it is out of sight, object permanence develops. Object permanence is a critical component of parent–child attachment which is described in affect (outward manifestation of emotions and feelings) and is seen in the development of stranger anxiety at 6–8 months of age. At this age, they are able to tolerate some amount of frustration and delayed gratification. Great interest in mirror image develops at this age.

Fourth Stage – Coordination of Secondary Schemas and Their Application to New Situation (9–12 Months)

Concept of object permanence advances, and increased motor capability promotes exploration of the environment. They discover that the hiding object does not mean that it is gone forever. This makes for the development of intellectual reasoning. They begin to associate symbols with events (e.g. saying bye-bye), and the classification of these events are based on their experience. Common behaviours manifested are active searching for hidden objects, comprehending meanings of words and simple commands and trying to be away from parents to explore the surroundings.

Fifth Stage – Tertiary Circular Reactions (13–18 Months)

The child uses active experimentation to achieve previously unattainable goals and develops increased concept of object permanence. The child incorporates old learning of secondary circular reactions and applies combined knowledge to new situations. This manifests traces of memory. The child differentiates him/herself separate from the environment. The child develops rudimentary awareness of spatial, casual and temporal relationships and shows curiosity about the environment. The child can use building blocks for making different objects. The child can identify gestures such as go up and down and gain comfort from the parent's voice even if the parent is not visually present.

Sixth Stage – Mental Combinations (9–24 Months)

Invention of new means through mental combination develops during 19–24 months of age. The child can infer a cause while only experiencing the effect. Sense of time in terms of anticipation begins to develop during this stage. Symbolic imitation of household activities is common (household mimicry), e.g. producing sound of a mixer grinder. Egocentrism is another typical feature, and the baby can see anything without reference to them. This is evident in their attitude like 'mine is mine' and 'yours is also mine'. The toddler who sees a toy with another child tries takes away the toy and makes the other child unhappy. The ideal processes of representation and invention are basic development of this stage. At this stage, the child wishes to obtain some end for which he has no habitual available means and he/she invents one. This is done by internal experimentation and not by the overt trail-and-error process.

To put in a nutshell, this sensory motor period is characterized by lack of symbols – Do not conceive objects as having any permanent independent existence apart from children's own experience with them. They do not carry around in their head the image or symbols of these objects. They have no representational ability. The objects cease to exist when they are not in vicinity. Usually, this stays up to 6 months.

After 6 months, infants develop object permanence when they may search for missed objects. This shows the child has an understanding that an object continues to exist even when it is not directly available to the senses. The infant gets object permanence of the mother and/or caretaker and is in distress when they are not around. No exact reason has been identified for the same.

Second Phase – Preoperational Period (2–7 Years)

The next phase of cognitive development is the *preoperational period*. The representational abilities become more sophisticated, and the child is capable of communicating his/her needs with language. The child becomes a social being but still does not understand the use of symbols and basic operations, hence the name preoperational stage. This phase consists of the following two substages:

Preconceptional Stage (2–4 years). This is a transient period which bridges the self-satisfying behaviour of infancy and rudimentary social behaviour of latency. This is the period of beginning of symbolization in thinking. The baby is only capable of making concept of a single object and not a class of objects. The principal characteristics of this stage are egocentric use of language and indulgence in make-believe play. The child begins to develop imagery and distinguishes between words and things. Play and imitation begin to develop. The child does not understand the nature of classes and class memberships. The preoperational membership implies that the child cannot think in terms of operations. The child views every object or situation as a single instance and will not understand the dimensionality of objects. For example, a child who picks up a blue pen picks it only as a pen. He will not understand that blue has a colour and also will not understand that a pen is one type of article that is used for writing. Preconceptional thought is extremely concrete and egocentric. Egocentric speech consists of repeating words and sounds for the pleasure of hearing oneself and not for communication. This collective monologue reflects the child's persistent self-centeredness. Egocentrism is a major hindrance to cognitive development. With egocentrism, the child is unaware of others' perspectives. Preschoolers do not realize that other people see things from a different viewpoint (perceptual egocentrism). For example, a young child playing hide and seek may close his/her eyes and may think that others cannot see him/her. Around 6–7 years of age, egocentric thought begins to give way to social pressure, and the child begins to accommodate others (cognitive egocentrism). Interaction with peers and playmates dissolve egocentrism. In the areas of language and thinking too, the child displays egocentric attitude and centrism. The child at this age will not be able to make speech interesting to his/her listeners. The preschoolers thinking is static and focussed at one feature at a time. They are unable to combine various features of an object. This is centration. For example, if you are serving food in a small plate and transferring the same food to a broader plate, the child will not agree that the second plate has the same amount of food as the first one. The child has only centred on the height of the food and failed to decentre the other dimension of broadness of the plate. A child of 4 years of age knows that 9 is greater than 7. But, if we put nine dots closer in a line and seven dots wide apart on another line, the child will invariably say that the line with seven dots is longer. This shows that the child is unable to decentre his/her perceptual evaluation. This pattern of behaviour continues up to the age of 6–7 years.

Piaget also used the transducive reasoning (a child proceeds from particular-to-particular centring on one salient aspect of an event and ignoring other aspects) to describe that a child during this stage fluctuates in reasoning without sequence and generalization. For example, 'I have not had my sleep, so it is not morning.' Here, the child argues by implication about the occurrence of morning. The child here can correlate the concept of time only with events of occurrence.

At this age, children are not aware of inconsistencies in thinking and there are two forms of transducive thinking. Piaget described this as juxtaposition and syncretism. In juxtaposition, he described indiscriminate relationship. For example, a child may draw various parts of a bicycle, putting them in a nonfunctional relationship. In syncretism, the child fails to relate various observations into a consistent whole. For a child of 4–7 years of age, the aeroplane flies because it is heavy and a bird flies because it has wings and is light.

At this age, children group items with similarity. For them, tall = big = more conveys the same meaning. (Children of this age also display irreversibility.). If A = B, then B must be equal to A. But the child of this stage cannot comprehend this concept. In other words, the child of this age does not develop a concept of invariance. Much of these changes in conceptualization are related to the child's language development, too. Conservation of number appears by 6–7 years of age. Conservation is the conceptualization of amount or quality regardless of any changes in shape or position. From 2 to 4 years, the child lacks speech. In egocentric speech, the child repeatedly uses 'I', 'I say', 'I have', 'I am', etc. in his/her communication with others. But at the age of 4–7 years, language becomes intercommunicative (socialized speech). Use of 'you', 'she', 'he', 'they', etc. is added to the conversation. According to Piaget, language serves three consequences to mental development. The child exchanges his/her ideas with other persons, which helps in the socialization process. There is beginning of thought, and the child thinks internally by using words and signs. There is internalization of action, and actions become more symbolic rather than perceptual motor. In essence, the child aged 2–4 years will have egocentric speech.

Concrete Operational (7–11 years). During this stage, the child's reasoning process becomes more logical and coherent. Children are able to sort, classify and order objects on the basis of similarities and use problem-solving abilities. The most important systems or concepts of classification the child uses at this stage are as follows:

1. Decentration: At the concrete operational stage, the child can simultaneously consider two kinds of classes or comparisons and makes the classification correct. For example, a child is shown box containing 15 marble beads of which 13 are red and two are white. The child is given two boxes and asked to put marbles in separate boxes. The child will classify the beads as per colour. The child at the age of 2–7 years will say more red beads. The child of 7–11 years of age will say more-red beads.
2. Seriation: Placing related objects in their correct order or succession. This is the mental ability of the child to arrange objects into increasing or decreasing order or size. Seriation of length is seen at the age of 7 years. Seriation of weight starts at the age of 9 years and seriation of volume is seen at the age of 12 years. Analogous concept of seriation is the concept of equivalence: A = B = C. Hence, A = C. This is the reason why much time is spend in primary school devoted to seriation exercises in

mathematics, sequence of dates in history, weather recording to geography and growth in nature study.
3. Reversibility: Concrete operational thought is reversible. The child after the age of 7 years acquires the ability for reversible operations, which indicates a higher level of intellectual functioning.
4. Conservation of area: Conservation of numbers develops towards the sixth year of age. Conservation of substance develops by the seventh year of age. Conservation of volume develops in the concrete operational stage. Conservation of area appears by 7–8 years of age and weight around 9–10 years of age. Conservation of volume remains until 11–12 years of age. This can be illustrated by the following example: Take two beakers of same size and pour equal amount water in both beakers (situation 1). In situation 2, pour the water from one of the beakers to a narrow beaker, the child under the age of 11–12 years invariably will say that more water is in the new beaker. Even with the child who has shown decentration and reversibility, the concept of conservation of volume remain to be developed.
5. Mental representation: Only during the age of 7–11 years, the child develops the capacity of internalization or mental representation. He/she can describe the whole sequence of events of every act, i.e. going to school, coming back, etc. This is not possible for a child of 4 years of age.
6. Casualty: The child until the age of 10–11 years will not understand the relationship between time and speed. For a child of 9–10 years of age, the speed is related to the finishing point, who reaches first and no consideration to the starting point.
7. Groupings: Concrete operational child gives evidence of grouping or ability to generalize. There are five such groupings mentioned as characteristics of concrete operational children.
   Law of combination: Two distinct classes may be combined to form another class. For example, all boys and all girls = all children in the class.
   Law of inversion: For each operation, there is an opposite operation that annuls it or two classes combined to form a comprehensive class may be separated. For example, all children, all boys = all girls.
   Law of association: If several operations are to be combined, then the order in which they appear is of no value. A + (B + C) + C.
   Law of identity: When the operation is combined with its opposite, it is annulled. For example, travel 5 miles east and then 5 miles back to the west means one is back to the starting point.
   Law of tautology: With the exception of a combination of numbers, e.g. 3 + 2 = 5, whenever a class is combined with the same class, it remains the same class. For example, all girls = all girls.

Formal Operational Stage (12 years and older). This child's cognitive structure reaches maturity during this period. After this period, there will not be any qualitative change in cognitive development. Only quantitative change takes place.

Concrete operational children cannot deal with complex verbal problems or problems involving future. But a child in the operational stage can deal with past, present and future. The child after 11 years of age can organize data, reason scientifically and generate hypothesis. They are capable of dealing with conceptual categories of problems as combinatorial thought, complex verbal problems, hypothetical problems, propositions and conservation of movement.

Combinatorial thought

Before 12 years of age, the child cannot visualize and understand part/whole relationships. He/she does not think of all possibilities. But a child older than 12 years thinks of all possibilities of a situation to get a desired result.

Verbal problems

Children younger than 12 years are unable to solve word problems of verbal nature. For example, Raj is fairer than Riju. Riju is darker than Shibu. Who is darker among the three? That is why in primary classes, word problems of this nature is not common.

Hypothetical problems

In formal operational stage, children are capable of deriving logical solutions from assumptions which have greater validity.

Propositions

Formal operational children understand the proposition, ratios, etc. For example, they understand an increase in both sides will keep the equation balanced. W/L = 2W/2L.

Abstract rules

Formal operational thought is rational and systematic. For example, what number is 20 less than 3 times itself? They are capable of systematically deriving this problem.

$$X + 20 = 3X$$
$$20 = 3X - X$$
$$X = 10$$

Conservation of movement

Movement conservation develops simultaneously with the concept of volume. For example, the child understands that the movement of pendulum can be made faster or slower by decreasing or increasing the length of the string. Shorter the length, the faster is the movement. By 15 years of age, the child becomes sure that it is not the only factor affecting the speed of movement of the pendulum.

Implications

Teachers in primary school can use the valuable contribution in planning curriculum and teaching strategy for primary school children. As Piaget stated, the teacher's duty is to provide opportunities. In designing audiovisual teaching materials, Piaget contribution has immense value. Nurses can ideally plan play materials at hospitals while caring sick children according to their cognitive development. Parents can help promote quality of their child's intellectual development.

MORAL DEVELOPMENT

Etymologically, the term 'moral' is derived from the Latin word *morea*, meaning manners, customs and folkways. Moral behaviour refers to the behaviour of the members of a given culture which has been accepted and followed. Much of the work on the concept of moral development was done by Piaget (1932) and Kohlberg (1964).

Moral development occurs in children through sociocultural conditioning. At birth, no child has a conscience or scale of values. There are a set of core behaviour which are considered to be moral and another set of behaviours whose tacit disapproval is also moral. For example, not stealing is moral. Disapproval of stealing is also moral. It is a feeling of personal responsibility, and true morality is a slow and gradual process of development and extends into adolescence. Moral development has two components, namely intellectual and impulsive aspect. It refers to what is called right and wrong.

According to Piaget, there are two clear-cut stages:
1. Stage of moral realism or morality by constraint
2. Autonomous morality or morality by cooperation or reciprocity

In the first stage, automatic obedience to rules without reasoning or judgement occurs. Parents and all adults are omnipotent. Here, children judge an act as right or wrong in terms of consequences rather than in terms of motivations behind it.

In the second stage, children judge behaviour in terms of underlying intent or purpose. This stage occurs between 7 and 12 years of age. By 5–7 years of age, concepts of justice begin to change. The rigid and inflexible right and wrong notions are modified. So, they start to take considerations of specific circumstances related to moral violations. To a 5-year-old, lying is bad but for an 8-year-old lying is justified in certain circumstances and is not always necessarily bad. This stage coincides with Piaget's stage of formal operations in cognitive development. They take many factors in consideration for solving a problem.

Theories of Development at a Glance

Age Group	Psychosocial Theory (Erik Erikson)	Cognitive Theory (Piaget)	Psychosexual Theory (Freud)
Infancy	Age 0–18 months Trust vs mistrust (consistency of needs being met allows the infant to predict responses)	Age 0–2 years Sensorimotor (cannot learn without doing; has reflexive behaviour)	Age 0–6 months Oral passive (id develops; biological pleasure principle) Age 7–18 months Oral aggressive (teething begins; whatever comes in contact an object, the infant will be put into the mouth; oral satisfaction decreases anxiety)

Theories of Development at a Glance—cont'd

Age Group	Psychosocial Theory (Erik Erikson)	Cognitive Theory (Piaget)	Psychosexual Theory (Freud)
Toddlerhood	Age 18 months to 3 years Autonomy vs shame and doubt (desire to do things independently)	NA	Age 18 months to 3 years Anal (bowel and bladder training occurs; the child projects feelings on to others; elimination and retention are used to express anxiety
Preschool age	Age 3–6 years Initiative vs sense of guilt (mimics more purposeful and active in goal setting)	Age 2–4 years Preoperational–preconceptual (egocentric, animistic, and possesses magical thinking)	Age 4–5 years Phallic (ego develops) objective conscious reality; possesses Oedipal complex – love for the parent of the opposite sex
School age	Age 6–13 years Industry vs inferiority (using hands to make things; tries to master tasks)	Age 4–7 years Intuitive–preoperational (begins to use cause–effect reasoning) Age 7–11 years (concrete operations (collecting; mastering facts)	Age 6–12 years Latent Superego develops morality–sexual repression
Adolescence	Age 13–18 years Identity vs confusion (defining self in relation to others)	Age 11–15 years Formal operations (abstract ideas; reality-based)	NA

Kohlberg's Stages

Kohlberg elaborated on Piaget's theory to include three levels of moral development.

Level 1 – Preconventional morality. Here, the behaviour is subjected to external controls. This level is divided into two stages. In stage 1, the child is obedience–punishment oriented. The morality is judged in terms of physical consequences. In stage 2, the child conforms to the social expectations to gain rewards. There is some evidence of reciprocity and sharing, but it is based on battering rather than on a real sense of justice.

Level 2 – Conventional morality or of conventional rules and conformity. This level also has two stages. In stage 1, a good boy morality develops. The child conforms to rules to maintain good relations. In stage 2, children believe if the social group accepts rules as appropriate for all group members, they should also follow to avoid social disapproval.

Level 3 – Postconventional morality or morality of self accepted principles. This level is again divided into two stages. In stage 1, the child believes that there should be flexibility in moral beliefs so that it is modifiable to make it useful or advantageous to group members as a whole. In stage 2, the child conforms to both social standards and internalized ideals to avoid self-censure. Here, morality is based on respect rather than on personal desire.

Phases of Moral Development

There are two distinct phases. They are development of moral behaviour and development of moral concepts.

Development of moral behaviour – The child behave in a socially approved manner through trial and error by direct teaching. Here, direct teaching and identification are the best methods.

Development of moral concepts – The child learns principles of right and wrong in an abstract verbal form. So, teaching in moral principles can be given only when mental capacity is developed to generalize and transfer three principles of conduct from one situation to another.

Preschoolers are capable of abstract thinking. Good behaviour comprises specific acts such as obeying mothers, helping others, etc. and bad behaviour is not doing these things. In children aged 8–9 years, the concepts are generalized. They understand that stealing is wrong. But they don't understand that stealing a ball is wrong. This is because they understand general principles but not to specific context. Generalized moral concepts reflect social values (moral values). They are not static. They tend to change as social horizons broaden. By adolescence, the moral values are fairly developed.

Relation of Moral Development and Discipline

Discipline comes from the word 'disciple' – the one who learns from or voluntarily from a leader. Parents and teachers are leaders. The goal is to mould behaviour to conform to social and cultural norms of the society.

To some children, discipline is synonymous with punishment. With this concept, when children violate social norms that are put forward by adults of the society, they need to be punished. But the wrong behaviour of children is related to faculty training imparted to them by adults.

There are negative and positive disciplines. Negative concept is controlled by an external authority. Control is exercised through a distasteful and painful activity. Positive discipline is synonymous with education and counselling for inner growth of self-discipline and self-control. Consistency in providing discipline must be maintained and so also with reward and punishment.

- Discipline is essential to children's development because it fills certain of their needs. There are variations in the rate of development in children. So, discipline gives children a feeling of security by telling them what they may and may not do.

- Discipline helps children live according to standards approved by the social group by helping children avoid frequent feelings of guilt and misbehaviour.
- Discipline helps children have successful adjustment and happiness.
- Developmentally appropriate discipline helps ego-bolstering motivations which encourage children to accomplish what is required of them.
- Discipline helps children develop a conscience.
- Discipline has certain rules. Rules are essential to proper discipline. Rules restrain undesirable behaviour. Such disciplinary techniques are essential. Rules have educational values. Rules serve as the basis for moral concepts which helps develop moral codes of behaviour.

Punishment plays an important role in moral development by deterring repetition of socially undesirable behaviours. It tells what social group will tolerate or will not tolerate and motivates children to behave in a socially approved way. Just as punishment, rewards also function in moral development, as it provides appreciation of attachment. Rewards serves as a good form of motivation. Contradictory to this is bribery, which is a promise of rewards to induce good behaviours and loses its effectiveness unless its strength is constantly increased.

Three types of techniques are used in disciplining children. These are authoritative, democratic and permissive. Out of these three, democratic discipline is most acceptable, as it produces better results in all-round development of children.

Discipline provided can be evaluated so that it provides guidance for parents and other adults in disciplining techniques. The criteria used are the effects that a child has on his behaviour, on his attitude towards those in authority and discipline used and on his personality.

In disciplining children, one must remember that discipline and punishment are not synonymous. Inconsistency in disciplining, use of bribe and discrepancies between moral concepts and behaviour may lead to maladaptive behaviour in children.

THEORETICAL FOUNDATIONS OF LANGUAGE DEVELOPMENT

Children learn the intricate system of language with amazing speed. To develop a language, children should be born with intact physiological functions of the respiratory system, speech control centres of cerebral cortex, articulation and resonance structures of mouth and nasal cavities along with an intact and discriminating auditory apparatus, and intelligence to communicate a situation adequately.

Language is a form of communication. Speech is a form of oral communication. Learning to speak is a long and complex process. Children are born with the mechanism and capacity to develop speech and language skills. There are four components of language.

Phenology
Semantics
Syntax
Pragmatics

1. Phenology: This is the basic units of sound which are combined to produce words. Here, children learn to hear and to pronounce the speech like sounds peculiar to their language. Next, children learn the semantics of language, i.e. that words and sentences which are expressed to convey a meaning. Semantics leads to syntax and then the form or structure of language as pragmatics.

There are five stages of language development. First stage is **prelinguistic** stage – the period before the child utters the first meaningful words. This period is for the first 10–12 months of age. The second stage is **holophrastic** stage, where the speech consists of one-word utterance and represents the meaning of entire sentence. This begins at about 1 year of age. The third stage is **telegraphic** stage, where the speech consists of only content words, omitting less meaningful parts of speech. It begins at about 18–24 months of age. The fourth stage is the **preschool** period. The child begins to produce some very lengthy sentences, and speech increases in complexity. The fifth stage is the **middle childhood** period where children modify and refine their language skills and increase linguistic competence.

Theories Related to Language Development

There are three major theories related to language development. They are the learning theory, nativism and interactional approach.

- *Learning theory*: Language is acquired as children hear and respond to speech of their companions. But some believe that language is developed through operant conditioning as adults reinforce children in their attempt to produce grammatical speech. Some others believe that children learn language through imitation.
- *Nativism*: Here, it is believed that human beings have an inborn linguistic processor or language acquisition mechanism specialized for language development. Proponents of this theory believe that there is a critical period in language development between 2 years of age and puberty.
- *Interactional approach*: Proponents of this approach acknowledge that children are biologically prepared to acquire language and there must be development and maturation of the central nervous system for language development.

Stage of Language Development

The following chart represents, on an average, the age-wise language development. This is only a guideline for nurses. Most children acquire these developments at the upper range of age. Much of the language development is closely associated with hearing.

Language Development at a Glance

Period at the End of	Vocalization and Language
Birth to 3 months	Makes pleasure sounds (cooing, going) Cries differently for different needs Smiles when sees familiar face (especially the maternal figure)
4–6 months	Vocalization with information Responds to his/her name Responds to human voices without visual cues by turning his/her head and eyes Responds appropriately to friendly and angry tones Makes gurgling sounds when left alone and when playing with others
7–12 months	Uses one or more words with meaning (it can be a fragment of a word) Understands simple instructions, especially if vocal or physical cues are given Practices inflection Imitates different speech sounds Is aware of the social value of speech
13–18 months	Has vocabulary of approximately 5–20 words Vocabulary is made up chiefly of nouns Some amount of echolalia (repeating a word or phrase over and over) Much jargon with emotional content Is able to follow simple commands Puts two together (more biscuits, no milk, etc.) Uses some one- to two-word questions (What dada? Where mamma?)
19–24 months	Names numbering of objects common to his/her surroundings Is able to use at least two prepositions, usually chosen from the following: in, on, under Combines words into a short sentence – largely noun–verb combinations Approximately two-thirds of what a child says should be intelligible Vocabulary of approximately 150–300 words Rhythm and fluency often poor Volume and pitch of voice not well controlled Can use two pronouns correctly: I, me, you, although I and me are confusing My and mine are beginning to emerge Responds to such commands as 'Show me your eyes, nose, mouth, hair, etc.'
25–36 months	Uses pronouns 'I', 'me', 'you' correctly Uses some plurals and past tenses Knows at least three prepositions, usually in, on, under Knows chief parts of the body and should be able to indicate these if not their name Handles three-word sentences easily Has a vocabulary of 900–1000 words About 90% of what a child says should be intelligible Verbs begin to predominate in speech and understands most simple questions Able to reason out such questions as 'What must you do when you are sleepy, hungry, cool or thirsty?' Should not be expected to answer all questions, even though the child understands what is expected
37–48 months	Knows names of familiar animals Can use at least four prepositions Names common objects in picture books or magazines Knows one or more colours Can repeat four digits when they are pronounced slowly Understand such concepts as longer, larger, etc. Readily follows simple commands Uses a lot of sentences
49–60 months	Can use many descriptive words spontaneously Knows common opposites: big–small, hard–soft, heavy–light, etc. Has the concept of numbers of 4 or more Can count up to 10 Speech should be completely intelligible Should have all vowels and the consonants Should be able to repeat sentences as long as nine words Able to define common objects Tells stories that stick to the topic Says most sounds correctly, except a few such l, s, r, v, z, ch, etc. Understands today, yesterday and tomorrow

Continued

Language Development at a Glance—cont'd

Period at the End of	Vocalization and Language
6 years	In addition to the aforementioned, consonants such as *f*, *v*, *sh*, *zh*, *th*, *l*, etc. should be mastered
	Should have the concept of 7
	Speech should be completely intelligible and socially useful
	Able to tell a story connected to a picture
	Should be able to see relationship between objects
7 years	Should have mastered consonants
	Should handle opposites, analogies: girl–boy, man–woman, fly–swim, etc.
	Should be able to tell time to the quarter hour
	Should be able to do simple reading and write or copy many words
8 years	Can relate accounts of events, many of which occurred at some time in the past
	Complex and compound sentences can be used easily
	Should have few lapses in grammatical constructions – tense, pronouns, plurals, etc.
	Social amenities should be present in his/her speech in appropriate situations
	Control of rate, pitch and volume is generally well and appropriately established
	Can carry conversation at the adult level
	Has well-developed time and number concepts

Factors Affecting Language Development

- **Gender**
- **Order of birth**
- **No. of babies in a single delivery**
- Girls are more advanced in language development than boys.
- Firstborn develops language earlier than the second born.
- Children of multiple births acquire language later than those of single births.

Causes of Delayed Speech

- Congenital structural defects of mouth and nasopharynx and auditory problems
- Mental retardation
- Maternal deprivation
- Emotional factors
- Physiological and anatomical defects of organs related to speech development

SPIRITUAL DEVELOPMENT

It is closely related to moral development. To develop meaning, purpose and hope in life, people believe that there must be faith.

Fowler (1974) identified seven stages in the development of spirituality, five of which are closely related to cognitive and psychosocial development in children.

- Stage 0 – Undifferentiated: This period is infancy, where babies have no concepts of right or wrong, no beliefs and no conviction to guide their behaviour. Beginning to faith comes with the development of basic trust that there is somebody for me when I am in need.

- Stage 1 – Intuitive–Projective: Toddlerhood is a period where a child starts imitating others' behaviour. Children start showing religious gestures of adults without understanding the meaning or significance of the religious rituals. Parental attitude towards moral codes and religious beliefs is conveyed to children.
- Stage 2 – Mythical lateral: Schoolage where spiritual development parallels with cognitive development. It is relied to experience and interact with others. The existence of deity is accepted. The internal control of conscience is very active. They develop reverence towards thoughts and matters, and articulate their faith.
- Stage 3 – Synthetic–convention: Adolescent become increasingly aware of the spiritual disappointments. They identify that prayers are not always answered. Children start to question parent's religious standards. They develop or modify religious practices.
- Stage 4 – Individualising reflexive: Adolescence become more sceptical. They rationalise religious activities in an attempt to determine which one to adopt by comparing the religious beliefs in scientific context. They develop insights only late adolescence or early adulthood.

DEVELOPMENT OF SELF-CONCEPT

Self-concept comprises all the notions, beliefs and convictions that constitute children's knowledge of themselves and that influence their relationship with others (Whaley L F & Wong D L, 1996). Self-concept develops as a result of child's life experiences with significant persons. It is affected by cognitive ability and dominant motives of individuals coming in contact with stage-related cultural expectations. A child through different stages of life experiences differences in situations and forms and shapes his/her self-concept.

Body image is a vital component of self-concept. A positive body image without defect contributes to the development of positive self-concept where the child feels that he/she has worth and people around him/her appreciate his/her presence and activity. Positive strokes are necessary for the development of an appropriate self-concept. Continuous negative strokes and negative attitude psychologically hampers the child, and the child develops a feeling of worthlessness, leading to a negative self-concept.

GENDER PREFERENCE

From the time of birth, children are treated differently by their families on the basis of their biological sex. They are given male and female names, as well as made to wear male and female dresses, thus providing a sex-related attitude. Parental attitude towards appropriate sex-related behaviour also provides the baby a specific role related to gender. This gender label is achieved early in life by children imitating their parents. For example, preschooler wearing parents dress and imitating parental activities. Sex role standards begin in toddlerhood, and the preschoolers have a definite impression of masculinity and femininity, which is reflected in their overt make-believe play.

STUDY QUESTIONS

1. What are the developmental tasks of children?
2. Explain the cognitive development in preschool children.
3. What are secondary circular reactions?
4. Explain the development of language in infants.
5. Discuss Freud's theory of psychosexual development.
6. What is Oedipal complex? Give examples.
7. What is castration complex? Give its effects on development.
8. What is impact of self-concept development on children's development?
9. How gender preference affect personality of an individual?
10. How development of sexuality affect the personality and further life in children as adults?
11. What is the importance of spirituality in development of personality in children?
12. What are the factors affecting language development?
13. What are the theories related to language development?

BIBLIOGRAPHY

1. Betz, C.L. (March/April 1981). Faith development in children. Paediatric Nursing, 7, p. 22.
2. Bayely, N. (1933). Mental growth during the first three years. Genetic Psychological Monographs, 14, 1.
3. Berk, L. E. (2003). Child development. *Pearson Education* (6th ed.). Boston: Allyn/Bacon.
4. Erikson, E.H. (1963). Childhood and society. 2nd Edn. WW Norton: New York.
5. Castiglia, P. T. (May/June 1987). Speech-Language Development. *Journal of Pediatric Health Care*, 1:165.
6. Frankenburg, W.K., Dodds, J.B. (1967). The Denver developmental screening test. Journal of Pediatrics, 71, p 181.
7. Illingworth, R.S. (1982). Basic developmental screening. 3rd Edn. Blackwell: Oxford.
8. Knobloch, H., Stevens, F., Malone, A. (1980). Manual of child development. Harper and Row: Hagerstown.
9. Kohlberg, L. (1968). Moral development. In: Sills, D.L. (Ed). International encyclopedia of the social sciences. Macmillan: New York.
10. Levine, M. D., Carey, W. B., Croker, A. C. (1999). Developmental-Behavioral Pediatrics. (3rd Edn). WB Saunders: Philadelphia.
11. Piaget, J. (1969). The theory of stages in cognitive development. McGraw Hill: New York.
12. Stuart, G.W., Laraia, M.T. (2000). Principles and practice of pediatric nursing. 7th Edn. Mosby: St. Louis.

CHAPTER 17

DEVELOPMENTAL AND BEHAVIOURAL PROBLEMS IN CHILDREN

LEARNING OBJECTIVES

At the end of the chapter, the learner will be able to:
- Describe various developmental and behavioural problems in childhood.
- Identify the various types of management including multimodal therapy,
- Provide family-centred care to children and family suffering from developmental and behavioural problems.

Diagnosing and treating behavioural and developmental problems in children are difficult owing to their developmental stages. A male child of 5 years may say that he is Superman and he can fly and will kill a dragon that harms human beings. A health care professional should be able to distinguish these verbalizations from delusions to the normal development of a preschooler in the make-believe play. When a child says that somebody is telling him/her to do bad things or not to do bad things, it must also be differentiated from the inner voice of conscience. One must be able to discern the differences of such symptoms.

ENURESIS (BED-WETTING)

The first reference on enuresis may be found in the Ebers papyrus of 1550 BC. In 1472, Paulus Bagellardus of Padua published the first book on diseases of children, including a chapter titled 'On Incontinence of Urine and Bedwetting'. Enuresis is a common and troublesome condition which needs a lot of patience on the part of parents and caregivers. It is defined as repeated voiding of urine during day or night into bed or clothes. The exact definition of enuresis has been revised over the years. Enuresis is located under intermittent incontinence by the International Children's Continence Society (ICCS) in 2014. The term 'enuresis' is used to describe night-time intermittent incontinence. 'Enuresis nocturna' is used to provide extra clarity.

Usually, enuresis is involuntary and sometimes intentional. Clinically, with regard to bed-wetting, the individual must reach an age at which continence is expected. Thus, the chronological and developmental ages must be at least 5 years. Enuresis is classified as primary or secondary. Primary enuresis is seen in children who have established urinary continence for a period and then develop incontinence. This incontinence is nocturnal (night-time sleep), diurnal (during waking hours) or both times of the day.

Monosymptomatic enuresis: This results in children without any other lower urinary tract symptoms and without a history of bladder dysfunction. Children who have never achieved a satisfactory period of night-time dryness have primary enuresis; children who develop enuresis after a dry period of at least 6 months have secondary enuresis.

Nonmonosymptomatic enuresis: This is common in children with other lower urinary tract symptoms (e.g. increased frequency, daytime incontinence, urgency, genital or lower urinary tract pain).

Incidence

Enuresis reported at the age of 5 years is 7% in male children and 3% in female children. At the age of 10 years, the prevalence is 3% in male children and 2% in female children.

Usually, enuresis do not coexist with other mental disorders but the prevalence of mental disorders in these children are little higher than that in the general population. Enuresis can cause mental and emotional problems in children, especially in adolescents, when it results in being ostracized from other children and adults.

Aetiology

Occasionally, enuresis can develop from physiological or structural abnormalities of the urinary tract rather than an emotional cause. However, in most of the cases, no clear aetiology is known. The causes of bed-wetting is hypothesized to be related to genetics, sleep arousal dysfunction, maturational delay, stress, poor toilet training, altered smooth muscle physiology and, occasionally, organic causes.

Predictive factors noted are as follows:
- Prolonged periods of sleep during infancy
- Positive family history
- Slower rate of physical development in children up to 3 years of age
- Monozygotic twins more prone to enuresis than dizygotic ones
- 75% of all children having functional enuresis have a first-degree relative who have or had this disorder

Pathophysiology

Enuresis is primarily an alteration of neuromuscular bladder functioning and is self-limiting without producing any consequences. For children, it is a temporary self-regulating behaviour, especially after the birth of a younger sibling. However, for others, it is an occasional accident. In some children, it may be related to problem of toilet training such as rigid training or too early training or even excessive dependence on parents.

Proposed Theories of Enuresis

- Sleep theory: This theory states that children with enuresis find it difficult to wake up from sleep and thus void during sleep. However, electroencephalographic monitoring of depth of sleep has disproved this theory.
- Functional capacity: Some children with enuresis have a smaller bladder capacity than nonaffected children.
- Nocturnal polyuria theory: It suggests that kidneys of these children fail to concentrate urine during sleep hours owing to insufficient amount of antidiuretic hormone. Research on this field shows some evidence of this, too.
- Dysfunctional detrusion theory: This theory proposes that an unstable bladder detrusor muscle spontaneously contract during sleep, leading to enuresis.

Clinical Manifestations

Most children experience an urgency that is immediate and distressing. Children express their inability to be wakeful to urinate during sleep. Spontaneous remission occurs in 15% of children.

Diagnosis

Routine physical examination rules out physiological and structural abnormalities. A thorough history taking reveals that familial tendencies are essential. Assess functional bladder capacity, too. A bladder volume of 300–350 mL is sufficient to hold a night's urine.

Therapeutic Management

For treating enuresis, a combination of techniques is used. Guidelines for the management of enuresis propose a two-step approach. If the basic workup is normal, it is recommended to treat constipation, regulate eating and drinking habits and reassure children and families that this is common and that there is no serious medical problem. These are all part of the initial management and the ICCS named it as urotherapy. If this unsuccessful, the second line of management is initiated. This includes a detailed day- and night-time urinary diary. This helps identify whether the patient has truly monosymptomatic nocturnal enuresis (with no daytime issues) and also provides more data about bladder capacity and night-time urine volume. For monosymptomatic enuresis, more aggressive therapy can be considered such as operant conditioning using alarms.

- Conditioning therapy: It involves training the child to awaken after a stimulus such as urine alarm is given. This alarm consists of a moisture-sensitive buzzer with a wire pad. The urine pad is kept inside the underpants. When the system detects urine, the buzzer sounds which fully awakens the child. A 75% success rate has been reported with this treatment. Alarm therapy increases nocturnal bladder capacity in those children who become dry. It is has a response rate of 60%, and the long-term success rate is reported to be 43%.
- **Desmopressin:** It is a synthetic analogue of arginine vasopressin, which reduces urine output. Desmopressin decreases urine volume at night. It is available as an intranasal spray and as tablet formulations for the treatment of primary nocturnal enuresis for many years. Now desmopressin lyophilisate (MELT) formulation is available as convenient, sublingual oral preparation. Desmopressin therapy has a response rate of 70% during the treatment period. Discontinuation of therapy causes a high relapse rate, which can reach up to 60%. Hypercalciuria is a cause for nonresponders and may become desmopressin responders after using a low-calcium diet. The children with a small bladder capacity may be treated with oxybutynin (anticholinergic) as the drug of choice.
- Retention control training (RCT): RCT was initiated for children with a reduced functional bladder

capacity. The child drinks fluids and delays urination as long as he/she can tolerate in order to stretch the bladder to accommodate increasingly larger volumes of urine. Along with this, the child practices pelvic exercises. Other modalities of treatment include drug therapy and walking schedule where children are awakened at different intervals at night to void. The common drugs used are tricyclic antidepressants and antidiuretics.

The management of secondary nocturnal enuresis involves addressing the underlying stressor. Most of the children with secondary enuresis have no identifiable cause and are treated like children with primary enuresis.

Nursing Considerations

Discuss with parents and children the problems related to enuresis, treatment plan and probable difficulties.

- The nurse should try to get the active participation of children in the treatment plan.
- Teach the use of alarms to children and parents. Inform the parents how to make children in charge of alarms and safety measures.
- Instruct the effects and side effects of desmopressin and oxybutynin.
- Keeping a diary of wet and dry nights helps determine the effect of interventions.
- The nurse should help the child to follow a schedule for voiding during day and just before going to the bed.
- Instruct to avoid high-sugar and caffeine-based drinks, especially during evening hours.
- See that the daily fluid intake to be divided as follows: 40% of the intake should be in the morning hours (7 a.m. to 12 noon), 40% in the afternoon (12 noon to 5 p.m.) and 20% in the evening after 5 p.m.
- Discourage the use of diapers and pull-ups, as it will interfere with the motivation to get up for urination.
- The nurse should try to reduce the emotional trauma of the parents, as most parents believe that enuresis is an emotional disturbance and may be related to their faulty childrearing practices. Parents must be given reassurance that bed-wetting is not a manifestation of emotional disturbance as such.
- Parents must be informed that scolding, shaming, threatening or punishing a child with enuresis will produce a negative emotional impact and must be avoided.
- Supportive and understanding nature of parents contributes to the success of management.
- The nurse should try to relieve the feeling of shame, fear and ostracizing from children with an attitude of compassion. The psychological effects of nocturnal enuresis are significant. It has been found that the children who do bed-wetting have low self-esteem and there is improved self-esteem after successful treatment.
- It is important for the nurse to identify the everyday dilemmas of the parents of children with enuresis. The parents of these children use two main patterns of coping: unworried 'wet-bed fixers' and anxious 'night launderers'. The latter group cannot talk about enuresis publicly, thereby avoiding the thought that their child has psychological problems. They require psychological support. The main reason for providing treatment of enuresis is to avoid the negative impact of enuresis on social life and psychological status and also to improve self-esteem.
- The nurse should motivate children who are willing to accept some responsibility for the treatment. They should be motivated to keep a record of their progress. They must be rewarded according to the amount of activities carried out based on promises made.

ENCOPRESIS

Encopresis is called faecal incontinence. It is the repeated, involuntary or intentional passage of faeces into inappropriate places, e.g. in clothing or on the floor. Encopresis is considered only when a child's development and chronological age is at least 4 years, and it must occur once in a month for 3 months. Encopresis can be primary or secondary.

1. Primary: This occurs when the child has never acquired bowel control by 4 years of age.
2. Secondary: This occurs after a period of established bowel continuance by children 4 years of age.

It can be frustrating for parents and embarrassing for children.

Aetiology

Constipation precipitated by environmental changes such as the birth of a new sibling, moving to a new house, changing school or unfamiliar situation. Voluntary retention usually takes place in this situation, followed by a fear–pain cycle. This results in a learned process of abnormal defecation patterns.

Some causes of constipation include:
- Withholding stool owing to fear of using the toilet (especially when away from home) or because stools are painful
- Not wanting to interrupt play or other activities
- Eating too little fibre
- Not drinking enough fluids
- Drinking too much cow's milk or, rarely, an intolerance to cow's milk – though research shows conflicting results on these issues

Psychogenic encopresis is caused by emotional problems usually related to a disturbed mother–child relationship, divorce of a parent, birth of a sibling, difficult and premature toilet training, etc.

Children with encopresis will have large-bored stools which are painful and that lead them to withstand stool in contrast to normal soft stools of other children. Hardness of stool results from withholding stool in the rectum and sigmoid colon, where it loses its water content. Additional pressure of schooling and fear of using school bathrooms also cause encopresis in certain children.

Clinical Manifestation

A period of voluntary retention, followed by painful stooling, results in blood in stools. Involuntary retention is associated with a history of abdominal pain, distention, moodiness, poor appetite and accumulation of stools with periodic passing of voluminous stools. Children display particular posturing during suppression of colonic signals to defecate such as stiffening, standing in a corner with straight legs, hiding behind furniture and bright face and doing less dancing (movement). Leakage of stool or liquid stool on underwear, which can be mistaken for diarrhoea; constipation with dry, hard stool; passage of large stool that clogs or almost clogs the toilet; avoidance of bowel movements; repeated bladder infections, typically in girls, etc. also are seen. Psychologically, they are ashamed and wish to avoid environmental changes that may lead to embarrassment. Encopresis may damage self-esteem and self-concept and is directly related to ostracism by peers.

Treatment

It is directed towards the cause of stooling. Diet, lubricants and toilet rituals are promoted for developing normal defecation habits. Faecal impaction is relieved by catharsis, suppositories and mineral oils. Customary dosages are usually insufficient. Diets containing high fibre are advised. Increased fluid and fruit intake is also recommended.

Nursing Considerations

A detailed history to find outcomes and nursing interventions are related to the cause. Education regarding physiology of normal defecation, toilet-training process and implementation of proper treatment regimen are important concerns. Proper counselling to reduce the parent–child conflict is also essential.

DISORDERS WITH BEHAVIOURAL COMPONENT

Conduct Disorder

Childhood psychiatric problems are on the rise. Conduct disorder (CD) is one of the common psychiatric illnesses seen in children. The most common hallmark of CD is evident callous disregard for societal norms, and children feel they get a thrill out of causing harm to others. They feel happy for their bad behaviour and that is gratifying to them. One needs to be very careful to decide whether the child has CD or not, as children and adolescence normally have some level of acting-out behaviours. This psychiatric syndrome occurs in childhood and adolescence. It is characterized by a long-standing pattern of violations of rules and antisocial behaviour. According to the *Diagnostic and Statistical Manual of Mental Disorders*, 4th ed. (DSM-IV), symptoms typically include aggression, frequent lying, running away from home overnight and destruction of property.

Aetiology

Aetiology is multifactorial, including biologic, psychosocial ad familial factors. An interaction of genetic/constitutional and familial factors is attributed to the aetiology. Children with CD inherit decreased baseline autonomic nervous system activity. So they require greater stimulation to achieve optimal arousal.

Hereditary factors account for a high level of sensation-seeking activity associated with CD. Current research is concentrating to identify the role of neurotransmitters in aggression behaviours.

Clinical Features

Four types of symptoms are identified:
(1) Aggression or serious threats of harm to people or animals
(2) Deliberate property damage or destruction (e.g. fire setting, vandalism)
(3) Repeated violations of household or school rules, laws, or both
(4) Persistent lying to avoid consequences or to obtain tangible goods or privileges

Other accompanying features are inability to appreciate the importance of others' welfare and little guilt or remorse about harming others. Associated features include:

Inability to appreciate the importance of others' welfare

Little guilt or remorse about harming others

Outwardly verbalizing remorse to obtain favour or avoid punishment

View others as threatening or malicious without an objective basis

Unprovoked aggression

Mild: Few if any conduct problems in excess of those required to make a diagnosis, and conduct problems cause only minor harm to others.

Moderate: Number of conduct problems and effect on others intermediate between 'mild' and 'severe'.

Severe: Many conduct problems in excess of those required to make the diagnosis or conduct problems cause considerable harm to others.

There are two subtypes of CD, namely childhood-onset and adolescent-onset CDs. Childhood-onset CD if remains untreated, it has a poor prognosis. Forty per cent of this subtype develop into antisocial personality disorder in adulthood. Adolescent-onset CD should be looked in a social context. Adolescents exhibiting CD for survival needs are often less psychologically disturbed than those with early childhood behaviour disorders.

Risk Factors

Family history: Children with a parent or sibling having CD are more likely develop CD

Biological parents with attention-deficit/hyperactivity disorder (ADHD), alcoholism, depression, bipolar disorder or schizophrenia

Children who are abused and maltreated

Harsh and inconsistent parenting

Exposed to witness violence in the neighbourhood and experienced peer delinquency or peer rejection

Diagnosis

The primary diagnostic features are aggression, theft, vandalism, lying and violations of rules. To conclude a diagnosis of CDs, these symptoms should occur for at least a 6-month period. Differential diagnosis includes oppositional defiant disorder (ODD), ADHD, mood disorder and intermittent explosive disorder. Diagnosis requires persistent multiple behaviours (at least three).

DSM-IV Diagnostic Criteria for Conduct Disorder

A repetitive and persistent pattern of behaviours in which the basic rights of others or major age-appropriate societal norms or rules are violated, as manifested by the presence of three (or more) of the following criteria in the past 12 months, with at least one criterion present in the past 6 months:

Aggression to people and/or animals:
1. Often bullies, threatens or intimidates others
2. Often initiates physical fights
3. Has used a weapon that can cause serious physical harm to others (e.g. a bat, brick, broken bottle, knife, gun)
4. Has been physically cruel to people
5. Has been physically cruel to animals
6. Has stolen while confronting a victim (e.g. mugging, purse snatching, extortion, armed robbery)
7. Has forced someone into sexual activity

Destruction of property:
1. Has deliberately engaged in fire setting with the intention of causing serious damage
2. Has deliberately destroyed others' property (other than by fire setting)

Deceitfulness or theft:
1. Has broken into someone else's house, building or car
2. Often lies to obtain goods or favours or to avoid obligations (i.e. 'cons' others)
3. Has stolen items of nontrivial value without confronting the victim (e.g. shoplifting, but without breaking and entering; forgery)

Serious violations of rules:
1. Often stays out at night despite parental prohibitions, beginning before the age of 13 years
2. Has run away from home overnight at least twice while living in a parental or parental surrogate home (or once without returning for a lengthy period)
3. Is often truant from school, beginning before the age of 13 years

The disturbance in behaviour causes clinically significant impairment in social, academic or occupational functioning.

If the individual is 18 years or older, criteria are not met for antisocial personality disorder.

(Diagnostic and statistical manual of mental disorders. 4th ed. Washington, D.C.: American Psychiatric Association, 1994:90–1. Copyright 1994)

Treatment

Management of CD is not so easy. Treatment requires a team effort for an effective support network. It will be manageable if there is a dedicated group of parents, teachers, peers and voluntary groups to provide support.

Psychotherapy

Children with CD usually present with a negative attitude. Psychotherapy and behavioural therapy are given for pronged periods of time. The entire family is brought into the loop. Parent management training can be given by the therapist to make parents learns better ways of communication to such children for desired behaviours. For younger children, treatment of CD is similar to ODD. Adolescents may be trained to develop better interactions with authority figures at school and ensure better peer relations that are not harmful. Pharmacological management may be required for associated conditions.

Nursing Management

A nurse is a team member in the treatment process. Encouraging parents and children to participate in psychotherapy and behaviour modification training and to administer pharmacotherapy as prescribed are very important nursing responsibilities. Along with this, the nurse may assist the parents in continuing treatment of their children. The nurse can be instrumental in assessing the severity of illness and can refer the children for further management. The nurse can help parents structure children's activities and implement consistent behaviour guidelines. Emphasizing parental monitoring of children's activities (where they are, who they are with) and encouraging the enforcement of curfew can be considered. The nurse can encourage children's involvement in structured and supervised peer activities (e.g. organized sports, scouting). The nurse can discuss and demonstrate clear and specific parental communication techniques, help caregivers establish appropriate rewards for desirable behaviour, and help establish realistic, clearly communicated consequences. For noncompliance, the nurse can help establish daily routine of child-directed play activity with parent(s). Consider pharmacotherapy for children who are highly aggressive or impulsive, or both, or those with a mood disorder.

Attention-Deficit/Hyperactivity Disorder

'Attention-deficit/hyperactivity disorder' is the term used to describe a persistent pattern of inattention or hyperactivity–impulsivity that is more frequent and severe than is typically observed in individuals at a comparable level of development. It is usually present before the age of 7 years and is more commonly identified in school children (3%–5%). Boys are more commonly affected than girls. Difficulties are related to schooling, behavioural or academic activities or even related to social relationships. Early identification of affected children is essential, as it interferes with normal life. Attempts to cope with attention deficit lead to maladaptive behaviour in these children, which evokes negative responses from others that adversely affect their behavioural development. Prompt identification and treatment of ADHD are a growing public health concern. The attention-deficit disorder is a disorder that can continue to adulthood (DSMV-IV). Children with ADHD have self-esteem, poor peer relationships, delinquencies and substance abuse disorder.

In sex chromosome disorders such as Turner syndrome, children show impaired spatial abilities and right and left directional senses. Children with Klinefelter syndrome have learning, behavioural and peer problems. A concept of developmental lag is attributed to these children. Distractibility, short attention span and impulsiveness are all normal characteristics of children at a much younger developmental level. Symptoms of ADHD do not change with age. Usual symptoms persist from adolescence up to adulthood in 50%–60% of children.

Biochemical aetiology of ADHD suggests a relationship with the effect of central nervous system (CNS) stimulant drugs. Studies have proved that epinephrine and neurotransmitters, which control activity level, mood and awareness, are insufficient in ADHD. CNS stimulants that increase epinephrine levels have proved to be effective in controlling such behavioural problems.

Clinical Manifestations

These children do not have normal behaviour like their peers. There is a difference in quality of motor activity, developmentally inappropriate attention, impulsivity and hyperactivity. Most behavioural problems appear at an earlier age, before entering the school. Clinically, there are three types of ADHD. In combined type, the symptoms are predominantly inattentive and hyperactive. In this type, six or more symptoms of inattention, hyperactivity and impulsiveness are persistent for more than 6 months. In predominantly inattentive type, six or more symptoms of inattentiveness will be present along with fewer symptoms of hyperactivity and impulsiveness. In predominantly hyperactive type, six or more symptoms of hyperactivity and a few symptoms of inattention are present.

Diagnosis

Symptoms of inattention and hyperactivity are present in varying degrees. A history of both medical and development is also of help. Physical examination with detailed neurological assessment and psychological testing is also required. To be diagnosed with one of the categories of ADHD, a person must have six of the nine symptoms in at least two settings such as school/classroom and home. The symptoms must be present for at least 6 months. It should not be explained by other psychiatric disorders, too.

Aetiology

Aetiology is uncertain, obscure and often speculative. It can be related to injury or trauma or illness affecting brain at any stage of development, before, during or after birth. Multiple causes including psychological factors are attributed. Sex-linked factors operate in this disorder. Children and adolescents who have survived encephalitis lethargica and von Economo disease have postencephalitic behavioural syndrome similar to ADHD.

It is a genetically transmitted neurobiological disorder of the dopaminergic and noradrenergic pathways. So they have a high genetic rate of 50% in concordance with first-degree relatives. ADHD affects 6%–9% of children, and one-third to two-thirds of children continue to have it as adults.

Treatment

A multiple approach is used (multimodal therapy):
- Family education
- Counselling
- Medication
- Proper classroom placement
- Environmental manipulation
- Behavioural and psychotherapy

Medications usually included are sympathomimetic amines – methylphenidate (Ritalin) or dextroamphetamines (Dexedrine). These drugs produce strong effect on CNS dopamine or norepinephrine. Methylphenidate is preferred, as it does not produce much effect on prolactin and growth hormone. Tricyclic antidepressants are also used. Regularly scheduled revaluation is necessary.

Psychosocial Therapy

The primary treatment is pharmacotherapy, and accessory symptoms are benefited from psychosocial interventions.

Nursing Considerations

The following points need to be considered:
- Family counselling
- Medication administration
- Environmental manipulation
- Appropriate classroom placement
- Psychiatric, psychological and social therapies

Oppositional Defiant Disorder

This disorder is difficult to distinguish from CD. Contrary to the features of aggressiveness in CD, these children show argumentativeness, noncompliance with rules and negativism. They are less likely to have a history of problems with the law. Parents of children with ODD often show mood disorders compared with an antisocial pattern common among parents of children with CD. But children with ODD can develop CD in due course of time.

Childhood Depression

It is a clinical syndrome characterized by a persistent mood disorder and dysfunctional behaviour. Findings include sadness or unhappiness, social withdrawal, eating problems, sleeping disorders, loss of interest in usual activities and decreased ability to concentrate.

Incidence

In the general population, the incidence rate is 2% and depression accounts for 30% of childhood psychological disorders.

Aetiology

Multifactorial. Certain specific disease states are associated with depression (e.g. epilepsy, hypothyroidism, adrenal insufficiency, migraine, etc.). Assessment should include a detailed history from home and school regarding cause of the symptoms, and degree of dysfunction should be elicited. Assessment for learning disabilities should also be done. History about social withdrawal, mood, appetite, sleep patterns and irritability should be taken. A family history of depression also needs to be elicited. A complete physical assessment to identify and rule out organic causes is essential.

Management

It includes psychotherapy for the child and family and administration of antidepressant medications as prescribed.

Childhood Schizophrenia

Schizophrenia is a chronic psychotic disorder, with a prevalence of 4.6% worldwide. It is a devastating, neuropsychiatric problem. Deficits in cognition, behaviour and social functioning are marked. The onset is between the ages of 14–35 years. In total, 50% of cases are diagnosed before 25 years of age. The onset of schizophrenia before the ages of 13 years is referred as childhood schizophrenia or prepubertal or early-onset schizophrenia.

It is a syndrome of grossly impaired behaviour characterized by disturbance of thought, perception and relationship to the external world. Deterioration from previous levels of functioning, duration of at least 6 months, often loose associations, delusions and hallucinations are the main features. Childhood schizophrenia typically occurs after the age of 7 years and increases in frequency up to adolescence.

Aetiology

Schizophrenia is multifactorial, involving social, environmental and emotional stressors in a child with a genetic predisposition or a biologic vulnerability, or both. Genetic risk is well established with a high prevalence among first-degree relatives. Certain medical conditions are associated with childhood psychosis such as Wilson disease, thyroid disease and systemic lupus erythematosus. The young relatives of patients with schizophrenia show an increased rate of Axis I psychopathology (e.g. ADHD, CD), soft neurological signs and a high level of outwardly expressed emotions.

Diagnosis

According to DSM-V, diagnosis of schizophrenia requires two of the following conditions: delusions, hallucinations, disorganized speech, grossly disorganized or catatonic behaviour or negative symptoms such as affective flattening or paucity of thought or speech. To meet diagnostic criteria, symptoms must be present for at least 6 months (including at least 1 month of active symptoms); must result in deterioration in social, school-related and self-care functioning; and should not be accounted for by a diagnosis of schizoaffective disorder, a mood disorder, a substance use disorder or general medical conditions. The clinician should also be aware of the developmental, cultural and intellectual factors for an accurate diagnosis.

Assessment should include an essential history to determine child's current status, evidence of delusions, hallucinations and a family history of mental illness. Physical assessment should be conducted for identifying the organic causes (drug ingestion, thyroid dysfunction, etc.). Laboratory investigations should include urine testing for toxic substances, liver function tests and serum levels of ceruloplasmin to rule out Wilson disease. Psychometric tests should also be included.

Management

Course of childhood schizophrenia is chronic, and a number of treatments should be included such as antipsychotic medications, psychotherapy, support to child and family and specific education programmes. The first-line management in pharmacotherapy is with neuroleptics. Agitated children with schizophrenia are given benzodiazepine to alleviate the anxiety. The child's weight must be monitored carefully, along with blood pressure, glucose and lipid levels. For adults with schizophrenia, there are definitive guidelines for monitoring, but it is not yet developed for children. Children treated with chlorpromazine and thioridazine should be monitored and checked for retinopathy and lenticular changes.

Psychosocial Care

Children with schizophrenia require multimodal care. These include social skills training, supportive environment and structured, individualized special education programmes to make them fit to live in the society. Supportive psychotherapy to encourage reality testing and help the child monitor warning signs of impending relapse is very important. Cognitive behavioural therapy that is highly successful for adults can be used with children to help them cope. Children and adolescents who have drug addiction should also be referred for de-addiction treatment. Psychosocial intervention involves altering the environment that is stress producing to minimize undue stress. Identify factors that deteriorate the child's condition, and remove or minimize such factors. Parents, teachers and relatives must be involved to identify the child's progression towards psychosis. Parents and caregivers should be empowered to simplify the environment that is stressful for the child.

A team approach should be followed including a psychologist, a geneticist, a nurse, a paediatrician and a psychiatrist. Because there is cognitive impairment, IQ test must be done. A child neurologist and a geneticist should be consulted to evaluate possible organic causes.

Diet

Typical and atypical antipsychotic medications increase appetite. This may cause excess weight gain. Low-calorie snacks and limitation of total intake of food at meals may help reduce appetite and thereby decrease weight gain. Weight and body mass index should be monitored regularly. Food-containing omega-3 polysaturated fatty acids have been found to have preventive effect on schizophrenia.

Long-term Care

Children with schizophrenia need to be followed up for recurrence of positive symptoms such as hallucinations and delusions. These may be signs of relapse or warning of negative symptoms. Monitor these children for maniac symptoms, as about 15%–20% of children with initial diagnosis of schizophrenia develop bipolar disorder.

SPECIFIC LEARNING DISORDERS

Learning disorders refer to a heterogeneous group of disorders manifested by significant difficulties in the acquisition and use of listening, speaking, reading, writing, reasoning or mathematical abilities.

These can be seen as maturational and developmental problems or can occur (despite a good educational foundation) even in a child who appears to have a normal intelligence. Learning disorders may occur as discrete disorders limited to one or more learning modalities such as reading, mathematics, expression or reception of language and coordination, which may be substantially lower than expected for that particular age. These disorders are intrinsic to the individual and presumed to occur as a result of CNS dysfunction. These disabilities are occasionally described with reference to academic performance they affect (e.g. dyslexia for difficulty in reading; dyscalculia for difficulty in mathematics, dysgraphia for difficulty in writing). It can also affect the psychological process, leading to deficits in the auditory processing, visual motor integration, sequential memory or executive functioning.

Aetiology

No specific aetiology has been identified. However, aetiological hypothesis includes CNS damage, individual human variation, toxins and environmental factors.

Management

A complete assessment, which includes review of the perinatal course, evidence of medical problems (chronic otitis media), early developmental history, family history and review of school functioning, should be conducted. Physical assessment should be done for probing minor neurological ailments; computed tomographic scan may be done in suspected cases of brain damage. A comprehensive battery of tests is needed to establish learning disorders. These include IQ test, hand–eye coordination, auditory and visual perceptions, comprehension and memory test, etc.

Special training programmes are needed for these children in school. The problem needs to be defined by a remediation teacher or psychologist. The nurse is required to explain to parents and the class teacher about the learning disorders that the child has, explain them about what sort of attention needs to be paid in such a case, instruct them to introduce home-based remedial teaching measures and provide emotional support to the child and family through counselling. Follow-up should be instituted.

SCHOOL PHOBIA

School failure is a very common presenting problem. There are many cases of school fear or separation anxiety as a result of which a child may not like to leave home. As a rule, children below the age of 13 years having school phobia are anxious about separation from loved ones at home.

Children with school phobia present a wide variety of physical and emotional problems. The physical symptoms include headache, nausea, vomiting, anorexia, dizziness, leg pain or even abdominal pain; 'absenteeism' will be quite common among these children. The typical scenario involves a passive and dependent child who encounters an additional stressor (e.g. illness, school problems or death of a loved one).

Aetiology

School phobia is caused by a variety of factors.
Fear of mismatched overcritical teachers; fear of failing in examination; separation anxiety
Physical limitations, such as hearing impairment or visual defect

Management

Children with school phobia are not delinquent children. They actually want to attend school. They are anxious, worried and discontented. They are unable to master the courage to face the school in a normal sense.

School in a normal sense. Children should be counselled to cope with mismatched, irrational or overcritical teachers. Once they get help to cope positively, the problems can be solved. Some children may need psychiatric consultation. Physical problems such as visual or hearing difficulty need to be rectified. Short-term use of anti-anxiety medications is found to be useful.

Nursing Considerations

The nurse should explain to the parents the necessity of keeping children at school. If a child is kept away from school for a longer period, more problems may arise for re-entry into the school. As soon as possible, children need to be encouraged to re-enter the school. Counselling of parents is essential. The attending physician and the nurse should insist on immediate return to school, to avoid the long gap that promotes absenteeism, once physical symptoms of the child subsides.

Children with severe symptoms may be allowed to attend school on a part-time basis (in-between) after counselling sessions.

Prevention

School phobia related to separation anxiety can be prevented if the child is separated for short periods in his/her early life. From infancy, the baby can be kept with a surrogate person (grandparents) for a few hours. A toddler can also be kept away from parents during daytime. Preschooler can be kept with others for a day. Sending children to nursery school also helps avoid fears of separation. Parents creating an interest in school activities also help reduce fears. Parents sharing their school experiences may resolve *first-day* problems at school.

RECURRENT ABDOMINAL PAIN

Recurrent abdominal pain (RAP) is defined as three or more separate episodes of abdominal pain during a 3-month period. It is one of the somatic complaints of childhood with a psychogenic aetiology. It can also be of psychometric or organic aetiology.

Incidence

In total, 10%–20% of school-aged children experience a peak incidence at 10–12 years of age. Girls are slightly more affected than boys.

Aetiology

Organic causes include bowel inflammation, appendicitis, lactose intolerance, peptic ulcer, pelvic inflammation or urinary tract infection.

Functional abdominal pain may result from dyskinesia Davidson M, 1987 or dymotility (Cloeman W & Levine M 1986) of multifactorial origin.

Multifactorial causes attribute to somatic factors, lifestyle, habits, diet and temperament.

RAP is usually seen in high achievers whose parents have high expectations from them.

Clinical Features

Children will have real pain initially in the periumbilical or epigastric region. Other symptoms to accompany include vomiting, flushing, pallor, dizziness and fatigue.

A complete physical examination, laboratory investigations and family history are required. A family history may show evidence of hereditary predisposition. A complete evaluation will help rule out organic causes. Pain needs to be assessed for location, quality, frequency and other exacerbating factors.

Treatment

Usually, hospitalization is necessary. If the pain is related to organic causes, treatment will be directed towards it.

Alleviating discomfort related to precipitating factors is also needed. Usual recommendations are high-fibre diet, antispasmodic drugs and reassurance.

Nursing Considerations

Assisting for investigations and taking history. Identifying predisposing factors, educating the parents and children, providing reassurance, etc. are few of the major considerations.

OTHER RECURRENT PAIN SYNDROMES

These include headache and limb pain.

Headache

It may be a result of medical causes such as infection, increased blood pressure owing to various reasons, neurological causes such as migraine, increased intracranial pressure (ICP), vascular abnormalities and psychological causes.

The more localized the pain, the less likely it is to be psychogenic. Determination of blood pressure, assessment of visual field and a thorough funduscopic examination are essential. If organic causes are detected, treatment should be directed to the cause.

Limb Pain

It can be a result of orthopaedic disorders (e.g. Osgood–Schlatter disease, Legg–Calvé–Perthes disease, trauma), collagen vascular disease, infection, neoplastic diseases, etc. The more localized the pain, the less likely it is to be growing pains. Physical examination should be conducted with a detailed assessment of the affected limb to exclude atrophy, swelling, weakness and effusion. If an organic disease is identified, treatment should be directed towards the cause.

PICA

It refers to eating nonedible substances such as earth, dust, clay, chalk, flakes of paint and plaster from wall, fabrics, etc.

Children are often anaemic and may manifest associated deficiencies of minerals and vitamins. Other associated problems seen in these children are parasitic infestation, lead poisoning and trichotillomania (swallowing of hair). Children with trichotillomania may have palpable lump in the upper abdomen (trichobezoar) as a result of collection of hair.

Pica can result from these associated problems in addition to psychogenic reasons. Thus, treatment should be directed towards treating the associated problems, too. Psychotherapy is administered in children with psychogenic pica.

SLEEP WALKING (SOMNAMBULISM)

Loafing around aimlessly while asleep is somnambulism. Its prevalence is 5%–10%. A large number of children have sleep struggles at bedtime. Many children use a special toy, night light and lullaby from parents to go to sleep.

Aetiology

Separation anxiety is considered to be the most important cause for somnambulism. Sleep disorders in infancy are usually a result of parental anxiety. Older children suffer from night-time fears resulting from fables, the books they have read or the story they have heard from people, or even the threats given by adults (buglers, punitive treatment, kidnapping, thunder, lighting, etc.), which develop into episodes of somnambulism.

Familial tendency is also noticed in somnambulism.

Treatment

Parental support, reassurance and encouragement are essential components of treatment.

Small doses of diazepam are also found to be effective in treating somnambulism.

Nursing Considerations

Treatment is directed towards developing proper sleep habits in children. Parents must be given reassurance. Bedtime should be set. A dim night light can be provided. Stimulating TV shows should be avoided.

Before going to bed, a warm bath, a light snack and a quite affectionate moment with parents are advised as conducive measures to develop a sound sleep.

Preventive Measures

These include locking the doors and windows, removing a handful of objects and correction of superstitions.

HABIT DISORDERS

Habit disorders in children include tension-releasing phenomena such as head banging, body rocking, nail-biting, nail pulling, teeth grinding, biting or biting parts of one's own body, body manipulations, breath holding, tics, etc.

Teeth Grinding (Bruxism)

It results from tension originating from unexpressed anger. It is usually seen during sleep as a manifestation of disturbing dreams, pent-up tension and aggression. Bruxism is also seen in children with mental retardation and those suffering from CNS infections.

Diagnosis

Help the child find ways to express his/her resentment. Bedtime enjoyments such as pleasant stories are found to be helpful.

Improving the environmental situation which is responsible for the tension and conflict is advisable. Praising and other emotional supports are useful during such times.

Breath Holding

It is otherwise known as infantile syncope. The incidence rate is 5%–13% of psychosomatic disorders in the paediatric age group.

Aetiology

Breath holding results from frustration of a disciplinary conflict between the parent and the child. The child tries to assert him/herself to express his/her anger.

Clinical Features

The child cries, hyperventilates and holds his/her breath. Cyanosis results after a few seconds, and there is a momentary loss of consciousness and convulsive twitching.

Diagnosis

The cry is classical. Cyanotic spells are accompanied by tonic–clonic convulsions that are required to be differentiated from epilepsy. The precipitating factor may help differentiate it from epilepsy.

Treatment

Psychotherapy. Drug therapy is insignificant. As the child grows, the frequency of breath holding decreases. Associated disorders such as temper tantrum and other behavioural disorders are high with these children.

Thumb Sucking and Nail-biting

These are normally seen during infancy as pertaining to the oral stage of development. It makes the older child appear immature and may interfere with normal alignment of teeth. *Thumb sucking* may be viewed as a way of securing extra self-nurturance. *Nail biting* is a phenomenon demonstrated by children older than 4 years. The common cause is insecurity, a conflict or hostility.

Management

Provide reassurance to parents and children. Parents should ignore the symptom and should not be fussy over it. The child must be given orientation to develop interest in other aspects of life and should be provided other forms of satisfaction.

Tics (Habit Spasm)

Tics are stereotyped, fast, repetitive movements that can be alterable at will. This is a form of discharging tension originated from physical and emotional reasons. These movements have no apparent functions. Parts of the body most frequently involved are face, neck, shoulders, trunk and hands. There may be lip smocking and grimacing, tongue thrusting, eye blinking, throat cleaning, etc. This must be distinguished from epilepsy, dyskinesia and dystonia.

Tics can accompany other psychiatric disorders or follow encephalitis.

A kind of tics accompanied by vigorous vocalization is called Gilles de la Tourette syndrome.

Treatment

Severe types of tics require psychiatric evaluation. Gilles de la Tourette syndrome is treated with haloperidol, 1–5 mg orally alone or with anti-parkinsonian drugs.

Stuttering

Stuttering typically develops during speech learning. It starts gradually as stammering with repetition of consonants. The most important cause for stuttering is the critical attitude of the mother.

Generally, no treatment is needed. Consultation with a speech therapist is advised.

STUDY QUESTIONS

- What are the common developmental problems in children?
- Explain the nursing management for a child who is suffering from enuresis.
- What are learning disorders? How will you care a child with dyslexia?
- Define the following:
  1. Temper tantrums
  2. Thumb sucking
  3. Teeth grinding
  4. Nail biting
  5. Pica, recurrent abdominal pain
  6. Stuttering

BIBLIOGRAPHY

1. American Psychiatric Association. Diagnostic and Statistical Manual of Mental Disorders. Fifth Edition. Washington, DC: American Psychiatric Press; 2013.
2. American Academy of Pediatrics. Diagnosis and evaluation of the child with attention-deficit/hyperactivity disorder (AC0002). Pediatrics. 2000;105:1158-1170.
3. American Psychiatric Association. *Diagnostic and Statistical Manual of Mental Disorders*, Fourth Edition, Text Revision. Washington, DC: American Psychiatric Press; 2000.
4. Austin PF, Bauer SB, Bower W, Chase J, Franco I, Hoebeke P, Rittig S, Walle JV, von Gontard A, Wright A, Yang SS, Nevéus T. The Standardization of Terminology of Lower Urinary Tract Function in Children and Adolescents: Update Report from the Standardization Committee of the International Children's Continence Society. J Urol. 2014;191:1863–5. doi: 10.1016/j.juro.2014.01.110. [PubMed][Cross Ref] http://f1000.com/prime/718270635.
5. Bakwin, H., Bakwin, R.M. (1972). Behaviour Disorders in Children. Philadelphia: Saunders.
6. Barnad, K.E. (Sept/Oct 1985). Studying Patterns of Behaviour. MCN, 10, p. 358.
7. Bender L. Childhood schizophrenia. *Am J Orthopsychiatry* 1947;17: 40–56.
8. Berry, A.K. (Aug 2006). Bladder Matters: Helping Children with Nocturnal Enuresis. American Journal of Nursing, 106(8), pp. 56–64.
9. Betz, C.L. (March/April 1981). Faith Development in Children. Pediatric Nursing, 7, p. 22.
10. Biederman J, Faraone SV, Spencer T, et al. Patterns of psychiatric comorbidity, cognition, and psychosocial functioning in adults with attention deficit hyperactivity disorder. Am J Psychiatry. 1993; 150:1792-1798.
11. Tekgul S, Nijman RJM, Hoebeke P, Canning D, Bower W, Von Gontard A. Diagnosis and Management of Urinary Incontinence in Childhood. http://www.ics.org/Publications/ICI_4/files-book/Comite-9.pdf
12. Goldman LS, Genel M, Bezman RJ, Slanetz PJ. Diagnosis and treatment of attention-deficit/hyperactivity disorder in children and adolescents. Council on Scientific Affairs, American Medical Association. JAMA. 1998; 279:1100-1107.
13. Levine, M.D., Carey, W.B., Croker, A.C. (1999). Developmental–Behavioral Pediatrics. 3rd Edn. Philadelphia: WB Saunders.
14. Loening-Baucke, V. (Feb 1996). Encopresis and Soiling. Pediatric Clinics of North America, 43(1), pp. 279–298.
15. Lovering JS, Tallett SE, McKendry JB. Oxybutynin efficacy in the treatment of primary enuresis. Pediatrics 1988; 82:104.
16. McClung, H.J., Boyne, L.J., Lensheid, T., et al. (1993). Is combination therapy for encopresis nutritionally safe? Pediatrics 91(3), pp. 591–594.
17. Mishra PC, Agarwal VK, Rahman H. Etiological aspects of nocturnal enuresis: An analytic study. Indian Pediatr 1982; 19: 333-337.
18. Nørgaard JP, Rittig S, Djurhuus JC. Nocturnal enuresis: an approach to treatment based on pathogenesis. J Pediatr. 1989;114:705–10. doi: 10.1016/S0022-3476(89)80885-6. [PubMed] [Cross Ref]
19. Parker, S., Zuckerman, B. (2000). Behavioural and Develop-mental Pediatrics: Handbook for Primary Care. Boston: Little, Brown.
20. Prugh, D.U. (1983). The Psychosocial Aspects of Pediatrics. Philadelphia: Lea and Febiger.
21. Salmon MA. An historical account of nocturnal enuresis and its treatment. Proc R Soc Med. 1975;68:443–5. [PMC free article] [PubMed].
22. Tudor, M. (1981). Child Development. New York: McGraw Hill.

NUTRITIONAL NEEDS AND CARE OF CHILDREN WITH NUTRITIONAL DISORDERS

Proper nutrition is essential for any age group, but it is particularly important for children as they are growing. Growing children require more nutritious food to grow stronger. They require right vitamins, minerals and other nutrients for vital processes. Because children are growing, they require different nutrients in different amounts. Developing a wide range of tastes as a young child can prevent children from becoming fussy eaters as adults.

NORMAL NUTRITION IN CHILDHOOD

LEARNING OBJECTIVES

At the end of the chapter, the learner will be able to:

- Describe the nutritional requirements of children (0–12 years).
- Describe nutritional assessment in children.
- Explain nutritional requirements of children of various age groups.
- Explain the importance of breastfeeding.
- Discuss complementary feeding.
- Describe different feeding techniques.
- Explain total parenteral nutrition.

nutritional assessment, nutritional problems and their management.

Nutritional vulnerability of children is mainly a result of their high demands related to growth. The nourishment children require per unit body size is greatest in infancy because of their rapid growth during this period. The rate of energy requirement for growth during childhood is given as follows:

Age	Percentage of Energy Requirement
4 months	30
1 year	5
3 years	2

The risk of failure to thrive from decreased energy intake is greater during the first 6 months of life. The brain grows rapidly during the last trimester of pregnancy and throughout the first 2 years of life. Ninety per cent of brain growth completes by 2 years of age. Development of interneuronal connections during this period is also sensitive to undernutrition. Moreover, at birth, the brain accounts for two-thirds of basal metabolic rate and is 50% at 1 year of age. Protein–energy malnutrition along with inadequate psychosocial stimulation causes delayed development. The

NUTRITION IN CHILDREN

Paediatric nurses must balance their young patients' disease-specific nutrient needs with the ongoing dietary demands of growth. This dual criterion is an important clinical challenge for paediatric nurses, especially with seriously ill children. Paediatric nurses should have a thorough understanding of the nutritional vulnerability of infants and children, normal nutritional requirement, nurses need to remember that preterm infants have poor stores of fat and protein. Smaller children will have less caloric reserve, and they are not able to withstand starvation for prolonged hours. This is the reason why children are not permitted to starve for many hours preoperatively.

The conditions that can compromise nutrition are acute and chronic diseases and surgery.

Children who had poor nutrition during infancy have a tendency to have poor linear growth and are prone to develop certain diseases such as non-insulin-dependent diabetes, coronary artery diseases, hypertension, stroke, etc.

NUTRITIONAL ASSESSMENT

For thorough management of nutritional problems, nurses should conduct a proper nutritional assessment.

Nutritional assessment includes the following:

Anthropometry:
- Weight
- Height
- Mid-arm circumference
- Skinfold thickness

	Normal	Wasted	Stunted
• Weight for age %	100	70	70
• Weight for height %	100	70	100
• Height for age %	100	100	84

Laboratory data:
- Low plasma albumin
- Low concentration of specific minerals and vitamins

Food intake:
- Dietary recall
- Dietary diary

Immunodeficiency:
- Low lymphocyte count
- Impaired cell-mediated immunity

Dietary assessment:
Assess dietary intake by a detailed history of food consumed and its quality and quantity. Interview parents and the child to obtain the following data:
- Child's age
- Present diet:
  - Formula
  - Breastfeed/formula feed
  - Infant foods
- Present eating patterns
- Meals, snacks, etc. and who feeds the child
- Utensils – bottle, cup and spoon and techniques
- Medical problems/treatments
- Symptoms depressing intake:
  - Anorexia nervosa

- Decreased appetite
- Altered taste
- Sore mouth
- Loose teeth
- Trouble swallowing
- Reaction to medication
- Medical treatment
- Excessive appetite
- History of fever
- Activity level

Regular anthropometric measurements are valuable to determine malnutrition. The parameters have already been stated previously. The World Health Organization recommends that nutritional status is expressed as height for age – a measure of stunting and an index of chronic malnutrition. Weight for height is considered as a measure of wasting and an index of acute malnutrition. The skinfold thickness along with upper-arm circumference is an indication of skeletal muscle mass.

NUTRITIONAL REQUIREMENTS

Energy – Daily Requirements

0–3 months	120 kcal/kg
3–5 months	115 kcal/kg
6–8 months	110 kcal/kg
9–11 months	105 kcal/kg
During first year	112 kcal/kg
1–3 years	1300–1400 kcal per day
4–6 years	1800–1850 kcal
7–9 years	2150–2200 kcal
10–12 years	2600 kcal for boys
	2500 kcal for girls
16–19 years	3000 kcal for boys
	2300 kcal for girls

Protein Daily Requirements

0–3 months	2.4 g/kg per day
3–6 months	1.85 g/kg per day
6–9 months	1.62 g/kg per day
9–11 months	1.44 g/kg per day
1–3 years	16 g per day
4–6 years	20 g per day
7–9 years	25 g per day
10–12 years	30 g per day (male)
	29 g per day (female)
13–15 years	37 g per day (male)
	31 g per day (female)
16–19 years	38 g per day (males)
	30 g per day (females)

Mineral Requirements

Age (Years)	Calcium (g)	Phosphorus (g)	Iron (mg)	Iodine (mcg)
Infants and children (years)				
0–1	0.6	0.2–0.3	1.0/kg	40–50
1–3	0.5	0.8	20–25	70
4–6	0.5	0.8	20–25	90
7–9	0.5	0.8	20–25	120
Adolescents				
10–12	0.5	0.8	20–25	140
13–15	0.7	1.2	20–25	140
16–18	0.6	1.2	35	140

Fluid Intake at Different Ages

Age	Fluid Intake
Infants (>4 weeks)	100–120 mL/kg per 24 hours
Children (1–2 years)	90–120 mL/kg per 24 hours
Children (2–15 years)	50–90 mL/kg per 24 hours
Adults	20–35 mL/kg per 24 hours

Consequences of Malnutrition

Severe malnutrition leads to impaired immunity and poor wound healing after surgery. Malnutrition worsens the outcome of other illnesses. Malnutrition and infection form a vicious circle. Children with malnutrition develop infection easily. Diarrhoea also leads to malnutrition.

BREASTFEEDING

Infants can obtain most essential nutrients from breast milk or modified cow's milk formulas, although iron and fluoride supplements may be required by the breastfed infants. Breastfeeding is highly recommended for the first 6 months exclusively. It is recommended to continue breastfeeding for 2 years even with complementary feeds.

Advantages of breast milk are as follows:
- It contains optimum percentage of carbohydrates, protein and fat.
- It has a low renal solute load (determined by the concentration of protein and electrolytes).
- It has an easily digestible protein component (whey to casein ratio of 60:40 compared with 18:82 in pure cow's milk).
- It contains an easily digestible carbohydrate (lactose) in a higher concentration than that present in cow's milk.
- It has a rich source of linoleic acid, an essential fatty acid that helps in improved digestibility and absorption of fats.
- It is the ideal nutrition for the baby. The calcium to phosphorus ratio is 2:1.
- It protects against infections and allergies. It contains 90% humoral secretory IgA that provides mucosal protection. Bifidus factors promote growth of *Lactobacillus* that metabolizes lactose to lactic acid. Lysozyme has bacteriolytic enzyme. Lactoferrin is an iron-binding protein that inhibits the growth of *Escherichia coli*. The presence of interferon provides antiviral property. Lymphocytes may transfer delayed hypersensitivity responses.
- The first milk immediately after delivery is rich in nutrients and has special protective properties. This yellowish milk is called colostrum.
- It is hygienic, safe and readily available at the right temperature, needs no preparation and comes free of cost.
- It provides close physical contact and hence fosters strong emotional bond.
- Sucking process helps in the development of the facial muscles of the baby.

For the mother, breastfeeding has certain advantages:
- Helps in rapid involution of the uterus
- Helps lose extra weight
- Helps breast to return to the normal shape and size
- Helps in natural birth spacing
- Reduces the risk of breast cancer

In addition, human milk contains protective factors against infection and may contain a 'mucosal growth factor', which facilitates early maturation of the gastrointestinal (GI) system.

CONTRAINDICATIONS OF BREASTFEEDING

- Mothers suffering from HIV infection
- Mothers with open pulmonary tuberculosis

DISADVANTAGES OF BREASTFEEDING

- Transmission of drugs through breast milk is possible (e.g. antithyroid drugs, cathartics, antimetabolites)
- Transmission of infections such as CMV infection, HIV infection and hepatitis
- Development of breast milk jaundice
- Prolonged breastfeeding without complementary feeding can result in poor weight gain and deficiency disorders such as rickets, vitamin K deficiency, iron deficiency, etc.
- Smoking and alcohol intake of mothers during breastfeeding can pose threat to the child

Cow's Milk Formulas

If breastfeeding is not possible owing to some reasons, modified cow's milk formulas can be used. When choosing a formula, particularly for an infant whose metabolism has been altered by illness, consider the following factors:
- Digestibility and absorption of carbohydrate, protein and fat
- Percentage of calories from carbohydrate, protein and fat
- Renal solute load (concentration of protein and electrolytes)

Pure cow's milk should be avoided during the entire first year of life because it is a poor source of iron; it is associated with GI bleeding and contains excessive proteins and minerals, which increase the renal solute load.

Dietary Management of Preterm Infants

Premature babies (preemies) are born with an immature system, though they have more nutritional needs. Premature infants lack lipase and bile salts needed for the breakdown of fat, lactase needed for the breakdown of milk sugar and certain enzymes for the conversion of amino acids to proteins.

Preemies are prone to hypoglycaemia, metabolic acidosis and vitamin and mineral deficiencies (particularly vitamins D and E, folate and iron). Breast milk contains appropriate forms of nutrition for preemies. Preferred feeds for preemies should contain a decreased percentage of lactose, whey to casein ratio of 60:40, medium-chain triglycerides, a low renal solute load and an increased calorie per volume.

Composition of Different Milks (per 100 mL)

	Breast Milk	Cow's Milk	Infant Formula
Protein (g)	1.3	3.3	1.5
Casein:whey	40:60	60:40	Variable
Carbohydrate (g)	7.0	4.5	7.0–8.0
Fat (g)	4.2	3.6	2.6–3.8
Energy (kcal)	70	65	65
Sodium (mmol)	0.65	2.3	0.65–1.1
Calcium (mmol)	0.87	3.0	1.4
Iron (μmol)	1.36	0.9	10
Vitamin D (pg)	0.6	0.03	1.0

ORAL FEEDINGS

Oral feedings are indicated when the child's mouth, oesophagus and the entire GI system are intact and function well. Infants must be alert with an adequate suck and a coordinated sucking and swallowing reflex. This promotes oral feeding and avoids aspiration of milk. Remember that oral feeding should not be avoided just because it takes a long time to feed a child.

Bottle-feeding

Bottle-feeding is not advocated nowadays as a result of many of its ill effects. But sometimes it is necessary to maintain adequate nutrition and to provide sucking pleasure to the baby.

Special implements for feeding children with special needs can be used when fed orally. Syringe with latex tubing or medicine dropper can be used for children with postoperative cleft palate and lip surgery, plastic surgery or fracture where the jaw is wired, a mental or neurologic deficiency who can swallow but who cannot get fluid into their mouth using a regular cup.

Use spoons – when suture line trauma is not a factor or that are rubber coated for children who bite.

Use covered spouted cups – for older infants and children who are learning to drink from a cup.

Use flexible straws – when a child cannot sit upright to drink and also just for fun.

It is advisable to consult a physiotherapist for special implements when needed for special purposes according to the baby's needs.

Childhood Nutritional Needs

Protein and caloric requirements are high at the beginning of life when most rapid growth occurs, level off during the slower growth of school-age stage and increase again in the adolescence growth spurt. The sources of nutrient can be changed as the maturing infant gradually learns to take solid foods, develops fine motor skills and develops likes and dislikes. Therefore, each age group has specific nutritional and feeding needs. Additional calories are necessary for premature infants and children who are very active. During illness, children need additional proteins.

Age-Appropriate Feeding Approaches and Techniques

Infants

It is a period of rapid growth and rapid improvement in feeding ability.

First 3 Months

Involuntary rooting, sucking and swallowing reflexes dominate.

After 3 Months

The extrusion reflex (pushing out with the tongue) decreases and sucking becomes more voluntary.

By about 5–6 Months

The infant can grasp some objects and bring them to the mouth; chewing movements begin in this period, and lip coordination enables the child to drink from the rim of a cup.

After 6 Months

Chewing and swallowing improve, and teeth come in, enabling the child to take more textured foods.

Feeding schedules and volume of feeding should be individualized; the infant will regulate the volume, if allowed. Bottle-fed infant should not be forced to finish the bottle if they are satiated with less feeds. Infants will regurgitate the formula if their stomach capacity cannot accommodate the volume.

Encourage breastfeeding mothers to continue breastfeeding in the hospital as well when children are admitted because of sickness, if their condition permits. Emphasize on the following points:
- Feed infants on demand as much as possible.
- Keep the feeding schedule flexible.

- Use a nipple, bottle or cup familiar to the infant to facilitate feeding in hospital.
- Hold the bottle up so that the nipple is always filled with formula.
- Burp small infants frequently, after every ounce; older infants may need to burp halfway through the feeding and at the end.
- Hold the infants who cannot sit alone in a semi-upright position.
- Always keep children in safe positions while feeding – sitting upright, on the side or in a prone position.
- Involve parents or caretakers in the feeding process; perhaps, even share their techniques.
- Introduce cup at 5–6 months of age for feeding.
- Delay solid feeding until the infant has the developmental ability to control mouth and tongue movements (4–6 months).
- Add foods one at time and observe the child for allergies.
- A recommended sequence is rice, cereal, fruits, vegetables and meats.
- Avoid eggs and orange juice (frequently allergy producing) until late in the first year.
- Plain strained baby foods are best nutritionally compared with other foods.
- Textured foods can be introduced at 4–5 months of age, starting with strained foods, advancing to mashed foods (7–8 months) and finally cut foods (12 months) as tongue and mouth movements become more mature.

Remember the following while giving complementary feeds:

- Offer solid foods before the formula or breast milk.
- Place solids in the centre of the tongue, using a small spoon and press downward slightly to facilitate swallowing.
- An infant will push out solid foods when first learning to eat them.
- This does not mean dislike; it is just inexperience.
- Allow older infants as much independence as possible – holding their own bottle or cup and feeding themselves with fingers.
- Offer finger foods.

Precautions for feeding infants and toddlers are as follows:

- Avoid tiny, easily aspirated foods (e.g. nuts, hard candies, popcorn).
- Do not give foods that expand upon ingestion (e.g. popcorn, groundnut).
- Avoid raw vegetables or root tubers (e.g. carrot sticks), as they are difficult for most toddlers to chew well; pieces are often aspirated.
- Avoid shred, grind or finely diced meat.
- Observe for allergic reactions to food stuffs.

Dietary expansion is a key indicator of developmental progress, and the developmental status may be considered in the dietary management of young children.

Complementary Feeding

Nowadays, this term is used instead of weaning. The complementary feeding should be started at the beginning of the fifth month. Introduction to other foods besides breast milk before the fifth month is dangerous because the baby's stomach and digestive system are not ready for it. But after completing 4 months of life, mother's milk must be supplemented for good growth. Delay in starting complementary feeds beyond the fifth month can cause malnutrition and will make the baby vulnerable to diseases and infections, as after 6 months, the breast milk is highly inadequate to meet the nutritional needs of infants.

Age Group with Activities and Preferred Foods for Introduction

Activities	Preferred Foods for Introduction
1–4 months	Give only breast milk
5 months Starting to kick	Rice and oats
5–6 months Cooing and booing Crawling around	Vegetables and fruits make baby healthy
7–8 months Sitting up	Chicken and fish and yellow parts of egg
9–10 months Stands up	As above
11–12 months	Can give the 'family pot'
	Remember to continue breastfeeding along with all complementary feeds

Starting foods include the following:

- Cooked rice and oats make a good first solid food.
- Start with one to two teaspoons of rice twice daily and gradually increase the amount.
- Increase the amount slowly to three to four tablespoons per day for 5–7 days.
- After 5–6 days, start oats.

Introduction of Solids

Age	Feeding
6 months (not less than 4 months)	Smooth purees (fruit, vegetables, rice, meat, dairy products — avoid gluten)
6–9 months	Thicker consistencies and finger foods (fruit, vegetables, rice, meat, dairy products, cereals)
9–12 months	Mashed, chopped and minced consistencies (encourage variety of tastes and textures)
12 months	Mashed and chopped foods (encourage finger foods; can introduce whole cow's milk)

Foods to be avoided are as follows:

- Do not give wheat until after 6 months, as protein present in wheat (gluten) can cause allergy.
- Do not give any powered or liquid cow's milk.
- Do not add spices, salt, sugar or any other sweetener. Babies do not need them.

- Do not use a feeding bottle for feeding. Use a cup and a spoon. They need to learn to chew and swallow.

Age-wise Nutritional Needs

Toddlers (1–3 Years)

Toddlers can eat most table foods but may have problems chewing tough meat or vegetables. But these foods are essential source of iron, folate and zinc. Use a variety of foods to meet nutritional needs of toddlers. Toddlers prefer plain foods. Independence-seeking behaviour in the form of negativism, always eating the same foods and variable appetite may be frustrating for adults. Varying the colour, shape and texture of foods helps maintain interests in eating. The toddler may be ritualistic and want foods in special ways or in certain places on the plate.

Points to remember:
- Place appropriate portion on a small plate, as large trays are overwhelming.
- Allow independence in eating.
- Expect a mess and spills; do not scold the child for the mess.
- Set limits with this age group.
- Do not offer choices when there is no choice.
- Do not use force and do not use food as a bribe, punishment or reward.

Preschoolers (4–6 Years)

This period is characterized by a slow and steady growth with increased nutrient requirement because of their increased activities. Continue to encourage milk intake for adequate calcium and vitamin A, but not fully a milk diet because there is a chance for iron deficiency if the baby takes a large amount of milk. Preschoolers will imitate adult behaviour, avoiding foods they have seen adults avoiding. Hence, the responsible adults should be role models and should avoid food fads and grumbling over foods at least in front of preschoolers.

School-aged Children

Nutritional habits of school-aged children are affected by the school, peers, advertisements and the outside world and less by the family habits. Growth spurts and plateaus characterize this period. Appetite is generally good during this period. Loose and lost teeth present problems in eating.

Important points to be remembered include the following:
- Involve school-going children in nutritional planning and selection of food to spark interest in eating.
- Allow school-aged children to count their calories by food intake so that they will get an idea of their own needs of nutrition.
- Offer simple nutritional information and guidelines to promote understanding.
- Have children of similar ages eat together, as peers are important at this stage of development.
- Allow children to eat in an unhurried manner.

Adolescents

Adolescents experience dramatic body image changes, as growth and maturational changes occur rapidly. Diet and body image are closely related, and the peer group frequently influences choices of food. It is important to remember that diet is an adolescent's personal choice. Flexibility is the key point in planning and making adolescents to eat. Use a variety of foods to meet the nutritional needs of the adolescents.

Important points to be remembered while planning adolescents' foods include the following:
- Include favourite, popular foods in the diet, if possible.
- Teach and provide guidelines for food selection and allow independence in deciding meals.
- Serve food that looks pleasant.
- Avoid confrontation for compliance.
- Allow the adolescent to eat with peers.

Special Diets for Illness

Ill infants and children may require dietary changes because of altered metabolism of nutrients. Consult with a dietician before making any diet modification. Include lists of foods permitted on special diets in the nursing care plan. Common special diets are as follows:

SODIUM-RESTRICTED DIET

Sodium-restricted diets are prescribed for children with cardiac, renal, hepatic and oncologic diseases with complications. Sodium-restricted diets are ordered in milligrams or grams as 250, 500 or 1000 mg of sodium diets. In general, foods are to be cooked without salt and then the prescribed amount of salt can be added to the food. Preserved foods should be avoided, as it contains more salt than ordinarily prepared foods.

PROTEIN-RESTRICTED DIET

Protein-restricted diets are used for renal diseases to prevent accumulation of uremic waste from protein breakdown. In hepatic diseases, too, protein restrictions are needed to reduce accumulation of ammonia, thus reducing the severity of hepatic encephalopathy. It is also used in patients with inborn errors of metabolism. Electrolytes such as sodium and potassium are also restricted with this diet. When planning protein-restricted diet, remember that the included protein must be of high quality. High-calorie/low-protein diets are used to increase the calories. Many readymade diets are available from different manufactures.

HIGH-CALORIE/HIGH-PROTEIN DIET

High-calorie/high-protein diets are used for paediatric patients with disorders such as cancer and cystic fibrosis and for malnourishment in cases of failure to thrive or malnutrition. There is no restriction on these diets as long as all metabolic systems are functioning well.

Calories and protein are increased by adding milk and cream content of foods. Example of one such diet is high-calorie cereal milk. This is prepared with milk, coconut oil, groundnut flour and rice flour.

DIABETIC DIET

This is a calorie-controlled diet necessitating specific amounts of carbohydrate, protein and fat. Exchange lists for meats, vegetables, fruits and breads are used to plan three meals and two snacks per day. The goal is to distribute calories throughout the day to prevent hyperglycaemic episodes. Juvenile diabetic children should be allowed to use some of their favourite foods in their diets.

LACTOSE INTOLERANCE DIET

Lactose deficiency produces intolerance of sugar lactose, which is found in milk and dairy products. For infants, many lactose-free formulas are available in the market. Soya milk is an example of lactose-free milk.

KETOGENIC DIET

This type of diets is used in children younger than 5 years to control seizures. The diet is low in carbohydrate and high in fat content. The goal is to produce ketosis which affects the nervous system, thus decreasing seizure activity.

ALTERNATE FEEDING METHODS

There are different methods of alternate feeding techniques usually for children with difficulty in oral feeding.

Tube Feedings

Tube feeding or enteral feeding is indicated when the adequate nutrients cannot be provided by oral feedings. The common indications are given in Table 1.

Types of Patient	Examples
Physically impaired	Dental problems
	Facial fractures
	Head and neck surgeries
	Burns
	Upper GI surgeries
Neurologically impaired	Head injury
	Paralysis
	Loss of consciousness
Mentally disabled	Depression
	Anorexia nervosa
Weak	Premature
Other indications	Chemotherapy
	Radiation therapy
	Hypermetabolic states
	Malabsorption

Types of Tubes

Polyvinylchloride and newer polyurethane and silicone tubes (5–10 Fr) can be used for orogastric and nasogastric (NG) feedings.

Procedure

- Use a clean procedure.
- Obtain equipment: proper feeding tube (check size and length), tape, emesis basin (kidney tray), appropriate size syringe, stethoscope, pH test paper, water for older children to sip.
- Position child at an angle of 45° or on the right side.
- Explain the procedure to the child if he/she is old enough to understand it.
- Tear tape and place it where it can be easily reached.
- Measure length of tube (for NG tube, tip of the nose to the ear lobe to just below the sternum at the stomach, and for the nasojejunal (NJ) tube, NG tube measurement plus 4–6 inches).
- Mark measurements with a pen or tape.
- Have an assistant if the child needs restraining.
- Lubricate the tip of the tube with water.
- Insert the tip in a nostril, push gently up and back to pass the nasal ridge and continue pushing until desired length is inserted.
- Tell the child to swallow while the tube is passing or provide sips of water to swallow if not contraindicated to facilitate easy passage of the tube.
- Remove the tube at once if there is any respiratory difficulty, resistance, gagging and vomiting.
- Temporarily tape the tube in position.
- Check the back of the throat for kinking or curling of the tube.
- Inject 2–5 mL of air while listening with the stethoscope over the right upper quadrant for NG tube placement and the right lower quadrant for NJ tubes.
- Aspirate the contents; observe and test for semi-digested food for gastric contents or the formula – greenish colour and pH below 6; jejunal contents will be golden yellow and pH 6 or above.
- If no aspirate is obtained from the NJ tube, leave it open in air and check again in half an hour.
- Always replace aspirate because not replacing contents consistently can lead to fluid and electrolyte imbalances similar to those occurring with persistent vomiting.
- Tape the tube securely to patient's nose. DO NOT tape the tube UP against the nares. It may erode skin, causing permanent disfigurement.
- Place the child on the right side with the head of the bed elevated, and allow gravity and peristalsis to assist movement of the tube if the NJ tube has not passed the pylorus and is not kinked behind the throat.
- Allow the child to be calm before starting feeding.

Tube Maintenance

- NG tubes can be kept in place for 5–7 days provided that there is no complication.
- Change the tubes every 3–5 days. Use alternate nostrils.

- Alternate positions of the tape on the skin.
- Rinse the tube with sterile water or saline after intermittent feedings and medications.
- Tape all connections to tubing or syringes securely.

Nasojejunal/Gastrostomy Tubes

- Secure the tube in situ with tapes.
- Clean the skin around the tube with Betadine (povidone-iodine) or peroxide as per hospital policy.
- Change tapes daily and, as necessary, alternate positions of the skin.
- Use gauze dressings or Stomahesive around the tube if the child's skin breaks down.

Procedure for Bolus Feeding

- Use clean technique.
- Obtain and measure the correct formula in a sterile container.
- Warm the formula up to the room temperature if it is refrigerated.
- Check the tube placement.
- Aspirate and note the type and amount of residual contents. Always replace aspirated contents.
- Position the child upright at an angle of 45°, on the side or in a prone position.
- Explain the feeding to the child if old enough to understand.
- Add the room temperature formula to the feeding tube, start the flow and observe the flow. Never push the feeds. Permit gravity-assisted flow.
- Check the tubing's for kinks.
- Stay with the child during entire feeding; observe for gagging and vomiting.
- Keep suction equipment nearby to clear airways if vomiting occurs.
- Flush the tubing with 10–15 mL of water after feeding, if permitted.
- Remove the feeding syringe.
- Secure the tube in place.
- Rinse and reuse or discard the administration set as per hospital policy.

Procedure for Continuous Infusion Feedings

Continuous infusion pumps are used to administer small volumes of food to children over extended periods. This method is used for jejunal feedings.

- Connect the administration set to infusion pump tubing and attach to a pump.
- Use different types of pumps for feedings and intravenous fluids to avoid confusion and clearly label which are feeding tubes and which are intravenous tubes.
- Label feeding sets and tubes with the type of formula infusing and set the rate of the pump.
- Check the pump and reservoir hourly for progress.
- Rinse feeding sets and tubings every 4 hours.
- Change sets and tubings every 24 hours to prevent build-up and clogging and to prevent bacterial growth along the line.

- Always use clean technique when handling feeding equipment.
- When beginning, start slowly with a low volume and strength. Never advance both at the same time.
- Start with half-strength, advance to three-fourths and finally to full strength, as tolerated.
- Determine a schedule for advancing feeding volume and strength for the nursing care plan.

Formulas

Consider the following factors while selecting formulas for tube feeds:

- Nutritional completeness
- Content and types of carbohydrate, protein and fat
- Viscosity
- Osmolality
- Specific needs of the patient

TOTAL PARENTERAL NUTRITION

Total parenteral nutrition (TPN) is indicated when GI function is inadequate and nutrient needs cannot be met via the enteral route.

There are four groups of patients who require TPN (Harvey, K B, 1983)

- Malnourished and need nutritional requirement before surgery
- With prolonged postoperative complications
- With inflammatory bowel diseases when bowel rest is needed
- With inadequate oral intake

TPN can be administered by the central or peripheral route. Peripheral TPN is used in children when the need for parenteral nutrition is short term (5–7 days). If more than 7 days are required, a central venous access is sought. Central routes are preferred, as a high concentration of glucose irritates peripheral veins. Glucose concentration greater than 12.5% should be given through central veins. Broviac or Hickman catheters are used for the central line. The catheter is passed from the external site through the jugular vein into the subclavian or superior vena cava. The central line is always sutured in place and covered with sterile, occlusive dressing. TPN solutions are always administered by a pump or by adjusting drop rate to maintain constant rate of flow. TPN lines should not be used for other purposes. A second intravenous line or use of a multiple-bore catheter is recommended for medications, blood drawings and blood administration.

Nurses' Responsibility in Administering TPN

- Before starting TPN, the nurse needs to assess the nutritional status and physical growth in children below 3 years of age including head circumference for comparison information to monitor the response of the child to TPN.
- Determine the baseline – vital signs and activity level, hydration status, venous access route as central or peripheral.

- Review indications of TPN.
- Prepare the family for procedure like any other procedure.
- Assemble and prepare equipment and supplies as needed – infusion pump, if available, as it may not be available in many government hospitals, intravenous tubings with filter and Y connections, fluids – glucose 10%–20%, fat emulsion (10%–20%).
- Ascertain preparation schedule with order/prescription.
- Prepare solution as per directions with strict aseptic technique.
- Administer TPN using a strict aseptic technique. The preliminary steps include the following: connect tubing, filter and Y connections; connect tubing to solutions and prime tubing with solution. If intralipid (IL) or fat emulsion is to be added, purge the tubing of air and connect the same to Y connection below the filter.
- Insert tubing into the infusion pump and set the flow rate if the infusion pump is available. If not, calculate the drop rate and adjust the flow rate.
- Verify the patency of venous access and check the site hourly for signs of infiltration.
- Monitor vital signs and activity level 4 hourly.
- Monitor intake and output.
- Monitor and plot growth every day in terms of weight gain in a chart; height and head circumference are also indicated.
- Obtain laboratory values to see the level of serum electrolytes.
- Stimulate normal feeding and sucking in infants with pacifiers.
- If discontinuing, taper the infusion rate 1 hour before discontinuing. If the rate is 100 mL/hour, reduce the rate to 50 mL/hour for 30 minutes and then to 25 mL/hour for next 30 minutes.
- Flush the central venous access device after discontinuing TPN.
- Maintain accurate records of administration of TPN with its composition and rate of flow.

N.B.: Nurses should be vigilant not to use TPN line for blood and medication administration, to obtain Central Venous Pressure (CVP) and blood samples.

Common Complications of TPN

- Temporary phlebitis – Responds well to warm soaks. If infiltration, stop infusion and inject hyaluronidase into the swollen area and protect the site with a bulk dressing.
- Hydrocephalus and pulmonary oedema.
- Jugular and superior vena cava thrombosis.
- Catheter-related sepsis as a result of host factors and exposure to possible contaminations.
- Cholestatic jaundice – Study liver enzymes, as TPN can cause irreversible liver damage.
- Most common metabolic complications seen in low-birth-weight babies and older children include renal and hepatic diseases and central nervous system diseases.
- Monitor sugar and acetone level in the urine to follow tolerance of TPN.

- Monitor the child's temperature immediately after a new bottle of solution is hung. Temperature spikes indicate possible infection. If this occurs, discontinue the infusion and replace with fresh solution and intravenous tubing as prescribed.
  Two types of solutions are used:
- Hyperalimentation (HAL) solution
- Intralipid
  The TPN used in Paediatric Surgery Department of IMCH (Calicut) is given as follows:

	Day 1	Day 2	Day 3	Day 4	Day 5
Isolyte P	100 mL/kg	120 mL/kg	130 mL/kg	140 mL/kg	165 mL/kg
25% dextrose or	–	20 mL/kg	30 mL/kg	40 mL/kg	65 mL/kg
50% dextrose	–	10 mL/kg	15 mL/kg	20 mL/kg	33 mL/kg
Multivitamin injection	1 mL	1 mL	1 mL	1 mL	1 mL
KCl	1 mL/kg	1 mL/kg	1 mL/kg	1 mL/kg	1 mL/kg
Astymine 3	10 mL/kg	15 mL/kg	20 mL/kg	30 mL/kg	40 mL/kg

NUTRITION ALTERATION LESS THAN BODY REQUIREMENT

The major nursing diagnosis concerned with nutritional requirement in a paediatric set-up is nutrition alteration less than body requirement.

Common aetiological factors concerning this diagnosis with its nursing interventions are as follows:

Aetiology

- Metabolic deficiencies – juvenile dermatomyositis (JDM), hypoglycaemia, phenylketonuria (PKU), disorders of carbohydrate metabolism and cystic fibrosis
- Congenital defects of the GI tract, cleft lip and palate, gastroesophageal reflux, tracheoesophageal fistula, fistulas/atresia, biliary atresia
- Inadequate intake as a result of several reasons
- Increased metabolic needs – prematurity, burns infections
- Anorexia, loss of appetite, anorexia nervosa
- Congenital anomalies such as heart diseases, renal diseases and mental retardation
- Diarrhoea and chronic infections

Clinical Manifestations

- Body weight 20% (or more) less than height percentage on standard growth grids
- Loss of weight with appropriate food intake
- Poor muscle tone
- Lack of energy
- Hyperactive bowel sounds
- Lack of interest in food

Multidisciplinary Management

- Replacement of deficient nutrients/hormone/enzyme
- Surgical correction of a GI defect
- High-calorie/protein diet
- Administration of vitamins and minerals as required
- Behaviour modification and health education to improve compliance with treatment
- Psychological counselling

Nursing Management

Assessment

- Weight checking to identify abnormalities
- Food intake history and assessment
- Muscle weakness/apathy, mood changes
- Sucking reflux of infants to find out whether it is poor
- Bowel elimination pattern
- Colic/skin breakdown
- Serum albumin to find out whether there is any decrease in its level
- Lymphocyte count to find out decrease in count
- Heart rate, respiration (dyspnoea, tachypnoea)
- Causative factors of nutritional deficit
- Number of teeth for infants and children
- Food intolerance

Nursing Interventions

- Estimate the child's daily caloric requirements for maintenance and growth.
- Give small frequent feedings.
- Offer solid feedings.
- Record and describe food intake and bowel movements.
- Weigh the child daily.
- Encourage adequate rest.
- Promote relaxing, nonstressful meal times.
- Promote low-cost diet or diet as per financial capacity.
- Teach the parents principles of good nutrition and food groups and substitution values.
  Other common nursing diagnoses related to nutrition and health include the following:
- Activity intolerance
- Alteration in bowel elimination
- Fluid volume deficit
- Impairment of skin integrity
- Knowledge deficit

STUDY QUESTIONS

1. Why is it important to think about nutrition in children?
2. How will you perform a nutritional assessment in children?
3. Why is it important to measure anthropometrics in nutritional assessment?
4. What is the significance of measuring haemoglobin in nutritional assessment?
5. What are the biochemical parameters involved in nutritional assessment?
6. What is body mass index (BMI)? How will you calculate BMI?
7. What are the advantages of breastfeeding?
8. What are the contraindications of breastfeeding?
9. What factors are to be considered while an infant is put on formula feeding?
10. State the types of feeding.
11. Explain the age-appropriate feeding techniques.
12. What is complementary feeding?
13. Differentiate between weaning and complementary feeding.
14. Discuss the age-wise nutritional needs of children aged 1–7 years.
15. What are the preferred foods of infants ranging from 1 to 12 months of age?
16. What is a protein-restricted diet and when will you use such a diet?
17. What is high-calorie/high-protein diet? When will you advise such a diet to children?
18. What are the alternate methods of feeding used in children? Explain gastrostomy feeding.
19. Explain parenteral nutrition with its importance and the nurse's responsibility when administering TPN.
20. Explain the following special diets:
    (a) Sodium-restricted diet
    (b) Protein-restricted diet
    (c) High-calorie/high-protein diet
    (d) Diabetic diet
    (e) Lactose-free diet
    (f) Ketogenic diet
21. What is weaning? What is the difference between weaning and complementary feeding?
22. Explain the age-wise nutritional requirements of children 3–12 years of age?
23. What are the important points that you will keep in mind while giving dietary advice for adolescents?

BIBLIOGRAPHY

1. AAP (American Academy of Pediatrics). 2009. *Pediatric Nutrition Handbook*, 6th ed. Elk Grove Village, IL: AAP.
2. Baker, J. L., L. W. Olsen, and T. I. A. Sørensen. 2007. Childhood body-mass index and the risk of coronary heart disease in adulthood. *New England Journal of Medicine* 357(23):2329–2337. [PMC free article].
3. Briefel, R. R., K. Reidy, V. Karwe, and B. Devaney. 2004. Feeding Infants and Toddlers Study: Improvements needed in meeting infant feeding recommendations. *Journal of the American Dietetic Association* 104(Suppl 1):S31–S37.
4. Ebbeling, C. B., and D. S. Ludwig. 2008. Tracking pediatric obesity: An index of uncertainty? *Journal of the American Medical Association* 299(20):2442–2443.
5. Fox, M. K., S. Pac, B. Devaney, and L. Jankowski. 2004. Feeding Infants and Toddlers Study: What foods are infants and toddlers eating? *Journal of the American Dietetic Association* 104(Suppl 1): S22–S30.
6. IOM. 2002/2005. *Dietary Reference Intakes for Energy, Carbohydrate, Fiber, Fat, Fatty Acids, Cholesterol, Protein, and Amino Acids*. Washington, DC: The National Academies Press.
7. NATIONAL INSTITUTE OF NUTRITION. (Indian Council of Medical Research). (2009). Nutrient Requirements and Recommended Dietary Allowances for Indians RDA. Jamai-Osmania (P.O), Hyderbad-500 604.

CHAPTER 19

FLUID AND ELECTROLYTE MANAGEMENT IN CHILD HEALTH NURSING

LEARNING OBJECTIVES

At the end of the chapter, the learner will be able to
- Discuss the differences in fluid compartments of infants and adults.
- Discuss the importance of electrolyte maintenance in children.
- Explain the hormonal influences in fluid electrolyte maintenance.
- Discuss the importance of fluid maintenance in paediatric surgical patients.

FLUID AND ELECTROLYTE MANAGEMENT IN CHILD HEALTH NURSING

Accurate fluid, electrolyte and nutritional therapy requires calculating maintenance requirements, estimating preexisting deficits and measuring ongoing abnormal losses. Fluid balance is a complex interaction of numerous physiological principles, with many additional and closely related concepts such as nutrition and acid–base balance. Fluid electrolyte imbalance usually involves a combination of several problems. Fluid calculation is based on physiologic principles and applying clinical and laboratory observations in the individual patients. Fluid balance is especially important in children because of major physiologic differences that increase the risk of imbalance. Children have a higher total body water percentage by weight which decreases by age. In a preterm infant, the water content is about 80%; in full-term infants, it is 75%–80%; by the age of 3 years, it is 63%; and by 12 years and older, it is 58%, depending on the body fat. The distribution of water between the intracellular and extracellular compartments also varies with age, as the major portion of water located extracellularly in infants gradually locates to the intracellular compartment in older children and adults.

Despite the greater water content, children are more vulnerable to imbalances because of the following reasons:
- They must ingest and excrete (turnover) a greater volume per day (up to one-half of the body water compared with one-sixth in adults) to excrete metabolic wastes produced with a metabolic rate twice that of adults.
- A child has a greater body surface area in relation to body weight than adults which results in greater insensible water losses.
- Functional renal maturity significantly contributes to the risk of fluid imbalances, especially in children younger than 2 years.
- A less efficient renal ability to concentrate or dilute urine or to retain or excrete sodium allows fluid deficit or overload and/or sodium imbalances to rapidly develop.

All requirements and dosages in infants and children including nutritional requirements are quoted and prescribed per unit size. It should be remembered that within the childhood age range, we may be dealing with an infant weighing 1 kg or an adolescent weighing 50 kg, i.e. a 50-fold difference.

COMPARISON OF FLUID COMPARTMENT IN INFANTS AND ADULTS

Infant's Fluid Distribution

Plasma	Interstitial Fluid	Cellular Water	Solids
5	30	40	25

Adult's Fluid Distribution

Plasma	Interstitial Fluid	Cellular Water	Solids
5	25	30	40

In a normal newborn, the total body water content is 75%. ECF is 35%–40%. By 1 year of age, the total body water is dropped to 60% and Extra cellular Fluid (ECF) to 27%. By adolescence, it is only 20%. Total blood volume of a neonate is 85% of body weight.

In neonates, the kidneys have a slow diuretic response to a water load and cannot maximally dilute urine until 5 days of age. The maximum urine osmolality is only 600–700 mOsm/kg as compared with 1200 mOsm/kg in adults. The urine volume increases in infants from a range of 0–68 mL on the first day of life to 40–302 mL by the seventh day of life. Seventy-two hours of fasting in a newborn takes 13% of body weight and an increase in blood urea nitrogen (BUN). If 50 mL of water is given per day, still there is a loss of 8% of weight. Even when infants are given unlimited amount of breastfeeds for the first few days, they will have a weight loss of 10%, minimal urinary output and negative nitrogen balance. A normal newborn is inactive and has no appetite and has minimal urine output. Newborns get interested in food only on the third or fourth day of life. The fluid volume taken by breastfeed increases slowly to 150 mL from the second day of life to the fifth to seventh days of life. A 150 mL of breastfeed will provide 110 cal/kg. Hence, a newborn in the first 2–3 days does not require much fluid, and small urine output should not be taken as an indication of dehydration. This is a natural mechanism for human infants as the breast milk will be little during the first 2–3 days, which increases from the third day onwards. Hence, 50 mL/kg of fluid is sufficient to prevent dehydration in the first 2 days of life to replace if there is no abnormal loss and stepwise increase up to 100 mL/kg by the fifth day.

Initial fluid is 10% glucose, especially to premature infants, as there are decreased glycogen stores.

Second day – Glucose needs to be given with 0.2% saline to replace sodium (Na) 2–3 mEq/kg. Additional supplementation of calcium (Ca) is to be given in order to prevent infants from tetany. Cold stress and exposure to heating lamp increase fluid requirement.

Losses with postnatal vomiting need to be accurately assessed and replaced. Likewise, all gastrointestinal losses need to be clearly monitored and replaced within 48–72 hours. Weight checking is essential. Usually, the infant should lose 10–15 g per day. Increase in weight other than that is produced by replacement is oedema. Water turnover is at its maximum in infancy and decreases with growth. Compared with the older child or adult, an infant has a larger surface area with a more permeable skin, a more rapid respiratory rate and a less mature renal function. Therefore, losses of fluid and electrolytes are large and continuous by these routes. There is also free and rapid exchange of water throughout the extracellular compartment from plasma to interstitial fluid to lymph, and there is a large enterohepatic circulation, with fluids being secreted into the gut lumen and reabsorbed into the portal system. The interstitial fluid is a large component of the easily exchangeable fluid.

The nurse should have knowledge of the application of the fundamental fluid balance concepts to allow meaningful observation, permit knowledgeable collaboration with the physician and provide basic principles of therapy to guide both independent and dependent nursing practices. A brief review of the major forces, electrolytes and hormones influencing fluid balance is as follows:

ELECTROLYTES

The major electrolytes of concern are sodium (Na^+) and potassium (K^+) (both cations), and chloride (Cl^-, an anion). Both Na^+ and Cl^- are primarily extracellular; K^+ is the major intracellular cation. For chemical neutrality of any fluid, anions and cations must balance in body fluids. Electrolytes in intravenous fluids also need to be balanced.

FLUID MOVEMENTS

The forces that move fluid in and out of the vascular compartment include osmotic forces, oncotic pressures, hydrostatic pressures and changes in capillary permeability (Hazinsky M F, 1988). Osmotic force is the result of a serum osmolality (concentration of solution measured in mOsmol) that influences the movement of fluids. Na^+ is the major action determining serum osmolality. Free water moves from an area of low osmolality to an area of high osmolality. A low serum sodium level causes fluid movement out of the intravascular space into interstitial tissues and a high serum sodium level causes water to move into the intravascular space. Glucose also contributes to serum osmolality, causing similar fluid shifts. Osmotic forces work at the vascular level; other forces work at the capillary level. Plasma proteins exert oncotic pressure, which tends to hold fluid in the capillary vascular spaces; decreased plasma protein levels allow fluid to escape. Hydrostatic pressure generated by myocardial function helps maintain fluid balance in the vascular spaces. Myocardial dysfunction may lead to increased venous pressure and a net filtration of fluid into the interstitial tissues. Capillary permeability is the last factor opposing fluid filtration; the membrane is normally impermeable to plasma proteins. If capillary permeability increases, as it commonly does with sepsis, the protein pass into the interstitial spaces, drawing fluid with them.

HORMONAL INFLUENCES

The two major hormones that influence fluid balance are antidiuretic hormone (ADH, secreted by the posterior pituitary gland) and aldosterone (a mineral corticoid produced by the adrenal cortex). Secretion of ADH is promoted by increased serum osmolality. It increases reabsorption of sodium and water in the renal tubules and collecting tubules. This causes increase in vascular volume by decreasing urine output. Aldosterone acts on the distal tubules to reabsorb sodium by excreting potassium in exchange, causing water and sodium retention.

IMPORTANCE OF FLUID MAINTENANCE IN PAEDIATRIC SURGICAL PATIENTS

Volume of the total body and the rate of fluid exchange vary with age. A child's metabolism is altered by trauma of surgery. Dehydration as a result of diarrhoea in a child can be corrected within 24 hours. But dehydration as a result of intussusception in a child needs to be corrected within few hours, as the child has to undergo surgery safely following a preanaesthetic check-up (PAC). Fever increases caloric and fluid requirements by 12% for each degree rise in temperature, and stress or trauma in surgery with consequent wound healing increases calorie, protein and vitamin requirements. The metabolic expenditure of 100 cal forms a basis for calculating water requirements in paediatric surgical patients. Maintenance of fluid provides insensible water losses – water lost through skin, lungs and urine. At normal environmental temperature, a newborn loses about 30 mL of water through the skin and 15 mL of water through respiration.

Gastrointestinal losses can be determined by observing the number of times the baby passes stool or vomits and monitoring the amount of loss. The electrolyte composition of the vomited fluid depends on the level of obstruction. In infantile hypertrophic pyloric stenosis, the vomitus approximately contains 120–140 mEq of chloride/L with 10–12 mEq of K^+/L and minimal quantity of Na^+. But if the vomiting is bilious, it contains more Na^+ as 120–140 mEq/L and 100 mEq of Cl^-/L. Hence, while calculating fluid losses, a physician or surgeon will see that these losses are corrected. K^+ losses are likely to occur in a long-standing gastrointestinal loss. K^+ loss in acute surgical cases is rarely related to tissue release. But any deficit noted needs to be corrected by adding KCl to intravenous fluids.

STUDY QUESTIONS

1. Differentiate the fluid requirements in infants and adults.
2. What are the hormonal influences in fluid balance?
3. Discuss the importance of fluid maintenance in children.

BIBLIOGRAPHY

1. Amini, A., Schmidt, M.H. Syndrome of inappropriate secretion of antidiuretic hormone and hyponatremia after spinal surgery. *Neurosurg Focus.* 2004;16:E10.
2. Jospe, N., Forbes, G. Fluids and electrolytes – clinical aspects. *Pediatr Rev.* 1996;17:395–403.
3. Hellerstein, S. Fluids and electrolytes: clinical aspects. *Pediatr Rev.* 1993;14:103–115.
4. Rabin, N., Reed, T., Vallino, L.M. Balance and imbalance of body fluids. In: M.J. Hockenberry (Ed.). Wongs's nursing care of infants and children. 7th edition. Mosby: St. Louis (MO); 2003:1171–1206.
5. Stark, J. A comprehensive analysis of the fluid and electrolytes system. *Crit Care Nurs Clin North Am.* 1998;10:471–475.

CHAPTER 20

COMMON FLUID AND NUTRITIONAL PROBLEMS AND THEIR MANAGEMENT

LEARNING OBJECTIVES

At the end of the chapter, the learner will be able to

- Describe the nursing diagnoses and its interventions related to nursing care of children with nutritional disorders.
- Describe the postoperative fluid management.
- Define malnutrition.
- Discuss the care of children with protein–energy malnutrition.
- Classify malnutrition.
- Explain the grading system for malnutrition.
- Differentiate between marasmus and kwashiorkor.
- Discuss various vitamin and mineral deficiencies.

Water, carbohydrates and electrolytes are the standard constituents of simple intravenous fluids, as well as for standard feedings. However, there is an order of priority for survival in nutritional requirements. The main order of priority is water, followed by the major electrolytes, particularly sodium, acid–base status and some carbohydrates. Hence, the initial problem, and often the only problem, in the short-term illness is to replace water and electrolyte losses that have occurred because of illness. Correct any acid–base imbalances, replace any ongoing fluid and electrolyte losses that occur during treatment and give some carbohydrates to prevent hypoglycaemia and ketosis. The body will make up quickly for the deficiencies of protein, fat and other constituents when adequate normal nutrition is established.

IMPORTANT NURSING DIAGNOSES AND ITS INTERVENTIONS

Nursing Diagnoses

- Fluid volume deficit related to excessive loss or failure of regulatory mechanisms
- Fluid volume excess related to excessive fluid intake/ sodium intake or compromised regulatory mechanisms
- Altered tissue perfusion related to hypovolaemia or hypervolaemia
- Altered thought process related to electrolyte imbalances

Nursing Interventions

- Determine age and developmental level.
- Review physician/practitioner orders.
- Assess preexisting conditions, present status and current therapies for factors influencing fluid balances.
- Determine present and recent weight measures, if known, including date of measurement.
- Assess for physical signs of hydration status.
  - In infants, the anterior fontanel should be flat and soft.
  - Eye globes and orbits should be firm.
  - Conjunctivae and mucous membranes should be moist, with salivary bubbles under the tongue. Tearing should be noted with crying (over 6 years).
  - Assess skin turgor by pinching the skin over the abdomen and inner thigh; the skin should quickly recoil (within 1 second) on release.
  - The skin should be firm and smooth, the abdomen should be soft and nondistended, hands and feet

should not be puffy and the scrotum should be normal and not oedematous.

- Breath sounds are normal and clear; respiratory effort should be minimal. Fluid overload may give wet breaths or rales.
- Neck veins should have normal filling. If central monitoring is available, measure central venous pressure (CVP).
- Liver should not be palpable below the right costal margin.
- Assess for behavioural changes such as irritability, lethargy, confusion, seizures, etc.
- Assess systemic perfusion:
  - Capillary refill should be brisk (1–2 seconds), extremities should be warm and peripheral pulses should be strong.
  - *Urine volume:* Minimum acceptable by weight — infants 2 mL/kg per hour; children 1 mL/kg per hour and adolescents 0.5 mL/kg per hour.
  - Urine specific gravity (normal: 1.005–1.020).
  - *Skin colour:* Consistent colouring and pink mucus membrane.
  - *Acid–base balance:* pH, 7.35–7.45; pCO_2, 32–48; HCO, 21–28 mEq/L.
  - *Vital signs:* Normal limits for age (see the normal values).
- Assess intake and output – Assess the amount and character of recent intake and output.
  - Intake should include all types of fluids administered by different routes.
  - Check output through urine, stool and other aspirations.
  - Insensible losses through respiration and evaporation; perspiration is not an insensible loss; usual insensible losses include skin and lungs, 45 mL/100 cal; urine, 50–75 mL/day/100 cal; sweat, 0–25 mL/100 cal; stool, 5–10 mL/100 cal.
  - Asses abnormal losses such as sweat, vomitus, nasogastric suction, chest tube and wound drainage.
- Review laboratory data:
  - *Serum sodium:* 135–145 mEq/L
  - *Serum glucose:* 60–105 mEq/L
  - *Blood urea nitrogen (BUN):* Normal, 5–22 mg/dL; and creatinine: infants, 0.2–0.4 mg/dL; children, 0.3–0.7 mg/dL; adolescents, 0.5–1.0 mg/dL
  - *Serum osmolality:* Normal, 272–290 mOsm/dL; it can be calculated as follows: (2 × serum sodium) + (serum glucose ÷ 18) + (BUN ÷ 2.8) (mOsm/dL serum osmolality)
  - *Total protein value:* Neonates, 4.6–7.4 mg/dL; children, 6.2–8 mg/dL
  - *Serum potassium:* 3.5–5.5 mEq/L
  - *Haematocrit:* Neonates, 48%–69%; infants, 28%–42%; children, 35%–45%; adolescents, 36%–49%
- Evaluate present fluid balance to determine the type of management to be followed as maintenance, deficit therapy and monitoring concerns.
- If fluid volume deficit is present, determine the severity, preferably by weight loss or comparison with clinical signs; determine the type by serum sodium levels, history and clinical signs.

- Types of dehydration can be classified as isotonic, hypotonic and hypertonic dehydration.
- Calculate maintenance fluid requirement based on one of the three methods: metabolic rate, body weight or body surface area.
  - Metabolic rate or body weight
  - Weight (kg) 24-hour fluid requirements
  - 0–10   100 mL/kg
  - 11–20   1000 mL + 50 mL/kg for each kg over 10
  - 21–30   1500 mL + 20 mL/kg for each kg over 20
  - 31–40   1750 mL + 10 mL/kg for each kg over 3

Body Fluid Compartments (as a Percentage of Body Weight)

Age	Total Body Water	Extracellular Fluid	Intracellular Fluid
Newborn	70	35	35
12 months	65	25	40
Adult	60	20	40

Isotonic Crystalloid Fluids: Composition

Fluid	Sodium (mmol/L)	Potassium (mmol/L)	Chloride (mmol/L)	Energy (kcal/L)
0.9% saline (resuscitation fluid)	150	0	150	0
0.9% saline/5% dextrose (maintenance and suitable in electrolyte abnormalities)	150	0	150	200
0.45% saline/5% dextrose (maintenance if electrolytes is in the normal range)	75	0	75	200

- Body surface area: Use the Dubois or West surface normogram to provide requirements of 1500 mL/m^2 body surface area.
  - Modify maintenance fluid requirement appropriate to conditions – decreased requirements in renal failure, cardiac disease with failure, increased intracranial pressure, increased antidiuretic hormone (ADH) release, hypothermia, hypernatraemia with fluid excess or increased fluid requirements in hypermetabolic states.
  - Calculate deficit therapy requirements based on severity of dehydration and type – mild isotonic dehydration up to 50 mL/kg over 24 hours; moderate isotonic dehydration 100 mL/kg over the next 24 hours; severe isotonic dehydration 150 mL/kg over the next 24 hours.

- *Hypotonic dehydration* – Use fluid formula appropriate to the degree of dehydration as mentioned earlier. Replace 50% of fluid losses in the first 8 hours of therapy and remaining 50% during the next 16 hours.

Degree of Dehydration

Clinical Signs	Mild	Moderate	Severe
Weight loss			
Infant	5%	10%	15%
Child	3%	6%	9%
Skin colour	Pale	Grey	Mottled
Skin turgor	Normal/ decreased	Decreased	Tenting
Mucous membranes	Damp to dry	Very dry	Parched
Blood pressure	Normal	Normal/ lowered	Lowered
Heart rate	Normal	Increased	Rapid and thready pulse
Capillary refill time	Brisk	Slow	>3 seconds
Urine output	Normal	Oliguria	Marked oliguria and azotaemia
Behaviour	Alert, thirsty	Irritable and lethargic	Sensorium changes such as confusion

- *Hypertonic dehydration* – Use fluid formula appropriate to the degree of dehydration. Replace 50% of losses during the first 24 hours and 50% during the next 24 hours.
- Monitor intake and output – Explain to the parents and children the need for measuring intake and output. Instruct collection of all outputs for measurement.
- Measure and record all oral, enteral and parenteral intakes and all measurable outputs including normal and abnormal losses. Report significant imbalances.
- Perform ongoing assessment of hydration status.
- Monitor serial laboratory measures.
- Monitor neurological status.

POSTOPERATIVE FLUID MANAGEMENT

A child should enter the postoperative period with fluid and electrolyte balance by optimum replacement and maintenance therapy before and during the operation. If a child enters with fluid and electrolyte imbalance, maintenance and replacement of ongoing losses are necessary to maintain a satisfactory urinary output.

Immediate postoperative drainage (serous or bloody) needs to be measured and replaced with blood or plasma. Dressing may be removed and weighed to assess losses. Plastic bags or bottles can be used for collecting drainage that promotes correct measurements of fluid loss. All gastrointestinal drainage needs to be collected, and a sample should be sent to the laboratory for electrolyte estimation and replacement. This must be replaced within 4–12 hours depending on the volume and clinical condition. The nurse should be vigilant to replace the amount of gastric drainage with Ringer's lactate or 4.5% saline with 15–20 mEq of KCl/L to intravenous fluids. Satisfactory oral intake can be established 5–7 days postoperatively. When complications such as continued leakage, postoperative intestinal obstruction, sepsis or malabsorption occur, the surgeon may order for total parenteral nutrition (TPN).

MALNUTRITION

Malnutrition results from relative or absolute deficiency or excess of one or more essential nutrients. In India, as in the rest of the developing world, deficiency of essential nutrients is the major problem rather than excess, which is a common problem in developed countries. The essential nutrients are as follows:
- Proteins
- Carbohydrates
- Fats
- Water
- Minerals and vitamins

The main functions are as follows:
- Proteins are integral parts of all tissues in the body and are essential for repairs and growth of all tissues in the body.
- Carbohydrates and fats are the main sources of energy for all body functions. Thus, they are called as the energy foods.
- Water is essential for life. Lack of water leads to dehydration, which, if not corrected, may lead to death.
- Minerals and vitamins are essential but are required in very small quantities. They are not the sources of energy production. A variety of disorders are known as a result of their deficiency.

PROTEIN–ENERGY MALNUTRITION (PEM)

A child whose food does not contain enough protein and energy does not grow well and becomes malnourished. Such a malnourished child is said to be suffering from PEM. Thus, 'protein–energy malnutrition' is the terminology used for all kinds of malnutrition as a result of lack of protein and energy foods.

Magnitude of the Problem

PEM is the most important nutritional problem among children in the developing countries. Most of the other nutritional problems accompany PEM and are rare in well-nourished children. PEM is the leading cause of mortality and morbidity among children in developing countries. Children with PEM are more susceptible to infectious diseases, which are still a major problem among children in the developing world. PEM and infectious diseases have synergistic effect; each contributes to the precipitation and severity of the other. The cycle of PEM and infectious disease is perpetuating. Infections weaken a malnourished child by reducing appetite and lead to further reduction of food intake and thereby worsening the malnutrition. Many of the deaths as a result of PEM are never recognized as such because the terminal event is invariably caused by an infection. PEM in early childhood can have debilitating mental and physical consequences that are carried into the adulthood, and this will have a negative impact on the growth and productivity of a nation.

Most children with PEM are not identified because their weights are not taken routinely and recorded in a growth chart. Very few children with PEM are brought to hospitals and that to with some other ailments. Thus, we see only the tip of the malnutrition iceberg. Studies in India and Africa have reported the incidence of malnutrition to be as high as 30%–40% in children younger than 5 years, and 7.6% of these children have severe malnutrition as marasmus and kwashiorkor. Thus, the majority of these children have mild-to-moderate PEM.

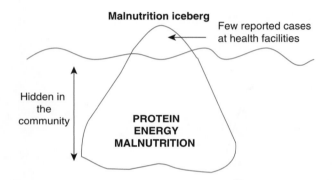

Causes and Risk Factors of PEM

- *Age:* Children between 6 months and 4 years of age are vulnerable, as this is the period of rapid growth. In infancy, the diet requirement is greater per unit body size because of their rapid growth. At 4 months of age, 30% of the energy intake is used for growth. By 1 year of age, 5% of the energy intake is used for growth, and by 3 years of age, only 2% of intake is used for growth. Hence, the risk of growth failure is more in the first 6 months of age.
- *Sex:* In India, boys are valued more than girls and girls may be consciously or unconsciously neglected.
- *Too many children in the same family:* If there are many children in a family, there is a chance of neglecting smaller children with respect to food and personal care, as the mother will be overburdened with many other responsibilities.
- *Lack of spacing between children:* If a mother becomes pregnant when her previous baby is still young (6 months), she may neglect that child. Her breast milk will get less and is not enough for the baby.
- *Low-birth-weight baby:* Babies who are born small for gestational age or premature have not enough food inside the womb of the mother. Many of them become malnourished subsequently. Children who are born

before the term have poor stores of fat and protein and hence less reserve to withstand starvation.
- *Twins/multiple births:* These children have a combination of high-risk factors. They are small and may receive only half as much milk and attention from the mother as a single baby, although there should be enough milk for both.
- *Poor growth in the first few months:* This can be judged only by weighing the baby regularly. Many children who gain less weight become malnourished. There may be many reasons for this, but the most important is the mother's failure to breastfeed. The reasons for poor growth may be a result of systemic diseases in children such as cardiovascular disorders or disorders related to ineffective feedings such as cleft lip and palate, oesophageal atresia, diaphragmatic hernia, etc.
- *Failure or stoppage of breastfeeding:* It may be as a result of sickness of the mother or as a result of ignorance or of certain problems with the baby.
- *Delay in introducing complementary feeds:* Although breast milk is given for 2 years, additional weaning foods need to introduce from the beginning of the fifth month, as the baby's requirement for growth and development increases with the advancing age. If complementary feeding is not given in time, it may lead to PEM.
- *Infectious diseases:* These may especially result from repeated diarrhoeas, acute respiratory infections or measles.
- *Chronic diseases and certain congenital disorders:* These may especially result from congenital heart diseases (CHDs), where failure to thrive or physical growth retardation is a common feature.
- *Lack of adequate care for the pregnant women:* Brain grows rapidly during the last trimester of pregnancy and throughout the first 2 years of life. Interneuronal connections also increase during this time. At birth, the brain accounts for approximately two-thirds of the metabolic rate and for about 50% at 1 year of age.
- Children's nutrition compromise follows acute illness or surgery. This may last for a week or so. If this is not considered and feeding is not appropriate, it can lead to malnutrition.

Infection and Malnutrition

The greater the severity and the longer an infection lasts, the worse is the effect on child's nutrition.

Hence, children at risk of developing PEM are as follows:

- Infants with low birth weight less than 2.5 kg
- Twin/multiple births
- Infants who are not breastfed
- Children with congenital defects (cleft palate and CHD, mental retardation, physical handicap)
- Children with high birth order
- Children with measles, pertussis and repeated diarrhoeas
- Children from a poor socioeconomic background
- Orphans or children living in special homes or foster homes and children of single parents
- Children with maternal deprivation

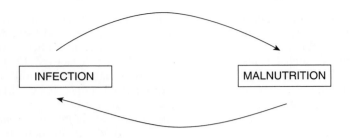

Malnutrition and early cessation of breastfeeding

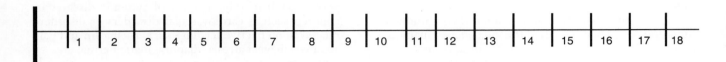

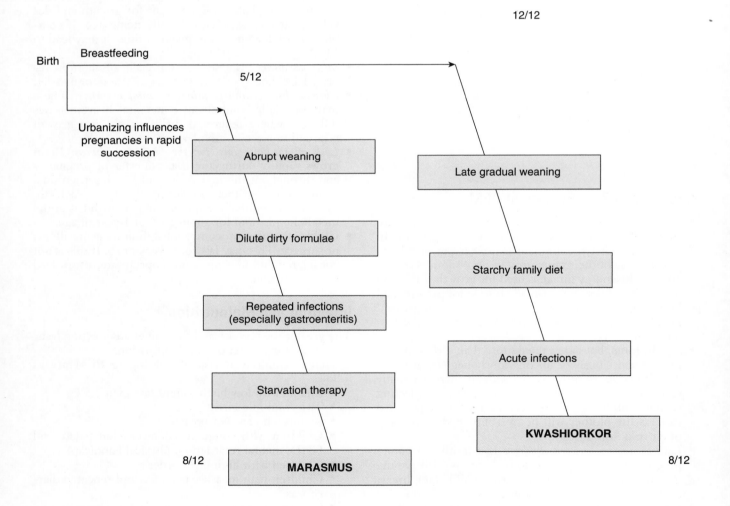

The long-term effects of nutritional deficiencies in childhood are decreased linear growth as adults and diseases in adult life (coronary heart diseases, stroke, non-insulin-dependent diabetes, hypertension and chronic airway diseases).

Classification of PEM

PEM is classified according to severity of the disease as mild, moderate and severe PEM.

1. **Mild PEM**
   Children whose weights are below the 3rd centile for their age but above the −3 standard deviation (SD). In a growth chart, the curves that are flat or tend to point downwards indicate mild PEM.
2. **Moderate PEM**
   Children whose weights are equal to or below the −3 SD line but above the −4 SD. Oedema is not a feature of moderate PEM, and children may not have skin and hair changes. Usually, these children are alert and their appetite is normal.
3. **Severe PEM**
   Children whose weights are equal or below the −4 SD line. Marasmus and kwashiorkor are two major forms of severe PEM. Another variety is marasmic kwashiorkor.

$$SD\,score = \frac{Observed\,value - Expected\,value}{SDs}$$

Those with weight for age is less than 60% without oedema have marasmus.

Indian Academy of Paediatrics (IAP) Classification of Malnutrition

Nutritional Status	Weight for Age (% of Expected Weight)
Normal	80%
Grade I PEM	70%–80%
Grade II	60%–70%
Grade III PEM	50%–60%
Grade IV PEM	<50%

Wellcome Trust Classification

Clinical Type of PEM	Oedema	Weight for Age
Kwashiorkor	+	60%–80%
Underweight	−	60%–80%
Marasmus	−	<60%
Marasmic kwashiorkor	+	<60%

McLean classification
- Dwarf children with less than 80% height
- Short stature of those with weight for age 80%–93%

WHO Classification

Features	Moderate	Severe
Symmetrical oedema	No	Yes
Weight for height (measure of wasting)	SD score −2 or −3	SD score <−3 (<70% of the expected weight)
Height for age (measure of stunting)	SD score −2 or −3 (85%–89% of the expected weight)	SD score <−3 (<85% of the expected weight)

- Normal more than 93%
- Marginal 90%–95%
- Moderate 85%–90% height
- Severe <85% height

Kanawati index = MAC/HC (where MAC and HC are mid-arm circumference and head circumference, respectively)
- Mild PEM 0.28–0.314
- Moderate PEM 0.25–0.273
- Severe PEM <0.25

Ponderal index
- Normal >2.5
- Borderline PEM 2–2.5
- Severe PEM <2

Marasmus is the severe nonoedematous malnutrition caused by a mixed deficiency of both protein and calories, with serum protein and albumin levels usually normal.

Grading of Marasmus

- Grade I – Loss of subcutaneous fat in the axilla and groin
- Grade II – Grade I + loss of abdominal fat and fat in the gluteal region
- Grade III – Grade II + loss of fat in the chest wall and the paraspinal region
- Grade IV – Grade III + loss of the buccal pad of fat

Kwashiorkor is the oedematous malnutrition as a result of low serum oncotic pressure that results from low protein intake compared with the overall intake. The children appear fat but with dependent oedema.

Grading of Kwashiorkor

- Grade I – Pedal oedema
- Grade II – Grade I + facial puffiness
- Grade III – Grade II + oedema of the chest wall and the paraspinal area
- Grade IV – Grade III + ascites

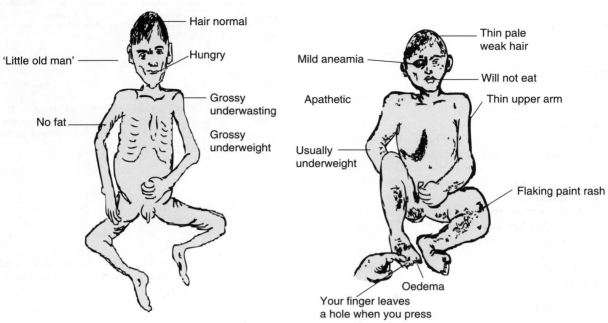

MARASMUS

Hair normal

Hungry

'Little old man'

Grossy underwasting

Grossy underweight

No fat

KWASHIORKOR

Thin pale weak hair

Mild aneamia

Will not eat

Apathetic

Thin upper arm

Usually underweight

Flaking paint rash

Oedema

Your finger leaves a hole when you press

Features of severe PEM.

Difference between Marasmus and Kwashiorkor

Features	Marasmus	Kwashiorkor
Growth failure	Marked, very low weight for age Weight < −4 SD	Marked, but masked by oedema
Muscle wasting	Marked; felt on the upper arm	Quite marked, sometimes hidden by oedema and fat; better felt than seen
Fat wasting	Marked; looks like an old man; especially, on buccal fat, groin, etc.	Fat is retained
Oedema	None	Most common in the feet, lower legs, lower back and face; pitting type
Skin	Normal usually	Pale skin prominent on the face, thick, scaly, cracked skin resembling crazy pavement, or flaky paint or ulceration beneath
Hair changes	Sometimes soft and straight	Soft, lighter, flag sign; can be easily pulled out and sparse
Appetite and behaviour	Often hungry, alert and anxious looking	Poor appetite, miserable face, feeble, whining cry
Vitamin deficiencies	Sometimes present	Usually present
Liver size	Normal	Enlarged because of accumulation of fat
Loose stools owing to poor digestion	Sometimes have constipation	Often loose stools
Infective diarrhoea	Sometimes	Often
Serum protein	Low in extreme cases	Always low
Anaemia	Sometimes	Always

ASSESSMENT FINDINGS

- *Nutritional assessment* includes history and clinical findings, 24-hour retrospective dietary recall, societal and environmental assessments to determine feeding skills, adequacy of eating, socioeconomic status and maternal interaction.
- Most important information can be obtained from a serially plotted growth chart.
- Anthropometric measurements (height, weight and head circumference) need to be compared with the population standard.
- Compare the actual with ideal body weight (IBW; average weight for height age). IBW is determined by plotting the child's height on the 50th percentile and recording the corresponding age. This is expressed as a percentage.
  - >120 = obese
  - 110–120 = overweight
  - 90–110 = normal
  - 80–90 = mild wasting
  - 70–80 = moderate wasting
  - <70 = severe wasting
- *Mid-arm circumference:* It gives information regarding subcutaneous fat stores and mid-arm muscle circumference. This value can be compared with standards for the patient's age and sex. In infants, subscapular skinfold thickness measurements are preferred.
- *Laboratory assessment:* Measurements of serum albumin (half-life 14–20 days), transferrin (half-life 8–10.5 days) and prealbumin (half-life 2–3 days) provide information about protein malnutrition. The ratio of albumin to globulin may decrease in protein malnutrition. The creatinine height index is a measure of lean body mass which decreases as muscle protein is used up as the energy source. Nitrogen balance may be obtained to determine the degree of protein anabolism or catabolism. Blood glucose level will be low in severe PEM developing into hypoglycaemia. Microbiologic investigation is the area indicated in sick children admitted with PEM. Blood, urine and rectal swab cultures are indicated according to the condition of the child. Mantoux's test is also done to rule out tuberculosis. Microscopic examination of urine and blood is also indicated.

Multidisciplinary Management

The major aims of treatment are as follows:
- To supply what has been lacking in the diet
- To prevent and treat infections and other diseases
- To teach parents how to prevent relapse

Mild PEM

- Rule out infections.
- Provide nutritional counselling to parents.

- Replace nutrients and breastfeed till 2 years of age, with the introduction of supplementary feeding at 4–5 months.
- Immunization screening should be done and immunize if required.
- Admission to hospital is required only if the parents need counselling and nutritional education with demonstration.

Moderate PEM

- Admit to hospital for a short period (5 days).
- Treat the underlying cause or problems.
- Diet is the most important part of treatment.
- Provide a reinforced milk diet.
- Teach preparation of a milk diet.

Severe PEM

- Admit to hospital.
- Watch for complications.
- *Dietary treatment:* Provide 4 g of protein/kg per body weight. Children with marasmus require about 150–200 cal/kg per day. Children with kwashiorkor need 100 cal/kg per day.
- Reinforced milk or high-calorie cereal milk can be given.
- Children should be fed with milk diet at the ratio of 125 mL/kg per day.
- Children with kwashiorkor will have more feeding problems.
- Severely ill children should be fed regularly, even at night, to prevent hypoglycaemia.
- Severely ill children should be fed through a nasogastric tube.
- Gradually increase the feeds.
- Continue till the baby could consume 1 L of reinforced milk per day.
- Usual schedule is eight feeds per day at 3-hour interval.
- By the second week, night feeds can be stopped.
- Supplement minerals and vitamins.
- Treat infections.

Nursing Diagnoses

- Alteration in nutrition less than body requirement
- Fluid electrolyte imbalances
- High risk for infections
- Potential for complications
- Knowledge deficit
- Parental anxiety
- Body image disturbances

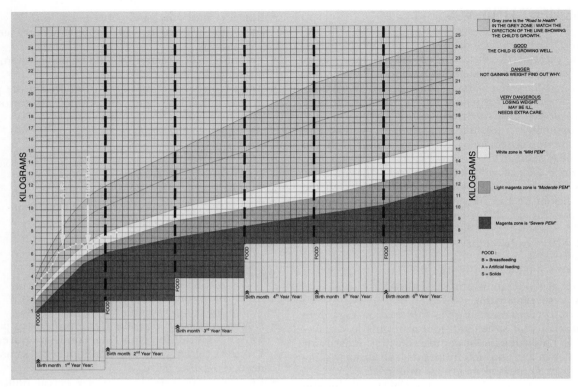

(A) Mild PEM.

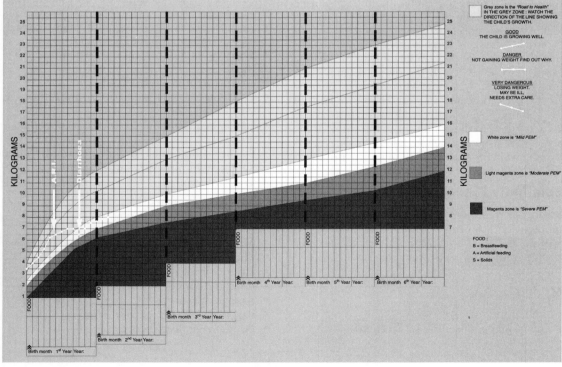

(B) Moderate PEM.

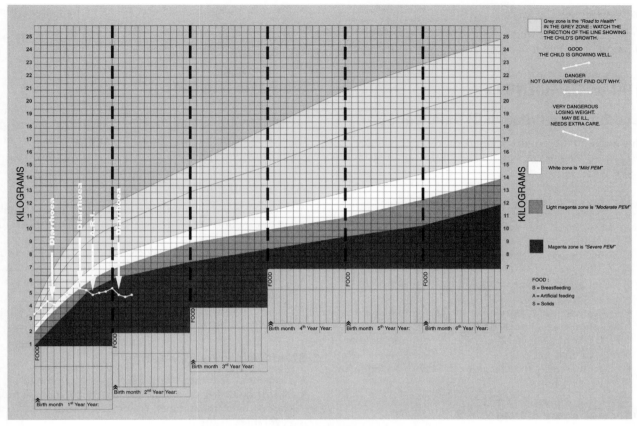

(C) Severe PEM.

Nursing Interventions

- Plan and provide a diet that contains 200 cal and 4 g of protein/kg of the current weight so that the child will receive a diet that contains 100 cal and 2 g of protein/kg of the expected body weight.
- Include first-class protein for supplementation (milk, egg, etc.).
- Start with 25% of the requirement or less depending on the tolerance and bring it up to 100% over a few days: on the second day, 50% of the formula, 75% on the third day, 90% on the fourth day and 100% on the fifth day.
- Very rapid increase should be avoided, especially in children with kwashiorkor, as it may cause unexplained sudden death. It can also cause nutritional recovery syndrome characterized by hepatomegaly, ascites, increased intracranial pressure, extrapyramidal signs, etc.
- Feeds should be given six to eight times a day.
- Breastfeed should be given only after scheduled feeds in breastfeed-addicted babies.
- Supplement electrolytes, minerals and vitamins as required according to serum studies – usually 2 g of potassium chloride and 2 g of sodium along with vitamins and minerals are added to the formula.
- If urine output is low, measure K+ levels.
- Administer $MgSO_4$ (50%) 0.1–0.2 mL/kg i.m. daily for 3 days as directed.
- If the child tolerates, give high-calorie cereal milk (100 mL of milk, 1 teaspoon sugar, 1 teaspoon coconut oil and 1 teaspoon cereal powder, e.g. rice flour).

- See that fat should not exceed 55% of the total daily calories.
- Iron and folic acid also can be added slowly to the diet (recommended dose of iron is 30–60 mg of elementary iron.
- However, postpone iron syrup till oedema disappears and the child is free of infection.
- Calcium phosphate and B complex vitamins also need supplementation.
- Slowly add family diet as the baby gains weight.
- Identify and treat occult infection.
- Administer antibiotics as prescribed.
- Prevent hypoglycaemia and administer 10% glucose 4 mL/kg stat to children with hypoglycaemia as prescribed.
- Prevent hypothermia by covering the body, including head, with a cap.
- If the temperature is at or below 35°C, there is hypothermia; keep the baby under 100-W bulb 45 cm above the baby's bed or by keeping hot water bottles in the crib with adequate precautions to avoid burns.
- Reassess the efficacy of warming by taking temperature, especially rectal temperature.
- Provide parental teaching on breastfeeding, weaning or complementary feeding, immunization, prevention of infections and diarrhoea, child spacing, personal and environmental hygiene, including food hygiene, utilization of locally available food for the child's diet and the need for supplementation of vitamins and minerals.

Evaluation

If the child regains weight as expected, then there is no infection or oedema.

VITAMIN DEFICIENCIES

Ascorbic Acid (Vitamin C) Deficiency

This is the first recognized micronutrient deficiency disease, and deficiency results in the clinical manifestations of scurvy.

Assessment Findings

Infantile scurvy is manifested by the following:
- Irritability
- Bone tenderness with swelling and pseudoparalysis of the legs
- Commonly seen in infants fed with unsupplemental cow's milk
- Persistence or progression of these deficiency leads to subperiosteal haemorrhage
- Hyperkeratosis of hair follicles and succession of mental changes
- Chronic scurvy may be associated with anaemia and folate deficiency

Multidisciplinary Management

- Administer vitamin C (250–500 mg).
- Provide nutritional advice to include citrus fruits and green leafy vegetables in the diet.
- Instruct that cooking destroys this vitamin.
- Amla is a rich source of vitamin, and cooking amla will not give away vitamin C.

Thiamine (Vitamin B₁) Deficiency

It functions as a coenzyme in biochemical reactions related to carbohydrate metabolism and other biochemical reactions. Thiamine is also involved in the decarboxylation of branched-chain amino acids. Deficiency produces beriberi.

Assessment Findings

- Infantile beriberi is seen in breastfed infants (1–4 months of age) whose mothers have thiamine deficiency and also in children with PEM.
- Other symptoms include polyneuropathy, calf tenderness, heart failure, oedema, ophthalmoplegia, etc.
- In severe cases, acute cardiac symptoms and signs are predominant.
- Anorexia, apathy, vomiting, pallor and progression to dyspnoea, cyanosis and death occur owing to heart failure.

Multidisciplinary Management

- Administer thiamine as prescribed. The usual dose is 5–25 mg.

- Provide nutritional advice as to include food items such as liver, meat, cereals, nuts and legumes.
- Inform parents that pasteurization and sterilization of milk destroy thiamine.

Riboflavin (Vitamin B₂)

It is a constituent of two coenzymes riboflavin 5′-phosphate and flavin adenine dinucleotide. Deficiency affects glucose, fatty acid and amino acid metabolism. Deficiency causes ariboflavinosis.

Assessment Findings

- Characterized by angular stomatitis, glossitis, cheilosis and seborrhoeic dermatitis around the nose and mouth.
- Eye changes include decreased tearing, photophobia, corneal vascularizations and formation of cataracts.
- Infants undergoing prolonged phototherapy are prone to develop ariboflavinosis.
- So also are diabetic children and children from a poor socioeconomic background.

Multidisciplinary Management

- Deficiency is treated with 5–25 mg of riboflavin.
- Nutritional advice should be given to include milk, cheese, liver, meat, eggs, whole grains and green leafy vegetables in the diet.
- It is decomposed by exposure to sunlight and strong alkaline solutions.

Niacin Deficiency

It is a compound of nicotinic acid and nicotinamide. Niacin is involved in multiple metabolic processes such as fat synthesis, intracellular respiratory metabolism and glycolysis. Niacin is stable in foods and can withstand heating and prolonged storage. Deficiency causes pellagra.

Assessment Findings

- Niacin deficiency is characterized by weakness, lassitude, dermatitis, inflammation of mucous membrane, diarrhoea, vomiting, dysphagia and, in severe cases, dementia.

Multidisciplinary Management

- Deficiency is treated with 25–50 mg of niacin.
- Nutritional advice to be give to include rich sources of foods in the diet such as meat, fish, liver, whole grains and green leafy vegetables.

Vitamin B₆ Deficiency

It includes three naturally occurring pyridines: pyridoxine, pyridoxal and pyridoxamine. Vitamin B₆ performs many metabolic functions such as interconversion reactions of amino acids, conversion of tryptophan to niacin and serotonin, metabolic reactions in the brain, carbohydrate metabolism, immune development and biosynthesis of haem and prostaglandins. Pyridoxal and pyridoxamine are destroyed by heat. Heat-stable pyridoxine-fortified formulas are now available.

Heat treatment produces deficiency. Seizures are common in infants fed with deficient vitamin B formulas. Deficiency causes many problems.

Assessment Findings

- Deficiency causes seizures, hyperacusis, microcytic anaemia, nasolabial seborrhoea and neuropathy.

Multidisciplinary Management

- Deficiency is treated with 5–25 mg of vitamin B_6.
- Nutritional advice to be given to include foods that are rich in vitamin B_6 such as meat, liver, whole grains, peanuts, soybean, etc.

Biotin Deficiency

It is a component of several carboxylase enzymes essential for fat and carbohydrate metabolism. It is synthesized by intestinal bacteria, and its deficiency is uncommon. But it is seen in children receiving biotin-deficient TPN.

Assessment Findings

- Deficiency is characterized by anorexia, nausea, glossitis, pallor, mental changes, alopecia and fine maculo-squamous dermatitis.
- Administration of antibiotics increases requirements.

Multidisciplinary Management

- Deficiency is treated with 0.15–0.3 mg of biotin.
- Nutritional advice must be directed to include yeast and meat in the diet.
- Biotin is also synthesized by the normal intestinal flora.

Vitamin B_{12} Deficiency

Vitamin B_{12} deficiency is a rare disorder. It produces irreversible neurological damage. The cause is a defect in absorption as that in pernicious anaemia owing to the absence of intrinsic factor or as a result of autoimmune juvenile pernicious anaemia and deficiency of transcobalamin II transport. Deficiency occurs in bowel resection, too. Breastfed infants get adequate vitamin B_{12} unless the mother is a pure vegetarian. Most cases of deficiency are not dietary in origin and require lifelong replacement.

Multidisciplinary Management

- Vitamin B_{12} is administered parenterally, as it is needed in micrograms.
- Dietary sources are meat, fish, cheese and eggs.

Vitamin A Deficiency

Basic constituent of vitamin A is retinol. Retinol influences the growth and differentiation of epithelia and serves as a cofactor in glycoprotein synthesis. Deficiency produces a group of ocular symptoms called xerophthalmia. Earlier symptom is night blindness, followed by xerosis of the conjunctiva and cornea. If untreated, it results in ulceration, necrosis, keratomalacia and permanent corneal scar. Urgent treatment is necessary.

Multidisciplinary Management

- Treatment includes administration of vitamin 5000–10,000 IU intramuscularly in severe cases. Doses may be repeated as needed.
- Prevention is aimed by administration of vitamin A prophylactically as a part of the national programme to control blindness in children.
- Nutritional advice to be give to include vitamin A-rich foods such as liver, milk, eggs, green and yellow vegetables and fruits in the diet.

Vitamin E Deficiency

There are eight naturally occurring compounds associated with vitamin E activity. The most active one is α-tocopherol (90%) of vitamin E in human tissues. Other important ones are β- and γ-tocopherol. It is a biological antioxidant which inhibits peroxidation of polyunsaturated fatty acids present in the cell membrane.

Assessment Findings

- Deficiency is seen in children with prolonged and profound fat malabsorption such as biliary atresia, cystic fibrosis, etc.

Multidisciplinary Management

- Deficiency is treated with administration of 100–1000 IU of vitamin in patients with malabsorption.
- Nutritional supplementation is by adding seeds, vegetable germ oils and green leafy vegetables in the diet.

Vitamin D Deficiency

Two major constituents of vitamin D are cholecalciferol (D_2) and ergocalciferol (D_3). These are produced by ultraviolet irradiation of inactive precursors in the skin. Vitamin D deficiency appears as rickets in children and as osteomalacia in prepubescent children. Rickets develops from defective bone growth, especially marked at the epiphyseal cartilage matrix which fails to mineralize.

Assessment Findings

- Deficiency manifestations are seen only after several months of deficiency and are most common during the first 2 years of life.
- Seen in children with a poor intake of vitamin D-rich food.
- Little exposure to direct ultraviolet sunlight is beneficial.

Multidisciplinary Management

- Deficiency is treated with 400–500 IU of vitamin D.
- Include fortified milk, cheese and liver in the diet.
- Appropriate parent and patient education must be provided.

Rickets in Children

Rickets is a condition that results from softening of bone owing to prolonged deficiency of vitamin D. The deficiency of vitamin D hinders the absorption of calcium and phosphorus from the gastrointestinal tract. So, the calcium–phosphorus levels in the bones are not maintained, leading to rickets.

Causes. Lack of vitamin D in the diet causes rickets. It may be a result of insufficient intake or problems in utilization of vitamin. The main sources of vitamin D are as follows:

- **Sunlight.** The skin produces vitamin D when it is exposed to sunlight. But children in developed countries spend much of their time indoors and are not exposed to sunlight. They also use sunscreen that blocks the rays that trigger production of vitamin D.
- **Food.** Fish oils, fatty fish and egg yolks contain vitamin D. Vitamin D is also added to some foods such as milk, cereal and some fruit juices.

Some children have problems with absorption of vitamin D such as those with coeliac diseases, inflammatory bowel diseases, cystic fibrosis and certain kidney diseases.

Risk Factors

- Dark skin: Dark skin may not react strongly to sunlight and may result in vitamin D deficiency
- Maternal vitamin D deficiency: If the mother suffers from vitamin D deficiency during her pregnancy, the baby may be born with rickets or develop it within a few months
- Children living in northern latitudes where sunlight is less
- Preterm babies
- Medications such as anticonvulsants and antiretroviral drugs
- Exclusive breastfeeding babies
- Hypophosphatic rickets occur as a rare genetic fault that prevents kidneys from processing phosphorus properly

Clinical Features

- Delayed growth
- Pain in the spine, pelvis and legs
- Muscle weakness
  It can cause skeletal deformities such as:
- Bowed legs or knock-knees
- Thickened wrists and ankles
- Breastbone projection

Prevention. Expose the baby to sunlight, as it is the best source of vitamin D. Give foods containing vitamin D such as fish, fatty fish, fish oil and egg yolks or foods that are fortified with vitamin D such as:

- Infant formula
- Cereal
- Bread
- Milk, but not foods made from milk, such as yogurt and cheese
- Orange juice
- All breastfed babies must be given supplemental vitamin D, as breast milk contains very less amount of vitamin D. The IAP recommends administration of vitamin D along with routine immunization at the age of 6 months. The usual dose is 400 IU.

Management. Perform blood investigation to check vitamin D, serum calcium, phosphorus, kidney function and bone turnover; perform urine test; and obtain photographs and X-rays. Children with a very low level of calcium need hospitalization for cardiac monitoring, as they may have rhythm changes.

Children with low levels of vitamin D require replacement. They require a calcium balance study. They also may need extra calcium and phosphate before administering a high vitamin D dose.

Children with a kidney problem require consultation with a nephrologist.

Children should be regularly followed up. X-rays and photographs should be taken at regular intervals to assess the progress of treatment.

Vitamin K Deficiency

It is essential for posttranslational carboxylation of clotting factors II, VIII, IX, X and proteins C, S and Z. Deficiency causes prolonged prothrombin time. Haemorrhage and elevated levels of protein are induced in vitamin K absence (PIVKA).

Assessment Findings

- Deficiency is observed in persons with impaired fat absorption caused by obstructive jaundice, pancreatic insufficiency and coeliac diseases. These problems are compounded by administration of antibiotics.
- Absorption can be inhibited by mineral oil and high intakes of vitamins A and E.
- Haemorrhagic disease of the newborn is more common in breastfed infants and occurs in the first few weeks of life. It is rare in infants who receive prophylactic vitamin K on the first day of life.
- Other features include generalized ecchymosis, gastrointestinal bleeding, bleeding from circumcision or umbilical stump and rarely intracranial haemorrhage.

Management

Management includes administration of vitamin K.

MINERAL DEFICIENCIES

Calcium Deficiency

Dietary calcium intake depends on the consumption of dietary products. There is no classical calcium deficiency syndrome as blood and cell levels are regulated. In total, 99% of calcium is in the skeleton and the remaining 1% is distributed to extracellular fluid, intracellular fluid and cell membrane. Body calcium mobilizes skeletal calcium and increases absorption ability of dietary calcium. Osteoporosis occurs in children with PEM, vitamin C deficiency, steroid therapy, endocrine disorders, immobilization and disuse. Poor mineralization of bones and teeth, osteomalacia, osteoporosis, tetany, rickets and impairment of growth are the common problems with calcium deficiency.

Management is by parenteral administration as per requirement.

Other Deficiencies

Chloride deficiency can cause hypochloraemic alkalosis. Cobalt deficiency causes hypothyroidism. Copper deficiency produces refractory anaemia. Magnesium deficiency occurs with malabsorption and may cause tetany. Fluorine deficiency causes dental caries. Phosphorus deficiency produces rickets. Deficiency of potassium causes muscle weakness, anorexia, nausea, tachycardia, etc. Iron deficiency is dealt along with haematological disorders.

STUDY QUESTIONS

1. Discuss the postoperative fluid management.
2. What is PEM?
3. What are the causes of PEM?
4. Explain the infection–malnutrition cycle.
5. What are the major classifications of PEM?
6. What is Kanawati index?
7. What is ponderal index?
8. How will you grade marasmus?
9. How will you grade kwashiorkor?
10. Differentiate between marasmus and kwashiorkor.
11. Prepare a nursing care plan for a preschool child with grade III PEM.
12. Write short notes on:
    (a) Vitamin C deficiency
    (b) Vitamin B_2 deficiency
    (c) Vitamin thiamine deficiency
    (d) Vitamin B_6 deficiency
    (e) Protein deficiency
    (f) Vitamin A deficiency
    (g) Rickets

BIBLIOGRAPHY

1. Macchlean, A., Williams, A.F. (1995). Optimising Infant Nutrition. Current Paediatrics, 5(1), pp 32–35.
2. Passmore, S.J., McNinch, A.W. (1995). Vitamin K Deficiency. Current Paediatrics, 5(1), pp 36–39.
3. Pipes, P.L. (1985). Nutrition in Infancy and Childhood. 3rd Edn. St. Louis: C.V. Mosby, CO.
4. Poskitt, E.M.E. Childhood Obesity. Current Paediatrics, 5(1), pp 49–51.
5. Singh, J., Moghal, N., Pearce, S.H.S. et al, The investigation of hypocalcaemia and rickets. *Arch Dis Child*. 2003;88:403–407.
6. Stephens, D., Jackson, P.L., Gutierrez, Y. (1996). Subclinical Vitamin A Deficiency: A Potentially Unrecognized Problem in United States. Pediatric Nursing, 22(5), pp 377–390.
7. Torun, B., Chew, F. (1999). PEM. In: Olson, J.A., Shike, M., et al. (Editors): Modern Nutrition in Health and Disease. 9th Edn. William & Wilkins: Philadelphia.
8. Walia, B.N.S., Singh, S. (1995). Protein-energy malnutrition. Current Paediatrics, 5(1), pp 39–43.
9. Wong DL., Wilson D. (1991) 'Whaley and Wong's Nursing Care of Infants and Children'. 5th Edn. Philadelphia: Mosby; 1228-1230.
10. Hazinski MF. 'Understanding fluid balance in the seriously ill child.' Pediatric Nursing, 14:231–236.

UNIT 5

NURSING CARE OF NEONATES

This unit encompasses a wide range of topics with five chapters that are related to newborn care. The chapters on review of genetics, embryology, chromosomal abnormalities and inborn errors of metabolism are given before going to the details of neonatal care. This is preceded by care of normal neonates, kangaroo mother care, essential newborn care and care of high-risk neonates including care of preterm infants.

CHAPTER 21

GENETIC CONCEPTS AND IMPORTANCE IN PAEDIATRIC NURSING

CHAPTER OUTLINE

- Cell Division
- Mutation
- Pattern of Inheritance
- Mode of Transmission
- Polygenic or Multifactorial Disorders
- Common Chromosome Abnormalities
- Down Syndrome
- Cri-du-chat Syndrome
- Turner Syndrome
- Fragile X Syndrome
- Klinefelter Syndrome
- Mosaicism
- Nursing Management of Children with Common Chromosomal Anomalies
- Inborn Errors of Metabolism (IEM)
- Long-term Treatment of IEM
- Newborn Screening for IEM
- Precautions to be Observed while Collecting Samples for Newborn Screening
- Galactosaemia

- Glucose-6-Phosphate Dehydrogenase Deficiency
- Phenylketonuria
- Albinism
- Genetically Lethal Disease
- Cystic Fibrosis
- VATER Syndrome
- Important Advancements in Genetics
- DNA Fingerprinting
- Sex Determination
- Reproductive Technology
- Eugenics
- Positive Eugenics
- Negative Eugenics
- Euphenics
- Euthenics
- Genethics
- Genetic Engineering
- Genetic Counselling

LEARNING OBJECTIVES

Upon completion of this chapter, the learner will be able to

- Review the foundations of heritance and terminologies, including patterns of inheritance.
- Discuss the common chromosomal abnormalities and inborn errors of metabolism.
- Describe the nursing management of chromosomal abnormalities.
- Identify the common investigations used to detect chromosomal and genetic abnormalities.
- Define DNA fingerprinting, sex determination reproductive technology, eugenics, positive and negative eugenics, euphenics, euthenics, genetics, genetic engineering, gene therapy and genetic counselling.

Rapid advancement in medical sciences has helped man to eliminate and control a majority of infectious diseases and nutritional disorders that were the major causes of childhood mortality in olden days. Now, disorders as a result of genetic factors account for half of all paediatric surgical cases in both developed and underdeveloped countries.

Genetics is defined as a branch of medical science concerned with the transmission of characteristics from parents to the child.

Genetic factors probably play a role in every disease and disorder. For example, certain diseases such as muscular dystrophy and cystic fibrosis result from specific genetic defects, whereas in diseases such as cancer, a genetic defect is suspected but not yet proved scientifically.

FOUNDATIONS OF INHERITANCE – A REVIEW

Cell division: All living beings begin their life as a single cell called zygote. The single cell reproduces either by mitosis or by meiosis.

A. **Mitosis** is the process of multiple divisions in which new cells are formed. These new cells have the same number and form of chromosomes as the parent cell. That is, 46 chromosomes comprising 44 autosomes and two sex chromosomes. Mitosis has five stages: interphase, prophase, metaphase, anaphase and telophase.

1. *Interphase*: Before cell division, DNA replicates itself so that the genes will be doubled.
2. *Prophase*: The chromatin shortens and thickens; the chromosomes reproduce; the spindles appear and the centrioles migrate to the opposite poles of the cell; the membrane separating the nucleus from the cytoplasm disappears.
3. *Metaphase*: The chromosomes line up along the poles of the spindle.
4. *Anaphase*: The two chromatids in each chromosome separate and move towards the opposite poles of the spindle.
5. *Telophase*: A nuclear membrane forms, the spindle disappears and the centrioles relocate to the outside of the nucleus; towards the end of this phase, the cell divides into two new cells with the same number of chromosomes as the parent cell.

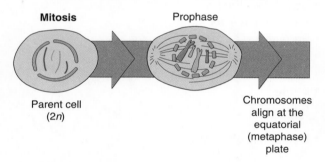

Mitosis — Prophase

Parent cell (2n)

Chromosomes align at the equatorial (metaphase) plate

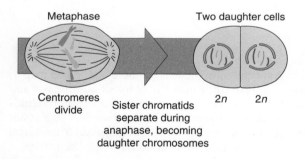

Metaphase — Two daughter cells

Centromeres divide

Sister chromatids separate during anaphase, becoming daughter chromosomes

2n   2n

B. **Meiosis** is the reduction division, where the maturation process of ova and sperm occurs (gametogenesis). This process of cell division occurs in two stages.

The first stage consists of four phases.

1. *Prophase*: Crossover of genetic materials takes place and accounts for a wide variety of features seen in same-parent siblings.
2. *Metaphase*: Spindle fibres attach to the separate chromosomes.
3. *Anaphase*: Chromosome pair migrates to opposite ends of the cell, with distribution of maternal and paternal chromosomes at random.

4. *Telophase*: The cell divides into cells, each with one-half (23) of the usual number of chromosomes (22 autosomes and one sex chromosome).

Meoisis I

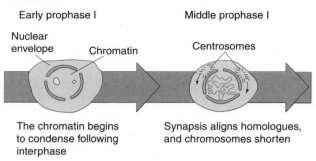

Early prophase I — Middle prophase I

Nuclear envelope — Chromatin — Centrosomes

The chromatin begins to condense following interphase

Synapsis aligns homologues, and chromosomes shorten

The second stage consists of two processes.

1. The chromatids of each chromosome separate and move to the opposite poles of each daughter cells.
2. This is followed by each of the cells dividing into two daughter cells, resulting into four cells (spermatogenesis and oogenesis). Spermatogenesis is continuous from puberty to senescence and oogenesis is noncontinuous.

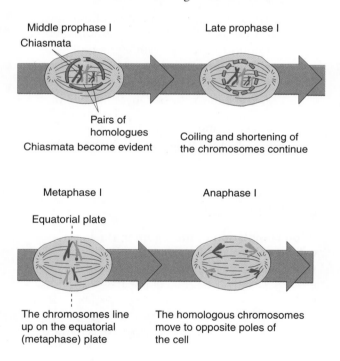

Middle prophase I — Late prophase I
Chiasmata
Pairs of homologues
Chiasmata become evident

Coiling and shortening of the chromosomes continue

Metaphase I — Anaphase I
Equatorial plate

The chromosomes line up on the equatorial (metaphase) plate

The homologous chromosomes move to opposite poles of the cell

During meiotic division, two chromatids may not move apart during cell division, resulting in autosomal nondisjunction or breakage to produce deletion leading to abnormal structure(s).

Genetic information is present on the chromosomes. Chromosomes are composed of DNA, a complex protein that carries the genetic material. (DNA and RNA, the molecules of life, were discovered by Friedrich Miescher in 1869.) DNA contains chemical ingredients called bases. There are four bases, namely thymine (T), adenine (A), guanine (G) and cytosine (C). These bases are arranged differently in each gene. Some have thousands and yet others have millions of them. Gene expresses through protein synthesis. Gene is a piece of nucleic acid which is responsible for a hereditary trait. Each gene is situated on a particular locus at one chromosome. A gene may have many alleles arising as a result of mutations. Genes also replicate semiconservatively so that they can be transmitted to the next generation. Each gene codes for a particular cellular function. Genes occur in pairs derived from the mother and the father during reproduction. Genetic errors can occur when there are changes in the location or products of genes.

The construction of a chart that uses standard symbols to designate family members, their relationships and their pertinent information is called a genome or pedigree or family tree. The complete set of genes for a human being is called **human genome**. It can be compared to a book of instructions, with each gene as a single instruction written in an unknown language. The international effort to learn the secrets of gene is called the **Human Genome Project**. They are valuable in demonstration of the various modes of inheritance for a gene disorder in a particular family. A **genetic disorder** is a disease caused by an abnormality in an individual's DNA. Abnormality can range from a small mutation in a single gene to the addition or substitution of an entire chromosome or set of chromosomes. In any pair, if one gene is **dominant** over the other, its instructions are followed. A **recessive gene's** instructions come into play only if neither gene in its pair is dominant; when a gene becomes active it produces a protein. Proteins are the basic chemicals of cells and genes direct their activities. Every protein has a different function, though with some overlapping of jobs. A gene in one person may carry a slightly different function from that of the corresponding gene in another person. Most variations in the same gene do not cause any health problems. For example, a person with blue eyes can see as well like that of a person with brown eyes.

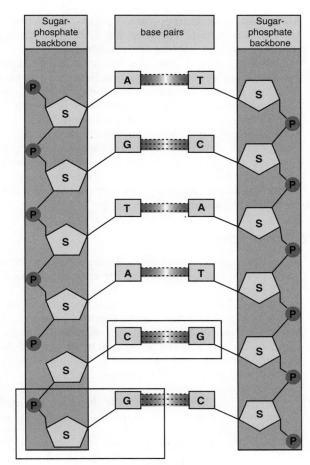

DNA strand.

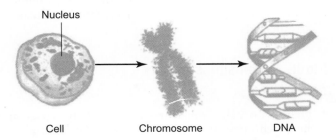

Cell   Chromosome   DNA

Mutation is a change that occurs in the order of the bases appearing in the DNA inside a cell. It can happen to any gene inside any cell of your body at any point in life. But most of it occurs when germ cells make copies of their chromosomes before dividing to form sperm or eggs. Usually, every copy of DNA has some errors. A base is put in a wrong place or is left out. Sometimes, extra copies are made of a string of bases or of whole

chromosomes. Many mutations happened to genes of people who lived long ago, and these mutations have been passed down through the generations. Some are new, occurring in a person during his/her lifetime. New mutation may be passed on to the next generation if it appears in the sperm or egg cells. Most mutations are harmless, and some trait is helpful to the survival of a species. Sometimes, mutations cause problems in body functions and are called disorders. For example, sickle cell trait. This gene variation is seen mainly in people living near equator. Inheriting one gene with this particular variation is helpful against malaria. People who inherit two copies of this gene variation are affected by the disorder sickle cell anaemia.

Three general pathways involved in the aetiology of genetic disease are as follows:
- Mendelian patterns of inheritance involving only one or two defective genes
- Multifactorial disorders related to genetic defects and environmental factors
- Gross genetic imbalances caused by chromosomal abnormalities

Chromosomes form a genetic blueprint that is made up of tightly coiled structures. Human beings have 46 chromosomes in each cell. (22 pairs of autosomes and a pair of sex chromosome.) The sex cells contain 23 chromosomes (haploid).

Abnormalities of chromosomes can be related to the number or structure of chromosomes. Abnormalities of the number of chromosomes are as follows:

- Nondisjunction: Paired chromosomes fail to separate during cell division. If nondisjunction occurs during meiosis (before fertilization), the fetus usually will have abnormal chromosomes in every cell and may result in trisomy or monosomy.
- If the nondisjunction occurs after fertilization, the fetus may have two or more chromosomes that evolve into more than one cell line (mosaicism), each with different numbers of chromosomes.

Abnormalities in chromosome structure are translocations, deletions and additions.

Pattern of Inheritance

1. Many diseases are caused by an abnormality of a single gene or a pair of genes, where the chromosomes are grossly normal.
2. Autosomal dominant inheritance: This disorder occurs when an individual has a gene that produces an effect whenever it is present (homozygous or heterozygous). This gene overshadows the other gene of the pair (the defect is limited to a single gene on one of the two paired autosomal chromosomes).
   ### Characteristics
   - Affected individuals generally have an affected parent and can be seen in multiple generations of individuals with the condition.
   - The affected individuals have 50% chance with each pregnancy to pass on the abnormal gene to the offspring.
   - Males and females have equal chance of being getting affected.
   - A mutation of a normal gene can result in a new case.
   - Autosomal dominant disorders produce a wide variety of manifestations in the same family itself.
   - An unaffected individual has no chance of transmitting the disorder.

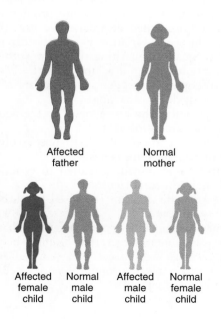

Affected father   Normal mother

Affected female child   Normal male child   Affected male child   Normal female child

3. Autosomal recessive inheritance: This disorder manifests only when there are two abnormal genes on the same chromosome pair (homozygous) in an individual.
   - A carrier state occurs when an individual who is heterozygous for the abnormal gene does not manifest obvious symptoms.
   - The condition occurs when individuals mate and pass the same abnormal gene.
   ### Characteristics
   - An affected individual has clinically normal parents, but they are carriers.
   - If both parents are carriers, they have 25% chance with each pregnancy to have an offspring with the disorder.
   - If the offspring of two carrier parents is clinically normal, there is 50% chance with each pregnancy being a carrier.
   - Consanguineous mating has an increased risk for autosomal recessive disorders.
   - Male and female have equal chance of being getting affected.
   - These disorders tend to be more severe in its clinical manifestations.
   - The presence of certain disorders can be detected in a carrier parent, e.g. sickle cell anaemia, Tay–Sachs disease and cystic fibrosis.
4. Sex-linked or X-linked disorders: These are disorders for which the gene is carried through X chromosome. The female may be homozygous or heterozygous for a trait carried on the X chromosome as she has two X chromosomes. A male has only one X chromosome, and the gene will be expressed and the disorders are manifested in the male who carries a gene.
5. X-linked dominant inheritance: In X-linked dominant disorders, females are affected if they carry a single abnormal gene on one of their X chromosomes. The inheritance pattern of an X-linked dominant trait resembles autosomal dominant inheritance with one exception – the trait is transmitted from an affected male to all his daughters but not to his sons. An affected female's offspring have 50% chance of being affected, whether male or female. In X-linked dominant disorders, usually twice as many females as males are affected.

Mode of Transmission

Characteristics

- There is no male-to-male transmission; fathers pass on their Y chromosome to their sons and their X chromosomes to their daughters.
- Affected males are related through the female line.
- There is 50% chance with each pregnancy that carrier mother will pass the abnormal genes to her sons and they will be affected.
- There is 50% chance for the mother to pass on the abnormal gene to her daughters, making them carriers.
- The affected father with X-linked condition cannot pass the disorders to his sons, but all of his daughters will be carriers.

- Rarely, a female carrier may manifest the symptoms as a result of random inactivation of the second X chromosome.

Polygenic or Multifactorial Disorders

Many common malformations are caused by the interaction of many genes and environmental factors such as the health status and age of the parents and exposure to pollutants and viruses.

Characteristics

- Malformations may vary from mild to severe.
- The severe the malformation, the more the number of genes involved.
- There often a sex bias in occurrence rates for a malformation. For example, congenital hip dysplasia occurs in females and pyloric stenosis in males.
- In the presences of environmental influences, it may take fewer genes to manifest the disease in the offspring.
- When more numbers of a family are affected, the severity of the clinical manifestations acts as the addictive influence of multifactorial inheritance.
- Risk factors are determined by the distribution in the general population.
- The risk of recurrence is usually 2%–5% for all first-degree relatives but is higher (10%–15%) if more than one member is affected.

COMMON CHROMOSOMAL ABNORMALITIES

Down Syndrome

This results from trisomy of the 21st chromosome. Trisomy is the product of the union between a normal gamete and a gamete that contains an extra chromosome. The individual will have 47 chromosomes; one pair will have three chromosomes instead of two. The overall incidence of Down syndrome is one in 1000 live births.

Maternal age of 35 years is considered as the cut-off point for recommending amniocentesis for chromosome analysis. It results from the well-known association between advanced maternal age and trisomy (XXY, XXX, trisomy 13, 18 and 21). The nondisjunctional event in meiosis that produces this anomaly increases in incidence with increasing maternal age, especially older than 40 years.

Maternal Age (Years)	Approximate Risk for Down Syndrome
30	1:1000
35	1:365
40	1:100
45	1:50

Advanced paternal age does not prove an increased incidence of Down syndrome until the paternal age of 55 years. But it is known that approximately 20% of all trisomy 21 cases derive the extra chromosome 21 from the father. The common syndromes associated with the increased paternal age are Apert syndrome, myositis ossificans, achondroplasia and Marfan syndrome.

A parent with 14–21 Robertsonian translocations is at risk for having multiple miscarriages. In total, 3.3% of all cases of Down syndrome result from unbalanced Robertsonian translocation in which a third copy of chromosome 21 is present.

Findings are upward palpebral slant, Brushfield spots, protuberant tongue, abnormal dermatoglyphics (Simian crease), clinodactyly of the fifth digit, generalized hypotonia and mental retardation.

Diagnosis

X-ray: Iliac index for those younger than 1 year and karyotyping will reveal trisomy 21.

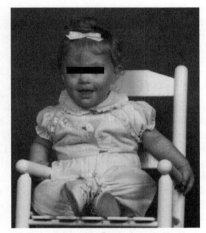

A baby girl with Down's syndrome.

Recurrence Rate

Females younger than 40 years have 1% chance of giving birth to a child with Down syndrome. Above 40 years of age, if the mother carries a translocation, the rate is 10%. If the father carries a translocation, the rate is 3%–5%. The expected IQ of a child with Down syndrome is between 35 and 65, with an average of 54. The trisomy of 18th chromosome is called **Edward syndrome,** where survival is only up to 6 months.

The external features of a neonate with trisomy 18 are subtle – a small face with micrognathia, small chest and low set ears.

This karyotype demonstrates trisomy 18 (47, XY + 18). It is uncommon for fetuses with this condition to survive, so the incidence is only one in 8000 live births. It is rare for babies to survive for very long if liveborn, because of the multitude of anomalies that are usually present.

Trisomy of 13th chromosome is known as **Patau syndrome.** Death occurs before the third month of life.

Cri-du-chat Syndrome

It is a structural abnormality of chromosome where there is deletion of one arm of the fifth chromosome. This syndrome is characterized by abnormal mental and physical development. When these children cry, they mew like a cat.

Myelogenous leukaemia is seen in those in whom there is a deletion of some portion of the 22nd chromosome known as **Philadelphia chromosome.**

Turner Syndrome

This is a condition where there is complete monosomy of a sex chromosome (X). This results in a sterile female with webbed neck, low set posterior hairline, shield chest with wide-spaced nipples, short stature, cubitus valgus, lymph oedema amenorrhoea, mental retardation and cardiac defects. It is diagnosed most frequently at puberty, with three outstanding features – short stature, sexual infantilism and amenorrhoea.

Karyotyping will yield XO sex chromosome pattern with 45 chromosomes. Buccal smear reveals the absence of Barr body.

Treatment is primarily hormone therapy. Psychological counselling for parents and children is also essential.

Fragile X Syndrome

The common features of children with this condition are prominent and elongated ears and face. Children of different ethnic backgrounds have similar features. No difference is seen in the physical appearance. This occurs in about one in 1500 males. Affected female carriers are typically normal. Affected male children usually have mental retardation and their testes are larger than normal.

Klinefelter Syndrome

There is trisomy of sex chromosomes. Features include a sterile male with gynaecomastia, cryptorchidism and sometimes mental retardation.

Karyotyping shows XXY chromosomes. Buccal smear shows an extra Barr body. The chromosome number is 47 instead of 46.

Mosaicism

It occurs when chromosomes fail to separate (mitotic nondisjunction) or fail to migrate (anaphase lag). If occurs in the early embryonic period, a greater number of cells are affected.

It is the presence of two or more chromosomally distinct cell lines, usually one normal and one abnormal. This type of nondisjunction occurs usually in postzygotic cell division. This anomaly may be either numeric or structural. Numeric mosaicism is the most common type. The percentage or level of mosaicism depends on the stage of embryonic development in which the cell division error takes place. If it occurs at the first cell division after fertilization, the level of mosaicism is about 50%. If the cell division errors occur in the later stage, the abnormality will be located to one cell type, such as brain tissue or germ cell.

NURSING MANAGEMENT OF CHILDREN WITH COMMON CHROMOSOMAL ANOMALIES

1. **Assessment**
   * Family history goes back at least three generations.
   * Evaluate physical findings, as chromosome abnormalities affect multiple body systems.
   * Diagnostic tests that may be performed are as follows:
     * Maternal serum α-fetoprotein (AFP) to screen for neural tube defects (increased serum levels) and Down syndrome (low levels)
     * Chromosomal analysis in chorionic villi sampling or amniocentesis
     * Developmental assessment of parents and siblings for possible risk rates
     * Fetal ultrasonography for suspected structural disorders such as omphalocoele or renal agenesis
     * Newborn screening for phenylketonuria (PKU), galactosaemia, hypothyroidism and sickle cell anaemia
     * Other laboratory tests as indicated by physical signs and symptoms
2. **Nursing diagnosis**
   * Knowledge deficit related to factors of heredity, infant potential and community resources
   * High risk for ineffective family coping related to physical and mental handicap of a family member
   * High risk for alteration in the family process related to diagnosis of a genetic disorder in the fetus or newborn
   * High risk for altered parenting related to genetic disorders and social isolation
3. **Common nursing interventions**
   * Explain appropriate genetic information to the family.
   * Discuss the implications of the condition to the parent, the infant and the siblings.
   * Refer the family to a genetics centre for a complete evaluation.
   * Explain diagnostic tests to the parents before the tests, with emphasis on its purpose, findings anticipated and possible side effects.
   * Encourage family members to verbalize their feelings.
   * Recognize grief is appropriate during a difficult decision-making process.

GENETICALLY LETHAL DISEASES

A genetically lethal disease is one that interferes with a person's ability to reproduce as a result of early death or impaired sexual function. The most common genetically lethal disease in human beings is cystic fibrosis.

Cystic Fibrosis

It is the most common autosomal recessive disorder in whites (1/600 births). About one in every 20 people is heterozygous for cystic fibrosis. It is characterized by dysfunction of exocrine glands, leading to chronic pulmonary disease, pancreatic insufficiency and intestinal obstruction. Males are azoospermia. The mean survival time is approximately 15–20 years. Patients with cystic fibrosis have mutations in one or more genes. These mutated genes give faulty instructions for the production of proteins that help retain more salts in the body. It causes lungs to be clogged with mucus, making hard to breathe and also make it difficult to digest food as a result of lack of pancreatic enzyme.

VATER Syndrome

VATER is an acronym used for Vertebral, Anal, Tracheo-Esophageal fistula and Renal or Radial abnormalities. Now, it is expanded to VACTERAL to include Cardiac and Limb abnormalities. All the defects included in these acronyms occur sometimes during embryogenesis. So, if one abnormality is found in a baby, a complete evaluation is recommended to rule out others.

Other acronyms used in paediatric practice include:
- STARCH – Syphilis, Toxoplasmosis, AIDS, Rubella, Cytomegalovirus and Herpes
- TORCH – Toxoplasmosis, Others (Syphilis) Rubella, Cytomegalovirus and Herpes
- CHARGE Association – Coloboma, Heart defects, Atresia choanae, Retarded growth, Genital and Ear anomalies

IMPORTANT ADVANCEMENTS IN GENETICS

Genetic Testing

There are different types of tests available. New ones are coming out all the time. It is helpful to diagnose disorders in children and adults. It is also helpful in predicting chances of developing a genetic disorder at a given period. Genetic tests are used by couples who want to learn their risk of passing genetic disorder to any of their offspring. It can be done during the prenatal period to see whether the fetus has any genetic problem.

What type of test a person should undergo depends on the type of disorder being looked for and what is known about a gene (location in the genome or its protein); in most cases, a genetic linkage study is passed down to the family (testing close relatives).

While conducting a genetic testing, a lot of ethical issues need to be taken care of. Prenatal test is often done when there is a risk for a disorder. These risks are a family history of genetic disorder, age of the mother and problems with earlier pregnancy.

Common tests used are as follows:
- **α-Fetoprotein (AFP) test:** A sample of the mother's blood is taken to measure the amount of a special protein produced by the fetus. The amount of AFP in large amount or too little indicates that the genes have problem. The brain or spine of the fetus may not be developing properly.
- **Enzyme studies:** In some diseases, the gene that gives instructions for producing an enzyme does not

work. This will affect production of the enzyme and some important functions do not occur.
- **Ultrasound imaging:** Sound waves are used to create an image of the fetus to identify position, size and congenital anomalies in the fetus.
- **Amniocentesis and chorionic villi sampling:** These tests check for defects in the fetus. Some cells around the fetus are removed and treated with a special dye and photographed using a microscope. The picture that is created is called as a karyotype. The karyotype makes it easy to view missing or broken chromosomes. Karyotyping helps locate the DNA marker.

DNA Fingerprinting

Inheritance of DNA is very stable. Every person has a specific pattern of DNA sequence which shows a combination of DNA sequences of both the mother and the father. DNA fingerprinting helps in identity establishment, identification of criminals and identification of the mother and the father of a child in case of disputed parentage. In this process, DNA is isolated from any cells of the body, stains of blood and semen or hair roots. In India, the first test of DNA fingerprinting was done in 1988 for settling a disputed parentage in Madras. This was done at the Centre for Cell and Molecular Biology, Hyderabad. Alec Jeffery developed DNA fingerprinting in 1985–1986 at Leicester University, United Kingdom. DNA typing has certain advantages such as to prove innocence, to uncover history, to study human evolution and to identify the remains of bodies.

With the advancement in the field of genetics, molecular biologists have identified several human genes. Genes for premature greying of hair have been identified, and a study conducted at Maine Centre, USA, suggested that these genes also control osteoporosis. Holt–Oram syndrome (HOS) is also identified to be gene abnormality that influences development of the heart. Genes of HOS is linked to chromosome 12.

Sex Determination

Sex of the individual can be determined at the time of fertilization. McClung (1902) gave the chromosome theory of sex determination. Barr and Bertram (1949) noted the presence of a darkly stained chromatin body in the nucleus of the nerve cells of a female cat. Later, this was found in all species of females. Of the two chromosomes of females, one X chromosome dissolves and is found to be present in the form of sex chromatin named the Barr body. The number of Barr bodies is one less than the number of X chromosomes. The sex is determined at the time of fertilization. The father is responsible for the sex of the child. It is estimated that if a family has four daughters, during fifth pregnancy, the chances of a son are 50%. In all individuals, sex chromosomes are present in all body cells according to the sex of the individual.

During pregnancy, amniotic fluid obtained through amniocentesis is studied to determine the sex of the unborn child and also chromosomal anomalies.

Reproductive Technology

It involves medically assisted ways of making babies. It helps people who face problems in conceiving children and also helps people to reduce the risk of having babies with genetic disorders. Artificial insemination is one of the reproductive technologies. Here, a sample of sperm is taken from the male, clean it up in a special way and inject into his partner's uterus. If the male of a couple carries a mutated gene causing a dominant disorder, a donor can be used to avoid the genetic disorder. A couple can make their choice if both of them carry the same mutated gene for a recessive disorder. Another way of assisted baby making is in vitro fertilization (IVF) – a common form is the test tube baby. IVF literally means 'in glass fertilization'. IVF with donated eggs is sometimes used when the female of a couple carries a mutated gene for a dominant disorder. Estrogenic testing is another new technology. The test is done after eggs and sperm have been mixed together using IVF.

Eugenics

It is the science of betterment of human race by application of law of inheritance. Sir Francis Galton in 1883 founded the science of eugenics. It has originated from a Greek word meaning *well born*. To many, it has got a bad connotation, as this has been used by people to claim superiority among races (e.g. Nazi Germany where thousands of people were killed in concentration camps and millions were sterilized). The study of such characters which lead to the degeneration of human race is called **dysgenics.**

Positive Eugenics

- By enlarging human opportunity. In 1963, Muller proposed artificial fertilization in females of desirable characters with sperms from a male of desirable characters.
- Protection against mutagens
- By the prevention of loss of good germ plasm, by avoiding wars and by the prevention of late marriages in genius persons
- By use of genetic engineering
- By sperm banks
- Genetic counselling

Negative Eugenics

- Restriction of marriage between blood relatives, as inbreeding causes recessive genes to become homozygous
- By controlling immigrations
- Sterilization of persons with serious hereditary defects and mental retardation
- Medical termination of pregnancy (MTP) of a seriously handicapped fetus by identification with amniocentesis

Euphenics

Euphenics involves elimination of defective gene or tissues by medical engineering.

Euthenics

Euthenics is betterment of human race by providing better living conditions. This aim can be achieved by the following:
- Proper arrangement of health facilities
- Proper housing and nutrition
- Proper utilization of talents
- Proper extracurricular activities for brilliant students

Genethics

Genethics is a new field of genetics. This new branch is a combination of genetics and ethics. With new discoveries in the field of genetics, new questions of morals and ethics are arising.

Genetic Engineering

The technology involves combining DNA from two different organisms to generate a recombinant DNA. This manipulation is called DNA recombinant technique. The application of these technique helps in understanding the structure and function of genes. It also helps in replacement of defective genes, thus curing heritable diseases and production of insulin and human growth hormone by this technique.

Gene Therapy

Treating disorders by altering genes is called gene therapy. Here, the new DNA will be inserted into some of the patient's cells. This new DNA will correct the gene's instruction for making the protein that directs the activity. Gene line therapy is the kind of treatment that could change the genes you pass on to your children. Here, genes could be corrected in the egg or sperm used for fertilization.

Genetic Counselling

Genetic counselling is the process by which patients or relatives at risk of an inherited disorder are advised on the consequences and nature of the disorder, the probability of developing or transmitting it and the options available to them in managing and planning in order to prevent, avoid or ameliorate that defect. Genetic counselling has diagnostic as well as supportive aspects.

Genetic counselling aims to provide the family with complete and accurate information about genetic disorders. The goals of genetic counselling include:
- Promoting informed decisions by involved family members
- Clarifying the family's options, available treatments and prognosis
- Examining alternatives to reduce the risk of genetic disorders
- Decreasing the incidence of the genetic disorder
- Reducing the impact of the disorder

To achieve these goals, genetic counselling must include an accurate diagnosis and nondirective counselling, which provides information in a nonthreatening, unbiased manner and reserves related decisions for the family. Such counselling must also be confidential and completely truthful, upholding the family's right to know what to expect. Also, it must be timed appropriately, preferably before pregnancy.

In a paediatric scenario, genetic counselling can occur:
- Before conception (as a part of planned parenthood) when one or both of the parents are carriers of a certain trait such as sickle cell trait
- During pregnancy when an abnormality is detected on an ultrasound scan, especially when the female is older than 35 years)
- After the birth if a birth defect is seen
- During childhood if the child has developmental delay

Prenatal genetic counselling is usually given by a counsellor at a high-risk or specialty prenatal clinic that offers prenatal diagnosis. Paediatric and adult genetic counselling is given at a genetics centre by a genetic nurse or a genetic counsellor.

In certain places, premarital genetic testing and counselling is advised (e.g. West Africa for sickle cell anaemia). In certain communities, premarital genetic counselling is mandatory and a legal requirement (e.g. Maine).

A team approach that involves physicians, nurses and social workers is essential. The nurse plays an important role in follow-up, clarifying information, providing continuous support to the family in the grieving process as appropriate. To decrease the risk of transmitting the disorder, a genetic counsellor can discuss with the family an alternative arrangement such as adoption, artificial insemination, surrogate pregnancy, prenatal diagnosis with selective abortion or prenatal treatment, curative treatment with gene splicing or fetal surgery.

Traditionally, nurses are information providers and genetic counselling is also considered to be one of her roles. A nurse who opts to be a genetic counsellor undergoes special training like other professionals who opt to be genetic counsellors (graduates of biology, genetics, psychology and nursing).

Paediatric nurses who work as a genetic counsellor work as a member of the health care team, providing information and support to families who have a member(s) with a birth defect or genetic disorder and families with risk for a variety of inherited conditions. They identify families at risk, investigate the problems present in the family, interpret information about disorder, analyse inheritance patterns and risks of recurrences and review available options with the family.

Genetic nurse counsellors also provide supportive counselling to families, serve as patient advocates and refer individuals and families to community or state support services. They also serve as educators and resource people for other health care professionals and for the general public. A study conducted by Torrance et al. (2005) among breast cancer patients found that genetic nurse counsellors can be acceptable and cost-effective alternatives to clinical geneticists for risk genetic counselling. This finding is true in other fields, too, as clinical geneticists are medical doctors with postgraduate qualification in genetics. The nurse graduates can also be trained as genetic counsellors at a lower cost.

STUDY QUESTIONS

1. What is Human Genome Project?
2. Describe pattern of inheritance.
3. Explain polygenic or multifactoral disorders.
4. What is Eugenics. Explain positive and negative eugenics?
5. Define: gene therapy, genethics, genetic engineering and euthenics.
6. What is reporductive technology?
7. What are the important advancements in genetics that contribute to improvements in human life?
8. What is DNA finger printing and what are the uses?
9. What is WATER Syndrome?
10. What are the important nursing interventions for caring the children with following conditions?
    1. Cystic fibrosis
    2. Downs Syndrome,
    3. Turners Syndrome
    4. Mosaicism
11. What is genetic counseling? Explain the role of a paediatric nurse in gentic counseling.

BIBLIOGRAPHY

1. American Association for the Advancement of Science. (1993). Benchmarks for Science Literacy. New York: Oxford university Press.
2. Baker, P. (1995). Genetics and society. New York: H.W. Wilson Company.
3. Buyse, M.L. (1990). The birth defects encyclopedia. Edn. Cambridge, Mass: Blackwell Scientific.
4. Cooper, Neca Grant. (1992). The human genome project. Edn. Los Alamos, NM: Los Alamos Science, No. 20.
5. Cutter, Mary Ann G., et al. (1992). Mapping and sequencing the human genome: science, ethics and public policy. Colorado Springs, CO: BSCS and American Medical Association.
6. Edelson, E. (1990). Genetics and heredity. New York: Chelsea House Publishers.
7. Gelehrter, T.D., Collins, F.S., Ginsberg, D. (1998). Principles of medical genetics. 2nd Edn. Baltimore: Williams and Wilkins.
8. Scricer, C.R., Beaudet, A.L., Sly, W.S., Valle, D. (1995). The Metabolic and molecular bases of inherited diseases. 7th Edn. New York: McGraw-Hill.
9. National Institute of Health Report on Causes of Mental Retardation and Cerebral Palsy. (1985). Task force on joint assessment of prenatal and perinatal factors associated with brain disorders. Pediatrics 76, p 457.
10. Torrance, N., Mollison, J., & Wordsworth, S., et al. (2006 Aug 21). Genetic nurse counsellors can be an acceptable and cost-effective alternative to clinical geneticists for breast cancer risk genetic counselling. Evidence from two parallel randomised controlled equivalence trials. *Br J Cancer*, 95(4), 435–444.

CHAPTER 22

CARE OF CHILDREN WITH INBORN ERRORS OF METABOLISM

LEARNING OBJECTIVES

Upon completion of this chapter, the learner will be able to

- Define inborn errors of metabolism (IEM).
- Identify the common clinical findings of IEM.
- Discuss the long-term management of children with IEM.
- Explain the newborn screening procedures.
- List the precautions to be followed while collecting samples for screening.
- Explain the medical and nursing management of neonates and children with galactosaemia, glucose-6-phosphate dehydrogenase deficiency, phenylketonuria, albinism and intellectually challenged children.

Inborn errors of metabolism (IEM) or Inherited Metabolic disorders (IMD) can cause disease manifestations in any organ at various stages of life, from newborn to adulthood. IEM are a group of inherited diseases in which a single gene defect causes a clinically significant block in a metabolic pathway, resulting in the absence of enzymes essential for cellular metabolism of protein, carbohydrates and fats. Advancement in medical technology and improved knowledge of the human genome had made significant changes in the diagnosis, classification and treatment of these inherited metabolic disorders. In normal situation, when a diet is taken, specific enzymes will convert a substrate (the substance on which enzymes act) into products. There will be many such enzymatic actions, called metabolic pathways. A food product that is not metabolized can build up in the body and cause a

wide range of symptoms. Several IEM cause developmental delay if not controlled. There is a wide range of IEM. If there is a blockage in enzymatic actions, it may lead to the following:

- Accumulation of substances as in galactosaemia or phenylketonuria (PKU).
- A deficiency of the enzyme may cause deficiency disorders such as familial hypothyroidism.
- Alternate metabolic pathway may lead to an increase in production of the product as in PKU where phenylketones are produced.

Common clinical findings include a history of consanguinity, mental retardation, symptom onset with institution of feedings or formula change; a history of growth disturbance, lethargy, recurrent emesis, poor feeding, rashes, seizures, hiccoughs, apnoea, tachypnoea, etc.

Physical findings include tachypnoea, apnoea, lethargy, hypertonicity, hypotonicity, hepatosplenomegaly, ambiguous genitalia, jaundice, dysmorphic or coarse facial features, rashes or patchy hypopigmentation, ocular findings (cataracts, lens dislocation or pigmentary retinopathy), intracranial haemorrhage, unusual odours, etc.

Laboratory investigations will show metabolic acidosis with an increased anion gap, primary respiratory alkalosis, hyperammonaemia, hypoglycaemia, ketosis or ketonuria, low blood urea nitrogen (BUN), hyperbilirubinaemia, lactic acidosis, high lactate/pyruvate ratio, non-glucose-reducing substances in urine, elevated liver function tests including prothrombin time (PT) and partial thromboplastin time (PTT), neutropaenia and thrombocytopaenia.

Initial approach include ruling out other causes of nonmetabolic disorders such as infection and asphyxia. The infant is usually subjected to a wide array of investigations prior to therapy such as blood test for glucose, newborn screen, complete blood cell (CBC) count with differential, platelets, pH and $PaCO_2$, electrolytes for anion gap, liver function tests, total and direct bilirubin, PT, PTT, uric acid and ammonia. Blood samples for ammonia, lactate and pyruvate levels should be collected without a tourniquet, kept on ice and analysed immediately.

Urine must be send for the analysis of colour, odour, pH, glucose, ketones, reducing substances (positive for galactosaemia, fructose intolerance, tyrosinaemia, etc.), ferric chloride reaction (positive for maple syrup urine disease [MSUD], PKU, etc.) and DNPH reaction (screens for α-keto acids).

Further management depends on the results of investigations.

Common management strategies include:
Provide hydration, nutrition and acid–base management.
- Rehydrate the infant.
- Stop all oral intakes to eliminate protein, galactose and fructose.
- Provide calories with intravenous glucose at 8–10 mg/kg/min (even if insulin is required to keep the blood glucose level normal).
- Give intravenous lipids only after ruling out a primary or secondary fatty acid oxidation defect.
- Withhold all protein for 48–72 hours while the patient is acutely ill and until an aminoacidopathy, organic aciduria or urea cycle defect has been excluded.
- Administer special enteral formulas and parenteral amino acid solutions as required.
- Treat significant acidosis (pH <7.22) with a continuous infusion of $NaHCO_3$.
- Treating hyperammonaemia as early as possible is essential to prevent neurological impairment.

Treat Co-existing Infections

Replace cofactor, as certain enzyme deficiencies are vitamin responsive.

Even if certain IEM are not completely curable, a specific diagnosis of the condition is essential for genetic counselling. So, the nurse being a team member should help in further investigations by collecting specimens and storing them. Also, if the child dies, a postmortem assessment of specimens may be needed. The nurse needs to act within the guidelines of the institutional ethics committee to get consent for such activities. The common investigations and specimens collected for children facing impending death or uncertain diagnosis (metabolic autopsy) are as follows:

1. Blood: 5–10 mL; frozen at −200°C; both heparinized (for chromosomal studies) and EDTA (for DNA studies) samples to be taken
2. Urine: Frozen at −20°C
3. CSF: Stored at −20°C
4. Skin biopsy: 3 × 2-mm full thickness in the culture medium or saline with glucose; stored at 4°C–80°C, not frozen
5. Liver and muscle biopsy: For histopathology, electron microscopy and enzyme studies
6. Kidney and heart biopsy: As indicated
7. Clinical photographs (in cases with dysmorphism)
8. Infantogram (in cases of skeletal abnormalities)

Long-term Treatment of IEM

Dietary management is the mainstay of treatment in PKU, MSUD, homocystinuria, galactosaemia, and glycogen storage disease types I and III.

Special diets for PKU and MSUD are commercially available in the other part of the world, which can be imported to India, too. These special diets are, however, very expensive and not affordable by most Indian patients. Based on the amino acid content of some common food products available in India, dietary exchanges are calculated and a low phenylalanine diet for PKU and a diet low in branched-chain amino acids for MSUD are being used in our country. But so far no research evidence exists to prove the efficacy of such diets being used in India. Urea cycle disorders and organic acidurias require dietary modification (protein restriction) in addition to other modalities. The ketogenic diet is the treatment of choice for glucose transporter 1 deficiency and pyruvate dehydrogenase deficiency.

Enzyme replacement therapy is available for some lysosomal storage disorders.

Cofactor replacement therapy for certain enzyme deficiencies is available as well.

Prognosis of IEM

Current prognosis of IEM for survival and normal neurological status is guarded. It is believed that outcomes will improve with presymptomatic diagnosis (by prenatal detection or neonatal screening), identification of genes and other factors that impact on phenotype, response to treatment, outcome and alternative novel approaches to therapy.

Prevention

Genetic counselling and prenatal diagnosis:
Most of the IEM are single gene defects, inherited in an autosomal recessive way, with a 25% recurrence risk. Therefore, when the diagnosis is known and confirmed, prenatal diagnosis can be offered and testing of chorionic villi and amniotic fluid will help identify the disorder.

Usual methods available are as follows:
- Substrate or metabolite detection (useful in PKU, peroxisomal defects)
- Enzyme assay: useful in lysosomal storage disorders such as Niemann–Pick disease, Gaucher disease
- DNA-based (molecular) diagnosis: Detection of mutation in proband/carrier parents is a prerequisite.

Newborn Screening for IEM

Newborn screening tests help identify serious developmental, genetic and metabolic disorders so that important treatment options can be taken during the critical time before symptoms develop. If detected early, most of these illnesses are treatable. Screening tests help identify which babies need additional testing to confirm or rule out illnesses. If further tests confirm a disease, appropriate treatment can be initiated before major symptoms appear and reduce neurological impairment. Tandem mass spectrometry (TMS) is used in some countries for neonatal screening for IEM. Disorders which can be detected by TMS include aminoacidopathies (PKU, MSUD, homocystinuria, citrullinaemia, argininosuccinic aciduria, hepatorenal tyrosinaemia), fatty acid oxidation defects, organic acidaemias (glutaric aciduria, propionic acidaemia, methylmalonic acidaemia, isovaleric acidaemia). The appropriate time for collection of samples is between 1 and 3 days of life. The cost of this procedure is very high, a potent disincentive for resource-poor countries such as India. Also, though the test is highly sensitive, the specificity is relatively low; there are difficulties in interpretation of abnormal test results in apparently healthy infants.

Usually, the screening tests help identify the following IEM. First investigation is a metabolic screen for all suspected cases of IEM. It includes:

1) CBC count (neutropaenia and thrombocytopaenia seen in propionic and methylmalonic acidaemias)
2) Arterial blood gases and electrolytes
3) Blood glucose
4) Plasma amonia (a normal ammonia level in newborn is less than 50 μmol/L. A blood ammonia level between 70 and 100 μmol/L should be viewed in conjunction with clinical findings
5) Arterial blood lactate (normal values: 0.5–1.6 mmol/L)
6) Liver function tests
7) Urine ketones
8) Urine reducing substances
9) Serum uric acid (low in molybdenum cofactor deficiency)

Second line or confirmatory tests include:

1) Gas chromatography–mass spectrometry (GCMS) of urine is used for the diagnosis of organic acidaemias.
2) Plasma amino acids and acylcarnitine profile are obtained by TMS for the diagnosis of organic acidaemias, urea cycle defects, aminoacidopathies and fatty acid oxidation defects.
3) High-performance liquid chromatography (HPLC) is used for quantitative analysis of amino acids in blood and urine for the diagnosis of organic acidaemias and aminoacidopathies.
4) Lactate/pyruvate ratio is used in cases with elevated lactate levels.
5) Urinary orotic acid is used in cases with hyperammonaemia for classifying urea cycle defects.
6) Enzyme assay: This is required for definitive diagnosis, but not available for most IEM. Available enzyme assays include biotinidase assay in cases with suspected biotinidase deficiency (intractable seizures, seborrhoeic rash, alopecia) and GALT (galactose-1-phosphate uridylyltransferase) assay in cases with suspected galactosaemia (hypoglycaemia, cataracts, reducing sugars in urine).
7) Neuroimaging: MRI may provide helpful pointers toward aetiology while results of definitive investigations are pending. Some IEM may be associated with structural malformations, e.g. Zellweger syndrome has diffuse cortical migration and sulcation abnormalities.

Agenesis of corpus callosum has been reported in Menkes disease, pyruvate decarboxylase deficiency and nonketotic hyperglycinaemia (NKH). Examples of other neuroimaging findings in IEM include:

- MSUD: brainstem and cerebellar oedema
- Propionic and methylmalonic acidaemia: basal ganglia signal change
- Glutaric aciduria: frontotemporal atrophy, subdural hematomas

8) Magnetic resonance spectroscopy (MRS) may be helpful in selected disorders, e.g. lactate peak is elevated in mitochondrial disorders, whereas leucine peak is elevated in MSUD.
9) Urine α-aminoadipic semialdehyde level is elevated in pyridoxine-dependent seizures. (The test is not yet available in India.)
10) Electroencephalography (EEG): Some EEG abnormalities may be suggestive of particular IEM, e.g. comb-like rhythm in MSUD, burst suppression in NKH and holocarboxylase synthetase deficiency.
11) Plasma very long-chain fatty acid (VLCFA) levels are elevated in peroxisomal disorders.
12) Mutation analysis is done when available.
13) CSF amino acid analysis: CSF glycine levels are elevated in NKH.

Precautions to be Observed while Collecting Sample for Newborn Screening

1. Should be collected before specific treatment is started or feeds are stopped, as it may be falsely normal if the child is off feeds.
2. Samples for blood ammonia and lactate should be transported on ice and immediately tested. Lactate sample should be arterial and collected in a preheparinized syringe after 2 hours' fasting. Ammonia sample is to be collected in EDTA vacutainer approximately after 2 hours of fasting. Avoid mixing of air. The sample should be free flowing.
3. Detailed history including drug details should be provided to the laboratory. (Sodium valproate therapy may increase ammonia levels.)

GALACTOSAEMIA

It is an IEM characterized by galactosaemia, galactosuria cataracts without mental deficiency or aminoaciduria. In galactosaemia, the body is unable to use or metabolize the simple sugar galactose. It is a rare autosomal recessive disorder affecting approximately 1 in 50,000 lives. It involves an inborn error of carbohydrate metabolism resulting from the absence of hepatic enzyme GALT (which catalyses the conversion of galactose-1-phosphate to uridine diphosphate [UDP] galactose).

There are three forms of this disease:

- GALT deficiency (classic galactosaemia, the most common and the most severe form)

- Deficiency of galactose kinase
- Deficiency of galactose-6-phosphate epimerase

Pathology

Accumulation of galactose in the blood affects general organs. Liver involvement results in cirrhosis leading to jaundice in the second week of life. Spleen gets enlarged as a result of portal hypertension. Cataract occurs by 1–2 months of age. Cerebral damage manifests by symptoms of lethargy and hypotonia. Infants with galactosaemia appear normal at birth. Symptoms persist for days after ingestion of breast milk which has high lactose content; they began to vomit and lose weight. Death during the first month of life is frequent.

Symptoms

Infants with galactosaemia can develop symptoms in the first few days of life if they are fed on formula or breast milk that contains lactose. The symptoms may be a result of a serious blood infection with the bacteria *Escherichia coli*.

- Convulsions
- Irritability and lethargy
- Poor feeding (the baby refuses formulas containing milk)
- Poor weight gain
- Yellow skin and the whites of the eyes (jaundice)
- Vomiting

Diagnosis

Blood studies show increased levels of galactose.
Tests include:
- Blood culture for bacterial infection (*E. coli* sepsis)
- Enzyme activity in the red blood cells
- Ketone in urine
- Prenatal diagnosis by directly measuring the enzyme GALT
- 'Reducing substances' in the infant's urine, and normal or low blood sugar level while the infant is being fed breast milk or a formula containing lactose

Treatment

Eliminate all milk and milk products from the diet. Lactose-free formulas are advised such as soya-protein formula, e.g. caselan.
Infants can be fed with:
- Soy formula
- Meat-based formula or Nutramigen (protein hydrolysate formula)
- Another lactose-free formula
- Calcium supplements

Prognosis

People who receive an early diagnosis and strictly avoid milk products can live a relatively normal life. However, mild intellectual impairment may develop even in people who avoid galactose.

Long-term complications are ovarian dysfunction, abnormal speech, cognitive impairment growth retardation and motor delay. Eliminating sources of galactose in the diet does not improve the outcome. New therapeutic strategies such as enhancing residual transferase activity, replacing depleted metabolites or undergoing gene replacement therapy are needed to improve the prognosis.
Possible complications are as follows:
- Cataracts
- Cirrhosis of the liver
- Death (if there is galactose in the diet)
- Delayed speech development
- Severe mental retardation
- Irregular menstrual periods, reduced function of ovaries leading to ovarian failure
- Severe infection with bacteria (*E. coli* sepsis)
- Tremors and uncontrollable motor functions

Nursing Considerations

Collect a detailed family history to identify genetic predisposition, as it is an autosomal recessive disorder. If there is a family history, advise genetic counselling. Genetic counselling will help you make decisions about pregnancy and prenatal testing. Once the diagnosis of galactosaemia is made, genetic counselling should be recommended to other members of the family. Instruct parents to stop promptly giving their infant milk and milk products once the diagnosis is made. Read labels of food items before administering as to find out the presence of lactose. The nurse must avoid administration of drugs such as penicillin, as it contains lactose as filler.

GLUCOSE-6-PHOSPHATE DEHYDROGENASE DEFICIENCY

Glucose-6-phosphate dehydrogenase (G6PD) deficiency is a hereditary condition in which red blood cells break down when the body is exposed to certain drugs or infections.

Causes

G6PD deficiency occurs when there is deficiency of an enzyme called glucose-6-phosphate dehydrogenase. G6PD deficiency leads to the destruction of red blood cells or haemolysis. In the active disease state, it is called a haemolytic episode. The episodes are usually brief, because the body continues to produce new red blood cells which have normal activity.
Red blood cell destruction can be triggered by infections, severe stress, certain foods (such as fava beans) and certain drugs, including:
- Antimalarial drugs
- Aspirin
- Nitrofurantoin
- Nonsteroidal anti-inflammatory drugs (NSAIDs)
- Quinidine
- Quinine
- Sulfa drugs

Other chemicals, such as those in mothballs (naphthalene balls), can also trigger an episode. This disorder is more common among:

- African American
- People of Middle Eastern decent, particularly Kurdish or Sephardic Jewish
- Male
- A family history of the deficiency

A form of this disorder is common in whites of Mediterranean descent. This form is also associated with acute episodes of haemolysis. The episodes are longer and more severe than in other types of the disorder.

Symptoms

Persons with this condition do not display any signs of the disease until their red blood cells are exposed either to certain chemicals in food or medicine or to stress.

Symptoms are more common in men and may include:

- Dark urine
- Enlarged liver
- Fatigue
- Pallor
- Rapid heart rate
- Shortness of breath
- Jaundice

Investigations

A blood test can be done to check the level of G6PD. Other tests that may be done include:

- Bilirubin level
- CBC count, including red blood cell count
- Haemoglobin – blood
- Haemoglobin – urine
- Haptoglobin level
- LDH test
- Methaemoglobin reduction test
- Reticulocyte count

Treatment

Treatment may involve the following:

- Medicines to treat an infection (if present)
- Stopping any drugs that are causing red blood cell destruction
- Transfusions, in some cases

Prognosis

Spontaneous recovery from a haemolytic episode is the usual outcome.

Nursing Management

Persons with G6PD deficiency must strictly avoid things that can trigger an episode. Explain parents and children about medications that are contraindicated in children with G6PD deficiency. Provide a list of medications that they should avoid. Provide medical alert cards to children so that they can be treated in case of emergencies.

Instruct them to avoid foods that may trigger an episode of haemolysis such as fava beans. Provide adequate instruction regarding genetic counselling or testing for those who have a family history of the condition.

Possible Complications

Rarely kidney failure or death may occur following a severe haemolytic event.

PHENYLKETONURIA

It is genetic disease of autosomal recessive trait caused by the absence of phenylalanine hydroxylase necessary for the metabolism of the essential amino acid phenylalanine.

Phenylalanine is found in foods that contain protein. Without the enzyme, levels of phenylalanine and two closely related substances build up in the body. These substances are harmful to the central nervous system and cause brain damage.

Incidence is one in 10,000–15,000 live births.

Pathology

Absence of phenylalanine hydroxylase results in the accumulation of phenylalanine in the bloodstream and increased urinary excretion of phenyl acids. The presence of phenylalanine in the urine gives the characteristic musty odour, which is a typical feature of PKU. In PKU, the amino acids produced by metabolism of phenylalanine are absent. One of the important amino acids is tyrosine, which is needed for the pigment melanin and the hormones epinephrine and thyroxin. Decreased melanin results in blond hair, blue eyes and fair skin as special features of PKU. These children are particularly susceptible to dermatological problems, especially eczema.

Accumulation of phenylalanine and decreased amount of dopamine and tryptophan lead to decreased myelination, cystic degeneration of grey matter and white matter and disturbances in cortical lamination. Mental retardation occurs usually before detection of metabolites in urine.

Clinical Features

- Affected infants are normal at birth
- Mental retardation, hypertonicity, tremors, behavioural disorders and hypopigmentation

Phenylalanine plays a role in the body's production of melanin, the pigment responsible for skin and hair colour. Therefore, infants with this condition often have lighter skin, hair and eyes than their brothers or sisters without the disease.

Other symptoms may include:

- Delayed mental and social skills
- Head significantly below the normal size
- Hyperactivity
- Jerking movements of the arms or legs
- Mental retardation
- Seizures
- Skin rashes

- Tremors
- Unusual positioning of hands

If the condition is untreated or foods containing phenylalanine are not avoided, a 'mousy' or 'musty' odour may be detected from the breath and skin and in urine. The unusual odour is as a result of a build-up of phenylalanine substances in the body.

Diagnosis

PKU is confirmed by Guthrie's test, plasma phenylalanine level >20 mg/dL, normal plasma tyrosine level and urinary phenylpyruvic acid.

Treatment

Restriction of dietary intake of phenylalanine and its serum level should be maintained between 2 and 9 mg/dL.

PKU is a treatable disease. Treatment involves a diet that is extremely low in phenylalanine, particularly when the child is growing. The diet must be strictly followed. This requires close supervision by a registered nurse, dietician or doctor and cooperation of the parent and the child. Those who continue the diet into adulthood have better physical and mental health. 'Diet for life' has become the standard recommended by most experts. This is especially important before conception and throughout pregnancy.

Phenylalanine is present in significant amounts in milk, eggs and other common foods. The artificial sweetener NutraSweet (aspartame) also contains phenylalanine. Any products containing aspartame should be avoided.

A special infant formula called Lofenalac is made for infants with PKU. It can be used throughout life as a protein source that is extremely low in phenylalanine and balanced for the remaining essential amino acids.

Taking supplements such as fish oil to replace the long-chain fatty acids missing from a standard phenylalanine-free diet may help improve neurological development, including fine motor coordination. Other specific supplements, such as iron or carnitine, may be needed.

Prognosis

The outcome is expected to be very good if the diet is strictly followed, starting shortly after the child's birth. If treatment is delayed or the condition remains untreated, brain damage will occur. School functioning may be mildly impaired. If proteins containing phenylalanine are not avoided, PKU can lead to mental retardation by the end of the first year of life.

Possible Complications

Severe mental retardation occurs if the disorder is untreated. ADHD (attention-deficit/hyperactivity disorder) appears to be the most common problem seen in those who do not stick to a very low-phenylalanine diet.

Nursing Considerations

- Educate the parents regarding dietary restriction.
- Older children and adolescents need special attention.

- High-protein diet needs to be eliminated.
- Foods with low-protein content are recommended.
- Control during infancy is not problematic, as the diet is controlled by adults.

Prevention

The nurse should educate parents regarding enzyme assay to determine if they carry the gene for PKU. Chorionic villus sampling can be done during pregnancy to screen the unborn baby for PKU. Inform women with PKU to follow a strict low-phenylalanine diet both before becoming pregnant and throughout the pregnancy, as build-up of this substance will damage the developing fetus even if it has not inherited the defective gene.

ALBINISM

It results from the deficiency of tyrosinase. Diminished or absent melanin in the skin, hair and eyes are usually present. Synthesis of melanin in melanosomes is defective. Depigmented skin does not tan but burns on exposure to sunlight. Photophobia, decreased visual activity and nystagmus are common symptoms. These children will have normal IQ.

MENTAL RETARDATION (INTELLECTUALLY CHALLENGED CHILDREN)

Intellectual disability was previously termed as 'mental retardation'.

Mental retardation refers to significantly subaverage general intellectual functioning existing concurrently with deficits in adaptive behaviour and manifests during the developmental period. This definition includes three facts: (1) a quantifiable intelligence test, (2) variable functional deficits in everyday living and (3) onset prior to 18 years of age.

The present definition of intellectual disability is as a disability characterized by significant limitations in both **intellectual functioning** and **adaptive behaviour**, which covers many everyday social and practical skills. This disability originates **before the age of 18 years** (American Association on Intellectual and Developmental Disabilities [AAIDD]). Intellectual functioning is the general mental capacity, such as learning, reasoning, problem solving, and so on, and is called intelligence. Intellectual functioning is measured with the IQ test.

The American Association on Mental Deficiency (AAMD; now AAIDD) defines retardation as occurring below an IQ of 68. Those with an IQ of 69–83 are not retarded as per definition but constitute a group with a high chance of educational problems and a very high potential for independent functioning. About 5%–10% of children with intellectual disability are profoundly retarded. IQ can be determined by dividing mental age by chronological age multiplied by 100. IQ is not a static phenomenon but can be changed depending on the developmental environment. Most commonly used IQ test is the Wechsler Intelligence Scale for Children–Revised (WISC-R) and the Stanford–Binet Intelligence Scale.

Aetiology and Incidence

Intellectual disability, the most common developmental disability, affects up to 3% of the population.

Causes are classified as idiopathic, acquired, inherited or genetic, and endocrine disorders.

a. Idiopathic: It includes all cases with an unknown cause.

b. Acquired: This includes all environmental and socioeconomic factors.

Environmental factors include:
- Perinatal infections (maternal infections such as rubella, toxoplasmosis, syphilis, cytomegalovirus infection), other maternal illness, teratogenic effects of prescribed and nonprescribed drugs used by the mother during pregnancy, maternal abuse of drugs and alcohol, birth injuries, pre-, peri- or postnatal hypoxia, kernicterus, trauma in infancy or childhood, lead poisoning, malnutrition, brain tumour, severe psychosocial or psychological deprivation
- Exposure to toxic teratogens. Postnatal complications of prematurity such as hypoxia and periventricular haemorrhage and brain injury
- Nutritional deficiencies
- Brain radiation
- Childhood brain infections

c. Inherited or genetic: This includes chromosomal abnormalities such as Down syndrome, Turner syndrome and Klinefelter syndrome; autosomal dominant disorders such as Huntington chorea and neurofibromatosis; autosomal recessive disorders such as PKU, Tay–Sachs disease and Hurler disease.

d. Endocrine: This includes congenital hypothyroidism.

Demographic Factors

- Age: Intellectual disability begins in the first two decades of life. But the onset depends on the cause of the disability and severity of neuropsychiatric dysfunction. Individuals with severe intellectual disability show delayed motor, language and social accomplishments within the first 2 years of life. Mild disability may not be evident till the child attends school where he/she may show learning difficulty.
- Sex: Male children are more affected than female children.
- Race: Coloured children are more affected than white children.
- Socioeconomic status: Children from poor socioeconomic background are more affected, may be owing to poor nutrition, as poverty is considered as a risk factor.

Comorbidity

According to the American Psychiatric Association (2013), many neurodevelopmental, psychiatric and medical disorders co-occur with intellectual disability, especially communication disorders, learning disabilities, cerebral palsy, epilepsy and various genetically transmitted conditions.

Classifications

According to severity, there are four degrees of severity: mild, moderate, severe and profound.

DSM-V also gives four categories of intellectual disability.

Diagnosis

History based on the following must be obtained:
- Health care during the pre-, peri- and postnatal periods
- A genealogical tree for at least three generations
- An intentional search for family antecedents of mental delay, psychiatric illnesses and congenital abnormalities

Physical examination should focus on:
- Secondary abnormalities and congenital malformations
- Somatometric measurements and neurological and behavioural phenotype evaluations
- High-resolution cytogenetic studies in addition to metabolic clinical evaluations

In the next step, if no abnormal data are identified, evaluate submicroscopic chromosomal disorders.

Other diagnostic modalities include:

a. Neurological examination including computed tomographic (CT) scans to rule out nervous system pathology

b. Radiological studies to detect lesions

c. Endocrine studies including urine screening for abnormal metabolites

d. Developmental screening tests such as the Denver Developmental Screening Test to identify apparent developmental delays

e. Intellectual evaluation with standardized tests such as the Stanford–Binet Intelligence Scale, the Wechsler Intelligence Scale for children and the Gesell Developmental Schedules

f. Adaptive behaviour evaluation using tools such as the AAMD Adaptive Behaviour Scale

g. Chromosomal analysis and genetic screening in cases of a family history of mental retardation or chromosomal abnormalities

Pathophysiology

Pathophysiology depends on the cause of mental retardation, and prognosis depends on early diagnosis.

Clinical Manifestations

Clinical manifestations vary according to the child's age and degree of impairment. General signs include developmental delays in motor, social, language and cognitive skills.

Treatment

Treatments of intellectual disability generally fall into three main categories:

(1) Treatments that address the underlying cause of intellectual disability; e.g. restricting phenylalanine in the diet of patients who have PKU

(2) Treatments of comorbid physical and mental disorders with the aim of improving the patient's functioning and life skills, such as targeted pharmacological treatments of behavioural disorders among children with fragile X syndrome

(3) Early behavioural and cognitive interventions, special education, rehabilitation and psychosocial supports

Nursing Diagnoses

- Impaired verbal communication
- Altered family process
- Altered growth and development
- Altered health maintenance
- High risk for infections
- Altered role performance
- Self-care deficit
- High risk for impaired skin integrity
- Impaired social interaction
- Social isolation

Planning and Implementation

- Support the family at times of initial diagnosis by actively listening to their feelings and concerns.
- Perform task analysis before attempting to teach the child any new task.
- Facilitate the child's self-care abilities by encouraging parents' participation in the care of the child and help parents to include their child in his/her own care.
- Promote optimal development by encouraging self-care goals by emphasizing the universal needs of children such as play, social interaction and parental limit setting.
- Promote anticipatory guidance and problem solving by encouraging discussion regarding physical maturation and sexual behaviour.
- Assist the family in planning for their child's future needs; refer them to available community agencies.
- Provide the patient and family education covering the following:
  - Normal developmental milestones and appropriate simulating activities including play and socialization activities
  - The need for patience with the child's for slow attainment of developmental milestones
  - Information regarding stimulation, safety and motivation
- Provide measures to ensure self-care activities and to prevent complication related to self-care deficit.
- Provide information regarding normal speech to the parents.
- Emphasize the need for discipline that is simple, consistent and appropriate to the child's developmental level.
- Adolescents need simple, practical sexual information including anatomy, physical development and conception.
- Use demonstration as a better method of education whenever possible.

- The benefits of motivating the child through positive reinforcement and shaping-and-fading principles must not be overlooked in handling children with mental retardation.

Evaluation

1. The child exhibits no evidence of infection or respiratory distress.
2. The child's skin remains intact and shows no breakdown.
3. The child participates in self-care activities appropriate to mental capacities.
4. The child and family actively participate in the health care programme of the child.
5. Parents verbalize understanding of appropriate recreation and discipline of their child.
6. Family members verbalize feelings regarding the child's limited mental abilities.
7. Family members express acceptance of the child into the family structures.
8. Family members verbalize realistic goals for care of the child.

STUDY QUESTIONS

1. Define Inborn errors of metabolism.
2. What are Inherited Metabolic Diseases (IMDs)?
3. Many IMDs can be treated successfully with early diagnosis. True or False?
4. Which 4 broad groups exist in the Pathophysiology/Clinical presentation of IMDs?
5. What are first and second line investigations in analysing IMDs?
6. Which first line investigation results may indicate the possibility of an IMD?
7. Explain the long term mangagement of IEM or IMD.

BIBLIOGRAPHY

1. AAIDD (American Association on Intellectual Developmental Disabilities). Intellectual disability: Definition, classification, and systems of supports. Washington, DC: AAIDD; 2010.
2. APA (American Psychiatric Association). Diagnostic and statistical manual of mental disorders. 5th ed. Washington, DC: APA; 2013.
3. Camp BW, Broman SH, Nichols PL, Leff M. Maternal and neonatal risk factors for mental retardation: Defining the 'at-risk' child. Early Human Development. 1998; 50(2):159–173. [PubMed]
4. Cooper B, Lackus B. The social-class background of mentally retarded children: A study in Mannheim. Social Psychiatry. 1983;19(1):3–12. [PubMed]
5. Fletcher RJ, Loschen E, Stavrakaki C, First M, editors. Diagnostic manual-intellectual disability: A textbook of diagnosis of mental disorders in persons with intellectual disability. Kingston, NY: NADD Press; 2007.
6. Hagerman RJ, Polussa J. Treatment of the psychiatric problems associated with fragile X syndrome. Current Opinion in Psychiatry. 2015;28(2):107–112. [PubMed]
7. Hudak ML, Jones MD Jr., Brusilow SW. (1985). Differentiation of transient hyperammonemia of the newborn and urea cycle defects by clinical presentation. J Pediatr. 107:712–719.
8. Moeschler JB, Shevell M. American Academy of Pediatrics Committee on Genetics. Clinical genetic evaluation of the child

with mental retardation or developmental delays. Pediatrics. 2006; 117(6):2304–2316. [PubMed]

9. National Institute of Health Report on Causes of Mental Retardation and Cerebral Palsy. (1985). Task force on joint assessment of prenatal and perinatal factors associated with brain disorders. Pediatrics 76, p 457.

10. Scricer, CR., Beaudet, AL., Sly, WS., Valle, D. (1995). The Metabolic and molecular bases of inherited diseases. 7th Edn. New York: McGraw-Hill.

11. Schalock, RL. & Luckasson, R. (2013). Clinical judgment (2nd ed.). Washington, D.C.: American Association on Intellectual and Developmental Disabilities.

12. Tassé, MJ. & Grover, MD. (2013). Normal curve (pp. 2059–2060). In F.R. Volkmar (Ed.), Encyclopedia of autism spectrum disorders. New York: Springer.

13. Waren, SA. & Taylor, RL. (1984). Education of children with learning problems. Symposium on learning disorders. Pediatric Clinics of North America. Philadelphia: Saunders.

CHAPTER 23

EMBRYOLOGICAL CONCEPTS IMPORTANT TO CHILD HEALTH NURSING

LEARNING OBJECTIVES

Upon completion of this chapter, the learner will be able to

- Describe fertilization and fetal development.
- Explain the uses of antenatal diagnoses and fetal therapy.

OVUM

Female germ cell with a large nucleus (germinal vesicle) and a nucleolus (germinal spot) is called ovum. The ovum is formed inside the Graafian follicle, which is a source of oestrogen for the ovum. The thick covering of the ovum is called zona pellucida.

Cytoplasm of the ovum is called yolk and the cell membrane is called vitelline membrane. The primary follicles in the cortex of the ovum are called oogonia which contain 46 chromosomes (44 + X + X). Only the mature ovum takes part in fertilization. Oogenesis is the process of forming an ovum by meiosis in specialized gonads called ovaries.

The oogonium during the sexual life is changed into an immature ovum called the primary oocyte containing 46 chromosomes. The primary oocyte undergoes reduction division and breaks into two unequal daughter cells, one large and another small. The larger one is called the secondary oocyte and the smaller one is called the first polar body. This first polar body occupies the space between zona pellucida and vitelline membrane called the perivitelline space. When this occurs, the Graafian follicle ruptures and liberates a secondary oocyte into the abdominal cavity. Secondary oocyte enters into the uterine tube for its fertilization by spermatozoa with the help of fimbria of fallopian tubes. Human male produces 200,000,000 sperms per day, whereas the female usually produces one egg in each menstrual cycle, with a total of 400–500 eggs during the lifetime.

After fertilization, it undergoes mitotic division and forms a mature ovum and a second polar body, followed by extrusion of the first polar body.

SPERM

The male sex cell called the sperm is produced in the seminiferous tubules of the testis. It is highly motile and consists of head, neck, body and tail. Sperms are produced from spermatogonia containing 46 chromosomes (44 + X + Y). During growth phase, the spermatogonium increases several times in bulk and is pushed towards the lumen of the tubules to form a primary spermatocyte containing 46 chromosomes. This primary spermatocyte undergoes at first reduction division (meiosis) and forms a secondary spermatocyte with 23 chromosomes (22 + X or 22 + Y). The secondary spermatocyte undergoes maturation division or equation meiosis or homotypical division to form spermatids. They are smaller and contain the same number of chromosomes (23). The spermatids, which remain in contact with the cytoplasm of Sertoli cells, undergo metamorphosis, which is the final step of maturation of sperms. The whole process of maturation of spermatozoa to form the spermatid is called spermiogenesis.

Sperm production begins at puberty and continues throughout life, with several hundred million sperms being produced each day. Once sperms are formed, they move into the epididymis, where they mature and are stored.

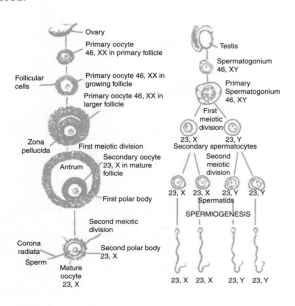

FERTILIZATION

The union of a mature ovum and a single mature sperm is called fertilization. It takes place in the ampulla of the fallopian tube where in order to fertilize an ovum, a sperm penetrates the zona pellucida of the secondary oocyte with its head. The other parts of the spermatozoa, i.e. the body and the tail, are passively engulfed by cytoplasm of the ovum where they are absorbed. After this, the secondary oocyte undergoes second maturation division of oogenesis and forms a mature ovum and a second polar body. The second polar body is then discarded. The head of the sperm swells up and forms male pronucleus. This unites with female pronucleus to form the zygote. It undergoes a series of mitotic division. Even though there are millions of spermatozoa in a single ejaculation, only one is required to fertilize an ovum, like

'survival of the fittest'. The zona pellucida prevents the entry of other sperms into the ovum.

During fertilization, there are certain processes that take place. These are as follows:
1. Segmentation
2. Restoration of the diploid number of chromosome characteristic to the species, i.e. 44 + X + Y in male and 44 + X + X in female
3. Determination of sex of the zygote
4. Prevention by zona pellucida of the entry of other sperms into the ovum

The zygote undergoes a series of mitotic divisions and forms a blastomere. The blastomere transforms to a morula comprising 16 blastomeres, looking like a mulberry fruit. This is formed when the zygote is traversing the uterine tube. After the morula enters the uterine cavity, a fluid-filled space appears inside it which is called blastocyst. The blastocyst has an outer layer called trophoblast and an inner formative or embryonic cell mass. The trophoblast along with primary mesoderm forms chorion and establishes a connection with the uterus of the mother to supply nutrition to the fetus.

After discharging the ovum, the Graafian follicle is called corpus luteum. If fertilization takes place, corpus luteum increases in size until the middle of pregnancy to provide oestrogen and progesterone for the maintenance of pregnancy. If pregnancy fails to occur, the corpus luteum degenerates. After the Graafian follicle ruptures and becomes corpus luteum, secretary changes are observed in the endometrium with regard to oestrogen and progesterone levels. These changes in the endometrium prepare the uterus for receiving fertilized ovum. If no fertilization occurs, the endometrium is shed as menstrual blood. Ovulation usually occurs on the 14th day, calculated from the first day of the menstrual cycle.

Cleavage is the process of formation of a number of small cells (blastomeres) from a large-sized zygote by mitotic division. With cleavage, the cytoplasm of the zygote is distributed to all cells. It increases the motility of the protoplasm by helping morphogenetic movements. It also helps in restoration of the cell size and the nucleocytoplasmic ratio characteristics of the specific species.

From the inner embryonic cell mass develops embryo proper and immediate covering called amnion. Differentiation of the inner cell into three primary germ layers – ectoderm, primary mesoderm and endoderm – is called gastrulation. Gastrulation is the process of formation of endoderm, the inner layer of the body. Invagination of the surface of the single-layered blastula at the pole forms a double-layered cup. The outer layer becomes the ectoderm and the inner layer becomes the endoderm. The cavity formed is lined with the endoderm and is called primitive gut cavity. Gastrulation is accompanied by the differentiation of an intermediate supporting layer that forms the mesoderm. So, it is during gastrulation that the process of differentiation takes place to form the three primitive layers of the embryo – ectoderm, endoderm and mesoderm.

Ectodermal vesicle (amniotic sac) is produced when the columnar cells of the ectodermal group arrange themselves to enclose a cavity. The primary mesoderm forms the covering of this cavity. The sac contains amniotic fluid. The amniotic cavity appears between the columnar cells of the primary ectoderm on the inner aspect of the amniogenic trophoblastic cells on the outer aspect. The roof of the primary yolk sac is formed by the primary endoderm. The circular bilaminar embryonic disc is formed from the columnar ectodermal cells present in the floor of amniotic cavity and cuboidal endodermal cells present in the roof of the yolk sac. Prochordal plate is formed from a few endodermal cells at one end of the bilaminar embryonic disc. Prochordal plate marks the future head of the embryonic disc.

As mentioned earlier, the blastocyst differentiates into an outer trophoblast and inner cell mass. Placenta and fetal membrane are developed from the trophoblast. It serves three important functions – invasion, nutrition and production of hormone for the maintenance of pregnancy. The endometrium of the pregnant uterus is known as decidua. Fetal membrane has two layers, chorion and amnion. The outermost layer is the chorion and contains two embryonic layers, an outer trophoblast and an inner primitive mesenchyme, which appears on the ninth day. Just before implantation, the trophoblast is further differentiated into an inner circular layer called cytotrophoblast (Langhans' layer) and outer multinucleated syncytium called syncytiotrophoblast (plasmoditrophoblast). At the beginning of the third week, the syncytiotrophoblast produces irregular projections called primary stem villi. After the appearance of primitive mesenchyme and the development of chorion, the primary stem villi are named chorionic villi. By 16th day, there will be insinuation of the primary mesoderm into the central core of the villus structure and forms the secondary villi. These villi are vascularized by the 21st day to form the tertiary villi.

Cytotrophoblastic cells penetrate into the overlying syncytium adjacent to the decidua. The cells become continuous, and a thin cytotrophoblastic shell is formed that surrounds the blastocyst. Decidua immediately near to this shell is called troposphere. Fibrinoid deposit that appears on the syncytiotrophoblast, outside the trophoblastic shell, is called Nitabuch's membrane. Maternal blood vessels pass through all the layers to reach the intervillous space.

DEVELOPMENT OF INNER CELL MASS

By the eighth day, the embryo blasts and differentiates into bilaminar germ disc, which consists of the dorsal ectodermal layer of tall columnar cells and the ventral endodermal layer of flattened polyhedral cells. The bilaminar germ disc is connected with the trophoblast by mesenchymal condensation called the connecting stalk or body stalk, which later becomes the umbilical cord.

Two cavities appear, one on each side of the germ disc. The fluid-filled space which appears between the ectodermal layer and up to the trophoblast is called amniotic cavity. The floor is formed by the ectoderm and the rest of its wall by primitive mesenchyme.

Extension of flat ectodermal cells occurs from the ectodermal disc or from the cytotrophoblast on either side to form the inner aspect of the mesenchymal lining. These two layers form the amnion. The cavity which appears on the ventral aspect of the bilaminar disc is known as yolk sac.

During the third week, primitive streak appears that invaginates and migrates between the ectodermal and endodermal layers to form the mesoderm layer. Embryonic stage extends from the fourth to eighth weeks. Individual differentiation of germ layers and formation of folds of the embryo occur during this period. By the eighth week, the embryo can be differentiated as human.

Primitive streak develops from the caudal end of the bilaminar disc by the end the second week by proliferation from the formative mass. Primitive streak confers a bilateral symmetry on the embryonic area. The primitive groove overlies the streak. The primitive node or the primitive knot develops from the cephalic end of primitive streak by enlargement. Primitive streak organizes the ectodermal cells and converges to the midline and insinuates itself between the overlying ectoderm and the underlying endoderm. It migrates into all directions. They differentiate to form the intraembryonic mesoderm or chorda mesoderm. It becomes the notochord. It is the forerunner of the vertebral column. The notochord consists of a tough notochordal sheath enclosing large stellate cells surrounded by intercellular fluid which imparts turgidity to it.

Neurula

Neural plate is formed from the ectoderm overlying the developing notochord. Formation of neural plate takes place under the inductive influence of prochordal plate, endoderm and chorda mesoderm. Forebrain and eyes are induced by the prochordal plate and cephalic end of the notochord. Hindbrain and associated structures are induced by the mid portion of the chorda mesoderm. The spinal cord and adjacent muscle masses are induced by the caudal part of the roof – the archenteron. Neural plate is destined to form the nervous system, and this entire stage is called neurula.

DERIVATIVES OF THE GERM LAYERS

With the appearance of primitive streak, the notochord and the mesoderm, the embryo develops a trilaminar outline with a broad cephalic and narrow caudal end. The mesodermal cells migrate cephalad in the midline and diverge sideways and separate the overlying ectoderm from the underlying endoderm. But the overlying ectoderm remains firmly attached at the endodermal prochordal palate. The mesodermal cells around the prochordal plate from both sides meet in the midline, beyond the plate, at the cephalic end to the prochordal plate in the cardiogenic area. Cephalic to cardiogenic area is the mesoderm of septum transversum. Further cephalic to the septum transversum is the extraembryonic mesoderm.

Derivatives of ectoderm

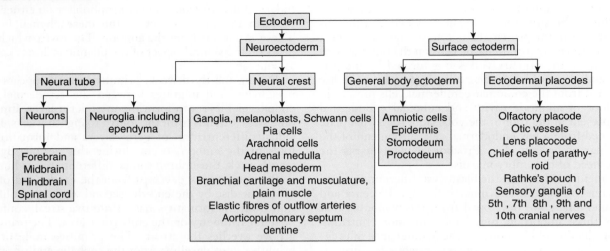

(Adapted from Bhatnagar et al. (2000). Essentials of human embryology. 3rd edition, Orient Longman.)

Derivatives of endoderm

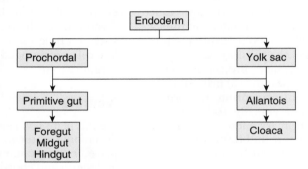

(Adapted from Bhatnagar et al. (2000). Essentials of human embryology. 3rd edition, Orient Longman.)

Derivatives of mesoderm

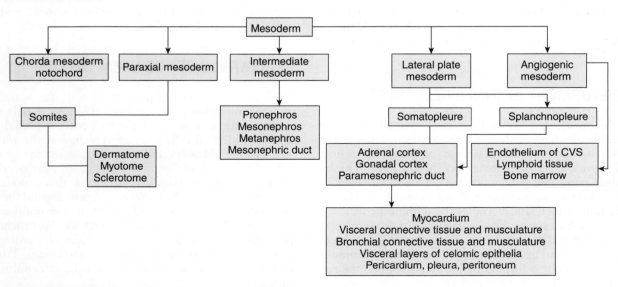

(Adapted from Bhatnagar et al. (2000). Essentials of human embryology. 3rd edition, Orient Longman.)

Ectodermal Layer

It differentiates into two lines as surface ectoderm and neuroectoderm. The surface ectoderm is further divided into the general body ectoderm and ectodermal placodes.

Important Events Following Fertilization

0 hour	Fertilization
30 hours	Two-cell stage (blastomere)
40–50 hours	Four-cell stage
72 hours	12-cell stage
96 hours	16-cell stage (morula in the uterine cavity)
Fifth day	Blastocyst
Sixth–seventh days	Zona pellucida disappears, interstitial implantation
Ninth day	Lacunar period, endometrial vessels tapped
10th–11th days	Implantation completed
13th day	Primary villi
16th day	Secondary villi
21st day	Tertiary villi
21st–22nd days	Fetal heart, fetoplacental circulation

HUMAN EMBRYO

Growth of a single cell measuring 130 mm and weighting a few micrograms to a full-term fetus composed of billions of cells and measuring 500 mm in length and 3000 mg in weight is the story of human embryology.

A miniature human can be recognized by the end of the eighth day after fertilization. The embryo measures less than an inch (23 mm) and weighs a few grams.

Age of the Embryo

The probable age of the embryo can be computed. This is equivalent to the duration of pregnancy. Determination of the age of an embryo is important for academic as well as medicolegal purposes.

- **Menstrual age** – From the first day of the last menstrual period
- **Coital age** – From the time of the last known coitus which led to the conception
- **Ovulation age** – From the time of release of the ovum from the ovary
- **Fertilization age** – From the time of fertilization of the ovum

Measurement of Embryo

Measuring the length of the embryo, a fetus or an infant can be a useful guide to its probable age.

- Total length in early embryos
- Crown–rump (CR) length or sitting height: Length between the crown of the head and the breech (buttocks); equivalent to the sitting height of an adult individual

- Crown–heal (CH) length: From the crown to the heel of the embryo; equivalent to the standing height of an adult individual
- Neck–rump (NR): From neck to rump in early embryos with a greatly flexed head

Other practical methods of measurement are as follows:

- Crown-to-heel length (in inches): For the first five lunar months, square the lunar months in centimetres. For example, at fourth month, the embryo measures $4^2 = 16$ cm; fifth month, $5^2 = 25$ cm. For the last 5 months, multiply the number of the month by five. For example, at the seventh month, the CH length is $7 \times 5 = 35$ cm.
- CR length (in mm):

15 days	1 mm
21 days	2 mm
32 days	5 mm (later add 1 mm per day)
55 days	28 mm (later add 1.5 mm per day)

Expected Date of Delivery

Expected date of delivery (EDD) is calculated from the first day of the last menstrual period by adding to it 1 year and 1 week and then subtracting 3 months.

Stages of Development

The various stages in development are as follows:

- Period of ovum or preembryonic period – first week. This is the prelude to the embryonic stage and extends from the formation of zygote to its subdivision into blastomeres and blastocyst. Implantation occurs by the end of this period.
- Embryonic period (2–8 weeks) – Embryo is the developing product of a fertilized egg from 1 week after fertilization to the end of the eighth week. This stage is further divided into the following:
  - Period of the two-layered embryo (second week)
  - Period of the three-layered embryo (third week)
  - Period of the embryo with somites (fourth week) – neurula stage
  - Period of the embryo completion (fifth–eighth week) – period of organogenesis

Fetal Period (9–40 Weeks)

Age	Characteristics
9–12 weeks	• Fetal size doubled (60 mm) • Organs assume definitive positions • Head is very large • Eyes become anterior • Eyelids are fixed • Ears ascend • Male and female genitals become evident • Gut returns to the abdomen • Nail furrows appear
13–16 weeks	• The brain is fully developed • Movements of the fetus are detectable on auscultation at about the 14th week • Fetal skin is transparent

Continued

Fetal Period (9–40 Weeks)—cont'd

- Scalp hair and later body hair (lanugo) appear
- Muscle tissue lengthens and bones become harder
- Glands, in general, differentiate
- Testis in iliac fossa is ready for descent through the inguinal canal
- The fetus can suck, swallow and make irregular breathing movements
- The fetus can feel pain
- Liver and organ produce appropriate fluids
- Eyelashes appear

17–20 weeks
- Quickening (the mother can feel the fetus moving) occurs
- Vernix caseosa formed (sebum, lanugo and the shed epidermal cells together form paste-like substance vernix) and acts as the protective covering
- Finger and toenails appear
- Lanugo covers the whole body
- Hears and recognizes the mother's voice
- Site of attachment of the umbilical cord moves up
- Development of the infraumbilical part of the abdominal wall

21–25 weeks (third trimester)
- Sex organs are visible on the ultrasound scan
- Dark hair appears on the scalp
- Eyelashes and eyebrows are prominent
- Lower abdomen is well formed
- Vernix covers the whole skin
- Fetus has a hand reflex and a startle reflex
- Footprints are forming
- Inhaling amniotic fluid as a practice of breathing
- Rapid brain development; the nervous system is able to control some bodily functions

25–28 weeks
- Subcutaneous fat develops
- Wrinkles disappear
- Contours become rounded
- Fused eyelids get detached
- Acquires viability
- At 25th week, there is 60% chance of survival

29–36 weeks
- Rapid increase in body fat
- Rhythmic breathing occurs, but lungs are immature
- The left testis is in the scrotum
- Nails reach the fingertips
- Large amount of vernix caseosa
- 95% of chance of survival

37–40 weeks
- Both testes are in the scrotum
- Umbilical cord is attached near the centre of the abdomen
- Lanugo disappears
- The fetus is considered full term
- Scalp hair is coarse and thicker
- The lungs are mature
- The average weight is 3 kg
- At birth, placenta detaches from the uterus
- At birth, breathing triggers changes in the heart and bypasses arteries, forcing all blood to travel through the lungs

Fetal Membranes and Placenta

The accessory structures essential for the normal development of the fetus until birth are called fetal membranes. They develop from the zygote but do not form any part of the embryo proper. These are as follows:
- Trophoblast and chorion
- Amnion or ectodermal vesicle
- Yolk sac, primary, secondary and tertiary or definitive sac
- Allantois
- Body stalk and umbilical cord

Trophoblast

It is the single layer of flattened cells derived from the outer cells of morula. It lines the blastocyst and nourishes the early embryo. It implants the embryo and forms chorionic villi. The roof of the blastocyst is formed by a plate of cuboidal cells that differentiate from the inner cell mass and arrange themselves to enclose a cavity known as primary yolk sac or archenteron. The trophoblastic cells become cuboidal and constitute the cytotrophoblast or Langerhans cell layer.

Chorion

It is thicker than amnion, friable and shaggy on both sides. It is attached to the amnion internally by loose areolar tissue and remnants of primitive mesenchyme and externally by vestiges of the trophoblastic layer and decidual cells. Chorion has no vessels or nerves. The syncytial trophoblast, the Langerhans cell layer and the primary mesoderm together constitute chorion. Original blastocyst cavity is filled with the primary mesoderm. Many isolated clefts are formed in this mesoderm and combine together to form a single cavity called extraembryonic coelom.

With the growth of chorion, its cavity also enlarges and the mesoderm arranges to form the inner lining of the chorionic wall, the outer covering of the yolk sac and the amnion around the rim of the embryonic area. The same mesoderm that also connects the chorion with structures described earlier is called the connecting stalk or body stalk and forms the basis of the umbilical cord.

At first, the syncytial trophoblast forms irregular knobs all over the chorionic surface called primary chorionic villi. Chorionic villi opposite to the connecting stalk enlarge and form finger-like projections called chorion frondosum that invades the decidua. The chorion frondosum and the adjacent decidua together take part in the formation of placenta. After complete embedding of the blastocyst in the decidua, the villi over the reminder of the chorionic surface disappear, giving it a smooth appearance. The smooth part of the chorion is called the chorion laeve.

Amnion

It is the inner layer of fetal membranes. Its internal surface is smooth, shiny and in contact with liquor amnii. Outer surface is a layer of connective tissue and is similar to the inner aspect of chorion. Fully formed amnion is 0.02–0.05 mm in thickness. Amnion has no blood, nerve or lymphatic supply.

Functions

1. Contributes the formation of liquor amnii
2. Intact membrane prevents ascending uterine infection
3. Facilitates dilation of the cervix during labour
4. Has enzymatic activities for steroid hormonal metabolism
5. Is a rich source of glycerophospholipids containing arachidonic acid, a precursor of prostaglandins E2 and F2

Amniotic Fluid

Surrounds the fetus everywhere except at its attachment with the body stalk.

Volume

Its volume is 50 mL at 12 weeks. The amniotic fluid is first produced by the activity of the cells of the amnion, either by filtration or by secretion. When fetal kidneys start functioning, fetal urine is added to the amniotic fluid. Other contributions are from tracheobronchial tree and the fetal surface of placenta. The fetus regularly swallows amniotic fluid, and the fluid is replaced approximately every 8 hours. At full term, the amniotic fluid measures about 1500–2000 mL; 400 mL at 20 weeks; reaches peak at 36–38 weeks (600–800 mL). Colour at early pregnancy: colourless; by term, colour becomes pale straw. Osmolarity: 250 mOsmol/L at fetal maturity.

Colour Abnormalities

- Green – Meconium stained
- Golden colour – Rh incompatibility
- Greenish yellow (saffron) – Postmaturity
- Dark-coloured – Accidental haemorrhage
- Dark brown (tobacco juice) — Intrauterine fetal death (IUD)

Functions

1. It acts as a shock absorber, protecting the fetus from possible extraneous injury.
2. It regulates excess temperature.
3. The fluid distends the amniotic sac and thereby allows for growth and free movement of the fetus.
4. The amnion and the chorion are combined to form a hydrostatic wedge which helps in dilation of the cervix.
5. During uterine contractions, it prevents marked interference with the placental circulation so long as the membrane remains intact.
6. It flushes the birth canal at the end of the first stage of labour and by its aseptic and bactericidal action protects the fetus and prevents ascending infection to the uterine cavity.

Yolk Sac

It is a vestigial structure and described in three stages as primary, secondary and tertiary or definitive. The primary yolk sac (archenteron) is a cavity enclosed in Heuser's exocoelomic membrane and is roofed by the primary endoderm.

Secondary yolk sac is much smaller than the primary yolk sac. At about 13 days of intrauterine life (IUL), an endodermal diverticulum arises near the caudal end of the roof of the yolk sac called allantois (allantoenteric diverticulum). The earliest blood cells develop in the mesoderm of the secondary yolk sac.

The tertiary or definitive yolk sac or vitelline sac is the remnant of the secondary yolk sac. As the embryo folds ventrally, it takes up the roof of the secondary yolk sac within it. This inclusion of the roof into the embryonic body forms the basis of the foregut, midgut and hindgut. The portion not included in the embryonic body remains as the definitive yolk sac.

It remains in communication with the midgut via vitellointestinal duct. With the growth of the vitelline duct and enlargement of the amniotic cavity, the yolk sac is pushed away from the body wall of the fetus. It grows separately and never reaches a size greater than 5 mm and is found at the placental end of the umbilical cord between the amnion and the chorion until the fifth month.

Allantois

It is again a vestigial structure which arises from the endodermal diverticulum from the primitive midgut. Its arteries vascularize the chorion. Its remnant is urachus that forms a part of the urinary bladder.

Umbilical Cord

It develops from the body stalk stretching between the embryonic disc and the chorion. It has got a covering of epithelium which shows stratification like the fetal epidermis.

Wharton's jelly consists of elongated cells in a gelatinous base. It is the connecting link and lifeline extending from the placenta to the fetus and is usually centrally attached to the placenta. The two arteries of the umbilical cord spring from the dorsal aorta of the fetus. The cord at full term is 50 cm in length (average). It contains the following parts:

- Wharton's jelly made up of the primary mesoderm
- Two umbilical arteries
- Single left umbilical vein
- Vitelline duct
- Allantois

Placenta

It has both maternal and fetal components. Placentation begins during the fourth week of IUL. Decidua is the highly modified uterine endometrium into which the blastocyst is implanted. The three regions of decidua are as follows:

- Decidua capsularis (decidua reflexa) – Thin compact layer facing the uterine lumen

- Decidua basalis (decidua serotina) – Made up of a compact spongy layer of chorion frondosum
- Decidua parietalis (decidua vera) – Reminder lining of the uterus

Chorionic villi develop in three stages—primary, secondary and tertiary villi. Primary villi consist of the syncytial trophoblast with an underlying cytotrophoblast. The core of the primary mesoderm is invaded by blood vessels to form the tertiary villi. The tertiary villi are divisible into two types, anchoring villi and floating villi.

Placental barrier – The barrier between fetal and maternal bloodstream is made up of the following:

- Syncytiotrophoblast and cytotrophoblast
- Basement membrane of the trophoblast facing the fetal membrane
- Endothelium of fetal blood vessels

Placenta thus:

- Attaches the fetus to the uterus
- Has dual origins
- Shows intimate contact between the fetal surfaces of chorionic villi and the maternal blood in the intervillous space
- Permits the passage of nutrient materials and oxygen from the mother to the fetus
- Allows excretion of nitrogenous waste and carbon dioxide from the mother to the fetus
- Produces hormones such as oestrogen, progesterone and gonadotrophins to sustain pregnancy
- Acts as a barrier to many harmful organisms and noxious substances, thus protecting the fetus

Perinatal Care

Perinatal care includes care of the fetus and the mother from conception until neonatal medical care. There are various modalities available that provide highly specialized technological care to identify many conditions during fetal life itself and to manage delivery without increasing perinatal mortality.

The successful outcome of a pregnancy depends on certain factors such as:

- Mother's state of health
- Nutrition status
- Higher socioeconomic living standard
- Educational level
- Quality of health care provided

Risk factors that affect the health and survival of the fetus in the womb and those that affect the neonate after delivery include the following:

- Medications taken during pregnancy – Drugs either prescribed or countermedications should be avoided because of the teratogenic effects to the growing fetus.
- X-rays – Exposure to X-rays for therapeutic purposes or otherwise can harm the growing fetus. Exposure to any type of radiation can be fatal, producing multiple anomalies in the fetus.
- Ingestion of alcohol and drug abuse – This may damage the fetus (see also the fetal alcohol syndrome).
- Smoking – Avoid not only active smoking but also passive smoking, as it reduces birth weight of the newborn. It is of critical importance in the case of

premature delivery. On an average, babies of smokers are 170 g lesser in weight than those of non-smokers. It is also associated with an increased risk of miscarriages and stillbirth among smokers. The infant born to smokers also have a high risk for sudden infant death syndrome (SIDS).

- Infections during pregnancy (TORCH infections) – Congenital rubella needs to be prevented by immunizing adolescent females before they become pregnant. Exposure to toxoplasmosis should also be avoided. This can be achieved by avoiding rearing pet animals (e.g. cats) and wearing gloves while handling pets and by avoiding eating undercooked poultry.
- *Listeria* infection can be prevented by avoiding eating unpasteurized dairy products, soft ripened cheese, etc.
- Eating liver during pregnancy also should be avoided, as a high concentration of vitamin A could harm the growing fetus.
- Any preexisting maternal condition, such as hypertension or obstetric risk factors that may lead to complications in pregnancy or delivery (i.e. bad obstetric history), e.g. miscarriages or previous preterm delivery, is a risk factor. Obesity increases the risk for gestational diabetes and pregnancy-induced hypertension (PIH).
- Couples with inherited disorders should be provided with genetic counselling before pregnancy in order to reduce the risk of genetic abnormality in their offspring.
- The following warning should be given to high-risk pregnant women:
  - The mother older than 35 years (risk of Down syndrome is greater than one in 380)
  - Previous abnormal child/children
  - Family history of inherited disorder
  - Parents who are carriers of autosomal recessive disorders
  - Parents having chromosomal rearrangements

Drugs Which are Harmful During Pregnancy

Cytotoxic Agents	Congenital Abnormalities
Diethylstilbestrol (DES)	Clear cell adenoma of vagina and cervix
Iodides/propylthiouracil	Goitre, hypothyroidism
Lithium	Congenital Heart Disease
Phenytoin	Hypoplastic nails and craniofacial abnormalities
Progesterone	Musculinization of the female fetus
Tetracyclines	Enamel hypoplasia of the teeth
Thalidomide	Limb shortening (phocomelia)
Valproate/carbamazepine	Neural tube defects
Vitamin A	Increased spontaneous abortions, abnormal facies
Warfarin	Interferes with cartilage formation – nasal hypoplasia, epiphyseal stippling; cerebral haemorrhage and microcephaly

Antenatal Examination and Care

The pregnant female should undergo regular antenatal check-up to prevent complications and to reduce perinatal, intranatal and neonatal mortality and morbidity.

Antenatal Diagnosis

There are many screening tests available to detect fetal abnormalities during pregnancy, thereby reducing risks and neonatal mortality. The main diagnostic tests for antenatal diagnosis are as follows:
- Maternal blood screening
- Ultrasound screening

Maternal blood is screened for the following:
- Blood group, Rh typing and other red blood cell incompatibilities
- Hepatitis B, VDRL, HIV, CMV and rubella
- Testing for neural tube defects (maternal serum α-fetoprotein [MSAFP]). It is raised in about 80% of neural tube defects and more than 90% of anencephalic cases. This is not done routinely in Kerala.
- Testing for Down syndrome – The risk is estimated by MSAFP with human chorionic gonadotrophin (HCG) and unconjugated oestriol (uE3) measurements. They are together called triple test adjusted for the maternal age. This is also not a routine test in Kerala.

Ultrasound screening is done for the following:
- Gestational age (estimated if performed within 20 weeks)
- Multiple pregnancy
- Structural malformations (70% can be identified)
- Fetal growth (identified by serial monitoring)
- Amniotic fluid volume (oligohydramnios results from reduced fetal urine production related to dysplasia of the kidney, obstructive uropathy [Posterior Urethral Valve (PUV)], absent kidney or from premature rupture of membrane [PROM]). It usually causes lung hypoplasia, limb and facial malformations owing to pressure on the fetus (Potter syndrome). Polyhydramnios is associated with maternal diabetes or gastrointestinal atresias in the fetus (tracheoesophageal fistula and atresia).

Structural Abnormalities Identified by Ultrasound Scanning

Body Systems	Anomalies
Central nervous system disorders	Anencephaly
	Spina bifida
	Hydrocephalus and microcephalus
Cardiovascular system	CHDs (a four-chamber view helps detect 60% of defects)
Thoracic	Diaphragmatic hernia
Facial	Cleft lip and palate
Gastrointestinal	Exomphalos and gastroschisis
Genitourinary	Dysplastic kidney, obstructive uropathy (PUV) and hydronephrosis
Skeletal	Skeletal dysplasia, achondroplasia and limb reduction deformities

Structural Abnormalities Identified by Ultrasound Scanning—cont'd

Body Systems	Anomalies
Hydrops	Oedema of skin, pleural effusion and ascites
Chromosomal	Down syndrome – Suspected from nuchal thickening, duodenal atresia or atrioventricular defect of the heart
	Other chromosomal abnormalities are suspected from multiple anomalies

Main diagnostic techniques used are as follows:
- Detailed ultrasound scanning is done to detect structural abnormalities.
- Amniocentesis is done to carry out the following:
  - Chromosomal analysis
  - α-Fetoprotein and acetyl cholinesterase for neural tube defects
  - Bilirubin estimation for Rhesus disease
  - Enzyme analysis for inborn errors of metabolism
- Chorionic villus sampling is done for the following:
  - Chromosomal analysis
  - Enzyme analysis for inborn errors of metabolism
  - DNA analysis (thalassaemia, haemophilia A and B, cystic fibrosis, muscular dystrophy)
  - Congenital infections (viral particles using polymerase chain reactions)
- Fetal blood sampling is done for the following:
  - Rapid chromosomal analysis
  - Severe Rhesus disease and platelet isoimmunization
  - Congenital infection serology
- Fetal tissue sampling is done to identify severe congenital skin disorders.

FETAL THERAPY

The fetus can be treated by giving medications to the mother. Glucocorticoid therapy administered to the mother before delivery helps accelerate lung maturity and surfactant production, which, in turn, reduce the incidence and severity of Respiratory Distress Syndrome (RDS) and severe intracranial haemorrhage. This therapy is given at least 24 hours before delivery for optimum results. But this may not be possible during most of the times. Digoxin or flecainide given to the mother for treating supraventricular tachycardia is also found to be effective.

Therapy given directly to the fetus includes:
- Rhesus isoimmunization – Severely affected fetus is treated by intrauterine methods (administration of anti-D to the mother has reduced the incidence of Rhesus disease)
- Perinatal isoimmune thrombocytopenia – A condition analogous to Rhesus isoimmunization

Following fetal surgeries are also performed:
- Aminoinfusion of saline for oligohydramnios
- Surgical correction by hysterotomy at 22–24 weeks for diaphragmatic hernia, spina bifida (efficacy is

uncertain; premature labour is common after this procedure)

- Catheter shunts inserted under ultrasound guidance for pleural effusion
- Intrauterine shunts for obstructive uropathies and also for hydrocephalus
- Dilatation of stenotic heart valves via a transabdominal catheter inserted under ultrasound guidance into the fetal heart

Multiple Births

Main problems associated with multiple births are as follows:

- Preterm labour – The median gestation for twins is 36 weeks, for triplets 34 weeks and for quadruplets 32 weeks
- Twin–twin blood transfusions – May cause discrepancy in growth, usually of monochorionic (identical) twins
- Preeclampsia
- Congenital abnormalities
- Intrauterine growth retardation (IUGR)
- Complicated deliveries

STUDY QUESTION

1. Explain fertilization.
2. Why is it important for a nurse to have knowledge of embryology?
3. What are the functions of umbilical cord, placenta and amniotic fluid?
4. What is perinatal care? why is it important to give perinatal care?
5. What are the common antenatal tests done?
6. What are the structural abnormalities that can be detected with ultrasound scanning?
7. Write short notes on:
   1. Fetal therapy
   2. Multiple births
   3. Antenatal screening
8. Harmful drugs during pregnancy.

BIBLIOGRAPHY

1. American Association for the Advancement of Science. (1993). Benchmarks for Science Literacy. New York: Oxford University Press.
2. Dias MS, McLone DG: Normal and abnormal early development of the nervous system, In McLone DG (ed): Pediatric Neurosurgery: Surgery of the Developing Nervous System. Philadelphia: W.B. Saunders, 2001, pp 31-71.
3. Moore, K.L.: The Developing Human. Clinically Oriented Embryology, 3rd ed. Philadelphia, W.B. Saunders Co., 1982.
4. Moore, K.L.: Before We are Born, Basic Embryology and Birth Defects, 2nd ed., Philadelphia, W.B. Saunders Co., 1983.
5. O'Rahilly, R.: Guide to the Staging of Human Embryos. Anal. Anz. 130:556, 1972.
6. A.D.M Software, Inc. Nine Month Miracle (CD ROM Software) 1600 River Edge Parkway, Suite 800, Atlanta, GA 30328, Georgia, USA.
7. The First Nine Months of Life, (brochure), Focus on the Family. Colorado Springs, CO, 1995.

NURSING CARE OF NORMAL NEONATES

NURSING CARE OF A NEONATE

Neonate is a baby of 0–28 days of age as per the World Health Organization (WHO) definition. The normal human gestational period is 280 days or 40 weeks, calculated from the first day of the mother's last menstrual cycle. Birth of a baby is a new experience, especially for a primigravid woman, and this must be considered while conducting delivery. Labour room is a place where lots of legal problems can arise. So, the nurse working in the labour room should be vigilant not to make any mistake while handling babies.

A nurse working in a labour room should prepare two identification bands and write the mother's hospital number, neonate's gender and time of delivery on them. Tie one band around the infant's wrist or ankle and the other band around the wrist of the mother. Check the birth records and identification before the neonate leaves the resuscitation area of the delivery room. When the neonate is handed over to the mother, ask her to verify her baby's gender with the information written on the band.

NEWBORN ASSESSMENT

A normal newborn should possess the following characteristics: weight should be greater than 2500 g, gestation above 37 weeks, birth weight between the 10th and 90th percentiles according to intrauterine growth charts, normal Apgar score, and absence of any maternal illness and no postnatal infections or complications.

IMMEDIATE ASSESSMENT OF THE NEWBORN

Care at Birth

Time of birth: Those who attend the labour should note the time of birth. Usual routine is to call out the time so that there will not be any inaccurate recoding of the time. This is essential, especially for people who believe in astrology and horoscope.

Universal precautions to be followed: Those who attend the labour should be vigilant to follow universal precautions or standard precautions. All fluids including amniotic fluid, blood, vaginal discharge, etc. should be treated as potentially infectious.

Protective eyewear or shields should be used during procedure to prevent either contact with fluids or potential flashing of fluids to the eye. One must be vigilant to follow five cleans to prevent infection such as clean hands (hand hygiene and wearing gloves), clean surface (use of a sterile towel to dry and cover the baby), clean cord (cord cutting with a sterile blade or scissors), clean thread or sterile clamp for clamping the cord, and keep the cord clean and not to apply anything to the cord.

Assess respiratory status, tachypnoea (the earliest sign of respiratory problem), nasal flaring, retractions and expiratory grunt.

Apgar Score

Apgar scoring, done at 1 and 5 minutes after birth, is based on the scoring method developed by Virginia Apgar.

Apgar Scoring

Sign	0	1	2
Heart rate	Absent	Slow, less than 100	Over 100
Respiratory effort	Absent	Slow, irregular	Good crying
Muscle tone	Flaccid	Some flexion of extremities	Active motion
Reflex irritability	No response	Crying	Vigorous crying
Colour	Blue or pale	Body pink, extremities blue	Completely pink

A score of 0–3 indicates severe asphyxia, and a score of 4–7 indicates mild-to-moderate asphyxia. The scoring done at 1 minute is a guide to the need for resuscitation. The score at 5 minutes is predictive of the outcome.

A score of 5 or less is a predictor of adverse outcome and indicates a need for assisted ventilation and possible cardiac support. A score of 5–7 indicates a need for stimulation and supplemental oxygen. A score of 8–10 reflects good oxygenation and ventilation and indicates no need for vigorous resuscitation.

ASSESSMENT OF GESTATIONAL AGE

A method of clinically estimating the gestational age, developed by Lubchenco in 1970 at the University of Colorado, can be safely used in the first few hours of life with little handling or exposure of the newborn. Completion of all the items on this assessment form yields a profile of the neonate's development and gestational age.

Dubowitz Scoring System

Dubowitz and colleagues (1970) developed a method of clinical assessment of the gestational age, which assigns a score of 0–5 to each of 10 neurological signs and a score of 0–4 to each of 11 external (physical) signs. The totals are added to yield a composite score which is correlated with weeks of gestation. This composite has a higher degree of correlation than does either the neurological or the external portion considered separately (±2 weeks with 95% confidence interval).

Newborn Maturity Rating (Ballard)

Ballard and co-workers (1979) developed the Newborn Maturity Rating, a simplified version of the Dubowitz tool. This version was later modified by Ballard in 1988 to assess neonates 20–44 weeks of age. The Ballard tool may be used from birth through the first 5 days, assigning a score of 0–5 to each of six neurological and six physical criteria. It requires less time and eliminates neurological assessment of active muscle tone which is difficult to assess in severely ill neonates. This tool is found to be reliable and is widely used in many countries.

Physical Maturity

Sign	Score						
	1	0	1	2	3	4	5
Skin	Sticky, friable, transparent	Gelatinous, red, translucent	Smooth, pink, visible veins	Superficial peeling and/ or rash, few veins	Cracking, pale areas, rare veins	Parchment, deep cracking, no vessels	Leathery, cracked, wrinkle
Lanugo	None	Sparse	Abundant	Thinning	Bald	Mostly bald	
Plantar surface	Heel to toe 40–50 mm: −1 <40 mm: −2	<50 mm No crease	Faint red marks	Anterior transverse crease only	Creases anterior two-thirds	Creases over the entire sole	
Breast	Imperceptible	Barely perceptible	Flat areola No bud	Slipped areola 1–2 mm bud	Raised are-ola 3-mm bud	Full areola 5–10 mm bud	
Eye/ear	Lids fused Loosely: 1 Tightly: 2	Lids open Pinna flat Stays folded	Slightly curved Pinna soft Slow recoil	Well curved Pinna soft but instant recoil	Formed and firm Instant recoil	Thick cartilage Ear stiff	
Genita-lia—male	Scrotum flat Smooth	Scrotum empty Faint rugae	Testis in the upper canal Rare rugae	Testis descending Few rugae	Testis down Good rugae	Testis pendulous Deep rugae	
Genita-lia—fe-male	Clitoris prominent labia flat	Prominent clitoris, small labia minora	Prominent clitoris, enlarging minora	Majora and minora equally prominent	Majora large, minora small	Majora covers clitoris and minora	

Neuromuscular maturity

- Assess for obvious signs of congenital malformations.
- Check the umbilical cord: two arteries and one vein.
- Look for meconium staining: skin, nails.
- Evaluate abnormal cry or no cry.
- Assess any injuries caused by birth trauma, i.e. dislocated shoulder, oedema of scalp, lacerations, etc.
- Assess neurological status: reflexes, tremors and twitching.
- Check for anal and nasal patency.

Maturity Rating

Total Score (Physical + Neuromuscular)	Weeks
−10	20
−5	22
0	24
5	26
10	28
15	30
20	32
25	34
30	36
35	38
40	40
50	44

Assessment of gestational age should accompany a detailed examination of the newborn which can be conducted at 2 hours of age, before the baby leaves the delivery room. Usually, the neonatologists use Parkin's method as a tool to assess the gestational age of the newborn or use simple physical criteria such as Usher's criteria as described for high-risk neonates.

The parameters used are skin texture, skin colour, breast size and ear firmness.

Skin texture is tested by picking a fold of abdominal skin between fingers and the thumb and also by inspection.
Score 0: Very thin, gelatinous
Score 1: Thin, smooth
Score 2: Smooth and of medium thickness
Score 3: Slight thickening, cracking, peeling, especially on hands and feet
Score 4: Thick, parchment like with superficial and deep cracking

Skin colour is estimated by inspection when the baby is quiet.
Score 0: Dark red
Score 1: Uniformly pink
Score 2: Pale pink
Score 3: Pale, pink only on ears, lips, palms and soles

Breast size is estimated by picking up the breast tissue between fingers and the thumb.
Score 0: No breast tissue palpable
Score 1: Breast tissue palpable on both sides; neither being more than 0.5 cm in diameter
Score 2: Breast tissue palpable on both sides; one or both being 0.5–1 cm in diameter

Score 3: Breast tissue palpable on both sides; one or both being more than 1 cm in diameter

Ear firmness is tested by palpation and folding of the upper pinna and looking for recoil when letting go.

Score 0: Pinna feels soft and folds into bizarre shapes without springing back into position spontaneously.

Score 1: Pinna feels soft along the edge and is easily folded but returns slowly to the correct position.

Score 2: Cartilage is felt up to the edge of the pinna, though it is thin at places; pinna springs back readily after being folded.

Score 3: Pinna is firm, with definite cartilage up to periphery; it springs back immediately after being folded.

Scoring clue: Add all the points allotted to get the gestational age. The following table can be used to assign gestational age:

Score	Gestational Age
1	27
2	30
3	33
4	34½
5	36
6	37
7	38½
8	39½
9	40
10	41
11	41½
12	42

Norms have been established for somatic growth at each week of gestation and are based on weight, length and head circumference. However, size per se should be used to infer gestational age or maturation. If an infant's growth parameters are between the 10th and 90th percentiles for a specific time of gestation, the infant's growth is said to be appropriate for gestational age.

CARE AT BIRTH

Lay the baby in the supine position on the table in a head-down position with a pad under the shoulder. Wipe the mouth and nostrils, and suck out with the mucus sucker or electric suction with precaution to clear the airway. In babies breathing spontaneously, wipe off the baby, dry and keep it well wrapped in a dry sheet to prevent hypothermia.

Immediate stabilization occurs in the first few hours after birth. Keep the healthy babies by the side of their mothers if possible even in the labour room. During this period also, observe the heart rate, temperature, colour, adequacy of peripheral circulation, level of consciousness and tone of activity.

Care of the Umbilical Cord

Clean the cord, and use sterile cord ties. Apply the first tie 2 cm away from the umbilicus; the second tie 2 cm away from the first tie. Crush the cord 2 cm away from the second tie and cut with sterile scissors at the crushed area.

Clean the stump as per hospital policy (whether using antiseptics or not). Avoid excessive exposure of the baby, as the body temperature is variable. Place the baby on its side or on a modified Trendelenburg position to facilitate drainage of mucus or blood. Suction the mucus as needed with a bulb syringe or mucus sucker. Identify the baby with ID bands.

Administration of Vitamin K

Vitamin K 1 mg i.m. should be given to all high-risk babies to prevent haemorrhagic disease of the newborn.

Care of the Eyes

Silver nitrate 1% solution is instilled to the eyes in certain hospitals as a routine procedure to prevent gonococcal ophthalmia neonatorum. The eyes must be washed off with normal saline or sterile water every 15 seconds after application.

Breastfeeding

It should commence as early as possible, preferably within 30 minutes after delivery. Early contact of the mother and the baby is essential for maternal and child bonding and successful breastfeeding along with incurring a very high anti-infective value of colostrums.

Care of the Skin

Clean the baby off blood, mucus and meconium before presenting to the mother. Baby bath is not recommended soon after birth. Sponge the baby the next morning with cotton and lukewarm water. No soaps are recommended. This procedure may be done according to the hospital policy.

Procedure

Procedure must be done near the mother's bedside for teaching her the procedure.

- Handle the newborn with clean gloves until after first bath as a precaution to prevent transfer of organisms that the baby might have received from the birth canal.
- Maintain measures to prevent injury to newborn (e.g. always maintain a secure hold and avoid rough fingernails or jewellery that can injure the baby).
- Position the baby comfortably in one arm or when lying in a radiant warmer or incubator.
- Adjust the water temperature by checking with a water thermometer or on outer aspect of own forearm. Water temperature should not exceed 100°F.
- Run water into a clean basin. Do not place the newborn in water until the cord is detached. Use water for sponging the body and bathing the head.
- At the beginning of bath, wipe eyes from the inner to outer canthus with sterile cotton swabs/cotton

Neurological sign	Score					
	0	1	2	3	4	5
Posture						
Square window	90°	60°	45°	30°	0°	
Angle dorsiflexion	90°	70°	45°	20°	0°	
Arm recoil	180°	90–180°	<90°			
Leg recoil	180°	90–180°	<90°			
Popliteal angle	180°	160°	130°	110°	90°	<90°
Heel to ear						
Scarf sign						
Head lag						
Ventral suspension						

balls and clean water. Use separate swabs for both eyes.

- Gently wash the face using plain water.
- Hold the newborn in the football hold and gently wet hair.
- Clean hair (shampooing is optional) with a cloth piece.
- Rinse hair completely and dry the scalp quickly and thoroughly.
- Wash external ears. Use clean part of a cloth rolled to a point to clean the external ear. Repeat with a different part of the cloth for the other ear.
- Wash the body extremities. After removing the newborn's blanket, wash the neck, chest, arms, legs and back in the same manner. Wash each body part with mild soap and water; gently rinse and dry the part before moving to the next body part.
- Clean the genitalia. For females, gently separate labia and carefully wash in posterior direction (front to back). For males, gently retract the foreskin only as far as it will easily go. Clean the tip of the glans in circular motion with a moistened cotton ball or

washed cloth. Replace foreskin immediately after cleaning.

- Wash and thoroughly dry the perineal area after rinsing.
- Avoid using powders, oils or lotions on newborn's skin.
- Liberally apply alcohol to the base of the umbilical cord; if policy permits, use a cotton-tipped applicator. Lift the cord if necessary to clean adequately.
- Apply diaper, folding the front below the cord so that the cord is exposed.
- Dress the newborn in clothes appropriate to the environmental conditions.
- Record the procedure and your evaluation of observation during bath.

Family Teaching Related to Newborn Bath

- When washing eyes, wipe from the inner canthus to the outer canthus.
- The family/mother may be instructed on applying or rubbing alcohol to the cord after discharge if

permitted and the method of application; not to apply any oil or other medications without prescription; signs and symptoms to watch for infection or delayed separation of the cord; and safety factors such as keeping cord dry, folding the diaper below the cord, etc.

- Teach the family to wipe female newborn's genitalia from front to back. Remind them to teach this principle to the child when she is being toilet trained.
- The family of the male child should be instructed to remove smegma from the infant's glans. In uncircumcised males, after the foreskin has naturally released and retraction is possible, the foreskin should be retracted for cleaning. The foreskin should be replaced to avoid tissue damage from swelling. Teach the child this procedure to incorporate it into his daily hygiene when he is cognitively able to learn it.
- Teach the family to avoid a cradle cap by gently scrubbing the infant's scalp after shampooing with a fine-toothed comb or soft-bristled brush.
- Reinforce checking the water temperature before giving a bath to the infant.
- Teach the family to avoid using soap on the face of the baby.
- Teach and demonstrate the family that bath time is an ideal time to play and interact with the infant.
- Instruct the caregiver that a towel may be placed in the baby bath tub to prevent the infant from slipping.
- Clarify to the family that sponge baths are given until the umbilical cord falls off. After that the infant can be given a full bath by placing the baby in the tub with adequate precautions and provided the container is filled up only a few inches.
- Reinforce avoidance of baby powder, which poses aspiration hazard.

GENERAL ASSESSMENT OF THE NEWBORN

Assessment of Respiratory Status

Good skin colour is the single most important indicator of cardiorespiratory function. Babies may have bluish tinge of the extremities called acrocyanosis and is benign. Check for central cyanosis, which is a danger signal. At birth, the negative pressure created by the first breath draws air into the lungs and an air–fluid interface is formed. The surfactant spreads along the epithelial lining of the alveoli and decreases surface tension at the end of expiration.

The infant's respiratory system must function immediately after birth when there is a loss of placental function.

At birth, the lungs contain 20–30 mL of fluid; approximately one-third of this is removed by the compression of chest wall during labour, and the remainder is carried to the circulation or to the lymph.

Surfactants are physiological phospholipids found in the lungs. They reduce surface tension in the alveoli and keep it from collapsing. They are also necessary to maintain lung expansion and prevent respiratory distress syndrome (RDS).

Normal respiration is about 40–60/min; above 60 or below 30 indicates a problem. Tachypnoea is a symptom of many neonatal problems. Respiration usually may be elevated during crying or shortly afterwards. Most infants are periodic breathers. They breathe rapidly for ½ minute and then stop for about 10 seconds. Hence, respiratory rate may be counted for a full minute.

Circulation

At birth, there is a rise in systemic vascular resistance that results from cessation of blood flow through the placenta. With first few breaths, pulmonary vascular resistance falls and the ductus arteriosus, ductus venosus and foramen ovale close. This allows all deoxygenated blood to return to the right ventricle to go into the lungs and become oxygenated.

Peripheral circulation may be sluggish; there may be mottling or acrocyanosis.

Pulse may be variable (normal 120–160). It will be higher than 160 during crying or below 120 while resting. Pulse, preferably peripheral, needs to be taken for a full minute.

Plethora will be visible, especially when the baby cries. Localize apex beat and find out whether it is heard on the left side or is there any shift; check for femoral pulse at the mid-inguinal region in the groin. Absence of femoral pulse may denote a coarctation of aorta. Check heart sounds and notify murmurs.

Transitory inability of the blood to clot leads to bleeding tendencies. This is attributed to lack of intestinal flora, necessary for the production of vitamin K, in the first few days after delivery. Hence, intramuscular injections of vitamin K are given routinely to prevent bleeding.

Thermoregulation

The baby staying at a temperature of 37.7°C in the uterus is suddenly exposed to the external environment with a much lower temperature. The baby suffers a large loss of body heat because it is wet at birth and may be because of the coolness of labour room. The infant may be wrapped in a warm blanket and given to the mother. The mode of heat loss in a neonate is by evaporation, radiation, convection and conduction. Evaporative heat loss in term babies is maximum in the labour room and after the bath. Heat loss through radiation is maximum when the baby is kept naked in cots or basinets. Convective heat loss occurs when the infant is kept exposed to cold and draughts. Conductive heat loss is negligible. The nurse needs to maintain neutral thermal zone (NTZ), which is defined as the thermal condition when heat production is minimum, with a minimum consumption of oxygen, and the core temperature of the baby is within the normal range. So, thermoneutral range of temperature is the one in which the baby maintains normal body temperature, with a minimum basal metabolic rate and least oxygen consumption. The range of neutral temperature varies according to the period of gestation and postnatal age. When NTZ is maintained, there will be minimal metabolic costs to the neonate. The following activities are advised to maintain NTZ:

- Prevent heat loss by drying and wrapping the baby in dry towels immediately after birth.
- Carry out all examinations of the baby under a radiant warmer or heat source such as under a 200-V bulb source.
- Avoid undue exposure of the body parts.
- Use a cap or head covering to prevent heat loss through the scalp.
- Mummify or swaddle the baby in a soft cloth.

The means of heat production such as increasing metabolism, shivering and consuming brown fat are not fully static. So, chilling can occur in a neonate if not adequately protected and will lead to cold stress. Cold stress increases the demand for oxygen and glucose. Usually, the glycogen store will be utilized for glucose demand.

The baby may become hypoglycaemic and may develop metabolic acidosis (products of incomplete metabolism accumulate with fatty acids from breakdown of brown fat).

Monitoring Temperature

It is not customary to measure the temperature of healthy newborn routinely if the warm chain is followed. In babies with serious illness, temperature should be monitored and recorded every 1–2 hours. It is advisable to record the temperature twice daily for babies weighing between 1500 and 2000 g, four times daily for babies below 1500 g and once daily for all babies who are doing well.

Methods of Monitoring Temperature

Touch Method. Temperature can be assessed by touch with the dorsum of the hand on abdomen. Abdominal temperature is representative of the core temperature. A baby's temperature can be accurately assessed with a human touch. This is an age-old practice, too.

When baby's hands and feet are warm, the baby has thermal comfort. When peripheries are cold and the trunk is warm, there is cold stress, and when both peripheries and trunk are cold, there is hypothermia. When using a thermometer, the WHO recommends low-reading thermometers that can read temperatures as low as 30°C. Thermister probe can be used to monitor skin temperature. The probe is attached to skin over the upper abdomen. The thermister will sense the skin temperature and display on the panel.

The concept of 'warm chain' practiced in the care of newborn reduces the chance of hypothermia in neonates. The delivery room should be clean and warm and prepared in advance. The temperature of the labour room should be 25°C–28°C and free from draughts from open windows, doors or fans. After birth, the baby's temperature falls at a rate of 0.1°C and 0.3°C. So the temperature of the room should be kept optimal through a radiant warmer or room heater if there is a chance for fall in temperature.

Other modalities to keep the baby warm are through immediate drying, warm resuscitation, skin-to-skin contact, breastfeeding, warm clothing and beddings, warm transportation, bathing and weighing with precautions and also through awareness training to health care professionals and families.

Nutrition. In babies, salivary glands are immature. Epstein pearls (raised white areas on palate) may be present owing to accumulation of epithelial cells. The baby may have circumoral cyanosis.

Sucking pads (fatty tissue deposits in each cheek that aid in sucking) are present. Abdominal muscles are not developed in newborns. Therefore, organs and masses are readily noted on observation. The liver is palpable 2–2.5 cm below the right costal margin. Spleen is not usually palpable. The gastrointestinal tract is immature to digest complex food items, and breast milk is the best food for the newborn. Regurgitation following feeding is common. It can be reduced by giving frequent burps during feeding. Infants usually loose 5%–10% of their weight during the first few days of life because of low fluid intake and excess loss from tissues and poor concentration capacity of the kidneys. (During the first week of life, extracellular fluid space contracts, resulting in a large reduction in body water. This water loss is responsible for 5%–10% reduction in weight loss.) Usually, they regain the lost weight within 10 days. Water loss through the skin and expired air is *insensible loss* and through urine and faeces is *sensible loss*.

Usual calorie requirement for the first few days are as follows:

1. The normal term infant needs 100–120 kcal/kg per day to meet the basal metabolic and growth requirements.
2. The infant also needs 2–3 g/kg per day of protein that is approximately 10% of the total calorie requirements. Forty per cent of the calorie requirements should be from carbohydrates.
3. The fluid requirement is 100 mL/kg per day in the first few days of life.

Babies who are unable to suck the breast may be fed artificially by the spoon-and-cup method. But neonates who have severe difficulty may be given parenteral nutrition. This will be discussed in the unit on Nutritional Needs of Children.

Elimination. Observe ability to concentrate urine and check to see if its specific gravity is elevated. Stools should be observed for colour, consistency and frequency. The normal colour of the infant stool is brown.

Infant stool: Meconium plug comes before meconium (thick grey-white mucus). Meconium is sticky, black, tarry-looking stools consisting of mucus, digestive secretions, vernix caseosa and lanugo and is usually passed during the first 24 hours after birth.

Transitional stool: On the second to fifth days, greenish yellow and loose (partly meconium and partly milk) stools are passed.

The number of stools varies. Breastfed babies have more stools than artificially fed babies.

Gender characteristics

Female genitalia: It may have heavy coating of vernix between labia and usually mucus discharge occurs.

The mucus may be blood-stained owing to elevated hormonal levels in the mother.

Male genitalia: Size of the penis and scrotum varies. Testicles should be descended or in the inguinal canal. Cremasteric reflex is present.

Skin. The skin is pinkish and may appear dry. Acrocyanosis may be present. Lanugo and vernix caseosa may be present. Petechiae may be present because of trauma during birth. Milia are common. Erythema toxicum neonatorum is transient in nature. Mongolian spots are present on the buttocks of babies. Mottling is seen in babies with chilling injuries.

PHYSIOLOGICAL JAUNDICE

Physiological jaundice is the jaundice attributable to physiological immaturity of neonates to handle increased bilirubin production. Visible jaundice usually appears between 24 and 72 hours of age. In term babies, total serum bilirubin (TSB) level usually rises to a peak level of 12–15 mg/dL by 3 days of age and then falls.

In preterm infants, TSB peak level occurs on the 3–7 days of age and can rise over 15 mg/dL.

This is usually seen in a normal neonate on the second or third day after delivery and is described along with problems of jaundice.

- Normal level is less than 1 mg/100 mL of blood.
- Jaundice may be visible on skin and sclera of the eyes.
- It does not become visible until the second or third day after birth.
- It is caused by impairment in the removal of bilirubin – a deficiency in the production of glucuronyl transferase, which is needed to convert indirect insoluble bilirubin to direct water-soluble bilirubin that is easily excreted.
- Jaundice begins to reduce by the sixth day.
- The baby should be watched carefully. Note if there is any jaundice. To estimate jaundice, the Kramer criteria can be used.
- Usual treatment includes exposure to sunlight or phototherapy when the bilirubin level is 13 mg/100 mL of blood.

Kramer's Criteria

Area of the Body	Range of Indirect Bilirubin (mg/100 mL)
Head and neck	4–5
Upper trunk	5–12
Lower trunk and thighs	8–16
Arms and lower legs	11–18
Palms and soles	>15

REFLEXES

Reflexes present at birth are the Moro and rooting reflexes in all babies.

MUSCLE TONE

Fists are usually kept clenched. The baby should offer resistance when a change in position is attempted.

Head should always be supported while lifting the baby. Normal movement of all limbs should be checked to rule out brachial plexus palsies and disorders of tone. Cry should be loud and vigorous. Note cry and suck of babies. The baby should cry when hungry and uncomfortable. A hungry baby is fretful and restless and may suck fingers.

Head

The normal head circumference is 33–35 cm. Look for cuts, bruises, caput succedaneum and cephalohaematoma. Check fontanels. Wide-open, large fontanels are significant, as they indicate hypothyroidism.

Mouth

Rule out hard and soft palate clefts by inserting the gloved index finger and gently palpating the palate. Look for micrognathia at the chin. Epstein pearls (small white cysts inside mouth) are a normal finding.

Sensation

Eyes

Light perception is present. Eye movement is uncoordinated. Usual colour is brown or dark. The baby may have subconjunctival haemorrhages, which disappear in a week. No tears are present in the first few days. The baby may gaze or follow bright objects. Examine the eyes by gently rocking the baby. Note subconjunctival haemorrhages, cataract and size of the cornea. Normal corneal diameter is 10.5 mm. Large cornea may indicate congenital glaucoma.

Nose

Babies are the obligatory nose breathers, with a sense of smell.

Ears, Taste, Touch

Hearing is present at birth. Taste is also present along with touch. The baby responds to stimuli and discomfort.

Sleep

The baby sleeps about for 20 out of 24 hours; it often stirs and stretches while sleeping.

Immunity

The baby may receive from the mother some passive immunity to infectious diseases such as diphtheria, measles and mumps. Capacity to develop its own antibodies is limited during the early period and thus has little resistance to infections.

ANTHROPOMETRY

Common parameters measured are weight, length, head circumference and chest circumference.

Weight

Take the weight with the baby naked. Weigh the baby at the same time every day before a feed. Use a scale capable of measuring up to 5 g of accuracy.

Length

Use an infantometer, if available. Otherwise, place the baby on a straight surface above a white cloth. Straighten the baby's limbs and head. Mark the point of the vertex at occipital protuberance and the heel. Measure the length. If using an infantometer, place the baby in a supine position. Stretch one lower limb of the baby and then measure the crown-to-heel length.

Head Circumference

Use a nonstretchable fibreglass tape or tailor's tape. Place the tape around the head over the most prominent part of the occiput and in front just above the eyebrows.

NEWBORN ASSESSMENT – SUMMARY CHART

Assessment	Normal	Abnormal
SKIN		
Note the skin colour and lesions	Pink, Mongolian spots	Cyanosis, pallor, beefy red
		Petechiae, ecchymosis or purpuric spots (haematological disorder)
	Capillary haemangiomas on the face or neck	Café au lait spots (patches of brown discolouration): Possible signs of neurological disorder
	Localized oedema in the presenting part	Raised capillary
	Cheesy white vernix	Haemangiomas on areas other than face or neck Oedema of the peritoneal wall
	Desquamation	Poor skin turgor
	Milia (small white pustules over the nose and the chin)	Yellow discoloured vernix
		Impetigo neonatorum
	Jaundice after 24 hours, gone by the second week	Jaundice at birth or within 24 hours
		Dermal sinuses (opening to the brain)
		Holes along the spinal column, low hairline posterioly (possible chromosomal anomaly)
Note colour of nails	Pink	Sparse or spotty hair: Congenital goitre
Note skin tone	Strong tremulous	
		Yellowing of nail beds (meconium-stained) Flaccid convulsions
HEAD AND NECK		
Note shape of the head	Fontanels: anterior open	Muscular twitching hypertonicity
	Until 18 months, posterior closed shortly after the birth with a maximum period of 6 months	Depressed, tense
		Bulging absent fontanels indicate hydrocephalus or dehydration
		Cephalohaematoma that crosses the midline
		Microcephaly and macrocephaly
Assess eyes	Slight oedema of lids	Purulent discharge, lateral upward slope of eyes with an inner epicanthal fold in infants not of Oriental descent
	Pupils equal and reacting to light by 3 weeks of age	Exophthalmos may indicate damage to the brain or cervical spine
	Intermittent strabismus	Constricted pupils, unilateral dilated, fixed pupil nystagmus
	Conjunctival or sclera haemorrhages	Continuous strabismus
	Symmetrical light reflexes off each eye in the same quadrant – sign of conjugate gaze	Absence of red reflex: Asymmetrical light reflexes
Note the placement of ears, shape and position		Low set ears may indicate chromosomal or renal system abnormality
Assess nose	Discharge, sneezing, sucking, rooting reflexes, retention cysts (pears)	Thick bloody nasal discharge
Assess mouth	Occasional vomiting	Cleft lip, palate, flat white spots (thrush), frequent vomiting (pyloric stenosis)
Vomitus with bile or faecal vomiting		

Continued

Assessment	Normal	Abnormal
Assess neck	Tonic neck reflex (Fencer's position)	Profuse salivation may indicate oesophageal atresia or tracheoesophageal fistula
		Distended neck veins, fractured clavicles, short neck, excess posterior cervical skin or resistance to neck flexion
Assess cry	Lusty cry	High-pitched or weak cry, horse cry (neurological abnormality) or cat-like cry (chromosomal abnormality)
CHEST AND LUNG		
Assess chest	Circular, enlargement of breasts, milky discharge from breasts	Depressed sternum, retractions and asymmetry of chest movements indicate respiratory distress and possible pneumothorax
Assess lungs	Abdominal respirations	
	Respiratory rate: 30–50	Thoracic breathing, unequal motion of chest, rapid grasping or grunting respirations, flaring nares, deep, sighing respirations, grunt on expiration: Possible respiratory distress
	Respiration movement irregular in rate and depth, resonant chest	
HEART		
Assess the rate, rhythm and murmurs of the heart	Rate: 100–180 at birth, stabilizes at 120–140	Hyperresonance of chest or decreased resonance
	Regular rhythm	Heart rate above 200 or less than 100
	Murmurs: Significance cannot usually be determined in newborns	Irregular rhythm
		Dextrocardia, enlarged heart
ABDOMEN AND GASTROINTESTINAL TRACT		
Assess abdomen	Prominent	
Assess the gastrointestinal tract	Bowel sounds present	Distension of abdominal veins: Possible portal vein obstruction
	Liver 2–3 cm below the right costal margin	Visible peristaltic waves, increased pitch or frequency: Intestinal obstruction
	Spleen tip palpable	Decreased sounds: Paralytic ileus
	May be able to palpate the kidneys	Distension of abdomen
		Enlarged liver or spleen
	Bladder perused 1–4 cm above the symphysis pubis	Midline suprapubic mass may indicate Hirschsprung disease
	Umbilical cord with one vein and two arteries	Enlarged kidneys
	Soft granulation tissue at the umbilicus	Distended bladder, presence of any masses
GENITOURINARY TRACT		
Assess genitalia	Oedema and bruising after delivery	One artery present in the umbilical cord may indicate other anomalies
	Unusually large clitoris in females a short time after birth	Wet umbilical stump or fetid odour from the stump
	Vaginal mucoid or bloody discharge may be present in the first week	Inguinal hernia
	Urethra opens on the ventral surface of the penile shaft	
Testis	Testis in the scrotal sac or in the inguinal canal	Hypospadias or epispadias
		Hydrocoele in males
SPINE AND EXTREMITIES		
Assess spine	Straight spine	Spina bifida, pilonidal sinuses: Scoliosis, asymmetry
Assess extremities	Soft click with thigh rotation	Sharp click with thigh rotations indicates possible congenital hip
		Uneven major gluteal folds indicate possible congenital hip
Assess anus and rectum	Patent anus	Polydactyl
		Closed anus, no meconium

BIRTH INJURIES

Most birth injuries are not serious. However, injuries to soft tissues in the abdomen (such as that of liver and spleen) are very serious.

The factors contributing to birth injuries are as follows:
1. Obstetrical factors:
   - Prematurity
   - Macrosomia
   - Cervical dystocia

- Abnormal presentations
- Prolonged labour
- Cephalopelvic disproportions
2. Instrumental delivery:
   - Mid-cavity forceps
   - Vacuum extraction

Usual Sites of Injuries

Skin

- *Petechiae:* Resulting from birth injuries are localized areas of pressure and bruising. Generalized one may be as a result of disseminated intravascular coagulation and not because of birth injuries.
- *Forceps marks:* These are linear depressed mark over both sides of the face or forehead.
- *Subcutaneous fat necrosis:* It is seen over the back of the neck, buttocks and shoulders and is seen around 6–10 days of age. The lesion feels hard. The skin over the lesion cannot be pinched. The condition does not require treatment. Observation for 6 weeks is advised along with parental reassurance.
- *Cuts:* Usually seen on the scalp, thighs and buttocks after caesarean section. Small cuts can be held together with adhesive. Bigger ones need suturing with 6–7.0 nylon. Usually, antibiotics are not needed.

Head

- *Caput succedaneum* (see disorders of the head) may be present.
- *Cephalohaematoma* may be present.
- *Subgaleal haemorrhage:* It is the collection of blood in soft tissue space between galea aponeurotica and periosteum of the scalp. It appears as diffuse swelling all over the scalp, even spreading behind the ears and neck. Babies can be sick and present with anaemia, shock and metabolic acidosis. The fluid replacement must be done.
- *Intracranial haemorrhage:* It is usually asymptomatic and needs no treatment. Epidural haemorrhage is very rare and difficult to diagnose. It requires surgical evacuation. Subdural haemorrhage is present with a full fontanelle and seizures. Tapping of fluid from haematoma is done as a treatment.
- *Skull fracture:* It is seen sometimes along with cephalohaematoma, and they are usually depressed in type. It needs further assessment with haematocrit, serum bilirubin, X-rays of the skull and computed tomographic (CT) scan.

Face

- *Facial nerve palsy:* It occurs secondary to compression of the facial nerve during a forceps delivery that affects the peripheral part of the facial nerve. On the affected part, the infant's eye remains open. The nasolabial fold is obliterated, the corner of the mouth droops and the skin is smooth. No specific treatment is required. But protection of the eyes with 1% methylcellulose drops is needed. The eyes must be kept shut by taping the lids with a nontraumatic plaster to avoid drying of the cornea.
- *Facial bones:* Fractures of the nose, mandible, maxilla and septal cartilage and dislocation of nasal septal bones can cause stridor and cyanosis. Confirmation of the fracture is done with X-rays and CT scan.

Eyes

- *Eyelids:* The common injuries are oedema, bruising and swelling. Eyelids need to be opened to check the presence of the eye balls. No special investigation or treatment is required, and the lesion resolves within 1 week. Lacerations may require microsurgery.
- *Orbit fracture:* It is usually rare but very serious. Death may occur. Orbit fracture is seen usually with exophthalmos.
- *Horner syndrome:* It includes miosis, partial ptosis, enophthalmos and anhydrosis of the ipsilateral side of the face. No treatment is necessary.
- *Cornea:* Haziness can occur secondary to oedema. It resolves within 2 weeks.
- *Intraocular haemorrhage:* Retinal bleed is seen as a streak bleed near the disc. It disappears within a week. Hyphaema is the gross blood in the anterior chamber. It resolves spontaneously within a week. Vitreous haemorrhage is seen as floaters in the vitreous with absent red reflex. If does not resolve even in a year, then surgery is required.

Ears

The common injuries are injuries resulting from forceps delivery; abrasion, haematoma, avulsions, and laceration or cuts during caesarean section.

Vocal Cord

Vocal cord injuries develop as a result of excessive traction on the head and neck during delivery, injuring the cervical sympathetic fibres of the first thoracic root. Unilateral paralysis presents with hoarseness and mild stridor. Feeding must be done carefully to avoid aspiration. The condition resolves within 4–6 weeks. Bilateral paralysis present with respiratory distress, stridor and cyanosis. Intubation, followed by tracheostomy, may be required.

Neck and Shoulder

- *Clavicular fracture:* This is the most common bone fracture that occurs during delivery. Greenstick fracture is noted 7–10 days after delivery. No treatment is required.

Brachial Palsy

- *Duchenne–Erb palsy:* The most common type involves the upper arm and occurs as a result of injury to the fifth and sixth cervical roots. Moro reflex is asymmetrical, but the grasp is intact. The arm is adducted and internally rotated. Treatment is immobilization.

- *Klumpke paralysis:* It results from the involvement of the seventh and eighth cervical roots. The hand appears 'dropped'. The wrist does not move, and there is no grasp reflex.
- *Total palsy:* It is characterized by a flaccid arm hanging limply with no movement and reflexes. Treatment is immobilization.
- *Phrenic nerve paralysis:* It is caused by phrenic nerve injury and is associated with Duchenne–Erb palsy. Paralysis may be bilateral or unilateral. In bilateral paralysis, the baby may present with cyanosis, tachycardia and thoracic breathing with no movement of diaphragm. Unilateral and mild bilateral phrenic nerve paralysis needs no treatment. Severe bilateral palsy needs prolonged ventilation assistance.

Sternocleidomastoid Muscle Injury

It is characterized by a well-circumscribed, immobile mass in the mid-portion of the sternocleidomastoid muscle. It enlarges after birth, slowly regresses and finally disappears. Upper brachial palsy may be associated with this, and the head may be tilted towards the affected side. Usually, conservative treatment is enough. However, surgical intervention is sometimes required.

Spinal Cord

Spinal cord injuries are rare but can occur owing to stretching of the cord. Respiratory problems are common with a higher level of injury. Lesions from the seventh cervical to the first thoracic region present with paraplegia, urinary and breathing problems.

Internal Soft Tissue

- *Abdominal injuries:* These may be suspected when there is a sudden shock with progressive abdominal distension, anaemia and irritability.
- *Liver rupture:* Liver is the most common organ affected. Sudden collapse is noticed when the haematoma ruptures through the capsule. Management is by evacuation of haematoma and reconstruction of laceration. Other injuries include spleen and head injuries and adrenal haemorrhage.

Limb

- *Humerus fractures:* Humerus is the second most common bone that fractures during delivery. Femur fracture is rarely seen and is common in breech extraction. All fractures are treated with immobilization.
- *Dislocation:* The common ones are hip dislocation and radial head dislocation.

Genitalia

The common injuries are bruise, oedema and ecchymosis. These do not require any treatment and resolve within 4–5 days. Testicular injury is a serious problem and requires urological consultation.

Most of the birth injuries do not require very sophisticated treatment. Parents need reassurance or a few days' observation and immobilization are needed as in the case of fractures. The nurse needs to be cognizant in preventing birth injuries by avoiding the cause of the same. If it happens, the nurse needs to be a psychological supporter to the parents. The nurse needs to educate the parents about the care of the baby with a birth injury based on the type of the injury.

KANGAROO MOTHER CARE

Kangaroo mother care (KMC) is a special way of caring of low-birth-weight (LBW) babies to foster their health and well-being. KMC promotes warmth, breastfeeding, infection control and infant–mother bonding.

Kangaroo care is different from KMC, though some of the aspects are same. Kangaroo care is a way of holding babies skin to skin with a parent irrespective of its gestational age and any parent or adult. Here, the baby is undressed down to the diaper and placed on a parent's bare chest. A blanket is placed over the baby for warmth. This type of care is given to any infant who is medically stable. KMC provides many benefits to LBW babies and their mothers. The babies will get warmth, breath better and sleep well. They also gain weight faster than other babies who are not cared for by KMC. Mothers who practice KMC are found to be having less episodes of depression and have more milk supplies. The major advantages of KMC are as follows:

1. Skin-to-skin contact
2. Exclusive breastfeeding
3. Support to the mother–infant dyad

Skin-to-skin contact is between the baby's front and the mother's chest. The baby is kept on the chest while wearing only a small nappy. Better to keep the baby day and night, but even shorter time periods will help the baby to regain warmth.

Exclusive breastfeeding is usually more possible with KMC. For very small or premature babies, some essential nutrients may need to be supplemented.

Support to the dyad. The infant and the mother feel much comfortable with KMC. The bonding is better. It is not only medically good for the baby but also provides emotional and psychological comfort for the mother.

Other benefits of skin-to-skin contact with KMC include:

- Temperature regulation
- Proper respirations
- Good oxygen saturation
- Weight gain
- Earlier discharge from hospital
- Ability to get colostrum/breast milk because the tactile situation improves oxytocin and prolactin levels
- Ability to stimulate a combination of hormonal responses (oxytocin/cuddling and prolactin/mothering) in the mother which increases bonding instincts during the first few hours after delivery which is considered a very critical period

Skin-to-skin contact reduces:

Apnoea

Hypothermia

Hypoglycaemia

How KMC improve the condition of premature baby?

1. Oxygenation – Oxygen saturation improves in KMC, as the heart rate and breathing stabilize with KMC.
2. Warmth – Because the mother's core temperature rises by 2°C, the baby gets a warm environment.
3. Nutrition – The mother's feel to feed increases, and the newborn's ability to utilize milk also increases. The vagal stimulation in the infant promotes better utilization of milk and thus the newborn grows faster.
4. Protection – Preterm infants experience prolonged severe stress, especially when exposed to cold that results in 10-fold increase in stress hormones. This level of stress hormones is neurotoxic. In KMC, the stress is less and thus improves immunity.

ESSENTIAL NEWBORN CARE

Essential newborn care (ENC) is a model of care designed to improve the health of newborns through specified interventions before conception, during pregnancy, at and soon after birth and in the postnatal period. ENC during pregnancy includes administration of tetanus toxoid, proper nutrition to the pregnant woman, iron/folate supplementation and treatment of maternal infections that affect the health of newborns. During labour, management of obstetrical complications and reducing risk of maternal and newborn infections by hygienic practices must be taken care of. Following is a brief discussion of ENC. The basic principles of ENC include:

- Resuscitate and maintain an airway.
- Keep the newborn warm, and avoid unnecessary hypothermia or cold stress.
- Encourage early breastfeeding, and feed high-risk newborns more frequently.
- Maintain hygiene during delivery and cord cutting; treat infections promptly.
- Ensure the newborn infant stays close to his/her mother, and the mother has open access to her newborn infant if he/she requires special care.

Care of the newborn at birth includes the following:

Four basic needs are thermal protection, normal breathing, mother's milk and protection from infection. It is essential to ascertain that these needs are met at birth.

Immediate care at birth according to ENC:

All babies including those who need resuscitation at birth require the following:

1. Call out the time of birth – It is important to announce the time of birth loudly to help accurate recording of the time of birth.
2. Receive the baby onto a warm, clean and dry towel and place on the mother's chest. If this is not possible, the baby should be kept in a clean, warm and safe place close to the mother.
3. Clamp and cut the umbilical cord.

The umbilical cord should be clamped using a sterile, disposable clamp or a sterile tie and cut using a sterile blade about 2–3 cm (1 inch) away from the skin.

4. Immediately dry the baby with a warm, clean towel or piece of cloth. The baby should be dried well off meconium and mucus but the vernix as it helps protect the baby's skin and gets reabsorbed very quickly.
5. Assess the baby's breathing while drying.

A normal newborn should be crying vigorously or breathing regularly at a rate of 40–60 breaths per minute. If the baby is not breathing well, then the steps of resuscitation have to be carried out.

6. Wipe both the eyes with a sterile gauze or cotton from the medial side to the lateral side using separate gauze for each eye.
7. Leave the baby between the mother's breasts to start skin-to-skin contact as explained in KMC to maintain temperature.
8. Place an identity label on the baby.
9. Cover the baby's head with a cap; cover the mother and the baby with a warm cloth to prevent loss of heat.
10. Encourage the mother to initiate exclusive breastfeeding.

Warm Chain

Immediately after birth, the newborn is at a maximum risk of hypothermia and early hypothermia may have a detrimental effect on the health of the infant. Special care should be taken to prevent and manage hypothermia. The temperature maintenance should be a continuous process, starting from the time of delivery and continued till the baby is discharged from the hospital.

Warm chain at delivery includes:

- Ensure the delivery room is warm (25°C), with no draughts.
- Dry the baby immediately; remove the wet cloth.
- Wrap the baby in a clean dry cloth.
- Keep the baby close to the mother (ideally skin-to-skin contact) to stimulate early breastfeeding.
- Postpone bathing/sponging for 24 hours.

Warm chain after delivery includes:

- Keep the baby clothed and wrapped, with the head covered.
- Minimize bathing, especially in cool weather and for small babies.
- Keep the baby close to the mother.
- Use kangaroo care for stable LBW babies and for rewarming stable appropriate for gestational age babies.
- Show the mother how to avoid hypothermia, how to recognize it and how to rewarm a cold baby. The mother should be taught to ensure that the baby's feet are warm to touch.
- Breastfeeding must be initiated at the earliest, preferably within 30 minutes.

Clean chain

A baby is protected in the womb of the mother before delivery. After delivery, the baby needs to be protected by explicit hygienic practices. Handwashing is the single most important step to be emphasized to both family members and health care workers.

WHO five cleans:

- Clean attendant's hands (washed with soap)
- Clean delivery surface
- Clean cord-cutting instrument (i.e. razor, blade)
- Clean string to tie the cord
- Clean cloth to wrap the baby and the mother

After delivery:

- All caregivers should wash hands before handling the baby.
- Feed only breast milk.
- Keep the cord clean and dry; do not apply anything.
- Use a clean cloth as a diaper/napkin.
- Wash your hands after changing the diaper/napkin.
- Cord care, care of the eyes and care of the newborn of a HIV-infected mother all have to be taken care of according to ENC.

If the baby needs resuscitation, this can be initiated after assessing the Apgar score.

STUDY QUESTIONS

1. What are the purposes of a newborn assessment?
2. What is an Apgar score? Explain its significance in a newborn assessment.
3. What is lanugo?
4. What are milia?
5. What are normal heart rate, respiratory rate and temperature in a newborn?
6. What is the normal head circumference? And how will you measure it? If head circumference is 4 or more cm larger than the chest, what is suspected?
7. What is normal newborn chest circumference? How do you measure it?
8. What is normal newborn length? How do you measure it? If a newborn is longer, what is this a possible sign of?
9. How much do normal newborns weigh? How much body weight do they lose, and for how many days? When do they regain it?
10. Why the first cry of a newborn is important?
11. How will you assess the gestational age of a newborn?
12. How will you assess the neuromuscular maturity in a newborn? Explain the tools used for it.
13. What is physiological jaundice? How will you care the baby with physiological jaundice?
14. What are Kramer criteria? Explain them.
15. Explain kangaroo mother care (KMC).
16. Discuss essential newborn care (ENC).
17. What are the common birth injuries? Explain their management.
18. What are the important points to be included in family teaching related to newborn care at home?

BIBLIOGRAPHY

1. Ballard, J., Khoury, J.C., Wedig, et al. (1991). New Ballard Score, Expanded to Include Extremely Premature Infants. Journal of Paediatrics, 119(3), pp 417–423.
2. Brazelton, T.B. (1973). The Neonatal Behavioural Assessment Scale. Philadelphia: J.B. Lippincott.
3. Brazelton, T.B. (1984). Neonatal Behavioural Assessment Scale in Planning Care for Parents and Newborns. 2nd Edn. St. Louis: J.B. Lippincott/Spastic International Medical Publishers.
4. Bryant, G.M. (Jan 1980). Use of the Denver Development Screening Test by Health Visitors. Health Visit, 53(1), pp 2–5.
5. Dubowitz, L.M., Dubowitz, V., Goldberg, C. (1970). Clinical Assessment of Gestational Age in the Newborn Infant. Journal of Pediatrics, 77(1), pp 1–10.
6. Kenner, C. (1990). Measuring Neonatal Assessment. Neonatal Network, 9(4), pp 17–22.
7. Kramer LI. Advancement of dermal icterus in jaundiced newborn. Am J Dis Child 1969;118: 454-8.
8. Marlow N: Do we need an Apgar score?. Arch Dis Child. 1992, 67: 765-767. 10.1136/adc.67.7_Spec_No.765. PubMed Central
9. Pediatrics AAo: Use and Abuse of the Apgar Score. Pediatrics. 1996, 98(1): 141-142. Google Scholar.
10. Pratinidhi A, Shah U, Shrotri A, Bodhani N: Risk-approach strategy in neonatal care. Bull World Health Organ. 1986, 64 (2): 291-297.
11. Suman RP, Udani R, Nanavati R. Kangaroo mother care for low birth weight infants: a randomized controlled trial. Indian Pediatrics 2008;45(1):17-23.
12. Kattwinkel, J., Denson, S., Zaichkin, J., & Niermeyer, S. Textbook of Neonatal Resuscitation (4th ed.). *American Heart Association: Dallas and American Academy of Pediatrics*, Elk Grove Village, IIL, 2000. pp 5.1–5.34.
13. Whaley, L., Wong, D. (1995). Whaley & Wong's Nursing Care of Infants and Children. 5th Edn. St. Louis: CV Mosby.
14. Worku B, Kassie A. Kangaroo mother care: a randomized controlled trial on effectiveness of early kangaroo mother care for the low birth weight infants in Addis Ababa, Ethiopia. Journal of Tropical Pediatrics 2005;51(2):93-7.

CHAPTER 25

NURSING CARE OF HIGH-RISK NEONATES

LEARNING OBJECTIVES

Upon completion of this chapter, the learner will be able to

- Define high-risk neonates.
- Classify high-risk neonates.
- Explain the problems faced by low-birth-weight babies.
- Discuss the methods of assessing gestational age.
- List the causes of preterm labour.
- Identify the risk factors of high-risk neonates.
- Differentiate the small for date and preterm infants.
- Discuss the care of preterm infants.
- Discuss the common problems of preterm infants with their medical and nursing management.
- Explain the nurse's role in planning of a neonatal intensive care unit (NICU).

Definition: A baby born with an increased risk for maintaining life like a normal newborn either because of prematurity or postmaturity or because of multiple factors leading to risk for life owing to maternal factors, fetal factors or environmental factors.

Classification: Three types of classification exist:

A. **According to size**
1. *Low-birth-weight (LBW) babies*: Infants whose birth weight is less than 2500 g regardless of gestational age
2. *Very low-birth-weight babies*: Infants whose birth weight is less than 1500 g
3. *Extremely low-birth-weight babies*: Infants whose birth weight is less than 1000 g
4. *Moderate low-birth-weight babies*: Infants whose birth weight is 1501–2500 g
5. *Appropriate for gestational age (AGA)*: Birth weight falls at the 10th percentile or above on intrauterine growth curves
6. *Small for date or gestational age (SFD/SGA)*: Rate of intrauterine growth is slowed, and birth weight falls below the 10th percentile on growth curves

7. *Intrauterine growth retardation (IUGR)*: Intrauterine growth is retarded and used as a more descriptive terminology for SGA
8. *Large for gestational age (LGA)*: Birth weight falls above the 90th percentile on the intrauterine growth chart

B. **According to gestational age**
   1. *Premature (preterm) babies*: Infants born before completion of the 37th week of gestation regardless of birth weight
   2. *Full-term babies*: Infants born between beginning of the 38th week and completion of the 42nd week of gestation regardless of birth weight

C. **According to mortality**
   1. *Live birth*: Birth in which the neonate manifests any heartbeat and breathes or displays voluntary movement regardless of gestational age
   2. *Fetal death*: Death of the fetus after 20 weeks of gestation and before delivery with the absence of any signs of life after birth
   3. *Neonatal death*: Early neonatal death occurs in the first 27 days of life; late neonatal death occurs in the first week of life; late neonatal death occurs between 7 and 27 days
   4. *Perinatal mortality*: Describes the total number of fetal and early neonatal deaths per 1000 live births
   5. *Postnatal death*: Death occurs between 28 days and 1 year

Any factors that contribute to a high-risk pregnancy may lead to the birth of a high-risk neonate. The factors that lead to the delivery of a high-risk neonate include the following:

- Poor socioeconomic background of the mother
- Maternal malnutrition with weight under 40 kg, height under 145 cm and haemoglobin (Hb) under 8 g%
- Maternal age less than 20 years, teenage pregnancy or maternal age 35 years or more
- Primigravida
- Grand multipara
- Bad obstetrical history with abortions, stillbirths, difficult labour or operative deliveries, perinatal deaths, LBW, congenital malformations, etc.
- Rh-negative mothers
- Hypertension during pregnancy (pregnancy-induced hypertension [PIH]), diabetes mellitus, thyrotoxicosis, heart disease complicating pregnancy, toxaemias of pregnancy, poor fetal growth, Anti-partum Hemorrhage (APH), hydramnios, Cephalo-Pelvic Disproportion (CPD) and other systemic illnesses in mothers
- Maternal infections
- Maternal drug addiction, alcoholism, smoking, etc.
- Exposure to radiation of different types and sources
- Drugs taken during pregnancy
- Factors related to delivery such as abnormal presentations (breech, shoulder, unstable presentations and cord prolapse), multiple-fetus pregnancy, fetal distress, meconium aspiration, premature rupture of membranes, early onset of labour, etc.

- All these high-risk factors during pregnancy and labour cause the paediatric nurse to warrant the birth of a high-risk neonate, which calls for the expertise of her nursing skills, to deliver and provide proper care to these vulnerable segments of neonates.

Important points to be remembered while caring a high-risk neonate include the following:
1. LBW babies: Babies weighing less than 2.5 kg regardless of the period of gestation can be called as LBW babies, and they usually constitute 25%–30% of all live-birth babies in India. They can be either preterm babies or SFD/SGA babies or babies with IUGR.
   It is essential to differentiate these two categories, as the severity of problems/handicaps is different, though some of the problems are same.

Problems Faced By LBW Babies

	Preterm	SGA/SFD
Asphyxia neonatorum	+	+ + +
Meconium aspiration syndrome (MAS)	+	+ + +
Infant Respiratory Distress Syndrome (IRDS)	+ + +	0
Apnoea spells	+ + +	0
Feeding difficulties	+ + +	0
Hypoglycaemia	+	+ + +
Hyperbilirubinaemia	+ + +	+
Infection	+ + +	+ +
Malformations	+	+ + +
Haemorrhage	+ + +	+
Immediate prognosis	Increased mortality	Better

2. Determination of gestational age: The main features of LBW babies can be differentiated by determination of their gestational age. For this purpose, a paediatric staff usually uses Usher's criteria.
Usher's Criteria

Characteristics	<36 Weeks	37–38 Weeks	>38 Weeks
Hair	Fine and fuzzy	Fine and fuzzy	Soft, silky
Ear cartilage	Pliable	Pliable	Springs back when folded
Breast nodule	<4 mm	4–7 mm	>7 mm
Genitalia	No scrotal rugae	Rugae present	Rugae present inferiorly and posteriorly
	Labia majora do not cover labia minora		Labia minora is covered by labia majora
Sole creases	None	Present on the anterior one-third	Entire sole is covered with creases

PRETERM INFANTS

Preterm infants are born before the beginning of the 38th week of gestation. The World Health Organization defines preterm babies as babies who have not completed 38 weeks of gestation. They are usually small, appropriate or large for the duration of time they spent in the uterus.

Incidence and Aetiology

Exact aetiology is unknown. Three groups of women are at a greatest risk for premature birth:
- Women who have had a previous premature birth
- Women who are pregnant with multiple fetuses (twins, triplets or more)
- Women with certain uterine or cervical abnormalities

Certain risk factors identified are as follows:
1. Low socioeconomic status of a pregnant woman, as an increased incidence is seen in low-income women.
2. Frequent closely packed pregnancies. Researchers have found that an interval of less than 18 months between birth and the beginning of the next pregnancy increases the risk of preterm labour, though the greatest risk is with intervals shorter than 6 months.
3. Premature rupture of the membranes (PROM)
4. Poor health and nutrition
5. Diseases during pregnancy. Certain medical conditions during pregnancy also may increase the likelihood that a woman will have preterm labour. These include:
   - Infections (including urinary tract, vaginal, sexually transmitted and other infections)
   - PIH, preeclampsia
   - Diabetes complicating pregnancy
   - Clotting disorders (thrombophilia)
   - Being underweight before pregnancy
   - Maternal obesity
6. Certain lifestyle factors may put a woman at a greater risk for preterm labour. These include:
   - Late or lack of prenatal care
   - Smoking
   - Use of alcohol
   - Drug abuse by mothers
   - Exposure to the medication diethylstilbestrol (DES)
   - Physical, sexual or emotional abuse
   - Lack of social support
   - Extremely high levels of stress
   - Long working hours with long periods of standing
   - Exposure to certain environmental pollutants

Characteristics

a. Appearance is frail and weak, and underdeveloped flexor muscle and muscle tone are present.
b. Extremities are limp and offer no resistance.
c. Extended fetal lie position is observed.
d. Head is larger than rest of the body.
e. Lack of subcutaneous fat makes their skin thin and appear red and transparent with visible blood vessels. Nipple and areola are barely perceptible.
f. Vernix caseosa and lanugo are abundant.
g. Plantar creases are absent in infants with less than 32 weeks of gestation.
h. Ear pinna appears flat when folded; ears are soft and may remain folded and return slowly to the original position as a result of less cartilage.
i. In female infants, clitoris and labia minora appear large and uncovered by small, departed labia majora.
j. Males have undescended testes, with a small, smooth scrotal sac.
k. Behaviour: Infants are easily exhausted from noise and routine care.
l. Cry: Their cry is feeble and seldom heard because they are too weak to cry.
m. Assessment of gestation can be done using either Parkin's method or Ballard's scoring as mentioned earlier.

COMMON PROBLEMS OF PRETERM INFANTS

Problems with Respiration

The presence of a surfactant in adequate amount is of primary importance for normal functioning of lungs. A premature infant also needs to do all the jobs as those of a full-term infant.

The surfactant reduces surface tension in the alveoli and prevents their collapse with expiration. Infants born before surfactant production are prone to develop respiratory distress syndrome (RDS).

Assessment

The lungs are assessed for adventitious sounds or areas of absent breath sounds. The Silverman–Andersen index is a useful tool for assessing respiratory distress.

Differentiate periodic breathing from apnoeic spells. Periodic breathing is the cessation of breathing for 5–10 seconds without other charges.

Apnoeic spells lasts more than 15 seconds or are accompanied by cyanosis, bradycardia or both. Apnoea without an identified cause in a preterm infant is called apnoea of prematurity.

The weak or absent cough reflex and very small air passages make the preterm infant susceptible to obstruction by mucus.

Being obligatory nose breathers, nasal obstruction in infants may cause respiratory distress. Respiratory effort and location and severity of retraction may need to be assessed. Excessive compliance of the chest cage during retraction may interfere with full expansion of the lungs. Special problems that require respiratory assistance include meconium aspiration, choanal atresia and progressive respiratory distress or cyanosis.

Grunting is the early sign of RDS. It closes the glottis and increases the pressure within the alveoli which keeps the alveoli partially open between breaths and increases the amount of oxygen absorbed.

Nursing Interventions

Assisting for Respiration. Sometimes, there may be need for endotracheal mechanical ventilation. Continuous positive pressure ventilation may be necessary to keep the alveoli open and improve expansion of the lungs. High-frequency ventilation may be used to provide very fast and frequent respirations with less pressure than that in other methods.

Liquid ventilation: Use of oxygenated fluid to let infants ventilate at low pressure is assumed to decrease lung damage associated with ventilator use.

Head hood (plastic box-like device that fits over the infant's head): Infants can breathe a high level of oxygen surrounding the head. There is no interference with access to rest of the infant's body for care.

Nasal cannula and nasal catheters are also used for delivering oxygen to preterm infants. Level of oxygen in the blood needs to be monitored. A noninvasive apparatus such as a pulse oximeter can be used for this purpose. Observe the infant's increasing or decreasing dependence on breathing assistance and need for oxygen. The infant's response to activity increases the demand for oxygen (handling, feeding, changing dress, etc.). Hence, the nurse should set the equipment to meet the increased oxygen demand before attempting such procedures. Administration of humidified oxygen is essential not only to prevent drying of the mucous membrane but also to reduce insensible loss of water.

Positioning Infants. Preferable positions include side-lying and prone positions, as these positions facilitate drainage of secretions and regurgitated feeding through the mouth. (NB: Prone position is not recommended for normal infants related to the increased chance of sudden infant death syndrome – SIDS.) In preterm infants, the prone position permits effective use of respiratory muscles and decreases respiratory effort that results in better oxygenation, lung expansion and compliance. In the supine position, head end of the bed needs to be elevated and then the head should be turned to one side. A rolled blanket or towel should be used to keep the head in the stable position. A small roll of towel under the shoulder will straighten the airway. Frequent changes of position will help air passages drain and prevent stasis of secretions, thus preventing hypostatic pneumonia.

Suctioning Secretions. Suction equipment must be available at all times. If no suction apparatus is available, a bulb syringe can be used for this purpose. Though it is less traumatic, it should not reach the deep respiratory tract mucosa. Suction should be performed whenever mucus is apparent. Always suck the mouth before the nose to prevent aspiration of fluids, as the infant gasps when the nose is suctioned. Suck gently to avoid trauma to the mucous membrane, as it may cause oedema, which predisposes the already small airway passage to further narrowing.

Chest Physiotherapy. Chest physiotherapy along with suctioning helps keep the airway clear. Chest physiotherapy includes postural drainage, percussion and vibration. Postural drainage helps affected areas of the lung to drain into the major bronchi. Percussion loosens the secretion and brings it to the bronchi for drainage. Percussion is not advisable in very low-birth-weight babies. Maximum time permitted for percussion is ½–1 minute at a time. Percussion is usually done with a special rubber instrument or a padded medicine cup. Percussion needs to be followed by vibration with fingertips. All this should follow with suction.

Complications. Low blood oxygen level, bradycardia and cyanosis are the common complications. Chest physiotherapy needs to be stopped immediately if any of these complications develop. Oxygen needs to be increased before, during and after the procedure.

Surfactant Administration. Surfactant is administered as an adjuvant to oxygen and ventilation therapy. By administering artificial surfactant, respiratory compliance is improved until the infant can generate enough surfactant on its own. Exogenous surfactant is manufactured from human, porcine or bovine amniotic fluid and is given in several doses via the endotracheal tube.

Side effects include patent ductus arteriosus (PDA) and pulmonary haemorrhage. Surfactant therapy has been shown to increase the rate of survival in premature infants.

Meconium Aspiration Syndrome. It is a multiorgan disorder with perinatal asphyxia, most commonly affecting postterm babies who are SGA. Usually, they have placental insufficiency. The fetal hypoxia as a result of placental insufficiency triggers through a vagal reflex where thick meconium passes to the amniotic fluid. The contaminated amniotic fluid is swallowed into the oropharynx and aspirated at birth with initiation of breathing, leading to hypoxia. The hypoxia affects the brain, heart, gastrointestinal (GI) tract and kidneys.

The diagnosis is confirmed with the presence of meconium in the trachea, leading to respiratory distress.

Therapy: The best way to prevent aspiration is by removing meconium by suctioning before initiation of breathing. In severe cases, babies need resuscitation.

Maintaining Hydration. Adequate hydration is essential to keep the secretion thin so that it can be removed easily. Dehydration will make the secretion thick and viscous that could obstruct the airway. (NB: Some physicians advocate administration of a small amount of saline through endotracheal tubes just before suctioning to dilute the secretions.)

Problems with Thermoregulation

Heat loss can occur even in normal newborn infants. However, it is more significant in preterm infants. The reasons for this include the following:

Thin skin, superficial blood vessels and less subcutaneous fat, especially brown fat are the reasons of heat loss. A normal newborn maintains heat by flexion of extremities, but the limp extended body of a preterm promotes heat loss as it exposes a large surface area. Term babies can increase metabolism to produce heat, but preterm babies are less able to do so. Hypoglycaemia and respiratory problems are more likely to develop. These limit the glucose and oxygen availability required to increase metabolism. Vasoconstriction, as a result of hypoglycaemia, leads to metabolic acidosis. Pulmonary vasoconstriction interferes with the production of surfactant, leading to more respiratory difficulty. Overheating produces increased oxygen and caloric demand. Therefore, an infant has trouble initiating breathing in hyperthermia as well. A neutral thermal environment (NTE) is essential. All newborns are homeothermic. But the ability to maintain the temperature is limited and highly dependent on the environment. Thermal protection of newborns is a set of continuing measures which starts at birth to ensure that they maintains a body temperature of 36.5°C–37.5°C through various activities.

Assessment

Monitor temperature every 2 hours or continuously with a skin probe connected to infant's abdomen using heat control mechanism of the radiant warmer or incubator. Maintaining thermoneutral environment is facilitated by monitoring the temperature from an overhead radiant heat source or an incubator with a servo-controlled mechanism. Temperature as shown on the monitor should be recorded at least every hour initially and then every 4–8 hours; compare it with the heat control reading to ensure that the machinery is functioning properly.

The axillary temperature should remain between 36.5°C and 37.5°C and the abdominal skin temperature should be 36.5°C (96.8°F–97.7°F).

Indicators of Inadequate Thermoregulation

- Poor feeding, intolerance to feeding, change in feeding behaviour, decreased intake or apathy towards feedings
- Lethargy or irritability, increased or decreased spontaneous activity, hypotonia, weak cry and difficulty in arousal
- Poor muscle tone
- Cool skin temperature – Skin (hands, feet, trunk) feels cold to touch
- Signs of hypoglycaemia
- Colour changes – Pallor, cyanosis (central – lips, mucous membrane, circumoral or orbital; peripheral – acrocyanosis of hands and feet), bright red skin or mottled skin
- Autonomic changes – Signs of respiratory difficulty (tachypnoea, slow rate or apnoea), bradycardia
- Axillary temperature <36.5°C or >37.5°C
- Abdominal skin temperature <36°C or 36.5°C.

Nursing Interventions

- Basic nursing care should be given as that to a normal newborn
- Hypothermia can be mild, moderate or severe
  1. In mild hypothermia, the core temperature will be between 32.2°C and 34.4°C (90°F–94°F). The baby will be conscious, but stumbling and shivering, and has ashen grey skin, with bradycardia and decreased blood pressure.
  2. In moderate hypothermia, the core temperature will be between 26.6°C and 32.2°C (80°F–90°F). There are signs of bradycardia, decreased blood pressure, decreased respiratory rate, decreased cough reflex and decreased urinary output.
  3. In severe hypothermia, the core temperature is between 21.1°C and 26.6°C (70°C–80°F). There are signs of hypotension, shock, cardiac arrest (at temperature <25°C), respiratory difficulty, i.e. difficult to discern because of extremely slow rate, apnoea (at temperature <24°C), deep coma, cold and stiffness, fixed and dilated pupils, metabolic acidosis and hyperglycaemia.

Activities to Prevent and Treat Hypothermia

Maintaining an NTE is essential to prevent the need for an increased oxygen demand to maintain body temperature (use of radiant warmers are preferred). NTE is the environmental temperature that enables a neonate's body temperature to remain normal with minimal metabolic efforts and therefore minimal oxygen consumption. NTE range is 32.5°C ± 1.4°C (90.5°F ± 2.6°F) for larger babies and 35.4°C ± 0.5°C (95.7°F ± 0.9°F) for smaller babies. Charts are available that indicate the appropriate temperature setting to maintain an NTE according to the infant's size and maturity. Smaller and less mature infants need more warmth, as they lose more heat and produce less heat. Some infants who require frequent care procedures are kept under open radiant warmers. Unclothed infant loses heat by convection despite the heat generated by radiant warmers. Only warm oxygen is given, as facial thermal receptors are very sensitive to cold. Cold oxygen could lead to cold stress. Insensible water loss is reduced by the use of transparent blanket that retains visibility of infant's body parts. When the infants are nursed in an incubator, the portholes and doors are kept closed as far as possible. On removal from incubators, infants should be placed in heated blankets and a head cover should be provided, as the large surface area of the head on exposure will lead to increased heat loss. When procedures are performed, the baby should be kept under heat lamps or hot water bottles wrapped in clothes can be kept on sides of the baby crib to ensure warmth. Overheating can also be a problem. It leads to increased metabolic rate, increased oxygen demand and increased water loss.

Weaning the Baby from Incubator. Preparation should start when the baby is in the incubator. Properly clothe the baby with a shirt, diaper and cap. When the baby is stable, this helps conserve heat and adjust him/her to variable temperatures on the face and the rest of the body. In the institution, the incubator temperature is adjusted by reducing 1°C–1.5°C each day. The temperature is increased if the baby's temperature falls below 36°C. When the infant can tolerate an incubator temperature of 28°C, he/she can be transferred to an open crib. If the temperature fall down, the baby may be returned to the incubator.

Use a servo-controlled device to prevent heat loss and maintain temperature. When using a servo-controlled device, attach skin probe with tapes to the upper abdominal quadrant. If a radiant heater is used, cover the probe with deflecting metal or a foam pad. Set the servo mechanism to the desired skin temperature (between 36°C and 36.5°C [96.8°F–97.7°F]). When non-servo-controlled devices are used (manual heating device), set them at the desired NTE. Block avenues of heat loss and apply external heat sources.

Trial the following activities as precautions to prevent heat loss and hypothermia in neonates:

1. *Avoid evaporative heat loss* – Keep the baby dry by removing wet clothes and linens and replacing with warm clothes, blankets and bed linens as many times as required. Keep hair/head dry and wrap/cover it with a dry towel or a cap.

2. *Decrease radiant heat loss and increase radiant warmth* – Use a heat shield or inner wall of a double-walled incubator that is warmed by the heated ambient air inside the incubator. Keep the incubator away from cooler surfaces (windows, air conditioners, etc.). Keep ambient room temperature between 22.2°C and 24.4°C/72°F and 76°F. Use radiant warmer which is preset to a control point (36.5°C), i.e. neonatal skin temperature. A radiant warmer provides easy access to an infant requiring frequent interventions. Use rapid rewarming (by setting servo control at 37°C) for more severe hypothermia. Drape a blanket of plastic wrap (e.g. Saran wrap) above, but not touching the infant, and over the sides of the warmer.

3. *Minimize conductive heat loss and increase conductive warmth* – Warm all objects that are in contact with the neonate's skin, such as examiner's hands, stethoscope, scales, X-ray plates, treatment tables, diaper/bed linen, etc. Place heated pads (hot water bottles) that do not exceed 40°C in the incubator or on the radiant warmer or in the basinet where the baby is nursed. Remember to cover the heating pads or bottles with a blanket or sheet. Place the infant on the coverings and not directly onto heated pads or bottles. When hot water bottles are used, take precautions to avoid spilling the hot water. Keep hot water bottles with a cover in the basinet on sides and ensure adequate precautions to protect the baby from burns. Replace the bottles as and when required. Use prewarmed blood and fluids (40°F–42°F). Minimize connective heat loss and increase connective warmth. Slowly rewarm the infant by maintaining incubator ambient temperature 1°C–1.5°C/2°F–2.6°F above the infant's skin temperature and increase every 2–3 hours until the temperature is within neutral thermal range. Decrease drafts over the infant's body surface by minimizing unnecessary opening of incubator portholes, organizing care, placing open warmers away from drafts and not blowing air/oxygen directly into the infant's face. Heat airway gases to 31°C–34°C (88°F–94°F). Measure the temperature of the heated gas at the delivery site. Warm endotracheal tube gases to 35°C–36.6°C. Swaddle the neonate in warmed blankets and put on clothing or wrap in insulating materials.

4. *Monitor body temperature frequently* – Every 2 hours in LBW babies (preterm and SGA) and sick neonates; every 2–3 hours after birth during neonatal transition from intra- to extrauterine life; every 3–4 hours in healthy term neonates; and every 30–60 minutes during rewarming of a cold stressed neonate.

5. *Monitor for signs and symptoms of systemic complications* of hypothermia, such as metabolic derangements.

    (a) **Hypoglycaemia** – Test blood with a reagent strip and/or obtain serum glucose level every hour until the neonate is stable. Observe for signs and symptoms such as tremors and jitteriness, respiratory difficulty, apnoea, lethargy or irritability, seizures and poor feeding.

    (b) **Hyperglycaemia** – Test blood with a reagent strip and/or obtain serum glucose level. Measure urinary output and test for glycosuria.

    (c) **Hyperkalaemia** – Draw blood for serum electrolytes. Monitor additives in intravenous fluids.

    (d) **Hypoxia and metabolic acidosis** – Interpret arterial blood gas values. Observe continuous pulse oximeter, administer oxygen and assist with ventilation as needed.

    (e) **Elevated blood urea nitrogen (BUN)** – Monitor intake and output (I&O) every hour. Test urine for blood, protein, pH, sugar and specific gravity.

    (f) **Hyperbilirubinaemia** – Observe for jaundice discolouration in head-to-toe progression. Interpret serum bilirubin values.

    (g) **Hypotension** – Observe vital signs, including blood pressure every 30–60 minutes.

    (h) **Seizures** – Observe for signs and symptoms of seizure behaviour. In neonates, it may be tremors, jitterness, opisthotonos, hypo- or hypertonia, chewing or boxing motions, apnoea, staring facial expression etc).

    (i) **Apnoea** – Observe respiration pattern. Provide continuous cardiorespiratory monitoring with alarms.

    (j) **Dehydration** – Observe urinary output, amount and colour. Test for specific gravity, protein, blood pH and sugar every hour. Evaluate skin turgor, mucous membrane moisture, arterial blood puncture, activity level and body weight.

    (k) **Pneumonia** – Observe respiratory effort, rate, rhythm and use of accessory muscles, and auscultate for breath sounds.

Problems with Fluid and Electrolyte Balance

Assessing and monitoring fluid balance are a significant part of nursing care. Fluid balance is especially important in preterm infants because of the increased amount of body water that decreases with age. The total body water content constitutes 80%–85% of the body weight in the preterm infants and 75%–80% in full-term infants. This decreases to approximately 63% and 58% by the ages of 3 years and ≥12 years, respectively. The distribution of water between intracellular compartments also differs by age, with the majority of water located extracellularly in infants and changing to intracellular content in the older children/adults. Though neonates have greater total water content, children are more vulnerable to imbalances because they must ingest and excrete (turnover) a greater volume per day (up to half of the total body water content as compared with one-sixth in adults) to excrete metabolic wastes produced with a metabolic rate twice that of adults. In addition, the greater body surface area in relation to the body weight results in a greater insensible loss of water. Functional immaturity contributes to the risk of fluid imbalances, with less efficient renal ability to concentrate or dilute urine or retain or excrete sodium, allowing fluid deficit or overload or sodium imbalance to rapidly develop.

Preterm infants loose water easily than term infants as a result of the following factors:

1. Thin skin
2. Little protecting fat
3. Greater water content of the body
4. More permeable skin than the skin of term infants
5. Large surface area in proportion to the body weight
6. Lack of flexion increases insensible loss of water
7. Use of radiant warmers and phototherapy (PTx) increases insensible loss
8. Water loss through the respiratory and GI tracts
9. Increased respiratory rate and increased fluid loss from the lungs
10. Loose stools if develop lead to rapid dehydration
11. Immature kidneys do not concentrate urine, causing a fragile balance between hydration and dehydration
12. Regulation of electrolytes by kidneys is also a problem

Signs of Fluid Imbalance

Dehydration
1. Urine output <1 mL/kg per hour
2. Urine specific gravity >1.015
3. Weight loss greater than expected
4. Dry skin and mucous membrane.
5. Sunken eyes and anterior fontanel
6. Poor skin turgor
7. Increased serum sodium, protein and haematocrit values

Overhydration
• Urine output >3 mL/kg per hour
• Urine specific gravity <1.005
• Oedema, weight gain
• Bulging fontanel
• Blood serum values decreases with decreases in serum sodium, protein and haematocrit values
• Moist breath sounds and breathing difficulty

Nursing Interventions

Measure Urinary Output. Do not use plastic bags to collect urine from the baby, as it injures the fragile skin. Weighing diapers before application and after urination is a reliable method. An increase in 1 g is equal to 1 mL of urine. Check specific gravity of the urine. Normal range is 1.005–1.015.

Check Weight. Weight can give an indication of fluid gain and loss. Undressed infant is weighed daily at a specific time each day with the same scale. Monitor for signs of dehydration and overhydration.

Preterm infants' needs increase as the kidneys do not reabsorb well. Normal urinary output is 1–3 mL/kg per hour per day for the first 2 days. Alert for fluid deficit and overload. Calculate I&O by all routes. Output from drainages should be measured. Urine output is <1 mL/kg per hour. Inadequate fluid >3 mL/kg per hour indicates overhydration. Keep a track of blood taken for laboratory analysis and also for fluid calculation.

Carefully regulate intravenous fluids, and use infusion pumps to prevent fluid overload. Use very little fluid to dilute intravenous medications consistent with safe administration of drugs and should be included in intake calculation.

Problems of Infection

A preterm infant's infection is 3–10 times greater than that of a normal newborn. There are several risk factors for infection. These are as follows:
• Mother's infection during labour
• Skin is fragile, permeable and easily damaged
• Use of adhesive on skin and its removal alert for signs of infection

Assessment

Temperature instability, respiratory problems, changes in feeding habits, etc. are the general symptoms of infections. Other system-wise symptoms include the following:

1. GI symptoms
2. Decreased oral intake
3. Vomiting
4. Gastric residual measuring over half of the previous feeding
5. Diarrhoea, abdominal distension
6. Hypoglycaemia or hyperglycaemia
7. Central nervous system (CNS) symptoms
8. Decreased muscle tone
9. Lethargy
10. Irritability
11. Bulging fontanel
12. Advanced infection shows jaundice, evidence of haemorrhage, anaemia, and enlarged liver and spleen
13. Respiratory failure
14. Shock
15. Seizure
16. Respiratory signs

17. Tachypnoea
18. Apnoea
19. Respiratory distress – Nasal flaring, retractions, grunting, etc.
20. Cardiovascular signs
21. Colour changes
22. Cyanosis
23. Pallor
24. Mottling
25. Tachycardia
26. Hypotension
27. Decreased peripheral perfusion

Prevention

Nursing interventions to prevent infection include the following:
- Explicit cleanliness and maintaining the infant's skin integrity are the important aspects.
- Maintain skin integrity.
- Use of adhesive dressings and bandages should be restricted to prevent possible skin damage.
- Use only the smallest amount of adhesive.
- Use special tapes that are less traumatic on removal and help protect the skin (e.g. pectin-based products).
- Carefully stabilize endotracheal tubes, skin probes and monitor leads.
- Avoid the use of chemicals that injure skin.
- Remove adhesives with water or diluted soap instead of chemicals.
- Frequent position changes are important but should be based on the infant's capacity to tolerate such changes.

Cleanliness of Personnel

Each special care unit should have its own policy/rules for preventing infection in its setting.

Follow universal precautions.

Gowning/special dress for personnel is recommended. Separate dress for permanent and part-time staff should be kept. Better to wear short-sleeved dresses or pant suits for personnel that need to be laundered daily by the hospital itself. Visitors to special baby care unit (SBCU) also should wear gowns before entering the unit.

Masks and sterile gloves should be used for procedures as far as possible, especially procedure such as lumbar puncture and suprapubic bladder aspiration, as also for umbilical vein catheterization, insertion of intercostal tubes and commencing total parenteral nutrition (TPN). Use sterile gloves for obtaining samples for blood cultures, thoracentesis and endotracheal suction.

Personnel should maintain good personal hygiene practices. They should not touch their hair, face or any other part of the body while providing care to the baby. If they touch their body parts, they need to wash their hands thoroughly well before handling the baby. Ornaments such as rings, watch, bangles and bracelets should not be worn in the SBCU. Personnel with diarrhoea, skin infection and respiratory tract infection should not enter the unit.

Handwashing. Handwashing to prevent cross-infection is very important, as even the normal flora on the hands of caretakers may cause sepsis. Although 3 minutes of handwashing is mandatory before entering the nursery, before performing invasive procedures and after providing care to infected babies, a half-minute washing is done before as well as after touching any baby. Instead of using soap cakes, liquid soap is preferred, as the former may promote colonization of bacteria.

Techniques of handwashing:
- Wash the hands and arms to a point above the elbows.
- Place a small amount of antiseptic preparation on the palm of the hand and soap the hands, wrists, forearms and elbows thoroughly.
- Cover all areas including between the fingers and the lateral side of the fifth finger.
- Give special attention to the thumb, as usually the thumb is not cared adequately by the people.
- Wash thoroughly under running water.
- Do not have long fingernails. Dirt may accumulate under these fingernails. If dirt is accumulated, use toothpick to remove it before cleaning.
- Dry hands with autoclaved towels or disposable sterile paper or allow them to dry spontaneously.
- Use of common towel is not a good practice and should be abandoned.

Minimal handling is recommended. Vaccination of caretakers is also recommended. Yearly vaccination of staff members against *Haemophilus influenzae* is practiced in Western countries.

Equipment

Equipment and articles used in the NICU need to be cleaned as per manufacturer's directions.

Use of disposable articles such as plastic masks and catheters is ideal if there is provision for disposal of biomedical wastes.

Cleaning with water and leaving the equipment wet are not good practices, as humidification promotes growth of microorganisms.

Thorough cleaning of the unit is also needed to prevent infection and sepsis in the NICU.
- Walls and sinks must be cleaned with 3% phenol (carbolic acid) or 5% Lysol at least once a day.
- Wet mopping of floors must be done three times a day.
- Do not sweep and dry dust the floor, as it may aid in transfer of organisms.
- Floors and walls can be vacuum-cleaned if possible.

Disposal of waste and soiled linen
- There must be adequate provision of closed bins to keep used materials and linen.
- The bin must be kept closed and to be emptied at regular intervals.
- The bins can be protected with plastic bags from inside, and these can be sealed before disposal.
- Dustbins used in the nursery need to be cleaned and washed properly under running water regularly.

The SBCU or nursery need not be fumigated routinely at regular intervals with excellent housekeeping techniques. But usually minimal cleaning is done by the workers, and fumigation is required only as an infection control procedure.

Procedure

- Scrub doors, windows, walls and floors thoroughly with soap and water.
- Shut off all central connections of oxygen and suction.
- Ventilator outlets, air conditioner vents and gaps in doors, etc. need to be sealed with adhesive tapes to make it airtight.
- All movable nursery equipment and furniture need to be moved and cleaned.
- Take 500 mL of formalin in a vessel and add 250 g of potassium permanganate and keep inside the closed room for 12 hours.
- The amount of formalin is decided by the area of the room to be fumigated.
- 500 mL of formalin is enough for a 30-m³ capacity room.
- If using a vaporizer, the fumigation time is only 6 hours.

Disinfection of equipment

Incubator

- The surface of the canopy and mattress should be cleaned with soap and water every day and dried.
- Alcohol cleaning is not advised, as the canopy may develop opacity.
- If a baby had stayed for 7 days or is awaiting discharge, the incubator needs to be cleaned thoroughly by cleaning every part of it.

  Cots and mattresses also need to be cleaned every day with 3% phenol or 5% Lysol. Mending of torn mattresses should be done routinely. Open care units also need routine cleaning by carbolization.

Thermometers

Thermometers need to be cleaned by wiping with alcohol after each use or with 40% Dettol by dipping it in for 3 minutes. After use, wash and dry the thermometer and keep it in bottle with dry cotton. Thermometers should not be stored in Dettol or Savlon.

Feeding utensils

Use disposable feeding tubes as little as possible. Cups, spoons and paladais used for feeding need to be cleaned and boiled for 30 minutes after each feed. Avoid use of feeding bottles. Autoclaving of articles is preferred if there is provision.

Suction apparatus

The tubes connected to suction apparatus need to be cleaned every day and disinfected in Cidex (activated glutaraldehyde solution) for 10 minutes.

Suction bottles need everyday cleaning with detergent and change them daily.

Add 3% phenol or 5% Lysol to the suction bottles. Use disposable suction catheters that can be discarded after a single use.

Cheatle forceps

Use of Cheatle forceps is not an ideal practice in the NICU or SBCU. If used, this must be cleaned and autoclaved or boiled for 30 minutes or kept immersed in 3% phenol.

Rubber items used in the NICU need to be cleaned with soap and water and disinfected using Cidex for 10 minutes.

Linen

Linen and cotton used in the NICU need to be autoclaved before use. No new linen should be used without washing and autoclaving.

Respiratory equipment

Disposable endotracheal tubes must be used as little as possible. If the tube needs to be reused, it should be disinfected in Cidex for 10 minutes. All resuscitation equipment should be cleaned and disinfected using Cidex. Laryngoscopes should be wiped with alcohol after each use. Oxygen hoods should be cleaned with detergent every day. Humidification chamber should be disinfected with Cidex for 10 minutes every day and autoclaved between patients. Use only distilled water in these chambers and change daily when in use. Air compressor filters should be cleaned every day. Cidex solution should be changed once in every 15 days or earlier if discolouration is noticed.

Intravenous equipment

Use disposable cannulae, needles and infusion tubes and bottles. Infusion sets should be changed every day and intravenous cannulae every third day. Do not use rubber tubings for infusion of calcium and sodium bicarbonate. All intravenous and arterial ports need to be wiped with alcohol before use. Top of all vials and neck of all ampoules must be wiped with alcohol before breaking or opening to prevent entry of microorganisms. Needle should not be kept vented to air in bottle stoppers. Flush solutions (normal saline) should not be kept at room temperature for more than 8 hours. It is better to prepare small vials of flush solutions by the hospital pharmacy.

Isolation at the NICU

Isolation rooms are not necessary in the NICU if adequate personnel are available to take care of the babies. Usually, the babies are kept 6–8 feet apart, and personnel caring for the infected neonate should not be posted for caring uninfected babies. The personnel should ensure explicit handwashing as described earlier.

Mothers who are infected should be provided special area for visiting their babies. A febrile woman who has no other problem can be permitted to feed her baby. Mothers should be provided with gown, mask and gloves, if needed, as per their disease condition.

Congenital viral infections such as cytomegalovirus infection are highly contagious. Adequate precautions must be taken in such cases.

Neonates born to hepatitis-infected mothers or HIV-positive mothers need special precautions, as there are chances for transferring the infections to their babies and also to others. Follow universal precautions in caring of such babies.

Problems with Pain

Infants in the NICU undergo many painful procedures. But caregivers give little attention to such painful act, as they believe that perception of pain in newborns is rudimentary. Preterm infants have well-developed pain perception mechanisms but do not have those required for pain modulation as in term infants or an adult. Preterm infants not only perceive pain but also have experience more pain intensity and their pain lasts longer. Pain has lasting bad effects on infant's brain development, which manifests later as abnormal pain perception, behavioural abnormalities, cognitive defects and learning disabilities. So, developmental supportive care is very important.

Common signs of pain in infants:
- High-pitched, intense or harsh cry
- Cry face, eyes squeezed shut, mouth open
- Grimacing, rigidity or flailing of extremities
- Colour changes, red, dusky, pale, increased or decreased heart rate, increased respirations, increased blood pressure, decreased oxygen saturation

Assessment

Assess infant's pain level and response to pain. A combination of physiological and behavioural changes needs to be noticed, as physiological changes alone are unpredictable. For this purpose, the Age Appropriate Pain Assessment Tool (APAT) developed by Dr Assuma for postoperative pain assessment can be used for the infants of 0–1 year of age. Other tool available is **Premature Infant Pain Profile (PIPP).**

Nursing Interventions

General measures to reduce pain are as follows:
- Assess level and degree of pain with pain scales.
- Prepare infants for painful procedures as per unit's policies.
- Wake them gently and slowly using containment (containment simulates the enclosed space of uterus and is comforting to the infant).
- Keep the extremities in a flexed position by swaddling or by blanket rolls or by the nurse's hands.
- Keep at least one hand of the baby near the mouth for sucking.
- Provide comfort measures to make the infant cope with mild pain and reduce agitation. For example, non-nutrient sucking, soft talking, restraining extremities to prevent flaring, stroking, holding and rocking. These measures should be adapted according to the infant's response.
- Administer pain medication for chronic and severe pain.
- The nurse should discuss the infant's pain responses with the physician concerned for getting appropriate prescription.

- Administer the medication before painful procedures.
- Prevent, limit or avoid noxious stimuli.·
- Avoid bright light, loud noise, etc.
- Limit the number of painful procedures and handling.
- Bundle up investigations and nursing interventions.
- Use tactile stimulation such as stroking, caressing, massaging, etc.

Nonpharmacological Measures. The environmental and behavioural interventions that do not use pharmacological agents are collectively called nonpharmacological measures. These include:
1. Sucrose/glucose solution-induced analgesia
2. Breastfeeding/breast milk supplementation
3. Skin-to-skin care
4. Non-nutritive sucking using pacifiers

Sucrose Analgesia. Sucrose administration is particularly useful for short procedures such as venipuncture, heel prick, etc. Oral administration of concentrated sucrose solution (24%–50%) acts by release of endogenous opioids such as β-endorphin. Analgesic effect lasts for 5–8 minutes.

Breastfeeding and Breast Milk Supplementation. These are almost as effective as sucrose analgesia in reducing pain in newborns undergoing single painful procedure.

Pharmacological Measures

The pharmacological measures can be broadly divided into:
Local anaesthetic agents
Systemic agents: Opioids, acetaminophen

Local Anaesthetics. Local anaesthesia is particularly useful for management of acute procedure-related pain with the exception of heel lances. It can be either topically applied on the intact skin or injected subcutaneously.

The common topical preparations marketed:
1. Eutectic mixture of local anaesthetics (EMLA): It is a mixture of two local anaesthetics, namely lidocaine and prilocaine, that comes as 5% cream. The dose of EMLA is 1–2 g, with a contact period of 30 minutes to 1 hour. Apply the cream over 2- to 3-cm area with 1- to 2-mm thickness and cover with transparent (Tegaderm) dressing.
2. Tetracaine (4%) gel preparation is used to prevent the risk of methaemoglobinaemia associated with repeated use of EMLA cream.
3. Use of liposomal lidocaine 4% cream.

Narcotic pain medications are opioids, mainly morphine and fentanyl.

Analgesia for specific procedures

The American Academy of Pediatrics (AAP) Committee on Fetus and Newborn recommends avoiding awake intubation of newborn babies except in emergent situations such as delivery room intubation and in cases where intravenous access is unavailable. Intubation of neonates in the awake state is associated with an increase in heart rate, greater fall in oxygen saturations/heart rate, increased intracranial pressure, increased risk of intraventricular haemorrhage (IVH), airway trauma and failure of procedure, especially in inexperienced hands.

The AAP recommends:

Analgesic agents or anaesthetic dose of a hypnotic drug should be given.

Vagolytic agents and rapid-onset muscle relaxants should be considered.

Sedatives used alone such as benzodiazepines without analgesic agents should be avoided.

A muscle relaxant without an analgesic agent should not be used.

Routine procedures that require analgesia:

Venipuncture

Heel puncture

Subcutaneous/intramuscular injection

Adhesive tape removal

Intravenous cannulation

The nurse must be able to provide developmental supportive care that is a set of actions such as reduction in noise and light, minimal handling, effective pain prevention and treatment aimed at reducing the stresses in the NICU and optimizing neurobehavioural outcome. Developmental care interventions are potentially beneficial to sick neonates, especially those born prematurely, to cope with the adverse external environment in the NICU.

Core measures of developmental supportive care or interventions:

1. Protected sleep
2. Pain and stress assessment and management
3. Developmentally supportive activities of daily living
4. Family-centred care
5. Creating a healing environment

Core Measures and Nursing Interventions for Developmental Supportive Care

Core Measure	Practice Points
Protect sleep	• All nonemergent caregiving is provided while the infant is awake and do not disturb the neonate while sleeping • Promote sleep by facilitative tuck, swaddling and skin-to-skin care • Light and sound levels are minimized. Day–night pattern is simulated by reducing lights in the night to facilitate nocturnal sleep • Family education on caregiving activities that promote safe sleep
Prevent and treat pain	• Assess if the baby suffers from pain once during each nursing shift and during all procedures using a validated score • Provide nonpharmacological and/or pharmacological measures to reduce pain for all stressful and/or painful procedures • Caregiving activities are adapted to minimize pain and stress • Parents are educated regarding infant pain and involved in its management
Provide developmentally supportive care	• Use boundaries around the infants to maintain them in flexed posture (similar to in utero posture) • Provide non-nutritive sucking while the infant is being fed by gavage or paladai by allowing the baby to suck on the mother's finger or breast • Provide lactation counselling and support to initiate and maintain lactation in the mother • Protect the integrity of skin during application and removal of adhesive products (minimize use, e.g. do not strap to achieve haemostasis after sampling; instead, just put a cotton swab and hold it for some time; adhesive should be removed only after 72 hours of application once it has loosened from the skin surface; wet the plaster before removal)
Provide family-centred care *(Do not consider the infant as a solo entity)*	• Disease has serious impact on the social fabric of a family Consider individuals beyond the infant and issues beyond the disease such as those related to financial condition and relationship within the family Consider cost–benefit ratio of treatment/investigation modality that you plan to employ • Allow the parents to visit the infant in the NICU and to have conversation with the treating team Involve parents in decision making regarding treatment of the infant Family observations and input regarding their infant are sought by the clinical care providers • Family is supported in parenting activities such as skin-to-skin care, holding the baby, feeding, dressing, diapering, singing and all infant care interactions • Babies in the NICU should be divided to available nurses on the shift so that all caregiving activities of a baby should be carried out by the allotted nurse of that baby The practice of 'task-specific' allotment of nurses (such as one nurse responsible for feeding, another for injections to all babies) must be avoided • Practice 'primary nursing' This means one nurse becomes 'primary nurse' of a baby and that baby always get allotted to the primary nurse in whatever shift duty she comes Her name should be recorded on the bedside identification tag and is communicated to the family 'Primary nurse' of the baby is responsible for keeping a close liaison with family and physicians for holistic care of the baby

Continued

Core Measures and Nursing Interventions for Developmental Supportive Care—cont'd	
Core Measure	**Practice Points**

Healing environment	• Minimize sound and lights
	  Do not place anything on incubators
	  Close the incubator doors gently. Cover incubators with a cloth sheet to minimize light
	  Do not use the procedure light unnecessarily
	• Make sure health care professionals follow caring behaviours such as adherence to hand hygiene protocols, cultural sensitivity, open listening skills and an empathic relationship with families
	• Do not perform investigation for a routine
	  Consider utility of an investigation before you do it
	  If it is unlikely to change your management, it is unnecessary and potentially harmful by causing pain and increasing the infection risk
	• Promote free and healthy communication between physicians, nurses and other professionals working in the NICU
	  A cohesive team is more likely to avoid errors and provide a healing touch

Adapted from: Coughlin M, Gibbins S, Hoath S. Core measures for developmentally supportive care in neonatal intensive care units: theory, precedence and practice. Journal of Advanced Nursing. 2009;65(10):2239–2248.

Problems with Parental/Maternal Separation

1. Allow parents to visit their baby frequently in the NICU.
2. Involve them in the care of the baby as early as possible to promote parent–infant bonding or attachment.
3. Answer questions openly; provide up-to-date information.
4. Help parents accept reality of the situation.
5. Explain specialized care to parents.
6. Allow the mother to feel confident in caring for her infant before discharge from hospital.
7. Explain to the mother about the infant's special needs.
8. Allow the parents to cuddle, hold or diaper the baby while in hospital.
9. Provide facility for the mother to breastfeed her baby if sucking is established.

Respiratory Distress Syndrome

This is also called hyaline membrane disease. It accounts for 30% of all neonatal deaths in preterm infants. It is more common in infants born at 26–28 weeks of gestation. It is also accompanied with birth asphyxia, infants of diabetic mothers (IDMs) and infants delivered by caesarean section, as this condition interferes with surfactant production. It is seen in neonates whose lungs are not fully developed. It can also be a result of genetic problems with lung development.

Risk factors for RDS:
• A brother or sister who had RDS
• Diabetes in the mother
• Caesarean delivery or induction of labour before the baby is full-term
• Problems with delivery that reduce blood flow to the baby
• Multiple-fetus pregnancy (twins or more) and rapid labour

Pathophysiology

RDS is caused by insufficient production of phospholipids that line the alveoli. Surfactant production starts at the 22nd week of gestation and by 32–36 weeks of gestation, the surfactant is usually mature enough to enable the infant to breathe normally outside the uterus. Function of surfactant is to decrease the surface tension to keep the alveoli remain open during exhalation. It needs to be continuously produced as it is being used. When there is too little surfactant, the alveoli collapse each time the infant exhales. The lungs become noncompliant or stiff and resist expansion. This makes the lungs to require a higher negative pressure for the alveoli to open each time the infant inhales. This creates a lot of struggle on the part of the infant owing to respiratory distress manifested by severe chest retractions, drawing the weak muscles of the chest wall inward. Because there is less expansion of alveoli, atelectasis and hypoxia may occur. This causes pulmonary vasoconstriction and pulmonary hypertension. Persistent pulmonary hypertension can result in return of fetal circulation pattern with opening of PDA. Respiratory and metabolic acidosis as well as alveolar necrosis can also develop.

A surfactant consists of lecithin, sphingomyelin and phosphatidyl glycerol. This can be detected by tests done on the amniotic fluid.

Clinical Features

RDS manifests right at birth, i.e. during the first hours after delivery, and becomes worse on the 10th day; it begins to improve within 72 hours after birth.

Signs and symptoms include tachypnoea, nasal flaring, retractions and cyanosis; grunting on expiration, wet breath sounds, acidosis and hypoxemia; bluish colour of the skin and mucous membranes (cyanosis), apnoea, grunting and decreased urine output.

Diagnosis

Chest X-rays: Ground glass appearance of bronchial air shades (air bronchogram pattern). This often develops 6–12 hours after birth.
• Blood gas analysis shows low oxygen and excess acid in the body fluids.
• Laboratory tests help rule out infection as a cause of breathing problems.

Multidisciplinary Management

Prophylactic treatment with surfactant replacement therapy to prevent RDS or as a rescue treatment is undertaken. It is instilled into infant's trachea soon after birth. Improvement takes place within minutes. Doses are repeated.

Prevention: RDS is diagnosed intranatally by testing amniotic fluids for culture and sensitivity ratio, fluid shake test, phosphatidyl glycerol for the presence and administration of injection betamethasone 12 mg or hydrocortisone on two occasions at a gap of 18 hours.

Other supportive measures include the following:

Mechanical ventilation, correction of acidosis, intravenous fluid administration and care of developing complications. Continuous positive airway pressure by a respirator is advised if the condition worsen.

Administer warm, moist oxygen. This treatment needs to be monitored carefully to avoid side effects from too much oxygen such as ROP. Administer extra surfactant to very sick children. It can be delivered directly into the baby's airway.

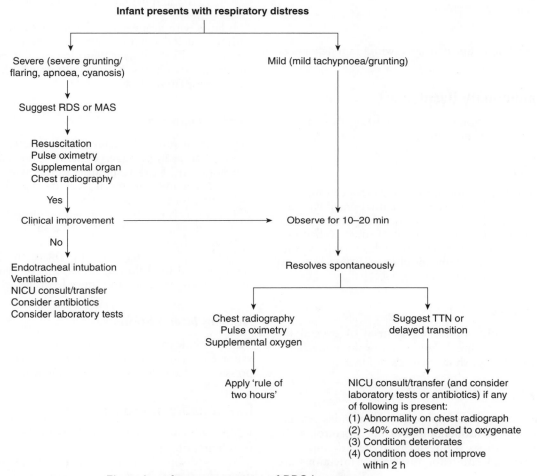

Flow chart for management of RDS in neonates.

Nursing Interventions

Supportive care include:
- Having a calm setting
- Gentle handling
- Maintaining at an ideal body temperature
- Carefully managing fluids and nutrition
- Treating infections right away
  - Observe signs of developing RDS.
  - Change in the infant's condition constantly assessed. For example, diuresis is an important sign of improvement.
  - Prevent cold stress (incubator care – Isolette or overhead radiant warmer can be used).
- Adjustment in ventilatory care as the improvement in condition occurs to increase the ability of the infant to oxygenate.
- Administration of oxygen to maintain PaO_2 at 50–70 mm Hg. The oxygen administered should be warmed and humidified.
- Observe for common complication such as PDA, bronchopulmonary dysplasia (BPD), etc.
- Indomethacin 0.2 mg/kg oral or intravenous twice daily used in certain hospitals as a routine therapy to promote closure of PDA.
- Implement general care of a preterm as mentioned earlier in this chapter.

Long-term complications may develop as a result of:
- Too much oxygen
- High pressure delivered to the lungs
- More severe disease or immaturity; RDS can be associated with inflammation that causes lung or brain damage
- Periods when the brain or other organs did not get enough oxygen

Other possible complications are as follows:
- Pneumothorax
- Pneumomediastinum
- Pneumopericardium
- Intraventricular haemorrhage of the newborn
- Pulmonary haemorrhage
- BPD
- ROP
- Intellectual disability associated with brain damage or bleeding

Bronchopulmonary Dysplasia

It is a chronic condition occurring in 30% of the infants treated with mechanical ventilation.

Pathophysiology

BPD results from a combination of factors including oxygen, high pressure of pulmonary ventilation, inflammation, infection and nutritional factors that cause damage to alveoli and lining of the respiratory tract. Inflammation, oedema and airway hyperactivity lead to thickening of the walls of alveoli and fibrotic changes. Atelectasis and pneumonia occur with these changes.

Clinical Features

Major sign of BPD is continuous need of oxygen for more than 28 days of life. Infant needs prolong mechanical ventilation. X-rays show changes in lungs.

Treatment

Usually, the treatment is supportive. It includes gradual decrease in oxygen, bronchodilators, corticosteroids, diuretics and antibiotics. Long-term oxygen therapy and frequent rehospitalization for respiratory infections are recommended.

The alveoli normally increase in number from 20–70 million at birth to as many as 300–400 million at 2–8 years of age when the lungs reach the adult size. Surfactant replacement therapy is also recommended.

Periventricular Haemorrhage and Interventricular Haemorrhage

These occur in 20%–30% of the infants of less than 32 weeks of gestation or weighing less than 1500 g.

Pathophysiology

The condition results from rupture of the fragile blood vessels in the general matrix located around the ventricles of brain. It is most often associated with hypoxic injury to vessels, increase blood pressure and cerebral blood flow and rupture of blood vessels. Haemorrhage is categorized into four grades according to the amount of bleeding:

Grade 1   Very small bleeds outside ventricle walls – few clinical changes
Grade 2   Haemorrhage extends to the lateral ventricle
Grade 3   Distends at least one ventricle
Grade 4   Haemorrhage causes ventricular dilation and damage to brain tissue

Infants with grade 1 and 2 haemorrhage may survive without much damage. Infants with grade 3 and 4 haemorrhage are likely to have neurological abnormalities and developmental delays. Infants with grade 4 haemorrhage have a poor survival rate.

Clinical Features

Periventricular haemorrhage (PVH) is determined by the severity of haemorrhage, lethargy, poor muscle tone, deterioration of the respiratory status with cyanosis or apnoea, drop in haematocrit level, decreased reflexes, full or bulging fontanel and seizure.

Diagnosis is usually confirmed by ultrasonography.

Treatment is usually supportive such as maintaining respiratory function.

Hydrocephalus may develop owing to blockage of cerebrospinal fluid flow. Lumbar taps or ventriculoperitoneal shunts are done to relieve hydrocephalus.

Nursing Interventions

These include measurement of head circumference, observation for changes in neurological status, control of blood pressure and avoiding excessive handling and crying.

Retinopathy of Prematurity

Retinopathy of prematurity (ROP) is otherwise known as retrolental fibroplasia.

It is a vasoproliferative disorder of the retina among preterm infants. Normally, neonates born at less than 32 weeks of gestation or infants weighing less than 1500 g are at risk of developing ROP. Preterm infants born at 32 weeks or later can also develop severe ROP if they had very rigorous NICU life or required prolonged oxygen therapy. Though a quarter of neonates in the NICU show signs of ROP, the majority heal on their own and not go for retinal detachment. Only a small percentage of neonates experience blindness, and timely screening and intervention can prevent blindness and reduce vision abnormalities.

Classification of ROP

The International Classification of ROP (ICROP) is used to classifying ROP. ICROP describes vascularization of the retina and characterizes ROP by its position (zone), severity (stage) and extent.

According to Location

Location	Zone 1	Circle with the optic nerve at its centre and a radius of twice the distance from the optic nerve to the macula
	Zone 2	Concentric circle from the edge of zone 1 to ora serrata nasally and equator temporally
	Zone 3	Lateral crescent from zone 2 to ora serrata temporally
Severity		
	Stage 1	**Presence of thin white demarcation line separating vascular from avascular retina**
	Stage 2	**Addition of depth and width to the demarcation line of stage 1 so that the line becomes the ridge**
	Stage 3	**Presence of extra retinal fibrovascular proliferation with abnormal vessels and fibrous tissue extending from the ridge to the vitreous**
	Stage 4	**Partial retinal detachment not involving the macula (4A) and involving the macula (4B)**
	Stage 5	**Complete retinal detachment**

Pathophysiology

ROP is caused by damage to immediate blood vessels in the retina. Exact cause of damage is unknown. This is thought to result partly from high arterial blood oxygen level. The level of oxygen in the blood is more important than the amount of oxygen infant receives. ROP develops even in babies who have not received oxygen. Therefore, accurate monitoring of the blood arterial oxygen level is important. Very low-birth-weight babies are more prone to ROP. In ROP, immature blood vessels in the retina constrict and become permanently occluded. New vessels proliferate, extending throughout the retina and into the vitreous of the eye; haemorrhage from the fragile vessels may cause scaring, traction on the retina and retinal detachment.

Treatment

LBW infants are screened between 4 and 8 weeks after birth to detect changes in the eye. Cryotherapy and laser surgery have been used to destroy the proliferating blood vessels or reattach the retina. In some infants, regression occurs with little or no impairment of vision. Peripheral retinal ablation is carried out either by cryotherapy or by diode laser. Diode laser ablation has largely replaced cryotherapy, as it is associated with a lower rate of postoperative ocular and systemic complications and lesser damage to the adjacent tissues.

Preoperative Preparation
- Discontinue all oral feeds 3 hours prior to the operation.
- Start intravenous fluids and put on cardiorespiratory monitors.

- Dilate pupil.
- Topical anaesthesia alone may not be sufficient for ROP treatment.
- Babies should be given general anaesthesia. This can be done in the NICU itself. Both eyes are treated together unless contraindicated with some other reasons.
- Monitor vital signs and oxygen saturation.

After laser therapy, the first examination should take place 5–7 days after treatment and should be continued at least weekly for signs of decreasing activity and regression. Retreatment should be performed usually 10 to 14 days after initial treatment when there has been a failure of the ROP to regress.

Postoperative Care
- The baby should be closely monitored. If condition permits, oral feeds can be started shortly after the procedure.
- Premature babies, especially those with chronic lung disease, may have increased or reappearance of apnoeic episodes or an increase in oxygen requirement. Therefore, they should be carefully monitored for 48–72 hours after the procedure.
- Antibiotic drops (such as chloramphenicol) should be instilled 6–8 hourly for 2–3 days.

Peripheral Ablation Therapy
- Take consent.
- Ensure good pupillary dilatation.
- Keep nil by mouth 3 hours prior to the procedure.
- Start on intravenous fluids.
- Put on a vital sign monitor/pulse oximeter.
- Keep a warmer for maintaining temperature.
- Arrange equipment and check functioning thereof:
  - Endotracheal tubes Nos. 2.5, 3, 3.5
  - Resuscitation bag and face masks
  - Oxygen delivery system
  - Syringes, infusion pumps, ventilator, etc.

Necrotizing Enterocolitis

It is a serious condition of the intestinal tract, with a 10%–50% mortality rate.

Pathophysiology

Exact cause of necrotizing enterocolitis (NEC) is unknown. It may be caused by interference with blood supply to the intestinal mucosa. During asphyxia, blood is diverted from the GI tract to the brain, heart and kidneys. Sepsis, polycythaemia and maternal cocaine use are among the other causes of decrease in intestinal blood flow. The resulting ischaemia makes the mucosa more susceptible to invasion with bacteria. When infants are fed, bacteria proliferate and gas-forming organisms may invade the intestinal wall. Eventually, necrosis, perforation and peritonitis may occur.

Clinical Features

These include distension, increased gastric residuals, decreased or absent bowel sounds, loops of bowel seen through the abdominal wall, vomiting, signs of infection and blood in the stools.

X-ray shows loops of bowel dilated with air and layers of gas in the intestinal wall. Free air in the peritoneum indicates that perforation has occurred.

Treatment

Antibiotics, discontinuation of oral feedings and use of parenteral nutrition to rest the intestines are the usual treatment modalities. Surgery may be indicated in perforation and lack of improvement.

Ostomy may be performed sometimes. Breast milk has some preventive effects on the development of NEC. Corticosteroids, slow advancement of feedings and oral immunoglobulins are also used as treatment modalities.

Nursing Interventions

Signs of NEC are essential to decrease mortality. Observation of early subtle signs leads to prompt treatment.

Postterm or Postmaturity

Postterm infants are born after the 42nd week of gestation. Approximately, 6%–12% of all pregnancies are considered to be postterm. They have two to three times higher perinatal mortality rate than infants born at term. In 20%–30% of postterm pregnancies, placental function deteriorates, causing interference with oxygen and nutrient supply. This results in hypoxia and malnutrition in the fetus called postmaturity syndrome.

Assessment

Signs may occur during pregnancy, labour or after birth. Diminished fetal growth or oligohydramnios may cause decreased uterine size during the last weeks of pregnancy. During labour, poor oxygen reserves may cause fetal distress. The fetus passes meconium as a result of hypoxia before or during labour, increasing the risk of meconium aspiration at delivery.

At birth the cord, skin and nails are stained. Hyperalert, wide-eyed, worried look are some of the signs of chronic intrauterine hypoxia. Inadequate oxygen causes the infant to have polycythaemia. Poorly nourished wasting, growth restriction, thin and loose skin with little subcutaneous fat, little or no lanugo and vernix caseosa, abundant hair on head and long nails, dry skin, cracked and peeling skin are also some of the features of postmaturity.

Hyperbilirubinaemia

Essential Concepts

The principal source of bilirubin is the haemolysis of erythrocytes. Haemolysis of red blood cells (RBCs) releases their components into the bloodstream to be reused by the body. The unusable residue is bilirubin that remains in the blood. Bilirubin released is unconjugated (indirect bilirubin) and is insoluble in water. Liver changes this into a water-soluble form to process excretion with the help of glucuronyl transferase. The soluble form is conjugated or direct bilirubin. The unconjugated bilirubin is fat soluble and is absorbed by subcutaneous fat, causing yellowish discolouration of skin called jaundice. If a large amount of unconjugated bilirubin is present in the blood, this may stain the tissues of brain causing kernicterus, resulting in bilirubin encephalopathy.

An abnormal elevation of bilirubin level (above 13–15 mg/100 mL) in the full-term infant can cause severe jaundice. The degree of jaundice can be roughly calculated by using Kramer's criteria described earlier. The major types are physiological jaundice, pathological jaundice and breast milk jaundice.

Physiological Jaundice

It results from transient hyperbilirubinaemia. It is never present during the first 24 hours of life but appears on the second or third day after birth. It will be visible when the serum bilirubin level reaches 5–7 mg/dL and is considered as a normal phenomenon in newborn babies.

The cord blood has an average bilirubin level of less than 2 mg/dL. In physiological jaundice, the serum bilirubin level rises rapidly, peaking at 5–6 mg/dL between the second and fourth days and then begins to fall below 2 mg/dL by the end of the first week.

Treatment
- Babies can be treated with PTx when the bilirubin level rises faster.
- Exposing the skin of the baby to sunlight is advisable.
- Administration of a small dose of phenobarbitone is also advisable.

Nursing Management
- Ensure good skin care.
- Provide protection of eyes and testes from harmful effects of PTx. (See also pathological jaundice.)
- Administer care similar to that of the preterm infant.
- Feed glucose as necessary, and infants may need intravenous therapy depending upon their condition.
- Start hypoglycaemia protocol regardless of weight if hypoglycaemia is present.
- See that the baby is not developing hypoglycaemia and respiratory distress and attaining normal growth and developing no infection.

Pathological Jaundice

Pathological jaundice occurs during the first 24 hours after birth, whereas physiological jaundice never occurs that early. A direct bilirubin level above 1 mg/dL or a total bilirubin concentration that increases by more than 5 mg/dL per day is higher than 12 mg/dL in a full-term infant or 10–14 mg/dL in a preterm infant or jaundice that persist after the second week of life is considered as pathological.

Any total serum bilirubin (TSB) value of 17 mg/dL or more should be regarded as pathological and should be evaluated for the cause and possible intervention such as PTx.

Pathological jaundice has the following features:
- Appears on the first 24 hours
- Presence of jaundice on arms and legs on day 2
- Yellow palms and soles anytime
- Serum bilirubin concentration increasing more than 0.2 mg/dL per hour or more than 5 mg/dL in 24 hours
- TSB concentration is more than the 95th centile as per age-specific bilirubin nomogram
- Signs of acute bilirubin encephalopathy or kernicterus
- Direct bilirubin more than 1.5–2 mg/dL at any age
- In preterm infants, clinical jaundice persisting beyond 2 weeks and in term infants for 3 weeks
- Haemolysis: Blood group incompatibility such as those of ABO, Rh and minor groups, enzyme deficiencies such as G6PD deficiency, autoimmune haemolytic anaemia
- Decreased conjugation such as prematurity
- Increased enterohepatic circulation such as lack of adequate enteral feeding that includes insufficient breastfeeding or the infant not being fed because of illness or GI tract obstruction
- Extravasated blood: Cephalohaematoma, extensive bruising, etc.

Causes

1. Excessive destruction of erythrocytes/haemolysis related to ABO incompatibility, Rh incompatibility, enzyme deficiencies such as G6PD deficiency, autoimmune haemolytic anaemia
2. Decreased conjugation such as prematurity
3. Increased enterohepatic circulation such as lack of adequate enteral feeding that includes insufficient breastfeeding
4. Extravasated blood as in cephalohaematoma, extensive bruising
5. Infection
6. Other metabolic disorders

Predisposing Factors

- History of anaemia/transfusion/liver disease/α_1-antitrypsin deficiency, galactosaemia
- Maternal history of unexplained fever/diabetes mellitus, drug intake during pregnancy, labour and delivery
- Whether the neonate had vomiting, formula feeds or delayed passage of meconium

Examination

- Look for head size – Microcephaly, cephalohaematoma or plethora – polycythaemia/pallor/omphalitis
- Hepatosplenomegaly – haemolytic diseases of newborn
- Umbilical hernia/optic atrophy and petechia
- Colour of urine and faeces
  Visual examination for jaundice include:
  Examine the baby in bright natural light. Alternatively, the baby can be examined in white fluorescent light. Make sure there is no yellow or off-white background.
  Make sure the baby is naked.
  Examine blanched skin and gums, as well as sclera.

Note the extent of jaundice (Kramer's rule).
Face 5–7 mg/dL
Chest 8–10 mg/dL
Lower abdomen/thigh 12–15 mg/dL
Soles/palms >15 mg/dL
Depth of jaundice (degree of yellowness) should be noted carefully. Karmer's criteria may be used to figure it out.
Measurement of serum bilirubin is usually done by transcutaneous bilirubinometry.
Methods of TSB measurements include biochemical methods and by micro method of estimation of TSB.
Neonates are at a higher risk of jaundice, if:
Gestation <38 weeks
Previous sibling with significant jaundice
Visible jaundice in the first 24 hours
Age-specific TSB level being above the 95th centile (if measured)
Laboratory investigations:
Maternal – Blood group/Rh/VDRL
Infant – TSB and direct
Blood group and Rh typing
Blood count – TC/DC/peripheral smear/reticulocyte count
If indicated, perform sepsis screen/thyroid function/urine for sugar/galactosaemia and gram-negative bacteria.

Usually, clinical jaundice is investigated to find out the total bilirubin value. If the level of bilirubin is ≥12 mg/dL or if the infant is less than 24 hours old, Coombs' test will be performed. If it is positive, identify the antibody for Rh or ABO. If it is negative, test for direct bilirubin is done. If the value is >2 mg/dL, hepatitis, intrauterine infection or sepsis is considered and treatment is directed towards this. If the value is <2 mg/dL, a haematocrit value is obtained. If haematocrit is normal or low, RBC morphology and reticulocyte count are noted. If these are normal, enclosed haemorrhage/increased enterohepatic circulation/hypothyroidism/asphyxia/infection or drug use may be suspected and treatment is directed towards the cause. Abnormal results are obtained if hereditary spherocytosis or ABO isoimmunization is suspected and treatment is administered accordingly. Newborns who have yellow discolouration below their thighs should be investigated.

Hyperbilirubinaemia is treated with PTx and exchange transfusion. Usually, the APP protocol is followed in treating jaundice in neonates, which provides two age-specific nomograms – one each for PTx and exchange transfusion. One each for lower-risk babies (38 weeks or more and no risk factors), medium-risk babies (38 weeks or more with risk factors, or 35–37 weeks and without any risk factors) and higher-risk babies (35–37 weeks and with risk factors).

Breast Milk Jaundice

Approximately, one of three normal breastfed infants has jaundice at 2 weeks of age. Most common cause of jaundice is insufficient intake of breast milk. Delayed feeds lead to delayed stool passage, and conversion of conjugated to unconjugated bilirubin state and absorption of bilirubin to blood also increase. A sleepy baby, one on an infrequent schedule, is a characteristic feature of this state. Pregnanediol hormone present in the mother's breast milk may contribute to jaundice, too. It inhibits conjugation of bilirubin by glucuronyl transferase.

Approach to an Infant with Jaundice

Perform visual assessment (VA) of jaundice every 12 hours during the initial 3–5 days of life.

VA can be supplemented with transcutaneous bilirubinometry (TcB), if available.

Step 1: Does the baby have serious jaundice?

If yes, start PTx. Measure TSB level and determine if the baby requires PTx or exchange transfusion.

Step 3: Determine the cause of jaundice and provide supportive and follow-up care.

If 'no', Step 2: Does the infant have significant jaundice to require TSB measurement? If yes, measure TSB level and determine if the baby requires PTx or exchange transfusion. If 'no', continue observation.

PTx remains the mainstay of treatment of hyperbilirubinaemia in neonates. PTx is highly effective and carries an excellent safety track record of more than 50 years. It acts by converting insoluble bilirubin (unconjugated) into soluble isomers that can be excreted in urine and faeces. The bilirubin molecule isomerizes to harmless forms under blue–green light (460–490 nm), and the light sources having high irradiance in this particular wavelength range are more effective than the others. A variety of light sources are available such as florescent lamps of different colours (cool white, blue, green, blue–green or turquoise) and shapes (straight or U-shaped commonly referred as compact florescent lamps, i.e. CFL), halogen bulbs, high-intensity light-emitting diodes (LEDs) and fibreoptic light sources.

Nursing Management

- Observe the infant for signs of increased jaundice.
- Observe for and prevent acidosis, hypoxia and hypoglycaemia which decrease binding of bilirubin to albumin and contribute to jaundice.
- Maintain adequate hydration and offer fluids between feedings as prescribed.
- Maintain skin temperature at 97.6°F. Avoid cold stress.
- **Provide PTx** (fluorescent light breaks down bilirubin into water-soluble products).
- Do not clothe infants.
- Cover the infant's eyes to prevent retinal damage.
- Cover the scrotum of male infants.
- Change position every 2 hours to ensure adequate exposure.
- Keep the distance between the baby and the light source to 30–45 cm.
- Remove the infant from light for feeding and remove eye pads at this time.
- Dress the baby when the baby is removed from the light to provide warmth.
- Carefully examine eyes for irritation from eye patches.
- Keep an accurate record of hours spent under PTx.
- Meet the emotional needs of infants.

- It is important that a plastic cover or shield be placed before PTx lamps to avoid accidental injury to the baby in case a lamp breaks.
- Monitor temperature of the baby every 2–4 hours. Measure TSB level every 12–24 hours.
- Discontinue PTx once two TSB values 12-hour apart fall below the current age-specific cut-offs.
- Institute care of a preterm baby with exchange transfusion when the bilirubin reaches high levels (20 mg/dL in full-term infants and lower levels in preterm infants).
- It is usually done in the operation room or delivery room.
- The infant is usually placed in a radiant warmer and restrained.
- Resuscitation equipment must be kept ready for use, and oxygen should be available all the time to meet emergency needs.
- Blood should be no more than 24 hours old and warmed.
- Aspirate stomach contents to prevent vomiting.
- Baseline vital signs are obtained and checked every 15–20 minutes.
- Transfusion is given via an umbilical catheter.
- **Exchange transfusion** is done by alternately withdrawing and adding blood.
- Maximum 500 mL of Rh –ve blood is given.
- Usual time taken for exchange transfusion is 45–60 minutes.

After Care

- Observe for bleeding from the umbilical cord.
- Observe vital signs.
- Maintain warmth.
- Administer oxygen if needed.
- Observe for signs of hypoglycaemia, sepsis and cardiac arrest.
- Resume feeding after 4–6 hours.
- Keep the umbilical cord moist if other transfusions are required.
- Provide exchange transfusion.

Exchange transfusion is indicted in preterm and term babies if they are suffering from hyperbilirubinaemia within the first 24 hours of life. An exchange transfusion soon after birth is indicated if:

- Cord blood bilirubin is ≥5 mg/dL.
- Cord Hb is ≤10 mg/dL, packed cell volume (PCV) is <30.
- Previous sibling history and positive Direct Coombs Test (DCT).

Double-volume exchange transfusion (DVET) is advised if the TSB reach the age-specific cut-off.

Indications for DVET at birth in infants with Rh iso-immunization include:

Partial exchange transfusion with 50 mL/kg of packed cells should be administered to quickly restore oxygen-carrying capacity of blood in the case of babies born with hydrops or cardiac decompensation.

Subsequent transfusions are indicated if:

- Bilirubin ≥10 mg/dL within 24 hours of age
- Bilirubin ≥15 mg/dL between 25 and 48 hours of age

- Bilirubin ≥20 mg/dL after 48 hours of age
- Rate of rise of bilirubin is 0.5 mg/dL per hour

On admission, even if the bilirubin level is in exchange transfusion state, PTx may be attempted and then repeat bilirubin count is obtained within 24 hours while preparing for exchange transfusion. If the bilirubin level is not declining at a rate of >0.5 mg/dl per hour, exchange transfusion is given.

Procedure. Route of transfusion is the umbilical vein. Rate is 4–5 mL/kg in a 2-minute cycle. Catheter tip and umbilical swab should be sent for culture after procedure. Stomach wash must be done prior to the procedure and nil orally 2–3 hours postprocedure. Maintain good hygiene. Treat underlying sepsis and hypothermia. Administer phenobarbitone 5 mg/kg per day.

Blood Group Used in Exchange Transfusion

Mother's Blood Group	Baby's Blood Group	Blood for Exchange
O	O	O
O	A	O
O	B	O
A	O	O
A	A	O/A
A	B	O
A	AB	O/A
B	O	O
B	B	O/B
B	A	O
B	AB	O/B
AB	A	O/A
AB	B	O/B
AB	AB	O/A/B/AB

If either the mother or the baby is Rh negative, then Rh-negative blood is given.

Type of Blood Used in Exchange Transfusion

Sl. No	Condition	Type of Blood
1	Rh isoimmunization	Rh-negative and blood group 'O' or that of the baby
		Suspended in AB plasma
		Cross-matched with the baby's and mother's blood
2	ABO incompatibility	Rh compatible and blood group 'O' (not that of the baby)
		Suspended in AB plasma
		Cross-matched with the baby's and mother's blood
3	Other conditions (G6PD deficiency, nonhaemolytic, other isoimmune haemolytic jaundice	Baby's group and Rh type
		Cross-matched with the baby's and mother's blood

NB: Volume of blood is twice the blood volume of the baby and to prepare the blood for double-volume exchange, use two-thirds of packed red cells and one-third of plasma.

Nurse Responsibility for Exchange Transfusion

Arrange equipment needed for the procedure:
- Mask, sterile gowns and gloves
- Complete resuscitation set
- Emergency medications
- Umbilical catheter pack
- Exchange transfusion set – A special four-way stopcock or two-way stopcock, two 20-mL syringes and two 10-mL syringes and a calibrated waste container
- Blood transfusion set
- Injection of heparin 5000 units in 5 mL
- Exchange transfusion records

Procedure
- Obtain an informed signed consent.
- Use full aseptic precautions.
- The neonatologist will insert the umbilical vein catheter. Obtain a pre-exchange sample for analysis.
- Help connect the stopcock (four-, two- or three-way) to the umbilical vein, donor blood, the waste container and the syringe.
- The paediatrician performs the procedure by withdrawing blood from the baby into a syringe and discarding it into the waste container. Equal amount of blood is filled into the syringe from the donor blood and injected into the baby.
- Each cycle should take approximately 5 minutes, withdrawing blood from the baby 1 minute and injecting into the baby 4 minutes.

Infants of Diabetic Mothers

Usually, the babies are big (macrosomia) and may be delivered early by caesarean section. Children with diabetic mothers have a higher incidence of congenital anomalies than the general population. Such babies are also at high risk of hypoglycaemia, respiratory distress, hypocalcaemia and hyperbilirubinaemia.

Assessment

- Assess for excess size, weight (as a result of excess fat and glycogen in tissues).
- Assess for high blood sugar levels (blood sugar in the mother cross the placenta and enters the baby's bloodstream, elevating the baby's blood sugar level; high blood sugar stimulates the infant's metabolic system to store glycogen and fat and increase the production of insulin).
- Check appearance of the infant (may be puffy in face and cheeks).
- Observe for signs of hypoglycaemia (twitching, difficulty in feeding, lethargy, apnoea, cardiac failure, seizure and cyanosis).

- Observe for signs of respiratory distress (tachypnoea, cyanosis, retractions, grunting and nasal flaring).

Hypoglycaemia in neonates can be defined as a true blood glucose level (BGL) less than 40 mg/dL (irrespective of gestation); if associated with symptoms of hypoglycaemia or if confirmed on repeat analysis in asymptomatic babies, it is indicative of hypoglycaemia. There are certain situations that require routine monitoring of neonates for glucose. These are as follows:

- Small for date babies
- Infants of diabetic mothers
- Rh haemolytic disease of newborn
- Babies with symptom suggestive of hypoglycaemia
- Babies with prolonged hypoxia, hypothermia, polycythaemia, septicaemia and cardiac failure or suspected metabolic disorders

Predisposing Factors

- Intrauterine growth retardation
- Maternal diabetes mellitus
- Immaturity
- Erythroblastosis fetalis
- Miscellaneous disorders.

Management

For symptomatic hypoglycaemia including seizures, a bolus of 2 mL/kg of 10% dextrose (200 mg/kg) should be given. This mini-bolus is advisable, as it rapidly increases BGL. The bolus should be followed by continuous glucose infusion at an initial rate of 6–8 mg/kg/min. BGL should checked after 30–60 minutes and then every 6 hours until blood sugar is >50 mg/dL. If BGL is still below 45 mg/dL after bolus infusion, continuous glucose infusion should be started in steps of 2 mg/kg/min every 15 minutes till it reaches 12 mg/kg/min. After 24 hours, monitor BGL and if it reaches >50 mg/dL, infusion can be tapered and oral administration can be continued. Once the BGL is within normal limits, infusion can be stopped. One should be very careful not to stop glucose administration abruptly, as it may cause severe rebound hypoglycaemia. Avoid using more than 12.5% dextrose infusion through a peripheral vein, as it may cause thrombophlebitis.

Nursing Management

- Assess serum glucose level.
- Administer intravenous fluids as indicated.
- Observe for signs and symptoms of hypoglycaemia.
- Record the progress and check the serum glucose level frequently as indicated.
- Report untoward symptoms such as convulsions, cardiac failure, etc.
- Monitor fluid administration.
- Maintain I&O.
- Weigh the baby every day on the same time using the same scale.
- Avoid hypothermia.

Outcome of Hypoglycaemia

Outcome of hypoglycaemia is determined by certain factors such as duration, degree of hypoglycaemia, rate of cerebral blood flow, cerebral utilization of glucose, and also comorbidities. Infants need to be evaluated for neurodevelopmental outcome, overall IQ, reading ability, arithmetic proficiency and motor performance. It is suggested to undertake vision/eye evaluation and hearing, too. Neurodevelopment will be assessed by using DASII 2. MRI at 4–6 weeks provides a good estimate of hypoglycaemic injury and is advisable to do so.

Care of Neonates with Hypocalcaemia

Calcium (Ca) is actively transferred from the mother to the fetus during the last trimester. This is the reason for high concentration of Ca in cord blood. Serum Ca in the fetus is 10–11 mg/dL at term which is 1–2 mg/dL higher than the mother's level. Hypocalcaemia is defined by different total serum calcium (tSCa) and iSCa cut-offs for preterm and term infants.

Causes of Early-Onset Hypocalcaemia

- Prematurity (termination of transplacental supply)
- Preeclampsia
- Infants of diabetic mothers (increased calcium demands of a macrosomic baby)
- Perinatal stress/asphyxia (delayed introduction of feeds, increased calcitonin production, increased endogenous phosphate load, renal insufficiency and diminished parathyroid hormone secretion – all may contribute to hypocalcaemia)
- Maternal intake of anticonvulsants (phenobarbitone and phenytoin alter vitamin D metabolism and predispose them to its deficiency)
- Maternal hyperparathyroidism (causes intrauterine hypercalcaemia, suppressing the parathyroid activity in the fetus, resulting in impaired parathyroid responsiveness to hypocalcaemia after birth)
- Iatrogenic (alkalosis, use of blood products, diuretics, PTx, lipid infusions, etc.)

Management of Early Neonatal Hypocalcaemia

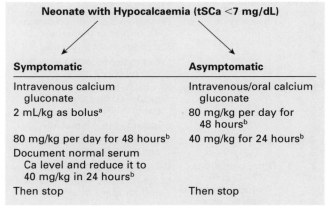

Neonate with Hypocalcaemia (tSCa <7 mg/dL)	
Symptomatic	**Asymptomatic**
Intravenous calcium gluconate	Intravenous/oral calcium gluconate
2 mL/kg as bolus[a]	80 mg/kg per day for 48 hours[b]
80 mg/kg per day for 48 hours[b]	40 mg/kg for 24 hours[b]
Document normal serum Ca level and reduce it to 40 mg/kg in 24 hours[b]	
Then stop	Then stop

Note: 1 mL of calcium gluconate contains 9 mg of elemental calcium
[a]Diluted 1:1 in 5% dextrose and administered under cardiac monitoring.
[b]Added to intravenous fluids and given as infusion. Be careful to prevent extravasation and sloughing.

Polycythaemia in Neonates

Polycythaemia is a condition caused by hyperviscosity of blood. When there is increased blood viscosity, it affects tissue oxygenation and perfusion. It also leads to microthrombi. Microthrombi in vital organs (cerebral cortex, kidneys and adrenals) can lead to fatal outcomes. It is not easy to measure hyperviscosity of blood. It is correlated with a high haematocrit value. Relationship between viscosity and haematocrit is almost linear up to a haematocrit value of 65% and exponential thereafter.

Polycythaemia is a condition that results when the haematocrit value is more than 65% and a venous Hb concentration is in excess of 22 g/dL. Hyperviscosity is defined as viscosity greater than 14.6 cP at a shear rate of 11.5 per second. The polycythaemia–hyperviscocity syndrome is confined to infants with haematocrit values of more than 65%; it is very rare for those with a haematocrit value of <60%.

Incidence

The incidence of polycythaemia is 1.5%–4% of all live births. The incidence is higher among both SGA (15%) and LGA infants. It is 2% for AGA infants. Neonates born at a high altitude also have a higher incidence of polycythaemia.

Risk Factors

Maternal smoking is a risk factor.
Delayed cord clamping may be a factor.
Infants born with caesarean section have lower haematocrit values.
Physiological changes in postnatal life and haematocrit – within first 24–48 hours of life, there are significant changes in haematocrit values. Haematocrit peaks in the first 2 hours of life (71%). It gradually declines to 68% by 6 hours and stabilizes by 12–24 hours.

Clinical features

There is a wide range of symptoms in neonates with polycythaemia.

Central nervous system
Early: Hypotonia and sleepiness, irritability, jitteriness, seizures and infarcts
Late: motor deficits, lower achievement and IQ scores

Metabolism
Hypoglycaemia, jaundice, hypocalcaemia

Heart and lungs
Tachycardia, tachypnoea, respiratory distress, cyanosis with plethora
Chest radiography: Cardiomegaly, pulmonary plethora
Echocardiography: Increased pulmonary resistance, decreased cardiac output

Gastrointestinal tract
Poor suck, vomiting, feed intolerance – abdominal distension, NEC

Kidneys
Oliguria (depending on blood volume), transient hypertension, renal vein thrombosis

Haematology
Mild thrombocytopenia, thrombosis (rare)

Miscellaneous
Peripheral gangrene, priapism, testicular infarction

Diagnosis

The following categories of neonates need to be screened for polycythaemia:

(a) SGA infants
(b) Infants of diabetic mothers (IDM)
(c) LGA infants
(d) Monochorionic twins, especially the larger twin
(e) Infants with morphological features of growth retardation such as many loose folds of skin around the buttock and thighs, loss of subcutaneous fat, difference between head and chest circumference >3 cm

Centrifuge venous blood in heparinized capillaries for 3–5 minutes

Schedule for testing should be 2, 6, 12, 24, 48 and 72 hours of age.

Capillary samples may be used for screening, but all high values should be confirmed by a venous sample for the diagnosis of polycythaemia as capillary versus venous blood. Capillary haematocrit values are significantly higher than venous haematocrit values.

Methods of haematocrit determination – Two types. *Automated haematology analyser and microcentrifuge*

Management

Before starting treatment, it should be ascertained that the baby is not suffering from dehydration, as dehydration increases haematocrit levels. Weight checking and comparing with birth weight may help distinguish this. Two important points must be considered in the management:

1. Presence of symptoms suggestive of polycythaemia and/or
2. Absolute value of haematocrit

Management is based on haematocrit values. If the haematocrit value is >65%, exclude dehydration (check for weight loss). If the baby is symptomatic, then partial exchange transfusion is provided. If the baby is asymptomatic and if the haematocrit value is more than 75%, partial exchange is preferred. If the haematocrit values is 70%–74%, dehydrate the baby with rigorous monitoring of I&O. If the haematocrit value is 65%–69%, monitor the baby for symptoms carefully.

Nursing management is basically developmental supportive care.

Neonatal Seizure

Neonatal seizure is the most common clinical manifestation of neurological dysfunction in the newborn infant and is at a high risk of neonatal death or neurological impairment/epilepsy disorders in later life. It is the paroxysmal alteration in neurological function, i.e. motor, behaviour and/or autonomic function. This includes epileptic seizures with corresponding electroencephalographic

(EEG) changes, nonepileptic seizures without corresponding EEG changes and EEG seizures with abnormal EEG changes with no clinical correlation.

Common Causes of Neonatal Seizures

Hypoxic-ischemic encephalopathy (HIE): HIE secondary to perinatal asphyxia is the commonest cause of neonatal seizures. It usually starts within the first 12 hours of life (about 65%) whereas the rest manifest by 24–48 hours of age. Associated problems are hypoglycaemia, hypocalcaemia and intracranial haemorrhage. Subtle seizures are the most common type of seizures following HIE.

Metabolic causes: These include hypoglycaemia, hypocalcaemia, and hypomagnesaemia. Rare causes include pyridoxine dependency and inborn errors of metabolism (IEM).

Infections: Meningitis is the most common infection in neonates with seizures. Meningoencephalitis secondary to intrauterine infections (TORCH group, syphilis) may also present as seizures in the neonatal period.

Intracranial haemorrhage: Seizures as a result of subarachnoid, intraparenchymal or subdural haemorrhage occur more often in term neonates. In preterm neonates, seizures secondary to IVH is common. Most seizures as a result of intracranial haemorrhage occur between 2 and 7 days of age. Seizures occurring in a term 'well baby' on days 2–3 of life is often a result of subarachnoid haemorrhage.

Developmental defects: Cerebral dysgenesis and neuronal migration disorders can also be the causes of seizures.

Miscellaneous: They include polycythaemia, maternal narcotic withdrawal, drug toxicity (e.g. theophylline, doxapram), local anaesthetic injection into the scalp and phacomatosis (e.g. tuberous sclerosis, incontinentia pigmenti).

Diagnosis

History – Antenatal history of exposure to infections, certain drugs, natal and postnatal history of drugs, labour, injury during labour, etc. need to be elicited. A family history of seizures in either parent or sibling(s) in the neonatal period may suggest benign familial neonatal convulsions (BFNCs).

General examination of vitals and other systems requires CNS examination including bulging of anterior fontanel and detailed neurological assessment.

Systemic examination for IEM and essential investigations including EEG and MRI are essential.

Management

Nurse the baby in a thermoneutral environment.

Ensure airway, breathing and circulation.

Administer oxygen as needed.

Intravenous access to be secured; blood should be collected to check hypoglycaemia and hypocalcaemia.

Achieve correction of hypoglycaemia and hypocalcaemia.

Administer antiepileptic drugs as prescribed such as phenobarbitone. The usual dose is 20 mg/kg i.v. slowly over 20 minutes (not faster than 1 mg/kg/min). If seizures persist after completion of this loading dose, additional doses of phenobarbitone 10 mg/kg may be used every 20–30 minutes until a total dose of 40 mg/kg has been given. The maintenance dose of phenobarbitone is 3–5 mg/kg per day in one to two divided doses, starting 12 hours after the loading dose.

Another antiepileptic used is phenytoin. The dose is 20 mg/kg i.v. at a rate of not more than 1 mg/kg/min under cardiac monitoring. This is given if phenol has no effect on improvement.

Benzodiazepams are also given. The commonly used benzodiazepines are lorazepam and midazolam. Diazepam is generally avoided in neonates because of its short duration of antiepileptic effect but very prolonged sedative effect, narrow therapeutic index and the presence of sodium benzoate as a preservative.

Nursing Management

Developmental supportive care

Care during seizure and proper administration of antiepileptic drugs

Careful monitoring of drugs, signs and symptoms

Prompt reporting and recording of the status

Maintenance of Airway, Breathing and Circulation (ABC) and accurate recording

Alleviation of parental anxiety

PLANNING OF A NEONATAL INTENSIVE CARE UNIT (NE. USUAL DOSE IN THE NICU)

Newborn intensive care is defined as care for medically unstable or critically ill newborns requiring constant nursing, complicated surgical procedures, continual respiratory support or other intensive interventions. Intermediate care includes care of ill infants requiring less constant nursing but does not exclude respiratory support. When an intensive care nursery is available, the intermediate nursery (step-down NICU) serves as a 'step-down' unit from the intensive care area. But all hospitals will not have this facility. For any hospital that has a birthing unit, it is always better to have a facility to care for critically ill neonates. The number of premature labour cases, complicated pregnancies and babies born after infertility treatment are all in the increase. These contribute to a major section of precious babies. All these factors warrant the requirements of neonatal intensive care units (NICUs) in hospitals. NICU plan is a teamwork, and the team should include, among others, health care professionals, families (whose primary experience with the hospital is as a consumer of health care), administrators and design professionals.

The nurse is an important person in the planning team of NICUs. The nurse should have working knowledge of the requirements and statutory regulations guiding the plan of any intensive care units. The nurse is responsible for planning nursing service in the NICU. There are set criteria and standards for the designing and developing an NICU. An NICU design should facilitate excellent health care for infants in a setting that supports the family needs and the needs of the staff.

In the last decade, remarkable changes have occurred in the 'landscape' of NICU design. The designing team should take into consideration the requirements of the hospital and the availability of newer technology and advanced treatments for proper planning of an NICU. The planners should look into the current evidence that supports excellent designing with state-of-the-art facilities at a affordable cost. For this, the program planning and design process should include research, evidence-based recommendations and materials, with objective input of experts in the field in addition to the internal interdisciplinary team. The program and design process should consider many factors such as vision and mission of the institution of which the NICU is going to be the part. The team should review articles on usual practice, conduct visits to classical NICUs of other places, learn space planning, operations planning including traffic patterns, functional locations and relations to ancillary services, interior planning, surface material selection, building construction, post-construction verification and remedying before actual occupation. It is better to have mock-ups before the actual occupation. The planning team has to decide what type of design (such as single- or multiple-occupancy design) is suitable. Private or single-family room designs are now so common and a primary feature of the most new construction projects in the developed countries and affluent hospitals in India. Evidence indicates that such designs are practical, popular with families and justified by an increasing awareness of the impact of the sensory input (emotional bonding) with premature and ill newborns.

Unit Configuration

The NICU design should be based on systematically developed program goals and objectives that define the purpose of the unit, service provision, space utilization, projected bed space demand, staffing requirements and other basic information related to the mission of the unit. Design strategies to achieve program goals and objectives should address the medical, developmental, educational, emotional and social needs of infants, families and the staff. The design should allow for flexibility and creativity to achieve the stated objectives. The NICU should be configured in such a way that it individualizes the caregiving environment and services for each infant and family.

NICU Location within the Hospital

The NICU should be planned at a distinct area within the health care facility, with controlled access and a controlled environment. The NICU should be located within the space designed for that purpose. The NICU should provide effective circulation of the staff, family and equipment. Traffic to other services shall not pass through the unit. The NICU should be in close and controlled proximity to the area of the hospital where labour rooms are located for easy transport of neonates. When obstetric and neonatal services are on separate

floors of the hospital, an elevator with priority call and controlled access by keyed operation should be provided for services between the birthing unit and the NICU. This is to provide safe and efficient transport of infants while respecting their privacy. So, the NICU should be a distinct, controlled area immediately adjacent to other perinatal services, except in those local situations (e.g., freestanding children's hospitals) where exceptions can be justified. Transport of infants within the hospital should be possible without using public corridors.

Size of the Unit

As a general rule, the intramural requirement is three beds for every 1000 annual deliveries in the health facility dedicated to the NICU. For extramural deliveries (deliveries taking place outside the hospital), the number of beds in the NICU will be 30% of the estimated beds. If a hospital has 3000 deliveries per year, that hospital should have nine beds for the NICU (intramural) and for outside neonates 30% of this will be three beds, and the hospital may need 12 beds altogether. But for planning size and equipment, one has to consider sustainability of the unit.

Space Requirements

Each infant space shall contain a minimum of 100–120 square feet (9.9–11.2 m²) of clear floor space, excluding handwashing stations, columns and corridors. Out of this 100–120 square feet, half of the space should be utilized for baby care area and half for general support and ancillary areas. There should be a corridor adjacent to each infant space, with a minimum width of 4 feet (1.2 m) for multiple bedrooms. When single-infant rooms or fixed-cubicle partitions are utilized in the design, there should be an adjacent corridor of not less than 8 feet (2.4 m) of a clear and unobstructed width to permit passage of equipment and personnel. In multiple bedrooms, there shall be a minimum of 8 feet (2.4 m) space between infant beds. Ideally, each infant space should be designed to allow privacy of the infant.

Baby care area may be divided into two interconnected rooms separated by transparent observation windows, with nurses' work station in between. This even promotes the purpose of isolation if required.

General Support Space

Distinct facilities should be provided for clean and soiled utilities, medical equipment storage and unit management services.

Clean utility/holding area(s): This is the area for storage of supplies frequently used in the care of newborns.

Soiled utility/holding room: It is essential for storing used and contaminated material before its removal from the NICU. Unless used only as a holding room, this room can contain a counter and a hands-free handwashing station separate from any utility sinks. The handwashing station shall have hot and cold running water that is turned on and off by hands-free controls, soap and paper towel dispensers, and a covered waste receptacle with foot control.

The ventilation system in the soiled utility/holding room should be engineered to have negative air pressure, with 100% air exhaust to the outside. The soiled utility/holding room should be placed to allow removal of soiled materials without passing through the infant care area. A designated area for collection of recyclable materials used in the NICU should be established. This area should measure at least 1 square foot per patient bed and be located outside the patient care area.

Charting/staff work areas: Provision for a charting space at each bedside should be provided. An additional separate area or desk for tasks such as compiling more detailed records, completing requisitions and telephone communication should be allowed in an area acoustically separated from the infant and family areas. Dedicated space shall be allocated as necessary for electronic medical recordkeeping within infant care areas. A clerical area should be located near the entrance to the NICU so that personnel can supervise traffic into the unit. Newborn charts, computer terminals and hospital forms can be located in this space. In addition, there should be one or more staff work areas, each serving 8–16 beds. These areas will allow groups of three to six caregivers to congregate immediately adjacent to the infant care area for report, collaboration and socialization.

Storage areas: A three-zone storage system is desirable. The first storage area should be the central supply department of the hospital. The second storage zone should be the clean utility area.

Routinely used supplies such as diapers, formula, linen, cover gowns, charts and information booklets may be stored in this space. There should be at least 8-ft³ (0.22 m³) space for secondary storage of syringes, needles, intravenous infusion sets and sterile trays for the care of each infant.

There should also be at least 18 square feet (1.7 m²) of floor space allocated for equipment storage per infant in intermediate care and 30 square feet (2.8 m²) for each infant bed in intensive care. Total storage space may vary by unit size and storage system. The third storage zone is for items frequently used at the infant's bedside. Bedside cabinet storage should be at least 16 square feet (0.45 m³) for each infant in the intermediate care area and 24 square feet (0.67 m³) for each infant in the intensive care area. Bedside storage should be designed for quiet operation.

Design of the NICU must anticipate use of electronic medical record devices so that their introduction does not require major disruption of the function of the unit or reduce space designed for other purposes. Design considerations include ease of access for staff, patient confidentiality, and infection control and noise control, both with respect to that generated by the devices and by the traffic around them.

Laundry room: If laundry facilities for infant materials are provided, a separate laundry room can serve the functions of laundry and toy cleaning within the NICU. Infant clothing and the cloth covers or positioning aids should be laundered on a regular schedule and as needed. In addition, toys utilized by infants or siblings (if permitted) are required to be cleaned on a regular basis for each infant and between infants. Space for an automatic washing machine with dryer promotes the aseptic cleaning process.

Staff Support Space

Space should be provided within the NICU to meet the professional, personal and administrative needs of the staff. Locker, lounge, private toilet facilities and on-call rooms are required at a minimum. These areas should include doctors' and nurses' changing room, support staff's changing room, etc.

Step-down Area (Rooming-in Facility or Family Transition Rooms)

Family–infant room(s) should be provided within or immediately adjacent to the NICU so that families/mothers and recovering neonates can stay together. This will release the pressure of NICU partially. The room(s) should have direct, private access to sink and toilet facilities, emergency call and telephone or intercom linkage with the NICU staff, sleeping facilities for at least one parent and sufficient space for the infant's bed and equipment. The additional space requirement should be about 40–50 sq ft per bed for this step-down NICU.

Family Support Space

Space should be provided in or immediately adjacent to the NICU for the following functions: family lounge area, lockable storage, telephone(s) and toilet facilities. Separate, dedicated rooms shall also be provided for lactation support and consultation in or immediately adjacent to the NICU. A family library or education area shall be provided within the hospital. Access to the internet and educational materials shall be provided via a computer station in the family lounge or at the infant's bedside.

Support Space for Ancillary Services

Distinct support space should be provided for all clinical services that are routinely performed in the NICU. Ancillary services such as (but not necessarily limited to) respiratory therapy, laboratory, pharmacy, radiology, developmental therapy and specialized feeds preparation are common in the NICU. Distance, size and access are important considerations when designing space for each of these functions. Satellite facilities (intranet) may be required for these services in a timely manner. Unless performed elsewhere in the hospital, a specialized feedings preparation area or room should be provided in the NICU, away from the bedside, to permit mixing of additives to breast milk or formula. (In some hospitals, this facility may be located near the central supply or pharmacy area. The facility supplies the prepared formula to the NICU according to requisitions.) This area should be equipped with a hands-free handwashing station, counter workspace and storage areas for supplies, formula and both refrigerated and frozen breast milk.

Isolation Facilities

An airborne infection isolation room should be available for NICU infants with the facility for data transmission to a remote location. A hands-free handwashing station for hand hygiene and areas for gowning and storage of clean and soiled materials should be provided near the entrance to the room. Ventilation systems for isolation rooms should be engineered to have negative air pressure, with 100% air exhaust to the outside. Airborne infection isolation room perimeter walls, ceilings and floors, including penetrations, should be sealed tightly so that air does not infiltrate the environment from the outside or from other airspaces. Airborne infection isolation rooms should have self-closing devices on all room exit doors. An emergency communication system and remote patient monitoring capability should be provided within the airborne infection isolation room. Airborne infection isolation rooms need to have observation windows with internal blinds or switchable (opaquing) glass for privacy. Placement of windows and other structural items should allow for ease of operation and cleaning. Airborne infection isolation rooms should have a permanently installed visual mechanism to constantly monitor the pressure status of the room when occupied by a neonate with an airborne infectious disease (e.g. meningococcal meningitis). There should be facility to monitor the direction of the airflow continuously. Airborne infection isolation rooms should have a minimum of 150 square feet of clear floor space, excluding the entry work area, family entry and reception area. This part of the NICU should have a clearly identified entrance and reception area for families. Families should have immediate and direct contact with the staff when they arrive at this entrance and reception area and handwashing stations.

Handwashing Facility

Where a single-infant room concept is used, a hands-free handwashing station should be provided within each infant room. In a room with multiple beds, every infant bed should be within 20 feet (6 m) of a hands-free handwashing station. Handwashing stations should be no closer than 3 feet (0.9 m) from an infant bed or clean supply storage. Handwashing sinks should be large enough to control splashing and designed to avoid standing or retained water. Minimum dimensions for a handwashing sink are 24 inches wide, 16 inches front to back, 10 inches deep (61 × 41 ×25 cm) from the bottom of the sink to the top of its rim. Space for pictorial handwashing instructions shall be provided above all sinks. There should be no aerator on the faucet. Walls adjacent to handwashing sinks should be made of nonporous material. Space also should be provided for soap and towel dispensers and for appropriate trash receptacles. Towel dispensers should operate so that only the towel needs to be touched in the process of dispensing. Separate receptacles for biohazardous and nonbiohazardous waste should be available. Sinks for handwashing should not be built into counters. Sink location, construction material and related hardware (paper towel and soap dispensers) should be chosen with durability, ease of operation, ease of cleaning and noise control in mind. Nonabsorbent wall material should be used around sinks to prevent the growth of mould on cellulose material.

Administrative Space

Administrative space shall be provided in the NICU for activities directly related to infant care, family support or other activities routinely performed within the NICU.

Electrical needs: The unit should have 24-hour uninterrupted power supply. Backup power supply is a must.

Electrical, Gas Supply and Mechanical Needs

Mechanical requirements, such as electrical and gas outlets, at each infant bed shall be organized to ensure safety, easy access and maintenance. There shall be a minimum of 20 simultaneously accessible electrical outlets. The minimum number of simultaneously accessible gas outlets is as follows: air: 3; oxygen: 3; vacuum: 3; and others for power supplies.

There should be a mixture of emergency and normal power for all electrical outlets per current supply.

To handle equipment, six to eight central voltage-stabilized outlets are required per bed: four of them should be of 5 amperes and 4–15 amperes. Two alternate sockets for mobile bedside X-ray equipment or Ultrasonogram (USG) machine need to be planned.

Lighting of the Unit

It should be well illuminated with adequate daylight. Panel of lights with cool white fluorescent tubes, preferably CFL or LED, will be required for adequate illumination.

Ambient Lighting in Infant Care Areas

Ambient lighting levels in infant spaces need to be adjustable through a range of approximately 1–60 foot-candles, as measured at each bedside. Both natural and electric light sources should have controls that allow immediate darkening of any bed position sufficient for transillumination when necessary. The lighting system should avoid unnecessary ultraviolet or infrared radiation by the use of appropriate lamps, lens or filters. Control of illumination should be accessible to the staff and families and capable of adjustment across the recommended range of lighting levels. Use of multiple light switches to allow different levels of illumination is one method that is helpful in this regard but can pose serious difficulties when rapid darkening of the room is required to permit transillumination; so, a master switch should also be provided. Perception of skin tones is critical in the NICU; light sources should be capable to provide accurate skin tone recognition. Light sources should be as free as possible of glare or veiling reflections. No direct light source or sunlight should be permitted in the newborn space, as this does not exclude direct procedure lighting.

Procedure Lighting in Infant Care Areas

Separate procedure lighting should be available to each infant bed. The luminaire should be capable of providing adequate illumination at the plane of the infant bed and must be framed so that no more than 2% of the light output of the luminaire extends beyond its illumination field. This lighting should be adjustable. Temporary increases in illumination necessary to evaluate a baby or to perform a procedure should be possible without increasing lighting levels for other babies in the same room. As intense light may be unpleasant and harmful to the developing retina, every effort should be made to prevent direct light from reaching the infant's eyes. Procedure lights with adjustable intensity, field size and direction will help protect the infant's eyes from direct exposure and provide the best visual support to the staff.

Illumination of Support Areas

Illumination of support areas within the NICU, including the charting areas, medication preparation area, the reception desk and handwashing areas, should conform to statutory specifications. Illumination should be adequate in areas of the NICU where the staff performs important or critical tasks.

Day Lighting

At least one source of daylight should be visible from infant care areas, either from each infant room itself or from an adjacent staff work area. When provided, external windows in infant care rooms should be glazed with insulating glass to minimize heat gain or loss and should be situated at least 2 feet (60 cm) away from any part of an infant's bed to minimize radiant heat loss. All external windows should be equipped with shading devices that are neutral colour or opaque to minimize colour distortion from the transmitted light.

Ambient Temperature and Ventilation

The NICU should be designed to provide an air temperature of 78.8°F–82.4°F (26°C–28°C) and a relative humidity of 30%–60%. A minimum of six air changes per hour is required, with a minimum of two changes being outside air. **The ventilation** pattern should inhibit particulate matter from moving freely in the space, and intake and exhaust vents should be placed to minimize drafts at or near the infant beds.

Air delivered to the NICU should be filtered. Filters should be located outside the infant care area so that they can be changed easily and safely. Fresh air intake should be located at least 25 feet (7.6 m) from exhaust outlets of ventilating systems, combustion equipment stacks, medical/surgical vacuum systems, plumbing vents or areas that may collect vehicular exhausts or other noxious fumes. Prevailing winds or proximity to other structures may require greater clearance. The airflow pattern should be at low velocity and designed to minimize drafts, noise levels and airborne particulate matter. A HEPA filtration system may provide improved infection control for immunocompromised patients. Supply-and-exhaust ventilation is a good choice for units with heating or cooling ducts, as it is an inexpensive way of providing fresh air.

Acoustic Environment

Infant bed areas (including airborne infection isolation areas), staff work areas, family areas, staff lounge and sleeping areas and the spaces opening onto them should be designed to produce minimal background noise and to contain and absorb much of the transient noise that originates within them. The combination of continuous background sound and transient sound in any of these areas should not exceed an hourly equivalent continuous noise level (Leq) of 45 dB and an hourly L10 of 50 dB (L10 is the sound level that is exceeded for only 10% of any specific hour). The acoustic conditions of the NICU should favour speech intelligibility, normal or relaxed vocal effort, acoustic privacy for the staff and parents, and physiological stability, uninterrupted sleep and freedom from acoustic distraction for infants and adults. Speech intelligibility ratings in infant areas, parent areas and staff work areas should be 'good' to 'excellent' as defined by the International Organization for Standardization (ISO) 9921:2003. Fire alarms in the infant area should be restricted to flashing lights without an audible signal. The audible alarm level in other occupied areas must be adjustable. Noise-generating gadgets and activities should be acoustically isolated. Telephones audible from the infant area should have adjustable announcing signals.

Mechanical Needs

The type of water supply and faucets in infant areas should be selected so as to minimize noise and should provide instant warm water to minimize time 'on'.

Floor Surfaces

Floor surfaces should be easily cleanable and minimize the growth of microorganisms.

Flooring material with a reflectance of no greater than 40% and a gloss value of no greater than 30 gloss units shall be used to minimize the possibility that glare reflected from a bright procedure or work area light will impinge on the eyes of infants or caregivers. Floors should be highly durable to withstand frequent cleaning and heavy traffic. Flooring materials should be free of substances known to be teratogenic, mutagenic, carcinogenic or otherwise harmful to human health. Although ease of cleaning and durability of NICU surfaces are of primary importance, consideration should also be given to their glossiness (the mirror-like reflectivity of a surface), their acoustic properties and the density of the materials used. Reduced glossiness will reduce the risks from bright, reflected glare; acoustic and density properties will directly affect noise and comfort.

Materials suitable to these criteria include resilient sheet flooring (medical-grade rubber or linoleum) and carpeting with an impermeable backing, heat- or chemically welded seams and antimicrobial and antistatic properties. Carpeting has been shown to be an acceptable floor covering in the NICU and has obvious aesthetic and noise reduction appeal, but it is not suitable in all areas (e.g. around sinks or in isolation or soiling utility/holding areas). Small floor tiles (e.g. 12-inch squares) have myriad seams and areas of nonadherence to the subfloor. These harbour dirt and fluids and are a potential source of bacterial and fungal growth. Additional efforts should be made to exclude persistent, bioaccumulative toxic (PBT) chemicals such as polyvinyl chloride (PVC) from health care environments. PVC or vinyl is common in flooring materials including sheet, goods, tiles and carpet. The production of PVC generates dioxin, a potent carcinogen, and fumes emitted from vinyl degrade indoor air quality. Dioxin releases are not associated with materials such as polyolefin, rubber (latex) or linoleum. Infants should not be moved into an area of newly installed flooring for a minimum of 2 weeks to permit complete off-gassing of adhesives and flooring materials. In India, the majority of hospitals use vitrified titles. Other floorings preferred are Kota stone or chip flooring, but they require thorough polishing.

Wall Surfaces

Wall surfaces should be easily cleanable and provide protection at points where contact with movable equipment is likely to occur. Surfaces should be free of substances known to be teratogenic, mutagenic, carcinogenic or otherwise harmful to human health. Specify low- or no-VOC (volatile organic compound) paints and coatings. Walls should be glazed up to a height of 7 feet.

Furnishings

Built-in and freestanding furnishings such as cabinets and carts, especially those in the infant care areas, should be easily cleanable with the fewest possible seams in the integral construction. Exposed surface seams shall be sealed. Furnishings should be of durable construction so as to withstand impact by movable equipment without significant damage. Furnishings and materials should be free of substances known to be teratogenic, mutagenic, carcinogenic or otherwise harmful to human health.

Furnishings in the NICU are often composite pieces, made of various parts and layers of materials that are assembled with glue or adhesives. Materials and substances typically used in these furnishings often contain VOCs, such as formaldehyde, which is frequently found in pressed wood products including plywood and particle board. Vinyl-based laminates, which often are applied to the surface of pressed wood products, also contain VOCs such as PVC. Specify low- or no-VOC materials, including urea–formaldehyde-free adhesives, for all furnishings in the NICU including ceiling finishes. Ceilings should be easily cleanable and constructed in a manner to prohibit the passage of particles from the cavity above the ceiling plane into the clinical environment. The ceiling construction should not be friable. As sound abatement is a high priority in the NICU, acoustical ceiling systems are desirable but must be selected and designed carefully to meet this standard. VOCs and PBTs such as cadmium are often found in paints and ceiling tiles and should be avoided. Specify low- or no-VOC paints and coatings.

Safety/Infant Security

The NICU should be designed as part of an overall security program to provide physical safety to infants, families and the staff in the NICU. The NICU shall be designed to minimize the risk of infant abduction.

Access to Nature and Other Positive Distractions

When possible, views of nature should be provided in at least one space that is accessible to all families and one space that is accessible to all staff members. Other forms of positive distraction should be provided for families in infant and family spaces and for the staff in staff spaces. Culturally appropriate positive distractions provide important psychological benefits to the staff and families in the NICU to avoid sensory deprivation as well as sensory overload.

Sample design of an NICU

Sample design of an NICU

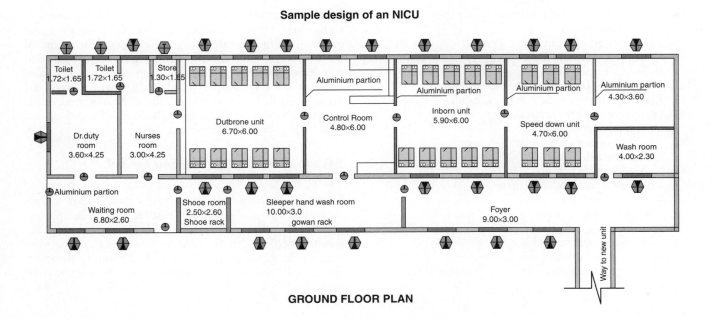

GROUND FLOOR PLAN

Equipment Required for the NICU

1. Open care system: Radiant warmer, fixed height, with trolley, drawers, O_2 bottles
2. PTx unit, single head, high intensity
3. Resuscitator, hand-operated, neonate, 250 mL
4. Resuscitator, hand-operated, neonate, 500 mL
5. Laryngoscope set, neonate
6. Pump, suction, portable, 220 V, w/access
7. Pump, suction, foot-operated
8. Surgical instrument, suture/SET
9. Syringe pump, 10, 20, 50 mL, single phase
10. Oxygen hood, S and M, set of three each, including connecting tubes
11. Oxygen concentrator
12. Thermometer, clinical, digital, 32°C–43°C
13. Scale, baby, electronic, 10 kg <5 g>
14. Pulse oximeter, bedside, neonatal
15. Stethoscope, binaural, neonate
16. Sphygmomanometer, neonate, electronic
17. Light, examination, mobile, 220–12 V
18. Hub cutter, syringe
19. Tape, measure, vinyl-coated, 1.5 m
20. Basin, kidney, stainless steel, 825 mL
21. Tray, dressing, stainless steel, $300 \times 200 \times 30$ mm^3
22. Stand, infusion, double-hook, on castors
23. Indicator, TST control spot/PAC-300
24. Irradiancemeter for PTx units
25. Monitor, vital sign, NIBP, HR, SpO_2, ECG, RR, Temp
26. Monitor, vital sign, NIBP, HR, SpO_2, ECG, RR, Temp
27. ECG unit, three-channel, portable/SET
28. Infantometer, Plexiglas, 3½ ft/105 cm
29. X-ray, mobile
30. Transport incubator, basic, with battery and O_2, w/o ventilator
31. Autoclave, steam, benchtop, 20 L, electrical
32. Laundry washer dryer, combo, 5 kg
    Equipment for disinfection:
1. Drum, sterilizing, 165-mm diameter
2. Electric sterilizer
3. Washing machine with dryer
4. Gowns for staff and mothers
5. Washable slippers
    Laboratory equipment:
1. Centrifuge, Hematocrite, benchtop, up to 12,000 rpm, including rotor
2. Microscope, binocular, with illuminator
3. Bilirubinometer, total bilirubin, capillary-based
4. Glucometer with Dextrostix
    General equipment:
1. Air conditioner (1.5 tonne)
2. Generator set 25–50 kVA
3. Refrigerator, hot zone, 110 L
4. Voltage servo-stabilizer (three-phase): 25–50 kVA
5. Room heater (oil)
6. Computer with printer
7. Spot lamps
8. Wall clock with second hand
    Renewable and consumable items:
1. Adaptor, meconium aspirator, disposable (for suction pump)

2. Line, infusion pump, sterile, disposable
3. Multistix, urine, five-parameter, Glu, Prot, Eryt, Spc Grav, pH
4. Cuvettes, Glu, box of 200
5. Cuvettes, Hb, box of 200
6. Vacuum tube, EDTA, 3 mL, set of 100
7. Vacuum tube, EDTA, 6 mL, set of 100
8. Vacuum tube, serum, 3 mL, set of 100
9. Vacuum tube, holder, set of 100
10. Vacuum tube, needle, 22 G set of 100
11. Lancet, safety, sterile, single-use/PAC-200 (1.8 mm)
12. Capillary tubes, box of 1000
13. Sealing compound, capillary tubes, pck 500 g
14. Mask, surgical, disposable, box of 100
15. Cap, surgical, disposable, box of 100
16. Cord clamp, disposable, set of 10
17. Extractor, mucus, 20 mL, ster, disp Dee Lee
18. Tube, suction, CH10, L50 cm, ster, disp
19. Tube, suction, CH12, L50 cm, ster, disp
20. Tube, feeding, CH05, L40 cm, ster, disp
21. Tube, feeding, CH06, L40 cm, ster, disp
22. Tube, feeding, CH07, L40 cm, ster, disp
23. Syringe, dispos, 1 mL, ster/BOX-100
24. Syringe, dispos, 2 mL, ster/BOX-100
25. Syringe, dispos, 5 mL, ster/BOX-100
26. Syringe, dispos, 10 mL, ster/BOX-100
27. Syringe, dispos, 20 mL, sterile/BOX-80
28. Needle, disp, 22 G, ster/BOX-100
29. Needle, disp, 24 G, ster/BOX-100
30. Needle, disp, 26 G, ster/BOX-100
31. Needle, scalp vein, 21 G, ster, disp
32. Needle, scalp vein, 25 G, ster, disp
33. Gloves, exam, latex, medium, disp/BOX-100
34. Gloves, surg, seven, ster, disp, pair
35. Infusion set, paediatric, with chamber 150 mL, ster, disp, with 22-G needle
36. Cotton wool, 500 g, roll, non-ster
37. Compress, gauze, 10×10 cm^2, n/ster/PAC-100
38. Compress, gauze, 10×10 cm^2, ster/PAC-5

Ethical Issues in the NICU

Ethical issues arise as a part of the rapid advancement of technology, economic changes, resource constraints and problems of health care delivery. Because of the nature of their career, health team members are constantly exposed to ethical issues and challenges such as end-of-life care, use of advanced technology and medical errors. Neonatal wards are filled with moral conflicts. Amazing advances in care of critically ill neonate challenge the established standards and clear procedures.

Essential Aspects of Care and Ethical Constraints

Skilled professional care: Do we have a trained team of professionals to give the skilled professional care? Skilled professional care in the NICU is the simple application of critical care technology such as ventilators/monitors, medications, invasive devices and a multiplicity of laboratory measurements to the sick and premature newborn. An effective team is essential, as no single person can do this alone.

Physical Constraints

Care is extended over a necessarily limited time period. The developmental needs of a growing infant cannot be met in the NICU environment from the standpoint of staffing, time use and patient access and interaction throughout the passing months.

Conclusion of Care

The care provided starts with stabilization of the newborn and facilitation of the transition to normal extrauterine neonatal physiology. This transition takes a longer time in some neonates and requires specific interventions and support. The reversal of acute disease process is considered as the end, e.g. RDS, MAS, infection, etc.

Iatrogenic Effects

These include minimizing chronic or debilitating sequelae of applied neonatal intensive care. The potential for negative iatrogenic effects needs to be identified such as effects of result from:
- Environment in which baby is managed (light, noise, touch)
- Mode of ventilation (conventional, synchronized, high frequency), types, doses and results of medication used
- Short- and long-term effects of certain painful procedures
- Foreign bodies or devices used
- How nutritional needs are met (enteral or parenteral nutrition)
  Expected outcome of ethical care
  Providing care that is reasonable for steady improvement is essential. Such care
- Should be with the absence of pain and avoidable suffering
- Develop care towards a capacity for the newborn to experience and enjoy human experience over a life prolonged beyond infancy

Parents

Maintain focus on the best interest of the child.

Parents are considered as spokespersons: Seek their opinions and provide care negotiated for the best interest of the child by the parents.

Shared decision-making is a commonly used process among relevant care providers and a willingness and capability to communicate effectively with the parents.

Medical futility of care must be determined in the context of goals and the likelihood, as well as appropriateness, of applied intervention achieving the desired ends. Availability of ethical guidelines for practice is essential in deciding on certain type of treatments. For example, 'do not resuscitate' orders developed and promulgated by professional societies and ethicists have assisted in day-to-day management of numerous difficult issues, including determining brain death and withdrawal or withholding of life-sustaining therapy.

Positive Aspects of Ethical Guidelines

- Ethical guidelines reflect experts' thoughts on different aspects. A group of experts will be involved in preparation of guidelines. They examine all positive and negative aspects of any intervention before reaching a conclusion of a guideline. So a guideline shows expertise.
- Ethical guidelines enable health care professionals from constraints of what to do in a particular situation.
- It encourages the health care team to make appropriate decision and promote teamwork, best strategies for communication and in confronting issues.
- It empowers the health care team and parents involved in a particular case.
- It is informative to all, especially novice, and helps mentor the novice by the experts or seniors.

Negative Aspects of Ethical Guidelines:

- They are incomplete in nature. Not all health care cases fall under the general guideline parameters. Consistency may not result in every case, even with the best-intended guidelines.
- Guidelines are sometimes imperfect. They stay only as a starting point. It requires much expertise and clinical judgement from the part of users, as they appear to be simple anecdotes of experience. One must remember that one cannot resolve the hurt associated with the emotional investment made toward patient care when outcomes are dismal.

Important point to be remembered while preparing guidelines:
- They should be based on facts and experience.
- They should be updated frequently to be based on currency of issues and based on current political and sociocultural practices. It should reflect the new paradigm (social, political, technological and fiscal influences).
- They should hold the responsibility to public when disclosure is necessary. Guidelines should stem from the principles of respect for persons, patient autonomy, avoidance of harm and maximizing benefit. This will keep the guidelines within their true nature of fiduciary, or trust-based, relationships between health care professionals and their patients.
- The guidelines should have the capacity for patient advocacy.
- They hold the concept of good and beneficence. So what is good for the critically ill neonate must be addressed in the guidelines. Health care professionals are considered as healers. So, the guideline should reflect faith, shared cultural heritage and image of health and health care.
- They should be based on the best interest of the patient and family.

Ethics and Communication Process at the NICU

All hospitals have protocols for practice. It is advisable to have guidelines for ethical practice, too. Parents look upon health care professionals as experts; they would like to get the opinion and explanation for any care provided to their newborns. So, in communicating the care needs to parents of neonates in the NICU, it is essential to develop consensus on care protocol between professionals before communicating them to the parents. The health care professionals should be able to discuss pros and cons of a particular intervention with the parents in a clear and understanding manner without using jargon. The health care members should be aware that parents may have difficulty in communicating, though they have their wishes about their neonate but the timing of premature deliveries may not afford them to express their wishes properly. The guidelines on communication should not dictate medical care but facilitate parent–health care professional communication for the decision-making process. They need to be **empowered** in decision making.

Health care professionals should **use a cautious approach** and should be aware that the resource they use for a very serious neonate may compromise the care of other less serious neonates such as late preterm or term infants who have better prognosis. **Allocating scarce resources** to provide the needs of all babies is difficult. The professionals should use such resources **judiciously** so that better use of resources should be made to benefit the most. One must remember that what is used for one neonate is unavailable to the other. While using available technologies and interventions, one should be aware that valuing the technology over human nature of the neonate, family and clinical staff to be curtailed. This may create burden of pain, suffering and moral angst among them.

STUDY QUESTIONS

1. Define a high-risk neonate.
2. How will you classify high-risk neonates?
3. What are the risk factors for high-risk neonates?
4. What are the common health problems faced by low-birth-weight babies?
5. Differentiate between LBW and SFD.
6. Explain Usher's criteria.
7. Explain the causes of prematurity?
8. List the risk factors of prematurity.
9. What are the lifestyle factors leading to preterm labour?
10. What are the physical characteristics of a preterm neonate?
11. What are the common problems of a preterm infant?
12. Define RDS. Explain the care of a preterm baby with RDS.
13. What is surfactant therapy?
14. Define ROP. Explain the medical and nursing management of a preterm with ROP.
15. What is meconium aspiration syndrome (MAS)? How will you treat and care a baby with MAS?
16. What is neutral thermal environment (NTE)? How will you maintain NTE?
17. What are the indications of inadequate thermoregulation?
18. How will you prevent and treat hypothermia?
19. What are the causes of hypoglycaemia in neonates? How will you manage hypoglycaemia in neonates?
20. What are the reasons of hypocalcaemia in neonates?
21. What are the causes of neonatal seizures?
22. How will you manage neonatal seizures?
23. What are the neonatal infections? How will you manage neonatal sepsis?
24. How will you prevent infection in the NICU?
25. What are the common signs of pain in neonates?
26. What are the nonpharmacological and pharmacological modalities of pain management in neonates?
27. What is hyperbilirubinaemia? Explain Kramer' criteria.
28. What is phototherapy? How will you use phototherapy for neonatal jaundice?
29. Differentiate between physiological and pathological jaundice.
30. Explain the role of a neonatal nurse in exchange transfusion.
31. Explain developmental supportive care.
32. What are ABO incompatibility and Rh incompatibility?
33. Explain breast milk jaundice.
34. What is NEC? Explain the clue of a neonate with NEC.
35. Explain the care of a neonate born to a diabetic mother?
36. Discuss the care of a neonate with polycythaemia.
37. Why is it important to differentiate hyperviscosity in polycythaemia and diarrhoea?
38. How will you manage a neonate with seizures?
39. What are the usual causes of neonatal seizures?
40. Explain the role of a nurse in planning an NICU.

BIBLIOGRAPHY

1. Anand, K.J.S., Hickey, P.R. (1987). Pain and Its Effects in Human Neonate and Fetus. *New England Journal of Medicine*, 317(21), pp 1321–1329.
2. Altimer L, Lutes L. Changing units for changing times: The evolution of a NICU. *Neonatal Intensive care*. 2000;13(6):23–27.
3. Apgar, V. (1953). A Proposal for a New Method of Evaluation of the New Born Infant. *Current Research in Anesthesia and Analgesia*, 32, pp 260–267.
4. American Academy of Pediatrics Subcommittee on Hyperbilirubinemia. Management of hyperbilirubinemia in the newborn infant 35 or more weeks of gestation. *Pediatrics*. 2004;114:297–316.
5. American Academy of Pediatrics, Committee on Fetus and Newborn and Section on Surgery; Canadian Paediatric Society, Fetus and Newborn Committee. Prevention and Management of Pain in the Neonate: An Update. *Pediatrics*. 2006;118:2231–2241.
6. Avery, G.B., Fletcher, M.A., MacDonald, M.G. (1994). Neonatology: Pathophysiology and Management of the New Born. 4th Edn. Philadelphia: J.B. Lippincott.
7. Bang, A. T., Bang, R. A., Baitule, S. B., Reddy, M. H., & Deshmukh, M. D. (1999). Effect of home-based neonatal care and management of sepsis on neonatal mortality: Field trail in rural India. *Lancet*, 354, 1955–1961.
8. Bang, A. T., Bang, R. A., Reddy, H. M., Deshmukh, M. D., & Baitule, S. B. (2005). Reduced incidence of neonatal morbidities: Effect of home-based neonatal care in rural Gadchiroli. *India Journal of Perinatology*, 25, S51–S61.
9. Berger, L.R., Schaefer, A.R. (Feb 1985). Review: The Premature Infant Goes Home. *American Journal of Diseases of Children*, 139, pp 200–202.

10. Brian S Carter. (2017). Ethical Issues in Neonatal Care Medscape. com. Pediatrics: Cardiac Disease and Critical Care Medicine. Updated: Apr 28, 2017

11. Carbajal R, Eble b, Anand KJS. Premedication for tracheal intubation in neonates: Confusion or controversy? *Seminars in Perinatology.* 2007;31:309–317.

12. Cignacco E, Hamers JP, Stoffel L, van Lingen RA, Gessler P, McDougall J, Nelle M. The efficacy of non-pharmacological interventions in the management of procedural pain in preterm and term neonates. A systematic literature review. *Eur J Pain.* 2007;11:139–52.

13. Cornblath M, Hawdon JM, Williams AF, et al. Controversies regarding definition of neonatal hypoglycemia: suggested operational thresholds. *Pediatrics.* 2000;105:1141–5.

14. Coughlin M, Gibbins S, Hoath S. Core measures for developmentally supportive care in neonatal intensive care units: theory, precedence and practice. *Journal of Advanced Nursing.* 65(10), 2239–2248.

15. Cuttini M, Casotto V, Orzalesi M, Euronic Study G. Ethical issues in neonatal intensive care and physicians' practices: a European perspective. *Acta Paediatr Suppl.* 2006;95(452):42–6.

16. Cornblath M, Ichord R. Hypoglycemia in the neonate. *Semin Perinatol.* 2000;24:136–49.

17. Dalal SS, Mishra S, Agarwal R, Deorari AK, Paul V. Does measuring the changes in TcB value offer better prediction of hyperbilirubinemia in healthy neonates? *Pediatrics.* 2009;124:e851–7.

18. Guedert JM, Grosseman S. Ethical problems in pediatrics: what does the setting of care and education show us? *BMC Med Ethics.* 2012;13:2.

19. Hall JH, Johnson BH. Design planning for newborn intensive care. Bethesda, MD, 1997, Institute of Family Centred Care.

20. Hall RW, Boyle E, Young T. Do ventilated neonates require pain management? *Seminars in Perinatology.* 2007;31:289–297.

21. Hall RW, Shbarou RM. Drug of choice for sedation and analgesia in newborn ICU. *Clin Perinatol.* 2009;36:15–26.

22. Halamek LP, Stevenson DK. Neonatal Jaundice. In Fanroff AA, Martin RJ (Eds): Neonatal Perinatal Medicine. Diseases of the Fetus and Infant. 7th ed. St Louis, Mosby Year Book 2002. pp 1335.

23. Hutton EK, Hassan ES. Late vs early clamping of the umbilical cord in full-term neonates: systematic review and meta-analysis of controlled trials. *JAMA.* 2007;297:1241–52.

24. Iype M, Prasad M, Nair PM, Geetha S, Kailas L. The newborn with seizures – a follow-up study. *Indian Pediatr.* 2008;45:749–52.

25. Kumar P, Denson SE, Mancuso TJ. Premedication for Nonemergency Endotracheal Intubation in the Neonate. *Pediatrics.* 2010; 125;608–615.

26. Kumar A, Bhat BV. Epidemiology of respiratory distress of newborns. *Indian J Pediatr.* 1996;63:93–8.

27. Kramer LI. Advancement of dermal icterus in jaundiced newborn. *Am J Dis Child.* 1969;118:454–8.

28. Kaur S, Chawla D, Pathak U, Jain S. Predischarge non-invasive risk assessment for prediction of significant hyperbilirubinemia in term and late preterm neonates. *J Perinatol.* 2011 Nov 17. doi: 10.1038/jp.2011.170

29. Lehr VT, Taddio A. Topical anesthesia: clinical practice and practical considerations. *Semi Perinatology.* 2007;31:323–329.

30. Lucas A, Morley R. Outcome of neonatal hypoglycemia. *Br Med J.* 1999;318:194.

31. Mackintosh TF, Walkar CH. Blood viscosity in the newborn. *Arch Dis Child.* 1973;48:54–53.

32. Kadivar, M., Mosayebi, Z., Asghari, F., & Zarrini, P. (2015 Feb 4). Ethical challenges in the neonatal intensive care units: perceptions of physicians and nurses; an Iranian experience. *J Med Ethics Hist Med,* 8:1. Published online

33. Manskopf, et al. (1995). Measuring Neonatal Assessment. Neonatal Network. 9(4), pp 17–22.

34. Streeter, N.S. Oehler, J.M., Goldstein, R.F., Catlett, A., Boshkoff, M., Brazy, J.E. (1993). How to Target Infants at High Risk for Developmental Delay. MCN. *American Journal of Maternal and Child Nursing.* 18(1), pp 20–23.

35. Madan A, Mac Mohan JR, Stevenson DK. Neonatal Hyperbilirubinemia. In: Avery's Diseases of the Newborn. Eds: Taeush HW, Ballard RA, Gleason CA. 8th edn; WB Saunders., Philadelphia, 2005: pp 1226–56.

36. Maisels MJ, Gifford K. Normal serum bilirubin levels in newborns and effect of breast-feeding. *Pediatrics.* 1986;78:837–43.

37. Mehta S, Kumar P, Narang A. A randomized controlled trial of fluid supplementation in term neonates with severe hyperbilirubinemia. *J Pediatr.* 2005;147:781–5.

38. Merenstein, G.B, Gardner, S.L. (1985). Handbook of Neonatal Intensive Care. St Louis: CV Mosby.

39. Mercurio MR. The role of a pediatric ethics committee in the newborn intensive care unit. *J Perinatol.* 2011;31(1):1–9.

40. National Neonatal Perinatal Database. Report for the year 2002–03. http://www.newbornwhocc.org/pdf/nnpd_report_2002-03. PDF (accessed Jan 8, 2012).

41. Numminen OH, Leino-Kilpi H. Nursing students' ethical decision-making: a review of the literature. *Nurse Educ Today.* 2007; 27(7):796–807.

42. Oden J, Bourgeois M. Neonatal endocrinology. *Indian J Pediatr.* 2000;67:217–23.

43. Oh W. Neonatal polycythemia and hyperviscosity. *Pediatr Clin North Am.* 1986;33:523–32.

44. Ramamurthy RS, Brans WY. Neonatal Polycythemia I. Criteria for diagnosis and treatment. *Pediatrics.* 1981;68:168–74.

45. Martin, G. I. (Ed.), (2003). Recommended standards for newborn ICU design [Theme supplement]. *Journal of Perinatology,* 23(n1s).

46. Rennie J, Burman-Roy S, Murphy MS. Guideline Development Group. Neonatal jaundice: summary of NICE guidance. *BMJ.* 2010 May 19;340:c2409. doi:10.1136/bmj.c2409.

47. Schauberger CW, Pitkin RM. Maternal-perinatal calcium relationships. *Obstet Gynecol.* 1979;53:74–6.

48. Stevens B, Johnston C, Petryshen P, Taddio A. Premature Infant Pain Profile: development and initial validation. *Clin J Pain.* 1996;12:13–22.

49. Stevens B, Yamada J, Ohlsson A. Sucrose for analgesia in newborn infants undergoing painful procedures. *Cochrane Database of Systematic Reviews.* 2004, Issue 3. Art. No.: CD001069.

50. Shah PS, Aliwalas LL, Shah VS. Breastfeeding or breast milk for procedural pain in neonates. *Cochrane Database of Systematic Reviews.* 2006, Issue 3. Art. No.: CD004950.

51. Sharma J, Bajpai A, Kabra M et al. Hypocalcemia – Clinical, biochemical, radiological Profile and follow-up in a Tertiary hospital in India. *Indian Pediatrics.* 2002;39:276–282.

52. Saarenmaa E, Huttunen P, Leppaluoto J, et al. Advantages of fentanyl over morphine in analgesia for ventilated newborn infants after birth: a randomized trial. *J Pediatr.* 1999;134:144–50.

53. Sundean LJ, McGrath JM. Ethical considerations in the neonatal intensive care unit. *Newborn Infant Nurs Rev.* 2013;13(3): 117–20.

54. van Imhoff DE, Dijk PH, Weykamp CW, Cobbaert CM, Hulzebos CV; BARTrial Study Group. Measurements of neonatal bilirubin and albumin concentrations: a need for improvement and quality control. *Eur J Pediatr.* 2011;170:977–82.

55. Volpe JJ, editor. Neurology of the newborn. 5th ed. Philadelphia: Saunders Elsevier, 2008. p. 203–44.

56. Wambach JA, Hamvas A. Respiratory distress syndrome in the neonate. In Martin RJ, Fanaroff AA, Walsh MC, eds. *Fanaroff and Martin's Neonatal-Perinatal Medicine.* 10th ed. Philadelphia, PA: Elsevier Saunders; 2015:chap. 72.

57. Wirth FH, Goldberg KE, Lubchenco LO. Neonatal hyperviscocity I. Incidence. *Pediatrics.* 1979;63:833–6.

58. Whaley, L., Wong, D. (1995). Whaley & Wong's Nursing Care of Infants and Children. 5th Edn. St. Louis: CV Mosby.

59. Young Infants Clinical Signs Study Group. Clinical signs that predict severe illness in children under age 2 months: a multicentre study. *Lancet.* 2008;371:135–42.

UNIT 6

CARE OF A HOSPITALIZED CHILD

Unit 6 deals with care of hospitalized children, their stresses, and parental and family issues along with care of a dying and critically ill child. The chapter on care of children undergoing surgery gives an account of pre- and postoperative care of children.

CARE OF HOSPITALIZED CHILDREN

LEARNING OBJECTIVES

At the end of the chapter, the learner will be able to:
- Discuss the reactions of children of different developmental stages to hospitalization.
- Explain the responses of children of various age group towards hospitalization.
- Discuss the nursing interventions to address the response to hospitalization.
- Describe the parental reactions towards hospitalization,
- Explain the factors influencing reactions of parents.
- Discuss the sibling's reaction towards hospitalization.
- Describe the coping strategies used by parents, children and siblings towards hospitalization.

LEARNING OBJECTIVES—cont'd

- Explain the nurse's role in reducing stress and anxiety towards hospitalization.
- Describe the age-appropriate nursing interventions to reduce anxiety and promote better coping among children of various age group, parents and siblings.
- Explain the modality of helping children to cope with death of a parent and family member.
- Explain the stages of death and dying.
- Explain the common frames of support for children of all ages.
- Explain how to break a bad news.
- Explain emotional labour.

Hospitalization of children is anxiety producing for children, parents, siblings and other family members. Children are considered as the most valuable assets by parents, and this creates more stress among parents. Because of the unique characteristics of children belonging to different developmental ages, their care requires additional skills on the part of caregivers.

RESPONSE TO HOSPITALIZATION

Hospitalization is a frightening experience for children who are striving to attain proper developmental tasks. Their response to hospitalization depends on the following:
- Developmental level and coping mechanisms
- Parent–child relationships
- Cultural and religious influences
- Previous experience with hospitalizations
- Nature of illness
- Children's perception and knowledge of the event

The major threats imposed by hospitalization in children include the following:
- Physical harm or bodily injury
- Separation from parents and the absence of trusted adults
- Strange and unknown environment
- Uncertainty about limits and expected acceptable behaviour
- Loss of control
- Autonomy and competence

Children at different developmental stages perceive these threats with different meanings. The fear of separation, physical harm or bodily injury and loss of control are discussed in detail as they apply to each age group. Fear of the strange and unknown and uncertainty about limits are included along with the discussion on coping with hospitalization.

INFANCY

At 0–5 months of age, infants are not yet attached strongly to the primary caretakers. But stress as a result of a change in caregivers or in the number of caregivers and change in the environment can be detected through altered sleeping, feeding and elimination patterns. Stranger anxiety surfaces between 5 and 7 months of age when the infant shows displeasure at the approach of unfamiliar people. Separation anxiety appears between 7 and 9 months of age. By this time, the infant is attached to the primary caregiver and is upset when separated.

EARLY CHILDHOOD

Separation anxiety peaks around 18 months of age. Separation from parents can be extremely traumatic for toddlers and preschoolers. The level of separation anxiety experienced by the child depends on development, previous experience with separation and the level of social contacts outside the family. Separation from parents or the primary caregiver threatens the feelings of autonomy and sense of initiative that the child is trying to achieve in the toddlerhood and preschool ages.

Robertson described three stages of separation anxiety in children if separated from their mother: protest, despair and denial. Some children who are hospitalized for only a short period of time do not advance beyond the stage of protest, but others reach the stage of despair. Children hospitalized for a long period of time and who are cared for by different nurses may progress to the stage of denial. Maccoby's research has demonstrated that although separation from the mother is more intense, the child begins to respond to separation from the father around 15 months of age.

Physical Harm or Bodily Injury

Toddlers and preschoolers are unable to understand the reason for hospitalization. They view hospitalization as punishment for wrongdoing. Children of preschool age may misunderstand the meaning of procedures. A child of this age is prone to fantasies of mutilation. This is specific to body parts that are developmentally important, such as the genitals, and to sensitive areas, such as the eyes and ears. (See guidelines for physical assessment.)

Loss of Control

Hospitalization threatens the feeling of mastery over basic tasks that children accomplish at each developmental age. Children who are placed in an environment with strangers are likely to regress to earlier stages of development to cope with the stress. The child usually gives up the most recently learned behaviour, such as toilet training or drinking from a cup. Children may react violently to restraining procedures by kicking, screaming and pulling away. Nurses who do not understand tend to increase physical restraint to perform a procedure. But more restraint leads to more intense rebellion and a no-win cycle is established. To cope with the threats of hospitalization, children regress to earlier stages of development. Children give up the most recently learned behaviour, such as toilet training or drinking from a cup.

MIDDLE CHILDHOOD

Separation

During the early school-age years, the child develops relationships with people outside the family. Although separation anxiety is not as obvious in this age as in the early childhood, separation from the family, friends and usual environment poses a threat to the independence and new relationships the child has begun to establish. Regression to an earlier stage of development is also common in this age group.

Physical Harm or Bodily Injury

School-aged children are cognitively able to understand about their illness. Their depth of understanding is limited, which frequently leads to misconceptions and the view that the hospitalization is a result of their own wrongdoings. These children are afraid of what will happen to their bodies in situations in which they are not in control, such as during surgery when they are under anaesthesia or during a major procedure when they are heavily sedated.

Loss of Control

Fear of loss of control intensifies in the middle childhood. As the child's sense of independence increases with new experiences, so also his/her sense of control. Hospitalization threatens the child's mastery over new skills. The young school-aged child fears loss of control in situations, such as surgery and anaesthesia. For example, the child may be afraid of what he/she might say while under anaesthesia.

NURSING INTERVENTIONS TO ADDRESS RESPONSE TO HOSPITALIZATION

Response	Expected Behaviour	Nursing Interventions
Infancy, 5–12 months		
Stranger anxiety	Cries when approached by the nursing staff and physicians; clings to parents.	Allow parents to remain present during procedures. Provide consistent caregivers.
Separation anxiety	Cries when parents leave, may reject attempts to comfort.	Encourage rooming in and liberal visiting hours.
Early childhood, 1–5 years	**Protest**	
Separation	Cries loudly when the mother leaves, may continue to cry for several minutes or hours, throws self about in the bed, rejects attempts to comfort.	Encourage rooming in. Permit liberal visiting hours. Suggest ways that parents can spend more time at the hospital, if appropriate. Allow child to bring toys, stuffed animals, blankets, etc. from home.
	Despair	
	Appears to have settled in, but really has increased hopelessness that parents will return, less active, cries intermittently, makes no demands on the environment; if parents return, may cry loudly releasing anger.	Have parents leave something of their own each time they leave. Keep pictures of family at bedside. Encourage family to make tapes with parents and siblings talking to child, singing favourite songs etc. Provide consistent caregivers.
	Denial	
	Hopeless of parents' return. Show more interest in the environment. Plays, smiles and does not cry if parents return and leave again.	Careful assessment of the child's response to separation through therapeutic play. Spend extra time with the child who is alone. Encourage play with other children on the unit.
Physical harm or bodily injury	Kicks screams and pulls away during procedures. May become upset and cry if the procedure is mentioned.	Explain all procedures carefully to the child old enough to understand simple explanations. Be truthful about whether or not the procedure is painful. Explain to the child why he/she must hold still and how to do so. Allow parents to be present during procedures to provide comfort and not to hold child down. Demonstrate the procedure on dolls when surgery is anticipated. Tell that he/she will be operated on only the problem area.
Loss of control	Regress to earlier stage of development (bottle, pacifier, bedwetting). Protest attempts to perform procedure.	Allow control when possible (e.g. choice about which leg for injection, which pill to be taken first). Allow child to wear underpants to surgery, if possible.
Middle childhood, 6–8 years and preadolescents, 7–12 years		
Separation	May be sad when parents leave. Cheerful when family and friends visit. Talks to friends on phone. May request a roommate.	Encourage family and friends to visit. Allow frequent phone calls. Assist if needed. Plan activities on the unit that encourage interactions with other parents. Assign to room with the same-age, same-sex patient if feasible.
Physical harm or bodily injury	May become upset during procedures. Express concern about what will happen to body, especially during surgery.	Assess understanding of all procedures. Clarify misconceptions. Explain exactly what body part will be affected and what it will look afterwards. Use models, pictures, body outlines, dolls with tubing, dressings, etc. Provide opportunity for therapeutic play.

Continued

Response	Expected Behaviour	Nursing Interventions
Loss of control	May regress to earlier stage of development (increased dependency on parents). Express fears related to anaesthesia. May ask about waking up during surgery, saying things while under anaesthesia.	Allow child to participate in decision making and self-care. Assess feelings about hospitalization and surgery through therapeutic play. Explain anaesthesia as a special sleep and assure he/she will not wake up during surgery. Explain purpose of side rails, dietary changes, etc.
Adolescent Separation	Like to be separated from parents for some time but prolonged separation produces stress.	Encourage parents to visit regularly. Provide consistent caregivers. Assist parents in understanding their adolescent's need to be in control while recovering. Support communication with peers by providing flexible visiting hours for peers whenever possible. Respect the adolescents need to conform to peers' expectations. Encourage verbalization of feelings with regard to peers, peer pressure, etc.
Physical harm or bodily injury		Provide privacy during procedures. Accept aggressive verbal behaviour without retaliating. Encourage verbalization of fears related to death or disability.
Loss of control		Encourage the adolescent's active participation in care. Consult the adolescent about the plan of care. Be flexible about hospital routines whenever possible. Promote cognitive mastery by asking the adolescent to explain what he/she knows. Be aware of intellectualization. Clarify misconceptions. Accept temporary withdrawal. Encourage expression of emotion by reflecting the adolescent's feelings. Respect the adolescent's need for independence.

PARENTAL RESPONSE TO HOSPITALIZATION OF CHILDREN

Reactions of parents to hospitalization of their child are unique. Individual personalities and coping styles, religious beliefs, cultural differences, previous experience in similar situations, the nature of the illness and the parents knowledge and understanding of the hospitalization all influence responses. Additionally, current life stresses play a very important role in their reactions, suggesting that the same parent might react differently on different occasions. For example, a mother might show much more emotion and difficulty with the hospitalization when her support people are unavailable than when they are able to accompany her to the hospital. Recent illness or death in the family, change in the family structure and financial difficulties are other examples of stresses that might affect parents' response to the hospitalization of a child. The nurse must assess parents' reactions during each hospital admission and must avoid preconceived notions regarding how they will respond.

The factors influencing the reactions of parents are as follows:

Whether admission is scheduled or not, most parents exhibit a certain level of anxiety. Behaviours that are observed in parents are crying, nervousness, asking numerous questions, impatience, aggression and anger. During emergency admissions, such as accidents, parents feel somewhat responsible and this increases parental anxiety, thus affecting other children at home. Parents may feel torn between waiting to stay with the hospitalized child and needing to be at home with other children. Parents who are not willing to leave their hospitalized child often find someone such as grandmother, relatives or friends to stay with other children. This also causes some level of anxiety. On the contrary, admission of an only child to the hospital can also be anxiety producing. Parents may fear that they will lose their only child, adding to the normal stress of hospitalization. The common stresses the parents face during hospitalization and pain of surgical interventions of their child are fourfold. They are as follows:

- Caring stress   Extra input of care
  - Neglect of other children's care in the family
  - Disturbed behaviour of the child
- Pain-induced emotional stress   Personal distress
  - Pain distress
  - Knowledge-deficit distress
- Social stress   Altered social life
  - Interpersonal problems
- Financial stress   Financial implications

The other commonly identified factors affecting parental reactions are fear of strange environment, fear that their child will suffer, fear of infection and contamination, fear of unbearable financial obligation and the fear that society's will look upon the illness as a reflection of some wrongdoing.

SIBLING RESPONSE TO HOSPITALIZATION OF CHILDREN

Hospitalization of a child disrupts the usual routine in the family. Other children in the family have to shoulder added responsibility at home, as parents spend more time at the hospital with the sick child.

Siblings also feel separation anxiety, especially from their mother who stays with the hospitalized child. There are many factors that intensify the effects of hospitalization on siblings. The children who have to stay at someone else home during hospitalization of their sibling experience more anxiety. Parents usually may not realize this. The nurse needs to alert parents about these effects so that potential behavioural changes in the siblings can be avoided.

COPING WITH HOSPITALIZATION

Coping is one's ability to deal with new situations and stressful experiences. Coping strategies are those mechanisms that a person uses consciously to manage stressful situations. The hospitalized child copes with the trauma of hospitalization in a variety of ways depending on age and prior experiences with similar stresses.

Common Age-wise Strategies Used by Children

Age	Coping Strategies
Infancy, 0–12 months	Increased motor activity, restlessness, crying, fussiness, and screaming, sucking, hand–mouth activity
Early childhood, 1–5 years	Regression, resistance, displacement Denial, aggression, protest, striking out, pushing away, making requests, temper tantrums, information seeking, withdrawal, trial and error, experimentation, familiarization, motor activity, play, clinging, comfort seeking, attempts to control and restructure
Middle childhood, 6–8 and 9–12 years	Avoidance, active participation, information seeking, cognitive mastery, rehearsal, repetition, problem solving, motor activity, support seeking, fantasy, denial, sublimation, repression, aggression, protest, resistance, withdrawal, quiet behaviour, sleeping, rejection of others, co-operation, attempts to control and restructure, diversionary thinking, humour, crying, regression, displacement and reaction formation

Many parents cope better with their child's hospitalization by staying with the child and actively participating in their care. Others stay with the child but assume a passive role, observing the hospital staff providing care. Some may not stay with their child. A study conducted by Mary Joseph (2003) to identify coping strategies used by parents of leukaemic children found that the majority of parents used problem-focused coping compared with emotion-focused coping.

Nursing Intervention – Role-related Activities

Though one of the major roles of a paediatric nurse is health maintenance, sometimes children get sick, making hospital admission a necessity. In such a situation, the nurse needs to prepare the child for hospitalization. Hospitalization is often a traumatic experience. But it has certain positive psychological experiences, too. Children who are properly prepared to experience hospitalization have a growth promotional impact as well.

Nurses need to prepare children at various stages of development for hospitalization. Very little can be done in an emergency situation to prepare children for hospitalization, so also in the case of young infants. But in a planned hospitalization, the child will be admitted after a few sessions of hospital visits. Here, the nurse, the physician or the physician assistant in the OPD gets a chance to prepare the child for hospitalization. This will help the nurse identify the particular behavioural characteristics of the child and help prepare the child according to his/her behavioural characteristics. Children who are vocal and mobile can be prepared by creative means if they do not require immediate admission. The common means used in the preparation includes the following:
- Booklets
- Films
- Puppet shows
- Role-play
- Tour to the hospital, etc.

In Western countries, school health nurses arrange programmes to educate parents and children about hospitalizations. The paediatric nurse who is working in a health care facility where children get admitted should practice based on certain ethical beliefs. They are considered as the core beliefs and key to successful nursing practice in a paediatric set-up. These are as follows:
- Children are a part of the family.
- Parents are the most important people for children.
- Children are unique and have needs based on their family environment, culture, stage of development and severity of illness.
- Children have the right to care and need love and security from adults.
- Paediatric nurses, as a professional, need to impart care to children based on their accepted different roles.
- Paediatric nurses are accountable to the care provided to their patients.
- Paediatric nurses should give explicit physical care and emotional support to children in a safe environment to children under their care.
- Paediatric nurses should promote growth and development of children and help promote free expression of feelings.
- Provision of adequate emotional support to children and their family is essential to promote dignity and feeling worthy of a dying child.
- Establishing trusting relationship with children and their family is the key to successful delivery of care.
- Assisting the grief process is a part of professional practice.

Nurses have a variety of interrelated roles to function when caring children at hospital. The amount of time spent in each of these roles also varies according to the age and severity of illness of children. As a caregiver, the nurse uses a wide range of knowledge, techniques and skills to provide the physical aspects of care essential during a child's hospitalization, viz. feeding, bathing, diapering, giving medications, checking vital signs, monitoring fluids, intravenous fluids, etc.

As an advocate for the child and family, the nurse has excellent opportunity to serve them. Nursing advocacy is demonstrated through efforts to reduce unnecessary interruptions of the infant's sleep, to promote optimal nutrition for the child, to promote normal growth and development of the child and to minimize separation from family and friends. The nurse also finds out the need for the parents to talk with doctors/physician regarding their child's condition.

As an educator, the nurse faces challenge of teaching parents whose level of understanding varies to a great extent. The nurse needs to teach and provide anticipatory guidance to the parents.

In nutshell, the nursing responsibilities are as follows:

Roles	Nursing Interventions
Caregiver	Hold the infant or the young child who is separated from his/her parents.
	Stay with the child during the painful procedure.
	Keep parents informed when the surgery is delayed.
	Facilitate communication between the family and health care workers.
	Provide physical care – feeds, bath, medications, etc. and encourage parents to involve in the child's care.
	Plan care to prevent interruptions.
Advocate	Listen attentively to parents who are upset because of their sick child.
	Keep parents informed when the surgery is delayed.
	Facilitate communication between the family and health care workers about the child's illness.
	Encourage siblings' and relatives' visit.
	Allow friends to visit.
Educator	Orient the child and family to the unit.
	Explain the policies of the unit.
	Provide teaching about related subjects.
	Answer their questions.
	Explain procedure appropriate to their age.
	Explain pre- and postoperative care.
	Plan for discharge.
	Warn potential hazards.

Facilitating Coping

Parental involvement in the care of children is important. Those who can provide care must be permitted to do so, as parents are the best person for their children. Parental participation in the daily care provides them an opportunity to find out what is happening to their child. Rooming in and liberal visiting hours help reduce tension and promote well-being in parents. Nurses must be careful not to take over. Nurses may have a feeling that they are the experts and parents may not know many things. For children, parents are the better people. Nurses help parents maintain discipline and provide adequate information to parents and children so that they will cooperate well. Providing safe and therapeutic environment is also important, as it promotes positive coping. Most paediatric wards must be arranged in such a way that it should be children friendly. Paediatric wards can be decorated with bright colours, murals and pictures. Special areas such as an aquarium, playroom and a TV room can be provided.

THERAPEUTIC PLAY

Play is essential in a child's development. Through play, the child achieves language skills, develops gross and fine motor skills, learns about the environment, expresses fears and fantasies, uses imagination and solves problems. Therapeutic play is an aspect of play through which the child can attain a sense of mastery and competency during hospitalization. Therapeutic play is used to assess the child's physical, emotional and developmental status to assess the child's understanding of hospitalization and procedures, to teach the child concepts and procedures, to provide diversionary activities for the child and to provide an outlet for expression of feelings. It is not a play therapy, as this is a technique used to treat emotionally disturbed children

PREPARING CHILDREN TO FACE DEATH OF A FAMILY MEMBER

Most of the time adults are hesitant to talk about death to children. Death and dying are inevitable and inescapable truth of life and everyone is destined to face it, so also are children. Talking about death to children is good to remove their misunderstanding and help them recover their fears, worries and misconceptions related to death. Providing needed information will help them improve comfort and understanding. Understanding about death and dying depends on the age and experience of children. It will also depend on their experiences, beliefs, feelings and the situations. Paediatric nurses need to be equipped with understanding of children's emotional reactions towards death. They need to guide parents to prepare children positively to face the loss through death. The nurses need to have necessary knowledge regarding different aspects of death and dying, children's perception on death and their developmental level. Nurses are usually not directly involved in preparing children. It is the responsibility of a nurse to prepare the parents in order to prepare their children to face death of a family member. Explain to the family that if a family member or a close relative or a friend is seriously ill, then this must be discussed with the child before death occurs. The nurse must understand that children are very sensitive to unusual happenings in their family. Based on this principle, the nurse must prepare family members. If adequate preparation is done, death will not be a complete surprise and the child can cope better, as the child is expecting something that is going to happen. If the child is not prepared adequately, the atmosphere of sadness in the family/home can be very frightening to the child. So, it is necessary for parents or responsible adults to explain what is going on and why they are sad and acting differently.

Talk to Children Soon after a Death Occurs

Long before adults realize it, children become aware of death. They see dead birds, insects and animals lying on the road. Children may see death at least once a day on television. The fairy tales which they hear also may give them an idea of death and act it out in their play. Death is a part of everyday life, and children, at some level, are aware of it.

Adults usually avoid telling children about death of a loved one. This is simply to save them from sadness. But children also must go through the effects of death in the family as a life process. So, early revealing of death by parents will help children deal with loss in a better way than hearing it at a later time. It is always better to reveal the loss by the parents than by other people. First-hand information from parents will promote trust and better coping. Many a time, adults are afraid to talk about things that upset them. Usually, they try to put a lid on their feelings and hope that saying nothing will be the best. But not talking about something does not mean that there is no communication. There are nonverbal communications that provide cues for emotional turmoil. Children are great observers. They read messages on adult faces and in the way they walk or hold their hands. The expressions that are shown by the adults are enough for children to understand something serious had happened. Children may not ask about it, as they find their parents are not talking about it. So, adults must be aware of the **communication barriers,** avoidance, confrontation and the delicate balance between all these. It is not wise to confront children with information that they may not yet understand or want to know. As with any sensitive subject, the adult must seek a delicate balance that encourages children to communicate – a balance that lies somewhere between avoidance and confrontation, a balance that is not easy to achieve. It involves:

- Trying to be sensitive to their desire to communicate when they are ready
- Trying not to put up barriers that may inhibit their attempts to communicate
- Offering them honest explanations when we are obviously upset
- Listening to and accepting their feelings
- Not putting off their questions by telling them they are too young
- Trying to find brief and simple answers that are appropriate to their questions, answers that they can understand and that do not overwhelm them with too many words.

Use Clear and Simple Terms

It is better to explain to children what death means. Parents should make sure that the children understood that the dead person would not be there with them and they will not be able to do any of the things they once did before. For example, they will not share their home, walk, talk, breath, play or bring toys or gifts for them.

No Casual Explanation

Simply telling them that someone has died because of sickness may cause stress and anxiety in children. They may feel that they will also die when they become sick. It must be explained to children that someone sick may not always die. After treatment, they may live for many years. Parents should provide reason on the cause of death in a clear way to the children. Parents also must not equate death with sleep. Children will develop fear going to sleep, as they may think that they will not wake up after sleep. 'Passed away' and 'gone to heaven' are other terms used by adults to explain death to children. Children may not understand these types of explanation. Religious explanations are most often confusing to children. Adults should use words that establish the fact that the body is biologically dead. The explanation given should fit with the developmental level of children. Adults should put their explanation into words that their children can understand and they should be available for answering queries.

Living with Death

Death is a reality that children, like all of us, can learn to live with. Even before the death of a close family member occurs, parents can begin to introduce the idea of death as a part of everyday life. The nurse can guide the parents to initiate talks about death with their children. The dead plant or a dead bird may spark a conversation about death. Start early, be honest and encourage children to talk about their feelings regarding death. Periodic conversations about death are important because understanding death is a gradual process. Children will take in the information as they are ready and increase their understanding as they develop.

Children's Reaction towards Death of a Parent

Children feel the loss of loved ones just as intensely as adults do, although this grief is often expressed in different ways – through play, art or even acting out. Children will cope with grief according to the stressors created by their relationship to the person (or animal) that has died. Death of a parent is usually a stress to children. Three stages of bereavement are observed in young children dealing with death of a parent:

- Protest
  - Anger and fear aimed at reattachment to the lost parent
- Despair
  - Sadness, distance, unresponsiveness
  - May result in psychosomatic symptoms (headaches, enuresis, etc.) or psychological problems (school phobia, depression, poor school performance)
  - Slowly processing the loss

- Detachment
  - Move from depression to increased activity and openness to new relationships

Reactions and Grief Strategies

- Regression to an earlier developmental stage
  - If denied the opportunity to openly grieve a lost parent, the child is likely to remain frozen in the regression.
  - With time and nurturance, the regression will subside.
- Hyperactivity
  - Increased activity to get attention is a common phenomenon.
- Emotional outbursts
  - Angry outbursts and irritability are symptoms of grief, and they may not know how to be poised.
- Overprotectiveness of the surviving parent
  - Preoccupation with the remaining parent's potential death and not even allowing any other people to talk with the remaining parent. They are really scared.
- Constructing the deceased parent
  - Locating, experiencing and reaching out to the deceased parent, waking memories of the parent or cherishing objects shared by the child and the dead parent. The children will not allow other people to touch the materials used by the deceased parent.

Death of a Sibling

- Bereaved siblings show significantly higher levels of behavioural problems and significantly lower social competence than normal children throughout the bereavement period.
- Siblings can tolerate and accept less parental attention and more anxiety if they know what is happening with the dying sibling.
- The anxiety level of children informed about terminal illness and loss is found to be significantly lower than that of uninformed children.
- Bereaved children need explanations, comfort and support.
- Pretense and avoidance can be frightening to anyone in a stressful and painful setting, especially a child.
- If children are involved in grieving of the family, it helps them learn coping strategies they can rely on in dealing with future losses.

Death and Dying – Ages and Stages

Newborn to 3 Years

Even the youngest children sense when their family routine is disrupted and those around them experience emotional upset. However, infants and toddlers have little understanding of death.

Child's Reaction. Elisabeth Kubler-Ross (On Children and Death) described the following reactions:

- 0–6 months:
  - Displays distress from loss by changing sleeping and eating habits
  - Reacts to grief reactions of others

- Needs continuous loving care
- Changes in sleeping, eating and mood
- 6 months to 2 years
  - Does not understand permanence of the loss and will ask for the missing parent
  - May become angry because the parent does not come back and is disinterested in play and food
  - Clinging to caregivers and refusal to let them out of sight
  - Constant loving care is the key

How to Support
- Keep routines and physical setting as familiar as possible.
- Provide constant nurturing. If the parent is too distraught, seek a caring adult substitute.

Ages 3–6 Years

Typically, a child aged 3–6 years will not understand the finality of death. The child may think of it as temporary or magically reversible or may even appear to be unaffected. Fears that dead people may be cold or hungry in the grave are common. Many children at this age may appear unaffected by the death of a loved one. They actually believe that the dead person will return. Some children will assume the responsibility for death. They may think that some of their acts resulted in death of the parent, as they hated them or they had ill feelings about the deceased.

Child's Reaction. They may have frightening dreams, repeat questions about death or revert to earlier behaviours. Children may play out the events surrounding the death. Children in this age will take words literally. Because children have limited experiences, they make sense of the world by connecting events that do not relate. For example, 'Aunt Shiela died from fever. Now mom also has fever. Maybe, she will die, too'. Parents should probe to find out their feelings and provide reassurance to remove guilt feelings. According to Elizabeth Kubler Ross, these children will:

- Ask questions concerning the absence of the parent
- Show anger reaction towards unfulfilled wish of parent's return
- Have magical thinking and thoughts about life in the cemetery
- Cling to their favourite toys

It is important to talk to the children and give them loving attention.

How to Provide Support for Children Aged 3–6 Years. While talking or discussing death with these children:
- Look into the child's eyes and touch the child gently when discussing a death.
- Shorten time away from the child. Be sure he/she knows where you are and how to reach you.
- Avoid words such as *sleeping, resting, loss, passed away, taking a long trip.*
- Talk about what it means to be dead in concrete terms such as *someone doesn't breathe, eat, go to the bathroom or grow.*

- Repeat simple, honest explanations as often as the child asks.
- Reassure the child of his/her own safety and your plan for continued presence. Share that most people die when they are older.
- Allow expressions of feelings such as drawing pictures, reading and telling stories about death or the loved one or re-enacting the funeral service.

Ages 6–9 Years

A child at this age begins to understand the finality of death but not completely. Children may think that death may occur to only old people or to other people. Children may not be able to understand the universality of death. Some children may still think that the dead person will return and take the responsibility of death to their wishful thinking.

Child's Reaction. The child may feel distressed, confused and sad or show no signs at all. Fear of abandonment by other family members is common. Often these children are obsessed with the causes of death, as well as the physical processes to the body after death. According to Elizabeth Kubler Ross, these children have:

- Beginning understanding of the finality of death
- Grieving manifest in changes in behaviour, school performance, anger reactions

It is important to have a trusting relationship which allows the child to talk about his/her grief and distress.

At the age of 9 years, with maturation of abstract thinking processes, most children have mature understanding of the concept of death.

How to Provide Support for Children Aged 6–9 Years

- Be a good listener. Correct any confusing ideas the child may have.
- Provide play opportunities and routine without interruption.
- Reassure the child that the death was not anybody's fault.
- Provide opportunities to open discussion with a quiet child by reading stories related to death.
- A child who chooses not to talk about the death may be comfortable writing or drawing his/her thoughts in a diary. So, help in keeping a diary.

Ages 9–12 Years

Preteens have a better understanding of the finality of death. On the surface, some children in this age range may appear to be unaffected by death. They may see death as a punishment for bad deeds. Some children at this age may take responsibility for death of someone else. They may handle most of the information that can be given to an adult.

Child's Reaction. Anger directed at a variety of people – self, parents, others, the person who died, siblings, etc. Guilt and grief stem from the anger, as do feelings of responsibility. These children also regress. So, some children may not be able to handle all details.

How to Provide Support for Children Aged 9–12 Years

- Assure him/her that the person did not die because he/she was 'bad'.
- Talk about the ways in which things are different and how they are the same.
- Reassure the child that he/she did not cause the death.

Teens

Teens have an adult-like understanding of the finality and irreversibility of death and realization that everyone will die. Even then they need support. They may inappropriately assume responsibility for adult concerns, such as family and financial well-being. Teens may assume the roles of the deceased person or deny feelings and express anger, which creates added pain.

Teens' Reaction. Teens may feel confused, responsible, helpless, angry, sad, lonely, afraid and guilty.

How to Provide Support for Teens

- Talk to the teen without criticizing or judging.
- Express your own feelings about the death.
- Guard against letting the teen assume adult responsibilities and reassure him/her of his/her roles.
- Reassure the teen that he/she did not cause the death.
- Continue to support and listen to the teen's feelings, although he/she may appear to be handling it.
- Allow time for solitude and reflection. Be available to talk within the teen's time frame.

Common Frames of Support for Children of All Ages

- Share information at the child's level of understanding. Find out what the child understands. Reassure the child.
- Talk about and accept feelings. Often, children are left out of the support network of relatives, neighbours and friends.
- Share rituals and do not send children away to stay with relatives or neighbours.
- Be available for ongoing discussions because mourning is a process. Admit that you do not have all the answers.
- Share information in doses the child can handle, small bits at a time. Let the child know it is okay to cry, okay to be angry or okay to be mad.
- Try not to alter daily routine.
- Try not to hide the adult's grief.
- Permit children to attend the funeral of loved one, especially family members.

Children's conceptions of death and personal mortality were studied in relation to age, cognitive developmental factors and life experiences with death or separation/divorce. Sixty children, ranging in age from 5 to 10 years, participated in the study. Children who had experienced the death of a significant other (parent, sibling, close relation or peer) were compared on a variety of measures with children who had experienced parental separation or divorce and with children from intact two-parent families with no experience of death or separation/ divorce. The results indicated that most children who were 6 years or older possessed some belief in the universality of death. A child's understanding of personal mortality was related both to the level of cognitive development and to death-related experience. Children did not differ systematically on measures of personality or adjustment.

Erik Erikson's Model of Lifespan Development on Death and Dying

- Stage 1: Trust versus Mistrust – Infancy
  The infant counts on caretakers to meet his/her basic physiological, social and belonging needs. Based on these experiences, the infant develops understanding of the world as a predictable place. Long-term unpredictable separation may lead to anxious, emotionally defensive reactions in infants. Maternal separation during this period has profound, bad effects on the child's life if there are no suitable surrogates.
- Stage 2: Autonomy versus Shame – Toddler
  A toddler learns what he/she can control (preference of food, preference of toys, excretory functions). Not regarding the child's efforts can lead to feelings of shame, self-doubt and a lasting sense of inferiority. So, toddler's efforts to understand the situation of death need to be considered.
- Stage 3: Initiative versus Guilt – Early childhood 3–6 years
  These children explore environment, initiate new activities and take on new challenges. Lack of encouragement may lead to self-negation, guilt, resentment and unworthiness.
- Stage 4: Industry versus Inferiority – 6 years to adolescence
  These children learn to function in an adult-like world and compare themselves with the standard or others. If the child does not learn strategies to overcome life's challenges and crises, it can, in most extreme cases, result in self-destructive and suicidal behaviours.
  People dealing with children should possess a humanistic perspective. They should remember that:
  - Each human being is unique and the child's reaction to loss depends on his/her unique personal experience, which goes beyond the child–parent bond and stages of cognitive development.
  - To understand a child's grief, his/her individual experience, environmental, familial and cultural backgrounds need to be taken into account.
  - Questioning of stage of theories of development is a key to understanding a child's concepts of death and grief reactions.

THE DYING CHILD

- Terminally ill children as young as 3 years old understand that they are dying and that death is a final and irreversible process. Children may not be able to talk about death but express an understanding of their approaching death in their behaviour.
  - Fear of wasting time, wanting to have things done right away
  - Dislike of talking about the future
  - Absorption with death and disease
  - Distancing from others but show acts of anger and silence
- Stages:
  - Initial awareness of the seriousness of the illness
  - Learn names of various drugs and medical procedures and perceive that they are seriously ill but will get better
  - Learn the purpose of various medical procedures and perceive that they are always ill but will get better
  - After a series of relapses, they perceive that they will never get better
  - After numerous relapses and remissions, they understand that they are dying (often associated with leaning about death of a peer with the same disease)
- Fear and anxiety
  - Separation from parents and other family members
  - Increasing anxiety of medical procedures
  - Increased anxiety because of feelings of fear and anxiety in their family members
- Anger
  - Loss of self-control and independence
  - Often results in developmental regression to an emotional level at which they are no longer independent
  - Some children overcompensate by refusal of help from family and hospital personnel
- Sadness
  - Grieving loss of what they had before the illness (decline in contact with friends, absence from social and other activities, pain, discomfort, decreasing mobility, alterations in body image, etc.)
- Loneliness and isolation
  - Because of the mutual presence of the approaching death, there may be no opportunity for parents and the dying child to truly share their concerns and fears and provide comfort, security and reassurance
  - Children's feelings about death sometimes become masked and repressed

Feelings of a Dying Child

- Often marked by mutual pretense of the approaching death.
- Children may want to maintain the pretense that they are feeling well because they are afraid of being abandoned or rejected.
- ' To let children talk about death, about their fears and feelings, their hopes and despairs, their certainties and uncertainties, their love, and hate, means we are allowing them to talk about life, *their* life, and we are providing them with the only possible help: the presence of another human being until the end.'
- Spiritual needs
  - Prominent in the lives of dying children
  - A positive image of what lies beyond death
  - Reassurance that they will be remembered

- Individual differences
  - Some children are resilient and playful even when their life is ending

BREAKING A BAD NEWS

Buckman (1992) defines breaking a bad news as 'any news that drastically and negatively alters the patient's view of her or his future'. Breaking bad news is one of the most difficult tasks faced by health care professionals. It is more common and difficult in paediatric emergency situations. There are different types of bad news. Even telling a patient that he/she cannot go home after consultation or need to have a blood arranged for transfusion. So, it is the little things that have an impact on day-to-day life and that can have the most profound effect on anyone.

Who will break a bad news?

From time immemorial, doctors have been in charge of delivering bad news to patients or their relatives. But nurses and other health care providers should also be a partner in this activity.

For adequate safety and care, it should be a person who has the best communication skills.

Emotional Labour

Emotional labour is dealing with feelings of others. When breaking a bad news, the health care providers should use emotional labour. So, people who are dealing with emotional labour need to learn to regulate the expression of emotions. The health care provider needs to be empathetic but not too involved in the emotions of others. The nurse or any other health care provider should maintain composure and calmness during breaking of a bad news. Breaking a bad news definitely brings an uncomfortable feeling, and one should learn distancing tactics.

Impact of bad news——, if it is a death

Death is the only irrevocable truth. Everyone knows this, but most of the time it is unacceptable.

Accepting the truth of universality of death is difficult when life is cut short in the bud without fulfilling the purpose of existence. Death is acceptable when it is anticipated. In emergency, it is not anticipated. Family needs to be prepared adequately and emotionally to accept the truth. Family should be informed with compassion and utmost care. Health care professionals must communicate death in no unmistakable terms that the child has died despite their best intentions and efforts.

Emotions of Parents

The common emotions that parents exhibit during breaking of a bad news include the following:

- Anger
- Hostility
- Shock
- Grief
- Guilt
- Denial
- Depression

What is the Nurse's Role?

The nurse must:
- Handle crises with poise, sympathy and empathy.
- Make them understand that this is the will of God or nature's ordain.
- Provide means if family wishes for religious support.
- Accompany parents to the rest room during the intrusive and life-saving procedure.
- Permit parents if they wish to take home the baby in anticipated death.
- Allow the parents to stay with their dying child.
- Do not shunt them away for medical reasons.
- Permit them to be near the child and talk to the child to allay the anxiety of the dying child by having his/her people near to him/her.
- Silently listen, as it is actually the best nursing care that you can provide in such a situation.
- Control your emotions and frustrations.
- Death punctures ego and teaches humility.
- Facing death provides strength to face reality and truth of life.
- Control emotions.
- Caregivers, especially novice nurses, need emotional support, guidance and advice from older nurses.
- Learn the art of detachment, imperturbability and poise in all odds of life.
- Assist autopsy if indicated.
- Do not give impression that autopsy is needed for making diagnosis.
- You may need to communicate that autopsy helps medical science and the family.
- After completing medical formalities, assist the parents in obtaining proper medical certificate (death certificate).
- Do not allow parents to wait because of your reasons.
- Show courtesy and profound respect for humanity and life.
- Every behaviour of yours should reflect this.

Whatever may be the situation, whether it is an emergency or otherwise, nurses who are working in a paediatric set-up should know the rule of the land to provide legal and ethical care to their client and to prevent possible litigations. They also should be cognizant about the implications of ethical principles to provide ethically acceptable care relating to nursing profession. They also should have good communication skills and emotional quotient to provide information to a critically ill child and his/her devastating parents!!!

STUDY QUESTIONS

1. What are the common reactions of children towards hospitalization?
2. What the responses of children towards hospitalization?
3. Discuss the nursing interventions to address the response to hospitalization?

4. Describe the parental reactions towards hospitalization?
5. What are the factors influencing reactions of parents?
6. What are the sibling's reactions towards hospitalization?
7. Describe the coping strategies used by parents, children and siblings towards hospitalization.
8. Explain the nurse's role in reducing stress and anxiety towards hospitalization.
9. Describe the age-appropriate nursing interventions to reduce anxiety and promote better coping among children of various age group, parents and siblings.
10. Explain the modality of helping children to cope with death of a parent or family member.
11. What are the stages of death and dying?
12. What are the common frames of support for children of all ages?
13. What is a bad news? How will you participate in breaking a bad news?
14. What is emotional labour?

BIBLIOGRAPHY

1. Alexander, D., White, M., Powell, G. (1986). Anxiety of Non-Rooming in Parents of Hospitalized Children. Child Health Care, 15, pp 14–20.
2. Algren, C.L. (1984). Role Perception of Mothers Who Have Hospitalized Children. Child Health Care, 14, pp 6–9.
3. Craft, M. J., Wyatt, N., Sandell, B. (1985). Behavior and Feeling Changes in Siblings of Hospitalized Children. Clinical Pediatrics, 24, pp. 374–378.
4. Curry, S.L., Russ, S.W. (1985). Identifying Coping Strategies in Children. Journal of Clinical Child Psychology, 14, pp 61–69.
5. Eberly, T.W., et al. (June, 1985). Parental Stress After the Unexpected Admission of a Child to Intensive Care Unit. Critical Care Quarterly, 8:57.
6. Erickson, E.H. (1968). Identify Youth and Crisis. New York: Norton.
7. Fagin, C. (1966). The effects of maternal attendance during hospitalization on posthospital behaviour of young children: A comparative study. Philadelphia: Davis.
8. Klein, C.B., et al. (1980). Preparation and Hospitalised Child. Journal of Association for the Care of Children's Health, 8:60.
9. Kubler- Ross, E. (1969). On death and dying. Macmillian. New York.
10. Lamontagne, L.L., et al. (Jan/Feb, 1984). Three Coping Strategies Used By School Children. Pediatric Nursing, 10:25.
11. Nelson, M. (May/June, 1981). Identifying the Emotional Needs of the Hospitalised Child. MCN, 6:181.
12. Meng, A.L. (1980). Parents and Children's Reactions Toward Impending Hospitalisation for Surgery. Maternal Child Nurs J, 9:83.
13. Pass, M.D., Pass, C.M. (Aug, 1987). Anticipatory Guidance for Parents of Hospitalised Children. Journal of Pediatric Nursing, 2:250.
14. Standiford, DA., Ahlrichs, J., Carmicle, C. (1993). Extended Day Programme: Bringing Preschool to Hospital. Pediatric Nursing, 19(3), pp 238–241.
15. Vipperman, J.F., et al. (March/April, 1980). Childhood Coping: How Nurses Help. Pediatric Nursing, 6:11.
16. Wong, D.L and Wilson David. (1995). Whaley and Wong's Nursing care of Infants and children. 5th edn. C.V. Mosby, St. Louis.
17. Young, R. (1977). Chronic sorrow: Parent's response to the birth of a child with a defect. American Journal of Maternal and Child nursing 1, 59.

CARE OF CHILDREN UNDERGOING SURGERY

LEARNING OBJECTIVES

At the end of the chapter, the learner will be able to:
- Explain the need for preoperative preparation for children.
- Identify the factors to be considered in preoperative preparation of children.
- Discuss the important developmental issues to be considered while preparing children for surgery.
- Prepare planned teaching programme for preoperative preparation.
- Identify the importance of consent and assent in children.
- Explain the postoperative care of children after surgery.
- Identify the common discomforts and complications of surgery.
- Explain the important nursing care needs of critically ill children.

INTRODUCTION

Hospitalization itself is stressful to children and their family. If a child requires surgery, this stress will be much more than for a usual medical care. A child undergoing surgical intervention creates undue tension among not only parents but also among other family members. It is an event of life and death for common a man. It always attributes an element of threat in surgical interventions. So, it is important for all health care professionals, especially for nurses, to prepare the parents, family members and children in a very comprehensive manner considering their developmental age. Studies have reported that 75% of children experience anxiety and 67% of children show negative behaviours after surgery. So, nurses

need to be cognisant about various aspects of pre- and postoperative care for children undergoing surgery. The factors that need to be considered include developmental age, duration of the procedure, current anxiety level, coping skills present and parents' role in the care of children.

PREPARATION FOR ADMISSION AND SURGERY

For nursing professionals, it is usual to prepare patients for surgery. But there are fundamental differences between children and adults who require a tailored approach to preoperative preparation. It is also important to find out whether the child is going to have an elective surgery or an emergency surgery. The preparation for elective and emergency surgery also varies. The children for elective surgery are considered only if they are systemically well and require little in the way of complex physiological assessment and investigation. However, some children present with a complex congenital disease or an unusual syndrome that requires specific preoperative investigation and preparation. Children requiring emergency surgery may become unwell very quickly, and these children must be recognized so that their conditions need to be optimized prior to surgery.

PREOPERATIVE CARE FOR CHILDREN

Main considerations for pre- and postoperative preparations are as follows:
Child's cognitive and social level of development
Family's perception of the child's health
During the preoperative period, the nurse, parents and the child must become acquainted so as to establish a trusting relationship.
Assess the following before starting preparation:
- Level of knowledge of parents as well as the child
- Anxiety of the child and parents

- Their coping mechanisms
- Pertinent history
- Physical findings
- Reasons for surgery
- Child's response to hospitalization
- Recent exposure to illness
- Previous surgical experiences, if any
- Developmental level
- Family's nature and habits
- Monitor and check vital signs
- Level of consciousness
- Level of hydration
- Blood workup
- Weight and height
- Respiratory status

Preoperative teaching must include their specific needs according to the assessment findings.

Routine interventions include the following:

- Orient the child and family to the unit and important places – place of postanaesthetic check-up (PAC), laboratories, operation theatre, etc. Usually, the child who is having elective surgery will be admitted to the hospital at least once prior to surgery. Preadmission programmes are now used in major corporate hospitals in India and aid in preparation of the child for surgery.

  These programmes may include a tour of the children's unit, videos, printed material and the use of play, including role rehearsal. The disadvantages of such programmes are that they are labour-intensive, expensive and time-consuming. Day case surgery provides the least disruption to the child's routine and has been shown to reduce postoperative behavioural problems; it should be encouraged where possible. In most developed centres, paediatric surgical procedures are done as day procedures if possible to reduce the emotional trauma associated with hospitalization.

- Discuss the surgical procedure in a nonthreatening manner with the child and family members according to their level of understanding. Preassessment should allow for a thorough explanation of the perioperative sequence of events to the child and parents. Preparation of the parents is crucial in reducing parental anxiety. Parents should be encouraged to ask questions about any concerns they may have. It has been shown that children with anxious parents are more likely to display signs of perioperative anxiety themselves. Explanation may be given through the use of videos, booklets and written instructions, as well as face-to-face. Use simple language and careful not to use jargon.

- Plan and provide preoperative teaching based on the level of comprehension of the child and family members.

  - Children younger than 2 years do not have the ability to grasp the details of surgery. Therefore, provide them reassurance that their parents will be waiting for them after surgery and they will be able to return home soon to join their dear ones. Toddlers do not understand the concept of time. So, they should be informed about surgery only few hours earlier or even only 1 day ahead. Allow them to have a sense of control by allowing their favourite toys, blanket, etc. Parents are the best medicine. Allow the parents to be there with the toddler, permitting them to comfort him/her with their routine, touch, voice, tec. Make the parents to reassure the child that his/her surgery is not a punishment but is a necessity for keeping his/her in good health. Provide therapeutic play with hospital equipment which is used in direct care of the child. For example, knee hammer, tongue blade, syringes without needles, stethoscope, etc. Be truthful about pain.

- Children aged 2–7 years can be provided with planned teaching sessions. Use play equipment (e.g. dolls) to provide teaching about their planned surgery. Clarify misconceptions about treatment. Draw body outline to explain. These children are capable of understanding body parts. Preschoolers may be concerned about body image and may fear that surgery may damage it. They also need reassurance that the surgery is not because of wrongdoing. Their power of imagination and fantasy thoughts may make them imagine worse about surgery. So, reassure and explain them about surgery 3–4 days in advance. This may give them some time to be prepared for surgery. Parents must be instructed to choose correct words while communicating, as the child will be curious. Parents as well as nurses should not use words having double meaning. This is particularly true about anaesthesia. The nurse should be able to quash the child's fears and encourage the child to express fears. Reassure the child and permit the child to cry if he/she desires so.

- Children aged 7–13 years can be provided with extended and science-oriented teaching. Dolls are not necessary as they have a feeling that dolls are immature. They have the concept of time, they can reason out their thinking and make generalizations. But they need clarifications of misconceptions and hearsays. They must be encouraged to ask questions. School children may fear about loss of control and may be worried about embarrassing things. They also fear about body image. It is better to prepare them adequately at least 1–2 weeks in advance. They should be provided with adequate details about surgery. Be supportive and honest in explanation. If possible, give age-appropriate reading materials. Check their understanding and involve friends and peers to visit them at the hospital or keep in touch with them.

- In adolescents, incorporate medical terminology in teaching. This group of children will be preoccupied with physical changes. They want to be in control of their care. Hence, involvement in care and proper explanation need to be given to encourage maximum self-care. Major points in preparing adolescents are as follows: involve them in their care and decision making, be truthful, encourage them to ask questions, involve their friends, give them privacy and be patient with them.

Other points in preoperative preparation include the following:

- Describe the postoperative experience according to the level of the child and readiness to learn.
- Do not overload with information; this will confuse children.
- Explanation should be in a nonthreatening manner; do not overwhelm the child and give only adequate information.
- For younger children, give information only on the evening before operation; older children can be prepared at different sessions.
- Teach children those activities that hasten recovery and prevent complications, e.g. deep breathing exercises, turning with care, walking, etc.
- Explain the activity schedule to children and their family:
  - Time of surgery
  - Need for Nil Per Oral (NPO) order and its duration
  - Approximate length of surgery
  - Anticipated postoperative activities
  - Anticipated postoperative hospitalization
- Explain preoperative discomforts, medication, treatment and postoperative discomforts and methods of relief available.
- Record specific teaching information or patient education.
- Permit self-expression of the child and family.
- Check and provide the following with a help of a preoperative checklist:
  - Monitor vital signs and report any abnormalities.
  - See that the child maintains the NPO status for the period prescribed prior to surgery.
  - Standard fasting guidelines for elective surgery are as follows:

Foods/Fluids	Time before Surgery
• Solids	• 6 hours
• Milk (breast)	• 3–4 hours
• Milk (formula)	• 4–6 hours
• Clear fluids	• 2 hours

- Infants and small children are less able to tolerate dehydration, especially in hot environments. Nausea and vomiting are more frequent in children who starve for a long period of time; hypoglycaemia can be avoided and there may be an increase in gastric contents through increased secretion if starvation is prolonged. In addition, pre- and postoperative behaviours can be improved by minimizing fasting times.
- Make sure that all preoperative procedures have been completed, e.g. bath, irrigations if needed, enemas, if prescribed, preoperative medications, etc.
- Dress the child with a clean hospital gown before sending to the operation room (OR) according to the hospital policy.
- Observe loose teeth, dental appliances and contact lenses; remove jewellery, nail polish, etc.
- Ensure that the consent forms for both surgery and anaesthesia are duly signed and witnessed.
- Ensure that all laboratory reports, radiology reports and results of any other tests are included in the patients chart before sending to the OR.
- See that the identification band is attached.
- Send the child to the OR with a familiar person (the primary nurse) and allow parents to accompany the child to the OR.
- Never leave the child unattended during transport to the operating area.
- Allow the child to a familiar object (security blanket or toy) to the OR to provide a feeling of security that something so familiar and is close to him/her.
- Psychological preparation: This requires special attention. Children are more likely to show behavioural problems if they are not prepared well before the surgery. They may even demonstrate problems during induction of anaesthesia. Behavioural differences can result in a stormy anaesthetic induction and postoperative psychological difficulties such as nightmares, phobias, fears and negativism. Postoperative psychological problems are more likely to occur in:
  - Children aged between 2 and 3 years
  - Children displaying a withdrawn affect preoperatively
  - A difficult, stressful induction
  - A child with a history of multiple procedures

So, the nurse must be vigilant on these aspects and prepare the child before surgery according to the cognitive level of the child. The nurse must remember that the perioperative experience of the child will also shape long-term attitudes of the child to health care.

Consent

Informed consent from parents and assent from children older than 7 years are required for surgery. Usually, nurses are responsible to check the details of the consent and verify whether the consent and assent are obtained before surgery. The nurse is responsible for sending all the documents related to the child's health condition including investigations, reports of investigations, medications, premedications, etc. The preassessment record should be reviewed, and any new findings such as a recent Upper Respiratory Tract Infection (URTI) gastroenteritis or change in medications should be reported to the concerned surgeon and the anaesthetist.

POSTOPERATIVE CARE

The major responsibility of the nurse in the postoperative room is to provide and meet the physical and postoperative needs of the child. The goal is safe emergence of the child from anaesthesia and an uneventful postoperative course. The nurse needs to help children cope with changed body image after surgery.

The nurse in the postoperative room should do the following:

- Receive the child to a postoperative bed.
- Place oxygen and suction near the bed and use it, as needed.
- Check airway and maintain a patent airway.
- See that necessary precautions are taken to prevent dislodging of intravenous lines, dressings, drains or chest tubes.

- Apply restraint, if needed.
- Check vital signs and blood pressure as often as necessary depending on the child's condition. Every 15 minutes for the first 1 hour; every 30 minutes for the next 1 hour and then hourly, until stable.
- Prevent hypothermia; keep the child warm. Observe skin colour.
- Assess breathing sounds (presence and character), equal air entry and signs of respiratory distress (retractions, grunting and nasal flaring).
- Monitor SaO_2 with a pulse oximeter.
- Provide pain medications, as prescribed.
- Check for signs of infection (systemic as well as local) elevated temperature, decreased blood pressure, increased pulse and increased respiratory rate.
- Maintain aseptic technique when handling intravenous lines, suctioning and dressing changes.
- Inspect surgical wound, intravenous lines, chest tube or other tube sites for signs of infection.
- Keep dressing dry, and diaper below the incision site to avoid wetting.
- Provide catheter care as and when required.
- Maintain occlusive dressing at vascular catheter insertion site.
- Assess bowel sounds, bowel patterns and frequency of bowel movements.
- Start with clear fluids as bowel sounds return and progress as tolerated.
- Monitor serum electrolytes and report abnormalities.
- Administer medications as ordered to compact metabolic problems.
- Monitor intake and output – Include urine output, nasogastric aspirations, and ileostomy, colostomy and chest tube drainages in the output.
- Check urine for blood, protein and signs of infection.
- Report and record all observations and care provided promptly and concisely.

Special Care Needs of Postoperative Children

In the Recovery Room

The nurses are supposed to closely monitor postoperative children. It is essential to monitor them closely for all vital functions.

- Monitor vital signs such as blood pressure, pulse, temperature and breathing.
- Monitor for any signs of complications and level of consciousness; check the drainage tubes, wound for bleeding, intake and output, intravenous lines, etc.
- Monitor pain and pain medications and comfort.
- Make sure that the child is fully awake before administering any oral feeds.

Postoperative Complications

Some of the discomforts children experience after surgery:

- Nausea and vomiting (from general anaesthesia)
- Soreness in the throat (if the patient needs artificial ventilation; caused by a tube placed in the windpipe to assist breathing during surgery)

- Soreness and swelling around the incision site
- Restlessness and sleeplessness
- Thirst
- Constipation and flatulence

Complications associated with surgery:

- **Shock.** Shock is most often caused by reduced blood pressure resulting from fluid and blood volume reduction as a result of surgery. Treatment may include the following:
  - Stopping any blood loss
  - Maintaining an open airway
  - Keeping the child in a prostrate position
  - Reducing heat loss with blankets
  - Intravenous infusion of fluid or blood
  - Oxygen therapy
  - Medication
- **Haemorrhage.** Rapid haemorrhage (blood loss) from the site of surgery can lead to shock. Treatment of rapid blood loss may include:
  - Infusions of plasma expanders such as saline and plasma preparation to help replace fluids
  - Blood transfusion
  - Stopping the bleeding with sutures (stitches), cautery (sealing damaged blood vessels with heat) or by repairing or removing damaged organs or tissues
- **Wound infection.** Infections can delay healing. Wound infections can spread to adjacent organs or tissue or to distant areas through the bloodstream. Treatment of wound infections may include:
  - Antibiotics
  - Draining of any abscesses (collections of pus under the skin caused by infection)
  - Opening the incision to remove the infected material
- **Pulmonary (lung) complications.** Pulmonary complications can arise as a result of lack of deep breathing in the first few days after surgery. Discomfort after an operation can make it hard to take deep breaths or cough to clear mucus out of the lungs. Make children do deep breathing exercise so that the air entry will be good and keep the lung healthy. Symptoms of pulmonary complications may include:
  - Wheezing
  - Chest pain
  - Fever
  - Cough
- **Urinary retention.** Temporary urine retention, or the inability to empty the bladder, may occur after surgery. Urinary retention is caused by the anaesthetics and is usually treated by the insertion of a catheter to drain the bladder until the child regains bladder control.
- **Reaction to anaesthesia.** Although rare, reactions to anaesthetics do occur. Symptoms may include:
  - Light-headedness
  - Wheezing
  - Rash
  - Low blood pressure
  - High temperature
  - Liver problems
  - Agitation and confusion

The nurse should closely monitor children after surgery and report any untoward symptoms noticed to the concerned surgeon. Preventing complications of surgery through quality care is essential to be child-oriented care. The nurse should keep in mind that the hospital stay should not be prolonged because of poor-quality care and the child should be discharged at the earliest to permit his/her emotional well-being.

CARE OF CRITICALLY ILL CHILDREN

Children who are critically ill require close or specialized monitoring and will spend time in the paediatric intensive care unit (PICU) or neonatal intensive care unit (NICU), depending on their age. Intensive care is needed for children who have had certain types of major surgery, such as heart operations, organ transplants or neurosurgery. After some surgical procedures, the child may remain on a breathing machine and have special monitoring lines that measure pressures in major veins or arteries. In the intensive care unit (ICU), the child will be closely watched 24 hours a day.

In the PICU or in the NICU, children who require continuous monitoring may be connected to a wide range of equipment. The nurse working at the ICU should be knowledgeable about working of such equipment.

Cardiorespiratory monitors, blood pressure monitors, pulse oximeters, transcutaneous oxygen/carbon dioxide monitors, respirator or mechanical ventilators, intravenous pumps, etc. are the common equipment used in the ICU for monitoring and for life support of critically ill children.

Care of critically ill children compounds ethical issues. Minors (children <18 years) are not legally competent to make responsible decisions. Hence, they are unable to create a living will or durable power of attorney before a life-threatening illness or injury. Decisions about resuscitation must be based on the substituted judgement of others, especially parents. Disagreements with the health care team may arise. Ethical resolution may need to be sought in the case of parental mental incompetency or even in the evidence of child abuse and neglect. When parents and caregivers have disagreements about treatment modality, a multidisciplinary meeting may be convened to proceed with interventions.

Removal of supportive therapy such as weaning from a ventilator may be sought by the family or recommended by the attending physicians when the child has a minimal chance of survival. Potential conflict may arise on discontinuation of treatment such as keeping on ventilator, as there may be no difference in the status of the child. A child who is not brain dead can be weaned from the supportive therapy through consensus of parents and physicians. Religious objections to therapy also can lead to conflict between health care professionals and parents. This is particularly true of children belonging to faith healers. Here, resolution can be sought with state or country laws, as an adult has the right to decline treatment but the child's right to treatment is safeguarded by the state, though it seems to be an infringement on the rights of parents to practice their faith or religion, especially in a secular country such as India.

No single formula is available that can be applied to the acute grief process. Health care professionals should ensure that family members receive support during the time of the child's death to help them understand and feel more comfortable with their grief. The following points may be considered as helpful while providing emotional support to the surviving family members:

- Immediate communication and support: Family members should be provided with adequate information regarding the health status of the child as they arrive. This will help them to deal with the shock of child's illness/injury.
- Provision of privacy: Certain amount of privacy may be helpful for the family members to express their grief, share their feelings and comfort each other in caring milieu.

STUDY QUESTIONS

1. Develop a preoperative teaching plan for parents of a toddler who is undergoing an elective surgery.
2. Explain the important points to be considered while planning a preoperative nursing care plan for a preschool child.
3. What is postoperative care and how will you set up your postoperative unit for receiving a child after surgery?
4. What are important observations to be made on a postoperative child?
5. Explain the common postoperative discomforts?
6. What are the common postoperative complications and their management?

BIBLIOGRAPHY

1. Aranha PR, Sams LM, Saldanha P. Preoperative preparation of children. Int J Health Allied Sci 2017;6:1-4.
2. Baker, C.F. (1984). Sensory Overload and Noise in the ICU: Sources of Environmental Stress. Critical Care Quarterly, 6(4), pp 66–80.
3. Betts, E.K., Downes, J.J. (1986). Anaesthesia. In: Welch, K.J., Randolph, J.G., Ravitch, M.M., O'Neill, J.A, Jr, Rowe, M.I. (Editors): Paediatric Surgery. 4th Edn. Chicago: Year Book. pp 50–67.
4. Elander, G., Hellstorm, G., Qvarnstorm, B. (1993). Care of Infants After Major Surgery: Observation of Behavior and Analgesic Administration. Pediatric Nursing, 19(3), pp 221–227.
5. Fassler, D. (1980). Reducing Preoperative Anxiety in Children. Information vs. Support. Patient Counseling and Health Education, 2, pp 130–134.
6. Kain ZN, Wang SM, Mayes LC, Caramico LA, Hofstadter MB. Distress during the induction of anesthesia and postoperative behavioral outcomes. Anesth Analg 1999;88:1042-7.
7. Kain A. Preoperative anxiety and postoperative nausea and vomiting in children: Is there an association? Pediatr Anesth 2000;90: 571-5.
8. Rayen R, Muthu MS, Chandrasekhar Rao R, Sivakumar N. Evaluation of physiological and behavioral measures in relation to dental anxiety during sequential dental visits in children. Indian J Dent Res 2006;17:27-34.
9. Shirley PJ, Thompson N, Kenward M, Johnston G. Parental anxiety before elective surgery in children. A British perspective. Anaesthesia 1998;53:956-9.
10. Wilson D, Hockenberry MJ. Nursing Care of Infants and Children. 8th ed. New Delhi: Elsevier Private Limited; 2007.

NURSING MANAGEMENT OF CHILDREN WITH COMMON MEDICAL–SURGICAL CONDITIONS

This unit discusses the nursing care of children with common medical and surgical conditions affecting various systems of the body. The different chapters of this unit discuss the embryonic and fetal development of the system along with consequences of abnormal development, followed by various medical and surgical conditions requiring special nursing care management.

UNIT OUTLINE

CHAPTER 28

NURSING MANAGEMENT OF CHILDREN WITH RESPIRATORY DISORDERS

LEARNING OBJECTIVES

At the end of the chapter, the learner will be able to:

- Explain the essential concepts related to development of the respiratory system.
- Identify the consequences of abnormal development.
- Explain fetal preparation for first breath and the respiratory events that occur at birth.
- Describe nursing management of common medical problems affecting respiratory function using the nursing approach.

FETAL DEVELOPMENT

The respiratory system is responsible for both transporting oxygen and carbon dioxide to and from the blood and helping with the regulation of the body's acid–base balance. Understanding dysfunctions of the respiratory system requires a fundamental grasp of the structure and function of the composite organs. This chapter reviews the embryonic development, consequences of abnormal development and nursing management of common medical and surgical conditions affecting the respiratory system.

EMBRYONIC DEVELOPMENT

The primary tissue layers constitute the primitive embryo. These are the endoderm or basal tissue layer, the mesoderm or middle layer and the ectoderm. The developing respiratory system is derived principally from the endoderm. The lungs, airways and the pleural cavity are structures rooted in endodermal tissues. But the support structures, such as tracheal cartilage, respiratory muscles, pulmonary vessels and pulmonary lymphatics, are generated from the mesodermal tissues.

Early Embryonic Period

Embryonic lung development occurs in five successive stages. The early embryonic period occurs 1–5 weeks after fertilization. The lungs initially appear as an outpouching on the ventral surface of the embryonic oesophagus or the foregut. This lung bud quickly divides into two bronchopulmonary pouches, giving rise eventually to the two main stem bronchi. By the fifth week of gestation, the common tube from which the lung bud rises differentiates into the oesophagus and the laryngotracheal tube.

The early embryonic period is one of rapid cell reproduction, and growth is evidenced by the remarkable development and differentiation of the bronchopulmonary buds. The left bronchial bud gives rise to two secondary buds, primitive upper and lower lung lobes. The right bronchus gives rise to three secondary buds, rudimentary upper, middle and lower right lobes. At the end of 5 weeks, the gross rudimentary lung structures are present.

Pseudoglandular Period (5–16 Weeks)

The second stage of lung development, the pseudoglandular period, begins at the fifth week of gestation and continues through the 16th week. This stage is so named because of the rudimentary lung which has the appearance of a gland. The fundamental structures for air conduction, the entire tracheobronchial tree, develop at this stage. This includes the main stem bronchi, their secondary bronchi and the bronchioles.

At 10th weeks, goblet cells appear within the bronchioles. In addition, 70% of the branching of the bronchi is complete. Towards the end of the pseudoglandular period (15th week), the bronchial arteries arise from the thoracic aorta and intercostal arteries. Rudimentary veins also appear. The embryonic lung is rich in glycogen, which provides nutrition for rapid development in this period.

Canalicular Period (16–25 Weeks)

The canalicular period marks the third stage of embryonic lung development. The fetal stage, 13–25 weeks' gestation, is marked by the formation of alveolar ducts and alveolar cells that eventually form alveoli. In addition, alveolar capillaries and the thoracic lymph system evolve and align closer to the alveolar ducts and primitive alveolar surfaces. The generation and multiplication of the alveolar capillaries are important steps necessary to facilitate oxygen and carbon dioxide transfer in the intrauterine life.

Terminal Sac Period (26–40 Weeks)

The fourth stage of lung development is termed the terminal sac period and spans from 24 weeks' gestation through birth. Structurally, the bronchioles give rise to terminal sacs or primitive alveoli. There will be progressive increase in the number of alveolar sacs, which creates a greater surface area for gas exchange. Although the alveoli are present, they are thick walled and narrow. The diffusion gradient or the distance that oxygen and carbon dioxide must transverse between alveoli and capillaries is so great that oxygenation is inadequate. Thus, the infant born prior to 36 weeks' gestation typically develops acute respiratory problems such as hyaline membrane disease (HMD) because of inadequate pulmonary structural development.

The production and storage of surfactant are not sufficient to support extrauterine life until the fetus has reached approximately 36 weeks' gestation. The surfactant is produced by a number of biochemical pathways. A predominant one in the developing fetus is the phosphatidylinositol (PI) pathway, which predominates until 32 weeks' gestation. This surfactant is unstable and quickly used. Hence, infants born prior to 32 weeks are more likely to suffer from HMD. The major function of the surfactant is to decrease alveolar surface tension and increase lung compliance. The surfactant prevents alveolar collapse at the end of expiration and allows for opening of the alveoli at a low intrathoracic pressure.

At about 32–34 weeks' gestation, a more stable form of surfactant, phosphatidylglycerol (PG), is synthesized, which is very stable and permits alveoli of differing sizes to inflate with an equal amount of pressure. Surfactant maturity has in the past been estimated by the measurement of lecithin to sphingomyelin (L:S) ratio. The L:S ratio is approximately equal to 1:1 until 35 weeks' gestation. With increasing age, lecithin increases so that an L:S ratio of greater than 2:1 suggests lung maturity.

Factors that Affect Fetal Lung Surfactant Production	
Increased Production	**Decreased Production**
Prolonged rupture of the fetal membrane	Combined fetal hyperglycaemia and hyperinsulinaemia
Maternal narcotic addiction	Acute hypoxia
Maternal steroid addiction	
Preeclampsia	
Chronic fetal distress	
Administration of theophylline	
Increase in thyroid hormone	

A third type of alveolar cell is called the macrophage or scavenger cell, and it can be compared with a chimney sweep. These cells are responsible for the engulfment and digestion of foreign materials, primarily bacteria that may find their way into the respiratory tract.

Alveolar Period

The final stage of lung development, termed as the alveolar period, occurs from late fetal development through 8 years of life. At this time, the primary developmental activity is growth of the terminal sacs (alveoli), thinning of the alveolar walls to the capillaries that will deliver fresh blood to the alveoli. A newborn has approximately 20,000,000 alveoli, and the number continues to increase until 8 years of life when anatomic development is completed.

NB: The major respiratory function is gas exchange that involves ventilation, diffusion and perfusion. The control of respiration involves neural and chemical processes.

CONSEQUENCES OF ABNORMAL DEVELOPMENT

Many factors may influence embryonic development of the lower respiratory tract. Either genetic or environmental condition may interrupt or distort the development of structures in the growing embryo. Some of the consequences of abnormal development are described in Table 28.1.

The biochemical maturation of the respiratory system also can be affected during embryogenesis. Some preterm infants of heroin-addicted mothers rarely develop HMD. Most mature infants have no respiratory problems at birth, but some mature infants such as those born to diabetic women are at the risk of developing HMD.

At-risk infants have one commonality, interference with biochemical development of surfactant. In fetuses exposed to chronic intrauterine stress as intrauterine infection or persistent malnutrition, accelerated fetal glucocorticoid synthesis and production are induced. These glucocorticoids have been shown to induce production of mature surfactant in lamb studies.

TABLE 28.1 Consequences of Abnormal Development

Fetal Age (Weeks)	Structure	Anomalies of Development
4–5	Trachea and oesophagus	Failure of fusion of the oesophageal and tracheal tubes into separate structures leads to tracheoesophageal fistula.
5–6	Lung lobes	Interrupted, delayed or interference with development leads to hypoplasia of lung lobes.
8	Diaphragm	Failure of closure of diaphragmatic canals leads to diaphragmatic hernia with hypoplasia of the lung on the herniated side.
8	Choanal atresia	Unilateral or bilateral obstruction of the posterior nasal airway by a membranous or bony septum. Results from failure of the buccal mucosa to rupture.

Developmental Differences

The primary differences in the respiratory system of a child as compared with an adult are shape, lung capacity, respiratory rate and pattern of breathing. The neonate chest is round, but it begins to change and become less barrel-shaped during the first year. By 10 years of age, the configuration is more elliptical, as in an adult, with a flattened anterior–posterior diameter.

Lung capacity is actually a reflection of the number and size of the alveoli. An infant has approximately 20,000,000 alveoli compared with 300,000,000 in an adult. Logically, it is expected that the increased lung volume would correspond with growth of the child and subsequent lung tissue growth.

Structurally, the conducting airways of the child (trachea, bronchi and bronchioles) up to the age of 8 years are narrower and shorter than an older child and an adult. This makes children more prone to respiratory infections. The smaller airways and the inability to clear the airway with coughing in a very young child (up to the age of 4 years) potentiate problems with mucous obstruction more readily than those in older children and adults. Poor tolerance of nasal congestion, especially in infants who are obligatory nose breathers until the age of 2–4 months, poses major threat in these age groups.

Infants breathing is characterized by abdominal rather than chest movement because the accessory muscles of respiration are poorly developed and do not contribute much to the movement of the chest wall during inspiration. In infancy, the ribs articulate with the spine at a horizontal slope rather than at an oblique slope that appears with later development. With inspiration and downward movement of the diaphragm, the abdomen becomes dome-shaped and the level of thoracic flaring appears minimal. By the age of 3 years, the respiratory pattern demonstrates the greater use of the chest muscles and less of the abdominal muscles. Increased susceptibility to ear infection as a result of shorter, broader and

more horizontally positioned Eustachian tubes is also a developmental issue with the respiratory system.

A final developmental difference is the change of respiratory rates with age. Respiratory frequency decreases as the body size increases. A newborn infant's respiratory rate fluctuates widely but becomes more stable within 1–2 days. The rate gradually slows down through the childhood.

Fetal Preparation for the First Breath

Prior to birth, the process of gas exchange is managed by the placenta. In the circulatory system, ductus arteriosus and foramen ovale shunt blood away from the fetal lungs. Only 10% of the fetal cardiac output reaches the lungs. Enough oxygen-enriched blood is available to keep the pulmonic tissue vitalized but not enough to initiate respirations.

The low volume of blood flowing to the fetal lungs contributes to the maintenance of a high pulmonary vascular pressure (PVP). This high PVP creates resistance to blood through the pulmonary vascular channels, forcing more blood to shunt away from the lungs. Low blood flow to the fetal lungs is essential to prevent the possibility of intrauterine respirations, respirations which could lead to aspiration of amniotic fluid. The fetal lungs are filled with approximately 50 mL of fetal liquid, a substance resembling plasma but with lower protein content. The purpose of the fetal lung liquid is to provide a slight distension of the alveoli, making the first breath at birth a little easier than it would be if the alveolar walls were collapsed on themselves.

Preparation of the respiratory system for extrauterine functions is demonstrated by the occurrence of fetal breathing movements in utero. This phenomenon, noticed first by Vesalius, is the fetus practicing for extrauterine existence. Nowadays, the presence or absence of fetal breathing movements is used by perinatologists as one of the criteria in the biophysical profile of the fetus for determining fetal well-being.

The newborn's first breath is the result of interplay of neurophysiological and environmental stimuli. The neurophysiological controls of respiration include respiratory centre (medulla), central chemoreceptors (vagus and glossopharyngeal nerves), peripheral chemoreceptors (aortic and carotid bodies), cervical sympathetics and reflex activity Environmental factors also influence the first breath.

The process of birth is asphyxiating, the fetal blood PaO_2 (the partial pressure of oxygen in the arteries) falls to >20 mm Hg and a drop in blood pH indicates acidaemia. The severe hypoxaemia (PaO_2 > 20 mm Hg) acts as a direct stimulant to the central respiratory centre (medulla) and the central chemoreceptors, causing the infant to gasp. A low pH also acts on peripheral chemoreceptors to stimulate respiration.

The passage of the infant through the vaginal canal during birth also facilitates the first respiration. The external pressure exerted on the descending infant's thorax increases the negative intrathoracic pressure. The vagus nerve also exerts control on respiration. Pulmonary stretch receptors located in the bronchioles stimulate the afferent pathways in the vagus nerve and stimulate respiration. Finally, the external environmental stimuli also activate respirations by stimulating the central nervous system in general. Noise, light, touch and temperature in the delivery room are examples of stimuli that may affect the initiation of respirations.

Respiratory System Overview

This includes a health history to determine whether the problem is acute or chronic, self-limiting or life-threatening. Other important points to look into are exacerbating factors and alleviating factors, family history of respiratory problems, etc. Physical assessment should concentrate on the following aspects:

- Alertness, changes in mental status
- Activity level and complaints of fatigue
- Skin colour changes, particularly cyanosis
- Respiratory rate and pattern, presence of apnoea
- Increased retractions (present or not)
- Adventitious lung sounds (wheeze, crackles, rhonchi, etc.)
- Cough (productive or nonproductive)
- Dyspnoea, stridor, grunting, nasal flaring, etc.

Laboratory and Diagnostic Studies

- Radiological examination may include chest X-rays to visualize internal structures and lung scans to visualize pulmonary blood flow
- Thoracentesis to obtain a pleural fluid specimen for analysis
- Pulmonary function tests (PFTs) to evaluate ventilatory function
- Blood gas analysis

NURSING MANAGEMENT OF CHILDREN WITH COMMON MEDICAL PROBLEMS AFFECTING RESPIRATORY FUNCTIONS

Choanal Atresia

Neonatal airway obstruction is a common problem among neonates admitted to neonatal intensive care units (ICUs). It can be a result of many disorders. Choanal atresia is one such problem.

Definition/Description

In Greek, the word *choana* means 'funnel'. It is the posterior nasal aperture by which air flows from the nasal cavity into the nasopharynx.

Choanal atresia is a congenital disorder in which the back of the nasal passage (**choana**) is blocked, usually by abnormal bony or soft tissue (membranous) as a result of failed recanalization of the nasal fossae during fetal development.

Aetiology

Normal embryology:

Between 4 and 6 weeks' gestation, one can see the formation of primitive nasal structures via neural crest cell migration such as the columella, philtrum and

upper lip. At about the same time, nasal pits form and burrow into the mesenchyme to create the primitive nasal cavities. These nasal pits sit atop the frontal portion of the stomodeum (i.e. primitive oral cavity), and the pits are separated from the stomodeum by the nasobuccal membrane. Once the nasobuccal membrane ruptures, the primitive nasal cavity and primitive choana are formed. The primitive choana matures and transforms into the definitive (i.e. secondary) choana. There is also an additional membrane known as the buccopharyngeal membrane which separates the stomodeum (ectoderm) from the primitive pharynx (endoderm).

Causes of Choanal Atresia

a) Problem with embryogenesis:
- Persistence of the buccopharyngeal membrane
- Failure of the buccopharyngeal membrane to rupture
- Medial outgrowth of the vertical and horizontal processes of the palatine bone
- Abnormal mesodermal adhesions forming in the choanal area
- Misdirection of the mesodermal flow as a result of local factors

b) Prenatal/maternal factors
- Use of antithyroid drugs (methimazole, carbimazole)
- High intake of vitamin B_{12}, zinc, niacin
- Low intake of methionine, vitamin D
- Cigarette smoking
- Coffee intake (≥ 3 cups per day)

Anatomic abnormalities are a narrowed nasal cavity, lateral impingement of the medial pterygoid plate, an abnormally thickened vomer and a membrane comprising most of the mucosa and/or bone extending across the choana.

Other potential causes of nasal obstructions that are to be ruled out are as follows:
- Fixed anatomic causes may include nasal pyriform aperture stenosis or septal buckling as a result of birth canal trauma; craniofacial abnormalities of all types may give rise to unfavourable nasal anatomy.
- Allergy and sinus disease are present with associated secretions and tissue swelling, especially in children with cystic fibrosis.
- Nasal masses such as haemangiomas and encephalocele must be ruled out in any child with nasal obstruction.

Incidence

Unilateral choanal atresia is more common than bilateral one (65%–75%) and most commonly affects the right side. Females are more likely to have it (2:1 ratio female to male). Bilateral choanal atresia has a high association with CHARGE syndrome, Treacher–Collins syndrome and Crouzon disease (75% of cases).

Clinical Features

Neonates are obligatory nose breathers for a period of 4–6 weeks after birth. The nasal anatomy comprising a relatively large tongue, superiorly placed larynx and floppy epiglottis contributes them to be nasal breathers. This complicates the situation. If it is unilateral, the neonate may be able to breathe through the opened nasal passage and the repair is not an emergency. Bilateral choanal atresia is a surgical emergency.

The neonate may present with:
- Cyanosis
- Notable chest retractions, which worsen with feeding
- Oxygen saturation improves with crying as air enters through the mouth

Multidisciplinary Management

Diagnostic evaluation: Clinical findings, imaging studies (rhinography, computed tomographic [CT] scan), procedures (failure of passage of an 8F catheter through the nostril more than 5.5 cm, acoustic rhinometry, lack of movement of thin cotton, absence of fog on the mirror)

Treatment is of two types: Emergent and elective.
- Bilateral choanal atresia is an emergency. An oral airway is inserted to break the seat formed by the tongue against the palate. Newborns are obligatory nose breathers, and immediate attention should be given for keeping a patent airway.
- An oral airway, McGovern nipple and intubation are viable options.

The ideal procedure should restore the normal nasal passage and prevent damage to the growing nasal structures that are important in facial development, should be technically safe and should take minimum time for surgery and comfortable recovery.

Surgical correction:
- Previously, transnasal puncture with or without a microscope was used (now not used).
- In trans-septal technique, a window is made in the septum anterior to the atretic plate.
- Transpalatal repair provides excellent exposure and has a high success rate but requires more time for the procedure.
- Endoscopic technique (nasal/retropalatal) with or without powered instrumentation offers excellent visualization and comparatively easy to remove bony choana.
- Combined transoral–transnasal technique is also a good alternative.
- Use of carbon dioxide and potassium titanyl phosphate (KTP) lasers provides minimal discomfort to the newborn and time of hospitalization is reduced. Mitomycin C used as an adjunct to surgical repair offers improved patency and reduces the chance of dilatations and repeated surgical procedures.

Nursing Management

Assessment: Cyanosis and retraction
   Noisy respiration
   Difficulty breathing during feeding
   Thick mucus
Nursing diagnosis:
- Impaired breathing pattern related to obstruction of posterior nares
- Ineffective tissue perfusion related to ventilation–perfusion mismatch
- Imbalanced nutrition less than body requirement related to breathing difficulty during feeding
- Parental anxiety
Interventions:
- Prone nursing/position with the head elevated
- Airway: Change in each shift to prevent infection
- Suctioning
- Intravenous fluids/orogastric feeds
Postoperatively:
- Vital sign monitoring
- Intravenous fluids/orogastric feeds
- Prevention of infection
- Watch for bleeding
Evaluation:
   Child maintains normal respiration and normal nutritional status
   Child remains free from infection

Epiglottitis

Definition/Description. Epiglottitis is characterized by swelling and rounding of the epiglottis, blunting of vallecula, hypopharyngeal ballooning and oedematous aryepiglottic folds.

Aetiology. It most commonly results from *Haemophilus influenzae* virus type B infection, and other possible organisms include *Pneumococcus* and group A streptococci.

Incidence. It most often develops in children 2–6 years of age, although it has been observed in patients from 5 months through adulthood.

Clinical Manifestations
- Sore throat
- Dysphagia
- High fever
- Hoarseness
- Drooling
- Respiratory distress
- Sitting in a tripod position
- Air hunger
- Anxiety
- Wheezy respiratory stridor, suprasternal and substernal retractions
- Tachycardia
- Late signs of hypoxia: Listlessness, cyanosis and bradycardia

Pathophysiology. Acute epiglottitis often preceded by minor upper respiratory tract infection of several days' duration. If untreated, it may rapidly progress to complex upper respiratory airway obstruction. Progressive obstruction resulting in hypoxia, hypercapnia and acidosis, followed by decreased muscle tone, altered level of consciousness and obstruction may lead to death.

Multidisciplinary Management
- Establish an airway (intubate, if necessary).
- Obtain lateral soft tissue neck X-rays, if condition permits.

- Administer antibiotics (racemic epinephrine is of no value).
- Perform laboratory studies, blood culture, arterial blood gases (ABGs), etc.
- Administer humidified oxygen.
- Provide observation in the ICU.
- Provide respiratory therapy.

Nursing Assessment
- Assess for signs and symptoms and obtain a history of prolonged upper respiratory tract infections.

Nursing Diagnoses
- Ineffective airway clearance
- High risk for injury
- Anxiety of parents and the child

Goal of Nursing Management
- The child will maintain a patent airway.

Nursing Interventions
- Maintain the child in a sitting position.
- Do not attempt to visualize epiglottis; under no circumstances place a tongue blade or other objects in the child's mouth.
- Monitor vital signs closely; be alert to indications of airway obstruction.
- Keep NPO (nil per os or nothing by mouth).
- Have intubation or tracheostomy set at the bedside.
- Monitor for side effects of antibiotics.
- Maintain care of the child during oxygen administration and other general care.

Evaluation
- The child is free from dyspnoea or other signs of respiratory distress.
  Vital signs return to normal.

Laryngotracheobronchitis

Definition/Description. Laryngotracheal bronchitis is a severe inflammation and obstruction of the upper airway characterized by subglottic oedema and variable tracheal bronchial inflammation as a result of a desquamating tracheitis.

Aetiology. It usually results from viral infection (parainfluenza virus, adenovirus, respiratory syncytial virus, influenza virus and measles virus) and rarely by bacterial infection from diphtheria and pertussis bacteria.

Incidence. It predominantly affects male children aged 3 months to 3 years. Peak incidence is seen in winter months.

Pathophysiology. This is usually preceded by an upper respiratory infection to laryngitis which then descends into the trachea and sometimes to the bronchi. The flexible larynx of a young child is particularly susceptible to spasm and causes complete obstruction. Airway oedema may lead to obstruction and seriously compromised ventilation.

Clinical Manifestations
- Coryza
- Barking cough
- Hoarseness
- Low-grade fever
- Stridor
- Respiratory distress
- Retractions
- Nasal flaring
- Cyanosis
- X-ray shows subglottic narrowing but a normal epiglottis

Multidisciplinary Management
- Use a high humidity oxygen tent.
- Provide intravenous hydration.
- Administer racemic epinephrine, steroids and antibiotics if bacterial infection is suspected.
- Perform tracheostomy or intubation if necessary
- Provide nursing assessment.
- Watch for the clinical manifestations.
- Use the clinical croup score that can be used for any upper respiratory airway disease.

Croup Score

Parameters	0	1	2	Score
Inspiratory breath sounds	Normal	Harsh with rhonchi/wheeze	Delayed	
Stridor	None	Inspiratory	Inspiratory and expiratory	
Cough	None	Hoarse	Bark	
Retractions and flaring	None	Flaring and suprasternal retractions	Same as score 1, plus subcostal retractions	
Cyanosis	None	Present in room air	Present in 40% oxygen	Total score

A total score of 4–7 indicates moderately severe obstruction in which administration of racemic epinephrine may be beneficial.

A score of 7 or more with a PCO_2 <70 mm Hg in room air, persisting for >30 minutes, despite intravenous administration of fluid and use of mist and racemic epinephrine indicates need for an artificial airway (Downes J & Raphael R, 1975).

Nursing Diagnoses
- Ineffective airway clearance
- High risk for injury
- Anxiety of parents and the child

Goal of Nursing Management
- The child will remain oxygenated.

Nursing Interventions
- Assess for airway obstruction by evaluating the respiratory status.
- Keep emergency equipment ready at the bedside.

- Increase atmospheric humidity with a mist, tent or head hood.
- Administer oxygen therapy as ordered to alleviate hypoxia.
- Administer intravenous fluids as prescribed to ensure adequate hydration.
- Administer prescribed medications that include racemic epinephrine via a nebulizer, antibiotics and sometimes corticosteroids. Corticosteroids administration is controversial.
- Help reduce the child's anxiety by maintaining a calm environment and supporting parents and clearing their doubts.
- Include parents as much as possible in the care of the child.
- Provide patient and parent education about medication usage, administration and possible side effects, and how to manage symptoms at home. (Usually, the child will get up from sleep with barking cough and other symptoms of croup. Put the child in the bathroom and run hot water to produce steam; if this facility is not available, provide steam to inhale via home-made inhalators.)

Evaluation

- The child will exhibit no signs of respiratory distress and will be afebrile and well hydrated.
- Parents and the child verbalize understanding of diagnosis, treatment and home management of the condition.

Bronchial Asthma

Definition/Description. Asthma is a chronic, episodic, reversible, obstructive disorder characterized by airway narrowing as a result of bronchospasm, increased mucus secretion and mucosal oedema. It is often manifested by paroxysmal smooth muscle spasms in the nonconducting small airways.

Aetiology. The most common cause of asthma is allergic hyperresponsiveness of the trachea and bronchi to irritants. The precipitating factors include viral infection, air pollution, animal dander, dust, moulds, pollens, certain foods, rapid change in environmental temperature and physical and physiological stress. A familial tendency is also noticed in the aetiology.

Incidence. It is the most common chronic lung disease in children and affects 8%–10% of children in the urban area and 5%–8% of children in the rural area. It affects boys more (twice more than girls) before puberty, and the reverse is seen at and after puberty. In India, one out of 10 children has asthma.

Pathophysiology. The hypersensitivity reaction results from histamine release that produces oedema of the respiratory mucosa causing obstruction as a result of bronchiolar narrowing, secretion accumulation and bronchial and bronchial smooth muscle spasm. This leads to air-trapping wheeze and respiratory distress. If not promptly treated, it will lead to status asthmaticus.

Clinical Manifestations

- Dyspnoea
- Air hunger
- Anxiety
- Cough (nonproductive, hacking cough which later becomes productive)
- Wheeze (expiratory in nature)
- Tachypnoea
- Complaints of chest tightness
- Costal retractions
- Diaphoresis
- Severe cases of cyanosis
- Barrel chest
- Assuming a tripod position

Diagnostic Evaluations

- History
- Clinical findings
- Chest radiography
- Bronchoprovocation test and skin prick test
- Peak expiratory flow rate
- Blood investigation – Complete blood cell (CBC) count (eosinophilia)

Multidisciplinary Management

- Oxygen
- Drug therapy:
  a) Prevention of exacerbation (inhaled corticosteroids, long-acting bronchodilators, leukotriene antagonists, methylxanthines, etc.)
  b) Rescue medications (intravenous corticosteroids, short-acting bronchodilators)
- Hyposensitization
- Bronchodilators, expectorant therapy, corticosteroids and antibiotics
- Respiratory therapy
- Occupational therapy

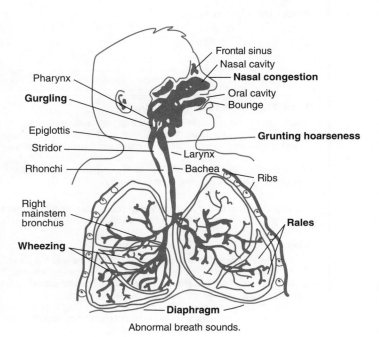

Abnormal breath sounds.

Abnormal Breath Sounds

Recommended Stepwise Management of Asthma in Children Under 5 Years of Age

Step	Symptom Relief	Maintenance	Additional/Alternate Therapies
1	Inhaled short-acting (β-2 antagonists as required (not more than once daily)		If inhaled β-2 antagonists are needed more than once daily, move to step 2
2a	Inhaled short-acting β-2 antagonists as required	Regular inhaled cromoglycate, e.g. powder 20 mg three to four times daily or 10 mg three times via a metered-dose inhaler (MDI) and a large-volume spacer	To gain rapid control, consider 5-day course of soluble prednisolone at 1–2 mg/kg per day or doubling the dose of inhaled steroids for 1 month.
2b	Inhaled short-acting β-2 antagonists as required	Regular low dose of inhaled steroids up to 400 mcg of beclomethasone or budesonide daily	To gain rapid control, consider 5-day course of soluble prednisolone at 1–2 mg/kg per day or doubling dose of inhaled steroids for 1 month.
3	Inhaled short-acting β-2 antagonists as required	Regular high dose of inhaled steroids up to 800 mcg of beclomethasone or budesonide daily via a large-volume spacer device	Additionally, consider adding regular long-acting β antagonists twice daily before going to step 4. Alternately, slow-release xanthene may be added, particularly for nocturnal symptoms, but side effects may be troublesome.
4	Inhaled short-acting β-2 antagonists as required	Regular high dose of inhaled steroids up to 1200 mcg of beclomethasone or budesonide daily via a large-volume spacer device	Additionally, consider adding regular long-acting β antagonists twice daily, or slow-release xanthene as in step 3 or nebulized β antagonists.

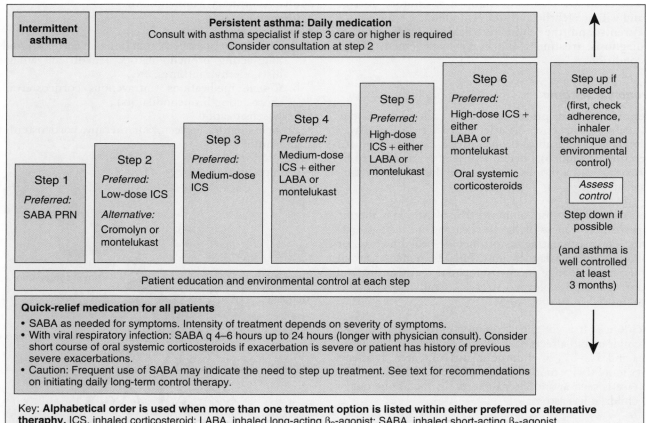

Stepwise management of asthma in children (0–4 years). (Adapted from: http://getasthmahelp.org/asthma-classification-infants.aspx)

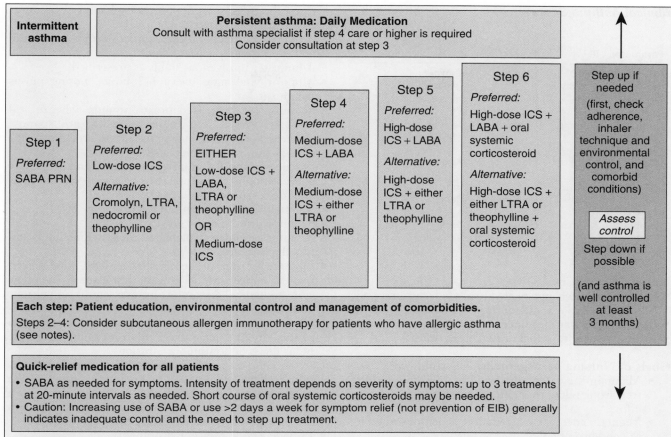

Intermittent asthma	**Persistent asthma: Daily Medication** Consult with asthma specialist if step 4 care or higher is required Consider consultation at step 3

Step 1
Preferred:
SABA PRN

Step 2
Preferred:
Low-dose ICS
Alternative:
Cromolyn, LTRA, nedocromil or theophylline

Step 3
Preferred:
EITHER
Low-dose ICS + LABA, LTRA or theophylline
OR
Medium-dose ICS

Step 4
Preferred:
Medium-dose ICS + LABA
Alternative:
Medium-dose ICS + either LTRA or theophylline

Step 5
Preferred:
High-dose ICS + LABA
Alternative:
High-dose ICS + either LTRA or theophylline

Step 6
Preferred:
High-dose ICS + LABA + oral systemic corticosteroid
Alternative:
High-dose ICS + either LTRA or theophylline + oral systemic corticosteroid

Step up if needed
(first, check adherence, inhaler technique and environmental control, and comorbid conditions)

Assess control

Step down if possible

(and asthma is well controlled at least 3 months)

Each step: Patient education, environmental control and management of comorbidities.

Steps 2–4: Consider subcutaneous allergen immunotherapy for patients who have allergic asthma (see notes).

Quick-relief medication for all patients
- SABA as needed for symptoms. Intensity of treatment depends on severity of symptoms: up to 3 treatments at 20-minute intervals as needed. Short course of oral systemic corticosteroids may be needed.
- Caution: Increasing use of SABA or use >2 days a week for symptom relief (not prevention of EIB) generally indicates inadequate control and the need to step up treatment.

Key: Alphabetical order is used when more than one treatment option is listed within either preferred or alternative theraphy. ICS, inhaled corticosteroid; LABA, inhaled long-acting β_2-agonist; LTRA, leukotriene receptor antagonist; SABA, inhaled short-acting β_2-agonist.

Notes:
- The stepwise approach is meant to assist, not replace, the clinical decision making required to meet individual patient needs.
- If alternative treatment is used and response is inadequate, discontinue it and use the preferred treatment before stepping up.
- Theophylline is a less desirable alternative because of the need to monitor serum concentration levels.
- Step 1 and step 2 medications are based on Evidence A. Step 3 ICS + adjunctive therapy and ICS are based on Evidence B for efficacy of each treatment and extrapolation from comparator trials in older children and adults – comparator trials are not available for this age group; steps 4–6 are based on expert opinion and extrapolation from studies in older children and adults.
- Immunotherapy for steps 2–4 is based on Evidence B for house-dust mites, animal danders and pollens; evidence is weak or lacking for moulds and cockroaches. Evidence is strongest for immunotherapy with single allergens. The role of allergy in asthma is greater in children than in adults. Clinicians who administer immunotherapy should be prepared and equipped to identify and treat anaphylaxis that may occur.

Stepwise management of asthma in children (5–11 years). (Adapted from: http://getasthmahelp.org/asthma-classification-children-five-to-eleven.aspx)

Nursing Assessment

- Rate and character of respiration, rales, rhonchi, retractions, expiratory and inspiratory effort, use of accessory muscles, grunting, flaring, cyanosis, diaphoresis, hydration, speech pattern, poor capillary refill, etc. need to be assessed. In addition, there may be carbon dioxide narcosis that may lead to anxiety in children.
- Use of asthma score is helpful for assessment.

Clinical Asthma Score

Parameter	0	1	2	Score
PO_2	70–100 in room air	70 in air	70 in 40% O_2	
Cyanosis	None	In air	Decreased to absent	
Inspiratory breath sounds	Normal	Unequal	Decreased to absent	
Use of accessory muscle	None	Moderate	Maximal	
Expiratory wheezing	None	Moderate	Marked	
Cerebral function	Normal	Depressed or agitated	Coma	Total score

Nursing Diagnoses
- Impaired gas exchange related to altered oxygen supply, decreased alveolar ventilation
- Ineffective airway clearance
- Anxiety related to actual or perceived death

Goals of Nursing Management. The child will:
- Maintain the patent airway with a decrease in rate, free from rales, rhonchi, wheezes and inspiratory effort.
- Maintain adequate oxygenation as demonstrated by the absence of pallor or cyanosis.
- Remain calm and participate in activities of daily living.

Parents and the child will be able to:
- Describe signs and symptoms of an impending attack, measures to be taken to avoid an attack and the follow-up measures.
- Describe proper administration of prophylactic medications, their side effects and signs of toxicity.
- Openly express their feelings about the disease, and realistically describe limitations on the child's activity.

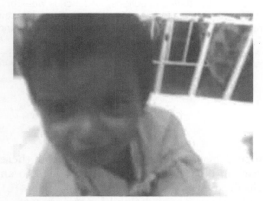

A baby on Fowler's position.

Nursing Interventions
- Set the patient in a high Fowler's position or sitting leaning forward.
- Use calm, reassuring approach, explaining procedures to the child and parents.
- Administer bronchodilators, corticosteroids, antibiotics and expectorants as prescribed.
- Administer intravenous fluids as prescribed.
- Monitor vital signs every 1–2 hours, noting pulsus paradoxus.
- Monitor for decreased breath sounds, wheeze and rhonchi. Progression to decreased breath sounds/absence of wheezing may signal severe bronchospasm/constriction and minimal airflow.
- Obtain sputum for gram stain, culture and sensitivity and eosinophil stain (presence of eosinophil indicates allergic response).
- Maintain intake and output (I&O).
- Monitor urine specific gravity.
- Monitor serum electrolyte and theophylline levels and blood gas values.
- Observe for signs of theophylline toxicity, noting fever, nausea, coffee-ground emesis, restlessness, hypotension, abdominal discomfort progressing to convulsions and coma.
- Observe for signs and symptoms of rapid metabolism of theophylline derivatives: failure to improve despite bolus doses or continuous infusions.
- If the child is near panic and able to follow instructions, tell the child to follow breathing pattern of the nurse; start with a rapid rate and then slow down gradually; encourage the child to breathe in through the nose and then exhale slowly through the mouth.
- Provide a cool, moist environment.
- Administer aerosol or nebulizer treatment as ordered.
- Perform percussion, vibration and postural drainage as indicated once airways have begun to open satisfactorily.
- Plan nursing care to allow for maximum rest.
- Administer sedatives for relieving anxiety.
- Encourage anxious parents to verbalize their fears and allow them to have small naps away from the child to see if the child relaxes.
- Discuss parents' sensitivity testing and eliminating allergic foods and other allergens.
- Reduce sensory overload by providing an organized, quiet environment.
- Review coping behaviours of parents and encourage adaptive coping to manage anxiety.
- Teach parents and the child signs and symptoms of an attack.
- Teach parents and the child to avoid contacts with allergens.
- Instruct parents and the child on proper administration of medication.
- Stress that medication should be taken even when the child is feeling well.
- Demonstrate correct use of the inhaler and ask for return demonstration.
- Instruct parents and the child on the proper use and side effects of prophylactic medications. Alert them to dangers of overuse.
- Encourage parents to be alert to possibility of the child's using his/her symptoms to manipulate his/her environment and to avoid parental rejection or overprotection.

- Encourage using exercise stop–start activity not requiring endurance.
- Discuss use of bronchodilators 20–30 minutes before exercise.

Evaluation
- The child's respiratory rate is within normal limits.
- The child is not anxious.
- Medications are within therapeutic limits.
- The child and parents describe signs of impending attack, prophylactic medications, their benefits and side effects.

Bronchiolitis

Definition/Description. Bronchiolitis is an acute viral infection with a maximum effect at the bronchiolar level.

Aetiology and Incidence. The infection occurs primarily in winter and spring and is rare in children older than 2 years. Respiratory syncytial virus is responsible for more than half of all cases of bronchiolitis. Adenovirus and parainfluenza virus may also cause acute bronchiolitis. The virus becomes epidemic in communities during the late fall and winter months and is easily spread by hand-to-nose transmission.

Pathophysiology. Bronchial mucosa is swollen and the lumen is filled with mucus and exudates, the walls of the bronchi and bronchioles are infiltrated with inflammatory cells and peribronchiolar interstitial pneumonitis is usually present. The variable degrees of obstruction produced in the small air passage by these changes lead to hyperinflation, obstructive emphysema resulting from partial obstruction and patchy areas of atelectasis. Dilation of bronchial passages on inspiration allows sufficient space for intake of air, but narrowing of the passage on expiration prevents air from leaving the lungs. Thus, air is trapped distal to the obstruction and causes progressive overinflation (emphysema).

Clinical Manifestations
- Nasal discharge
- Mild fever
- Respiratory distress with tachypnoea
- Paroxysmal cough
- Irritability
- Wheezing
- Respiratory excursions are rapid with flaring nares
- Suprasternal and subcostal retractions
- Hypercapnia that leads to respiratory acidosis
- Rales, diminished breath sounds

Investigations
- Chest X-rays, ABGs, virology (to identify the organism), etc.

Multidisciplinary Management
- Bronchodilators, expectorants, corticosteroids and oxygen administration
- Diet therapy

- Respiratory therapy
- Occupational therapy

Nursing Assessment
- Rate and character of respirations, breath sounds, rales, rhonchi, retractions, inspiratory and expiratory effort, use of accessory muscles, etc.
- Cyanosis, diaphoresis, hydration and poor capillary refill time

Nursing Diagnoses
- Ineffective breathing pattern
- Alteration in breathing
- Parental anxiety
- High risk for injury

Goals of Nursing Management. The child will:
- Maintain a patent airway with ease of respiration and free from rales, rhonchi, wheeze, etc.
- Parents describe the impending signs of attack and describe proper administration of prophylactic measures.

Nursing Interventions
- Set the child in a high Fowler's position or sitting leaning forward.
- Use calm reassuring approach, explaining procedures to the parents.
- Administer intravenous fluids.
- Administer bronchodilators, corticosteroids and expectorants as prescribed.
- Monitor vital signs every 1–2 hours.
- Maintain an I&O chart.
- Note specific gravity of urine.
- Provide a cool, moist environment.
- Administer aerosol or nebulizer treatment as indicated/ordered.
- Provide chest physiotherapy as indicated.
- Support anxious parents and allow them to take small break in between.
- Teach home care of children to prevent respiratory infections.

Evaluation
- The child's respiratory rate is within normal range and has no signs of respiratory distress.
- Parents express confidence in caring for their child.

Pneumonia

Definition/Description. Pneumonia, or inflammation of the pulmonary parenchyma, is common in childhood but occurs more frequently in infancy and early childhood.

Pneumonia can be classified according to morphology, aetiological agent and clinical forms. The most useful classification is based on the aetiological agent. In general, pneumonia is caused by four aetiological processes: viruses, bacteria, mycoplasmas and aspiration of foreign substances. Less often pneumonia may be caused by histomycosis, coccidiomycosis and other fungi. Morphologically, pneumonias are recognized as lobar pneumonia, bronchopneumonia and interstitial pneumonia. Clinically, pneumonia may be either primary or secondary as a complication of some other illnesses.

Aetiology and Incidence. It most commonly results from infection by viruses, bacteria, mycoplasmas or aspiration of foreign substances.

Viral pneumonia is the most common among these aetiological agents, and the most common virus responsible is respiratory syncytial virus. Other viruses include influenza and parainfluenza viruses, rhinoviruses and adenoviruses.

Among the bacterial pneumonias, the most common causative organisms are pneumococci, streptococci and staphylococci. *Pneumococcus* is the most common cause of lobar pneumonia and often affects children 1–4 years of age, with the highest incidence in late winter or early spring.

A streptococcal infection usually results in lobar pneumonia and commonly occurs as a complication of influenza or measles. *Staphylococcus* is the most common cause of bronchopneumonia and affects children younger than 2 years, with the highest incidence in winter. Pneumonia occurs in about 4% of children younger than 4 years, and its incidence decreases with advancing age.

Pathophysiology. Pneumonia typically begins as a mild respiratory infection and as the disease progresses, parenchymal inflammation occurs. Bacterial pneumonia produces lobar involvement and leads to consolidation. Viral pneumonia produces inflammation of interstitial tissue.

Clinical Manifestations. Clinical manifestations are according to the causative agents:
  1. **Viral pneumonia:**
     - Varying degrees of fever – mild to high
     - Severe cough and prostration
     - Nonproductive cough or productive whitish sputum
     - Rhonchi or fine crackles
  2. **Pneumococcal pneumonia:**
     - Manifestations vary with age
     - In infants – Vomiting, seizure, poor feeding, fretfulness, fever with bulging anterior fontanel, circumoral cyanosis, respiratory distress, diminished breath sounds, rales, pleural friction, rub, etc.
     - Older children – Headache, abdominal or chest pain, high fever with tachypnoea, hacking nonproductive cough, expiratory grunting, circumoral cyanosis, vocal fremitus, tubular breath sounds and disappearance of crackles indicating consolidation and copious blood-tinged mucus
  3. **Streptococcal pneumonia:**
     - Fever and chills
     - Signs of respiratory distress
     - Listlessness or extreme prostration
     - Rales
  4. **Staphylococcal pneumonia:**
     - High fever
     - Cough
     - Tachypnoea

- Cyanosis
- Anorexia
- Dyspnoea
- Intercostal retractions
- Nasal discharge
- Lethargy
- Diminished breath sounds
- As the condition deteriorates, signs of empyema or pneumothorax are visible

Nursing Diagnoses
- By clinical manifestations, radiological and laboratory findings
- Radiological findings show patchy infiltration with perbronchial distribution in viral pneumonia
- One or more areas of consolidation in pneumococcal pneumonia
- Disseminated infiltration in streptococcal pneumonia
- Patchy clouding in one or more lobes in staphylococcal pneumonia
- Laboratory findings include elevated blood cell count, identification of the causative agent in blood cultures and positive antistreptolysin-O titre in streptococcal pneumonia
- Thoracentesis may be performed if there is pleural effusion

Multidisciplinary Management
- Diagnostic tests—CBC count, sputum culture, chest X-rays and ABGs
- Antibiotics, expectorants
- Respiratory therapy
- Thoracentesis
- Chest tube insertion and closed chest drainage

Nursing Assessment
- Complete history
- Physical assessment
- Sputum culture
- Signs and symptoms

Nursing Diagnoses
- Ineffective airway clearance
- Alteration in breathing pattern
- Comfort alteration in pain
- Anxiety of parents and the child.
- Ineffective coping
- High risk for injury

Nursing Interventions
- Assess for respiratory distress by monitoring vital signs and respiratory status.
- Ease respiratory effort by:
  - Administering oxygen therapy as ordered
  - Creating a high humidity atmosphere using a humidifier or mist tent, if available
  - Performing chest physiotherapy every 4 hours and pre- and postural drainage
  - Using incentive spirometry
  - Suctioning if needed
  - Changing position frequently

- Encouraging breathing exercise for developmentally capable children: diaphragmatic breathing, side bending, pursed lips breathing, playing a wind instrument, blowing games with feathers or ping pong balls
- Changing position frequently and elevating head of the bed
- Help prevent dehydration by ensuring adequate oral or intravenous fluid intake; evaluate fluid status by monitoring I&O and weighing the child daily.
- Promote rest by maintaining bed rest and organizing nursing care to minimize disturbances.
- Ensure adequate nutrition by providing desirable high-calorie foods served in a pleasant, relaxed atmosphere.
- Support the child's family by answering questions and explaining all treatments and procedures.
- Teach and involve all capable family members to participate in the child's care, as appropriate.
- Administer prescribed medications as ordered, which may include antibiotics, expectorants, bronchodilators and antipyretics.
- Teach home care and need for close pulmonary monitoring and follow-up measures.

Evaluation
- The child exhibits no signs of respiratory distress.
- Oral fluids are taken and well tolerated, and the child is adequately hydrated; the urine output is 1 mL/kg of body weight.

STUDY QUESTIONS

- What are the stages of lung development?
- What is phosphatidylglycerol (PG)?
- What are the consequences of abnormal embryonic development of the respiratory system?
- Explain the fetal preparation for first breath.

- Plan and provide nursing care to children in the following medical problems:
  a. A 6-month-old baby with bronchiolitis.
  b. A 3-year-old brought with allergic asthma.
  c. A toddler with tracheolaryngeal bronchitis.
  d. An 8-year-old girl with pneumonia.
- State reasons for:
  1. Bronchiolitis is not treated with antibiotics.
  2. Artificially fed children get ear infections.
  3. Children are prone to respiratory distress.
  4. Children with respiratory difficulty are treated with nebulization.

BIBLIOGRAPHY

1. Brokgen, M.W., Gronkiewicz, G.A. (1995). Update Your Asthma: Care From Hospital to Home. American Journal of Nursing, 95(1), pp 26–35.
2. Consensus Guidelines on Management of Childhood Asthma in India. (1999). Indian Pediatrics, 36, pp 157–165.
3. Eisenbeis, C. (1996). Full Partner in Care: Teaching Your Patient How to Manage Her Asthma. Nursing, 26(1), pp 48–51.
4. Higgins, R.M., Stradling, J.R., Lane, D.J. (1998). Should Ipratropium Bromide be Added to Beta Agonists in Treatment of Acute Severe Asthma. Chest, 94, pp 718–722.
5. Nohoglu, Y., Dai, A., Barlan, I.B., Basaran, M.M. (1989). Efficacy of Aminophylline in Acute Asthma Exacerbation in Children. Annals of Allergy Asthma and Immunology, 80, pp 395–398.
6. Brown, OE, P Pownell, and SC Manning. (1996). Choanal Atresia: A New Anatomic Classification and Clinical Management Applications. Laryngoscope, 106, pp 97-101.
7. Flint, PW, BH Haughey, VJ Lund, JK Niparko, and MA Richardson. (2010). Cummings Otolaryngology Head and Neck Surgery. 5th. 2. Philadelphia: Elsevier, pp. 2694-2695.
8. Friedman, NR, RB Mitchell, CM Bailey, DM Albert, and SEJ Leighton. (2000). Management and Outcome of Choanal Atresia Correction. International Journal of Pediatric Otorhinolaryngology. 52, pp 45-51.
9. Gujrathi, CS, SJ Daniel, AL James, and V Forte. (2004). Management of Bilateral Choanal Atresia in the Neonate: an Institutional Review. Internal Journal of Pediatric Otorhinolaryngology. 68, pp 399-407.
10. http://getasthmahelp.org/asthma-classification-infants.aspx
11. http://getasthmahelp.org/asthma-classification-children-five-to-eleven.aspx
12. Downes J, Raphel. R. (1975). Paediatric intensive care. Anesthesiology. 43, pp 238-250.

ALTERATIONS IN GASTROINTESTINAL FUNCTIONS

LEARNING OBJECTIVES

At the end of the chapter, the learner will be able to:
- Describe the essential concepts related to gastrointestinal system development.
- Discuss the consequences of abnormal development.
- Describe the nursing management of common medical and surgical problems affecting gastrointestinal function using the nursing process.

This chapter discusses the care of children suffering from common gastrointestinal disorders that are important for a paediatric nurse.

ESSENTIAL CONCEPTS

Development of the gastrointestinal system proceeds in a series of orderly steps. By the fourth week of gestation, the primitive foregut is identified; by the sixth week, division for the foregut, mid gut and hindgut occurs. The malformations in the gastrointestinal tract result from failure in division, normal rotation or vascular accidents.

Embryology

Development of the primitive gastrointestinal system begins during the fourth week of gestation. But extensive developmental changes occur in the last few weeks of life before birth. The bronchial arches and the foregut, midgut and hind gut give rise to the gastrointestinal tract. During the fourth week of gestation, the primitive gut (foregut, midgut and hindgut) is formed as the dorsal portion of the yolk sac.

Oral Cavity

It is primarily developed from the brachial arches during the fourth week itself. The first brachial arch gives rise to the development of the face.

Oesophagus

The laryngotracheal groove becomes evident around 26 days after gestation. This groove divides to form the trachea and the oesophagus. The laryngotracheal groove begins as a very short tube and grows rapidly. At the same time, an increase in the thickness of the epithelial lining obliterates the lumen until around 8–10 weeks after the lumen is restored.

Stomach

The stomach first appears as a fusiform expansion of the caudal portion of the foregut (around 28 days), which then enlarges and broadens. The dorsal border grows faster than the ventral border during the next few weeks, creating the greater curvature of the stomach. The capacity of a newborn's stomach is 10–20 mL at birth. Peristalsis is rapid, causing frequent regurgitation.

Duodenum

The duodenum develops from the foregut and midgut. The junction where the foregut and the midgut fuse is just beyond the bile duct. This part of the duodenum grows rapidly and becomes a 'C'-shaped loop. As the stomach rotates, the duodenum rotates to the right. During the fifth and sixth weeks, lumen of the duodenum becomes temporarily obliterated because of the proliferation of epithelial cells. By the end of the embryonic period, the duodenum becomes recanalized.

Jejunum through the Mid-transverse Colon

This portion of the intestine is formed from the midgut. During the sixth week of gestation, the U-shaped intestinal loop herniates into the umbilical cord because of inadequate room in the abdomen. While this intestinal loop is out of the abdomen, it rotates 90°. During the 10th week, the intestinal loop returns to the abdomen, rotating another 180°. Like the duodenum, the other portions of the gut are obstructed because of the epithelial cells during the fifth and sixth weeks and then recanalize.

Large Intestine

The hindgut gives rise to the transverse colon through the superior portion of the anal canal. The inferior portion of the anal canal develops from the proctodeum. The cloaca (the caudal portion of the hindgut) is divided into the urogenital sinus and rectum by the urorectal septum. The inferior portion of the anal canal is initially separated from the superior portion by the anal membrane, but this membrane usually breaks down by the end of the eighth gestational week.

Biliary Tract

The liver bud is formed from an outgrowth of the foregut early in the fourth week. The liver bud extends into the septum transversum. The liver diverticulum rapidly enlarges and divides into two parts. Initially, both the left and right lobes of the liver are about the same size. Later, the right side becomes much larger. Haematopoiesis begins during the sixth week and is the main cause for the larger size of the liver. Bile formation begins during the 12th week. The pool size of bile acid of a premature infant of 32 weeks' gestation is about 50% of that in the full-term infant.

The caudal portion of the hepatic diverticulum expands to become the gallbladder and its stalk becomes the cystic duct. The stalk connecting the duodenum to the cystic duct and the hepatic duct becomes the bile duct. Initially, the extrahepatic biliary apparatus is occluded with endodermal cells, but it is later recanalized like the duodenum.

Pancreas

The pancreas develops from the dorsal and ventral pancreatic buds that arise from the caudal portion of the foregut as it is developing into the duodenum. As the pancreatic buds fuse, their ducts anatomize. The main pancreatic duct forms from the ventral bud duct and the distal part of the dorsal bud duct. The proximal portion of the dorsal bud duct often persists as an accessory pancreatic duct. There is frequently a communication between the two ducts.

Stool

The first stool of a newborn is called meconium. Normal newborn passes one to six stools a day.

Biochemical Development

Gastric functional development begins during the second trimester. Gastric acid activity starts after the 32nd week of gestation and increases in the first 24 hours of extrauterine life. Functional development of the small intestinal extends to postnatal life, too. The disaccharidase activity begins by the 12th week of gestation. Lactase activity is low till birth.

CONSEQUENCES OF ABNORMAL DEVELOPMENT

Disturbances in the normal pattern of development lead to congenital defects in newborn children. Oesophageal atresia with tracheoesophageal fistula (TEF) may occur when the tracheoesophageal septum deviates posteriorly or if the lumen is not recanalized by the end of the embryonic period. Malformations of stomach are uncommon except pyloric stenosis. If reformation of the duodenal lumen does not occur after 6 weeks, duodenal atresia may result. Failure of the gut to recanalize after the sixth week causes stenosis, atresia or duplications. Omphalocoele, malrotations or abnormalities of fixation result if the intestinal loop fails to return to the abdomen or rotates abnormally. Most anorectal abnormalities (rectal atresia, fistulas) are caused by arrested growth and/or deviation of the urorectal septum.

Consequences of Abnormal Development

Fetal Age (Weeks)	Structure	Anomalies at Birth
4	Branchial arches	Treacher–Collins syndrome
		Pierre–Robin syndrome
	Incomplete closure of lateral folds	Gastroschisis
	Division of the foregut into respiratory and digestive portions	Tracheoesophageal fistula
5–7	Two horizontal projections beside the tongue fuse to form the palate	Cleft palate
	Neural crest cells migrate into the wall of the colon	Hirschsprung disease
	Urorectal septum fuses with cloacal membrane	Anal stenosis

Continued

Consequences of Abnormal Development—cont'd

Fetal Age (Weeks)	Structure	Anomalies at Birth
8	Gastrointestinal tract becomes epithelialized	Oesophageal atresia
	Anal membrane ruptures	Imperforate anus, anorectal malformation (ARM)
10	Intestine returns to the abdomen	Omphalocele
		Umbilical hernia
	Intestines rotate as they re-enter the abdomen and become fixed	Malrotations of the midgut, volvulus
		Meckel diverticulum[a]
		Pyloric stenosis[a]

[a]Abnormalities not identified during fetal developmental periods.

Gastrointestinal disorders affect children of all ages. Most gastrointestinal problems can be effectively managed if identified early. Important nursing interventions used in the care of children with gastrointestinal disorders include careful monitoring after abdominal surgery, observation of feeding tolerance, implementation of specialized feeding regimens such as enteral feeding or total parenteral nutrition and education of the family about home care measures.

NURSING MANAGEMENT OF COMMON MEDICAL AND SURGICAL PROBLEMS AFFECTING GASTROINTESTINAL FUNCTIONS

Vomiting in Children

Vomiting is the forceful ejection of gastric contents. It is common during infancy and childhood. There are many reasons. It can result from a feeding technique, such as not breaking the wind (burping) after feeding an infant. There may be posseting and regurgitation (nonforceful return of milk after feeding). 'Posseting' is a term used to describe the return of milk that accompanies with swallowing of air. Regurgitation is larger and more frequent return of milk. Vomiting as a result of faulty feeding technique can be corrected by teaching parents the correct technique. But serious causes of vomiting need to be excluded if vomiting is bilious or prolonged. The common causes of vomiting can be divided under three headings as follows:

Medical Causes	Surgical Causes	Others
Gastroenteritis	Intestinal obstructions	Inborn errors of metabolism
Gastroesophageal reflux (GER)	Pyloric stenosis	Renal failure, congenital adrenal hypoplasia
Feeding problems	Duodenal stenosis/atresia	Coeliac disease
Infections	Intussusception	Cyclical vomiting
	Malrotation	Raised intracranial pressure
	Volvulus	

Medical Causes	Surgical Causes	Others
Respiratory tract infections	Hirschsprung disease	Anorexia nervosa/ bulimia
Otitis media		
Urinary tract infections		
Protein intolerance		
Meningitis		
Peptic ulcers		
Migraine		

The causes of vomiting need to be ascertained before attempting treatment. There are certain clues for identifying the causes of vomiting. Nonbilious vomiting may be a result of causes outside the gastrointestinal tract. If the vomitus is bile-stained, intestinal obstruction must be excluded. Projectile vomiting in the first few months of life suggests pyloric stenosis and later may be a result of increased intracranial pressure. Blood in the vomitus can be related to a bleeding oesophageal varices or peptic ulcer.

Multidisciplinary Management

This depends up on the cause of vomiting.
Rectify the cause.
Provide fluid replacement.
Administer antiemetics.

Nursing Management

1. Assess the type of vomitus.
2. Observe the colour and content of vomitus.
3. Measure the amount of vomitus.

Nursing Diagnoses

1. Fluid volume deficit
2. High risk for injury/complication
3. Alteration in nutrition
4. Parental anxiety

Nursing Interventions

1. Beware of the probable dehydration.
2. Evaluate the child for dehydration.
3. Assess the serum electrolyte and pH values.
4. Administer fluids on the basis of assessment.
5. Reassure the parents.
6. Report untoward symptoms.

GASTROESOPHAGEAL REFLUX

Definition/Description

GER is the involuntary passage of gastric contents into the oesophagus. These gastric contents irritate and sometimes cause mucosal damage in the oesophagus.

Aetiology

Infrequent GER is physiological and can occur in any child. When GER is frequent, it is a cause of concern. It results from the short intra-abdominal length of the oesophagus. It is common during the first year of life. By 12 months of age, nearly all symptomatic refluxes will be resolved because of maturity of the lower oesophageal sphincter. Severe reflux may be associated with cerebral palsy, bronchopulmonary dysplasia and also following surgery for oesophageal atresia.

Clinical Features

It may vary in different age groups.
Infants:
- Regurgitation
- Excessive crying and irritability
- May manifest as respiratory problems such as wheeze, stridor and cough
Older children:
- Abdominal pain
- Dysphagia
- Noncardiac chest pain
- Heart burn

Multidisciplinary Management

1. Perform 24-hour oesophageal pH monitoring.
2. Perform endoscopy with oesophageal biopsy.
3. Perform barium swallow and scintigraphy.
4. Mild reflux can be treated with the addition of inert thickening of feeds and upright positioning.
5. Elevate the head to 30° while positioning.
6. Keep the baby on its right side after feeding, with head in an elevated position or head up in a prone position.
7. Administer drugs that promote gastric emptying (e.g. domperidone) and H_2-antagonists (e.g. ranitidine) to reduce both gastritis and gastric acid secretion.

Surgery

- Fundoplication, in which the fundus of the stomach is wrapped around the intra-abdominal oesophagus, is performed if the symptomatic management fails.
- Perform fundoplication with pyloroplasty.
- Perform the Stretta procedure.

Nursing Management

1. Evaluate the child for frequency of vomiting.
2. Assess dehydration.
3. Observe for signs and symptoms.

Nursing Diagnoses

1. Alteration in fluid–electrolyte balance
2. Alteration in nutrition
3. Potential for growth retardation

4. Parental anxiety
5. Decreased parental coping

Nursing Interventions

1. Assess for dehydration.
2. Observe colour, consistency, type and frequency of vomiting.
3. Report any untoward symptoms.
4. Administer fluids as per prescription.
5. Encourage the upright position during sleeping.
6. Advise on avoidance of soft bedding.
7. Assess nutritional status (refer the chapter on nutrition).
8. Provide thickened feeds as per schedule.
9. Assess growth and development.
10. Provide parental support.
11. Instruct parents to reschedule the family routine (more frequent feeding time).
12. If surgical intervention is needed, provide pre- and postoperative care the same as for any gastrointestinal surgery.

GASTROENTERITIS

Definition/Description

Infection and inflammation of the gastrointestinal tract lead to gastroenteritis. Infective diarrhoea and vomiting are the main features of gastroenteritis.

Aetiology

The causes of gastroenteritis can be broadly categorized as viral, bacterial, fungal and environmental. Out of this, 60% of diarrhoeas are caused by virus, mainly rota virus, in children younger than 2 years. One needs to differentiate diarrhoea from gastrocolic reflex. There is passage of stools in small infants immediately after feeding. The most common and dreaded danger of diarrhoea is dehydration. Dehydration takes a heavy toll of precious life of children. Infants are at a high risk for losing their life as a result of dehydration related to their physiological constitution. The reasons for this are as follows:
- Increased surface area-to-weight ratio, leading to greater insensible water loss (300 mL/m^2 per day) equivalent to 15–17 mL/kg per day in infants
- Inability to gain access to water, related to the stage of development
- Higher basal fluid requirements (100–120 mL/kg per day, i.e. 10%–12% of body weight)
- Immature renal tubular reabsorption processes

There are many features of dehydration according to the degree of dehydration. As per the degree of dehydration, it can be classified as mild, moderate and severe. Correction of dehydration is the fundamental aim of treatment of diarrhoea. Degree of dehydration can be assessed for the proper management of dehydration.

Assessment of Dehydration

Parameter	Moderate Dehydration	Severe Dehydration
General appearance	Thirsty and restless	Drowsy, cold and sweating
Anterior fontanel	Sunken	Grossly sunken
Eyes	Sunken	Grossly sunken
Tears	Decreased/absent	Absent
Oral mucosa	Dry	Very dry
Pulse	Rapid	Rapid, weak and impalpable
Capillary refill	Normal/prolonged	Prolonged (>2 seconds)
Blood pressure	Normal/low	Low or nonrecordable
Urine output	Reduced	Marked oliguria
Weight	5%–10% reduction	>10% reduction

Dehydration can be assessed using the Child Survival and Safe Motherhood (CSSM) guidelines. These include restlessness,* increased thirst,* decreased skin turgor,* dry mouth and tongue, absent tears and sunken eyes. As per CSSM guidelines, dehydration may be diagnosed by the presence of two or more signs out of which one must be the asterisk-marked sign (*).

Treatment of Diarrhoea

Ask	Look	Decide	Classification of Dehydration	Treatment Plan

Ask the following: Does the child have diarrhoea?
• If the child has diarrhoea ask the following:
 • For how long?
 • How many times?
 • Is it accompanied by vomiting?
 • Is there any blood in stool?
	1. Look at the child's general condition:
	 • Is the child
	  • Lethargic or unconscious?
	  • Restless or irritable?
	2. Look for:
	 • Sunken eyes
	 • Skin turgor with a pinch of the skin – goes back promptly/ slowly/very slowly
	3. Offer the child fluid to drink – thirsty
	 • Not able to drink or drinking poorly?
	 • Drinking eagerly, appears thirsty?
	 • Drinking normally?
	4. Look at the eyes
	 • Normal eyes
	 • Sunken eyes
		Degree of dehydration:
		1. Some dehydration:
		 • Restless, irritable
		 • Sunken eyes
		 • Drinks eagerly, thirsty
		 • Skin pinch goes back 'slowly'
		2. Severe dehydration:
		 • Lethargic or unconscious
		 • Sunken eyes
		 • Not able to drink or drinking poorly
		 • Skin pinch goes back 'very slowly'
		3. No dehydration
			Severe dehydration
			Any of the two among the following signs:
			1. Unconscious or lethargic
			2. Sunken eyes
			3. Loss of skin turgor – skin pinch goes back very slowly
			Some dehydration
			Any two of the following signs:
			1. Restless and irritable
			2. Sunken eyes
			3. Loss of skin turgor – skin pinch goes back slowly
			No dehydration:
			No symptoms to classify
				PLAN C for SEVERE DEHYDRATION
				
				 PLAN B FOR SOME DEHYDRATION
				
				 PLAN A FOR NO DEHYDRATION

Plan A	Plan B	Plan C

Treat diarrhoea at home
Follow 4 rules while advising:
• Give extra fluid
• Continue breastfeeding if breastfed
• Advise mother when to bring the child to hospital
• Administer zinc for 14 days as prescribed
	Plan B is carried out at OPD in ORT corner of clinic/PHC
	• Treat 'some' dehydration with ORS (50–100 mL/kg)
	• Give 75 mL/kg of ORS in first 4 hours
	• If the child wants more, give more
		1. Start i.v. Fluid immediately:
		 • Give 100 mL/kg of Ringer's lactate
		 • Age under 12 months:
		  • First give 30 mL/kg in 1 hour
		  • Then give 70 mL/kg in 5 hours
		 • 12 months and older:
		  • First give 30 mL/kg in ½ hour
		  • Then give 70 mL/kg in 2½ hour

Treatment of Diarrhoea—cont'd

Plan A	Plan B	Plan C

1. Extra fluid:
  • Advice to the mother: breastfeed frequently and for longer period at each feed; if exclusively breastfed, give ORS for replacement of stool losses from each stool
  • If not exclusively breastfed, give one or more of the following:
    ◦ ORS, food-based fluid (such as soup, rice water, coconut water and yogurt drinks) or clean water
    ◦ Teach the mother how to prepare and give ORS
2. Amount of fluid to give in addition to the usual fluid intake:
  • Up to 2 years: 50–100 mL after each loose stool
  • 2 years or more: 100–200 mL after each loose stool
  • Continue usual feeding, which the child was taking before becoming sick 3–4 times
3. When to bring back the baby to hospital:
  • Advise mother to return immediately if the child has any of the following symptoms:
    ◦ Not able to drink or breastfeed or drinks poorly
    ◦ Becomes sicker
    ◦ Develops a fever
    ◦ Presence of blood in stool
	After 4 hours:
	Reassess and classify degree of dehydration:
	• Signs of severe dehydration
	Child not improving after 4 hours
	• Refer to higher centre – give ORS on way/keep warm/and breastfeed
	• When child comes back, follow-up like other children
		Fluid therapy in severe dehydration
		• Administer fluid either intravenous or intraosseous route
		• Ringer's lactate with 5% dextrose or ½ normal saline with 5% dextrose at 15 mL/kg/h for the first hour is usual fluid and dose
		• Never use dextrose alone
		• Monitor children continuously every 5–10 min
		• After 1 hour, if the condition is not improving or worsening, consider septic shock and report to the concerned physician immediately
		• If improvement is observed (pulse slows/faster capillary refill/increase in blood pressure), switch to ORS 5–10 mL/kg/h orally or by nasogastric tube for up to 10 hours

Adapted from World Health Organization "Manual for the Health Care of Children in Humanitarian Emergencies". Geneva: 2008.

Multidisciplinary Management

1. If the child does not have dehydration, there is no need for hospitalization.
2. Instruct the mother on preparation of homemade oral rehydration solution (ORS).
3. Give only homemade fluids to prevent dehydration.
4. Continue breastfeeding for breastfed babies.
5. Acute watery diarrhoea is usually self-limiting and there is no need of antibiotics.
6. If dehydration is present, give ORS as prescribed by the World Health Organization (WHO).
7. If vomiting is present, intravenous fluids may be needed.
8. No antimotility drugs required.
9. Administer zinc syrup and probiotics (such as Enterogermina).

CSSM guidelines for correction with intravenous fluids are as follows:

Age	30 mL/kg	Then give 70 mL/kg	Total 100 mL/kg
Infants	1 hour	Next 5 hours	6 hours
Older children	½ hour	Next 2½ hours	3 hours

Nursing Diagnoses

1. Fluid–electrolyte imbalance
2. Alteration in nutrition
3. Knowledge deficit
4. Parental anxiety

Nursing Interventions

Administer fluids as per prescription. Usually, ORS 100 mL/kg of body weight must be given within 4 hours orally. Other foods need not be given during this period. After correction of dehydration, foods can be given.

If the child vomits, ORS may be stopped for 10–15 minutes and restart the same.

If vomiting is persistent, start intravenous fluids. Remember vomiting is as a result of disturbed homeostasis and the treatment is fluids by the oral or parenteral route.

• Monitor serum electrolytes.

Check for hyponatraemia as evidenced by low serum sodium level (value less than 135 mEq/L as the lower limit of normal).

Administer normal saline for correction. The formula used for correction is deficit × 0.6 × body weight. The deficit can be measured by subtracting the measured serum level from normal (e.g. if serum level is 128 mEq/L, then the deficit is 135 − 128 = 7). Acute correction is done with the administration of 3% saline. If this is not available, the child can be treated with sodium bicarbonate 7.5% in normal saline. The bicarbonate thus administered corrects acidosis, too.

One millilitre of 7.5% sodium bicarbonate gives 0.9 mEq/L of bicarbonate and the same amount of sodium. One hundred millilitre of normal saline yields 15 mEq/L of sodium.

- Identify hypernatraemic dehydration as well. It is difficult to diagnose, as the obvious symptoms such as depressed fontanel and loss of skin elasticity are not seen. It is also very dangerous, as there will be fluid shift from the intracellular space to the extra-cellular space. This contributes to fluid shift from brain tissues, leading to cerebral shrinkage within the rigid cranium, causing multiple small cerebral haemorrhages and seizure. Associated hyperglycae-mia can also occur but may resolve by itself.
- Reduction of plasma sodium must be done with caution, as there is a chance of fluid shift leading to cerebral oedema. Correction should be done within 24–48 hours at a slow pace.
- Treat hypokalaemia. Administer potassium chloride (KCl) along with intravenous fluids. Addition of 1 mL of 15% KCl will give 2 mEq/L of potassium.
- NEVER administer potassium directly through the intravenous catheter. It should be added to the fluids that need to be infused.
- Maintain patency of the cannula; calculate the rate of flow.
- When diarrhoea subsides, the child needs to be fed properly to prevent malnourishment. Extra calories and protein need to be given to prevent malnutrition.
- Educate the parents regarding the causes and preventive measures of diarrhoea, such as need for proper personal and environmental hygiene, prevention of communicable diseases by immunization, breastfeeding for 2 years and introduction of complementary feeding by the fourth month with proper hygiene.
- If diarrhoea develops at all, then focus on how to prevent dehydration by giving homemade ORS.
- Teach preparation of homemade ORS or available fluids such as *kanji* water, lemon juice or coconut water.
- Prevent complications such as haemolytic uremic syndrome that can occur with *Shigella* dysentery. Other complications are ileus, shock, seizures, etc. that can be prevented if proper correction of dehydration is done.
- Lactose intolerance is a very serious complication of persistent diarrhoea. This needs to be treated with lactose-free formulas such as soya preparations.

COMMON TYPES OF GASTROENTERITIS

Cholera

This is a communicable disease caused by *Vibrio cholera* and is characterized by frequent passage of rice-water stools. Hardly any faecal matter may be present. Children will have severe fluid–electrolyte loss because of the secretary diarrhoea. Hence, fluid replacement needs to be increased from the usual recommended amount. Frequent assessment of dehydration to find out the

effectiveness of treatment is essential, as the losses are too high to be combated. Treatment is with drug tetracy-clines. But the use of tetracyclines in children younger than 8 years is not permitted. Doxycycline is less toxic among tetracyclines and is usually given to children with cholera in a dose of 6 mg/kg of body weight once daily for 3 days. Other drug used is erythromycin 40 mg/kg per day divided into four doses for 3 days.

As cholera occurs as an epidemic, proper public health measures need to be taken to prevent outbreaks and mass human loss.

Dysentery

It can be result from either bacterial invasion or proto-zoal invasion. Common bacteria that cause dysentery are *Shigella*, *Campylobacter* and *Salmonella*.

Essentially, treatment is with fluids and proper antibi-otics which may need a stool culture to isolate organisms and for sensitivity. Common antibiotics used are co-trimoxazole (8 mg/kg of body weight in two divided doses) and nalidixic acid (50 mg/kg of body weight per day in three divided doses).

The common protozoal dysentery is caused by amoeba and *Giardia*. Treatment is with metronidazole 30 mg/kg per day × 10 days for amoebiasis and 15 mg/kg per day × 5 days for giardiasis. A stool culture may be needed to confirm diagnosis. Treatment needs to be given with adequate precaution and prevent possible liver abscess.

Toddler Diarrhoea

This is a chronic nonspecific diarrhoea seen in toddlers and preschoolers. The stools in this type will vary in con-sistency, sometimes well-formed and sometimes explosive and loose. The presence of digested food particles, espe-cially vegetables, is a common feature. This characteristic of the stool gives diarrhoea the name 'peas and carrot syn-drome'. This symptom may subside by 5 years of age; see that children are not dehydrated. Hence, fluid replace-ment as per requirement needs to be considered.

Indian Childhood Cirrhosis

Indian childhood cirrhosis (ICC) of liver is a very serious condition affecting children in the Indian subcontinent. The word cirrhosis is derived from the Greek word *scir-rhus*, in which the surface of the liver appears orange or tawny at autopsy. It is one of the non-Wilsonian copper overload hepatic disorder. The first case in India was reported in the year 1880 in Kolkata.

Definition/Description

ICC is an autoimmune disorder characterized by fever, abdominal distension and hepatosplenomegaly.

Incidence

It is seen in children between the ages of 6 month and 4 years. Male children are affected more than female children, with a ratio of 4:1. There is a family predisposition for ICC. Siblings and twins are also affected. Among twins, the one who is fed with mixed feeds are more affected than those with exclusive breastfeeding for at least 6 months. It is commonly seen among middle-class families and among vegetarians. ICC has predisposition with diseases such as peptic ulcer, asthma and migraine in the pedigree. Decrease in the incidence of ICC has been observed in India because of decrease in the use of copper and brass vessels for cooking.

Aetiology

Exact aetiology of ICC is not known and believed to be autoimmune in nature.

Predisposing Factors

- Toxic (copper intoxication): Evidences shows that copper-binding proteins (orcein) are present in the liver of children with ICC. Addition of supplementary milk feeds before 3 months of age and use of copper and copper alloy vessels for boiling milk also contribute to ICC.
- Viral infection of the liver: Children who had infective hepatitis during the neonatal period also suffer from ICC.
- Immunological factors: High levels of circulating immune complexes cause insult to hepatocytes and result in immune-mediated injury to the liver.
- Nutritional factors: Malnutrition during young age may be a factor, but not much evidence is there to support this.
- Hepatotoxic agents: Some hepatotoxic agents such as aflatoxin, produced by *Aspergillus flavus* that grows on groundnuts, maize, and rice, can predispose to this disease. But the actual cause–effect relationship is not established.
- Familial history of the disease: A definite family predisposition is the hallmark of ICC. An increased prevalence of peptic ulcer, asthma, diabetes and migraine in the pedigrees affected by ICC has been observed.
- Metabolic factors: A child with inborn error of tryptophan metabolism, aminoaciduria, aminoacidaemia and disturbed lactose, zinc, copper and magnesium metabolism can predispose to the disease. So, a child at risk should be put on a low tryptophan diet.

It is possible that a genetically prone child suffers from one or more of the superadded factors (viral, toxic, metabolic and autoimmune) leading to ICC.

Pathophysiology

Aetiological factors contribute to marked damage to the hepatocytes leading to complete disorganization of liver architecture. This make changes in size, colour and formation of macro- and micro-nodules on the surface of the liver. The portal vein and biliary passages are patent and the lymphatics appear normal. Regenerating nodules in the liver are encircled by the bands of fibrous tissue. Absence of regenerative changes in the liver leads to degeneration, necrosis and fibrosis of hepatic lobules leading to cirrhosis. The necrosis of hepatocytes with ballooning, Mallory hyaline pericellular intralobular fibrosis and inflammatory cell infiltration along with cholestasis is present in the advanced stage.

Clinical Features

Clinical features depend on the type of onset. It can be insidious or acute onset.

I. **Insidious onset:** The insidious onset has two types, and type 2 has three stages as follows:
1. **The precirrhotic symptoms**
   - Irritability
   - Disturbed appetite
   - Chalky, pasty stools and distension of abdomen
   - Constipation or diarrhoea
   - Often slight irregular fever
2. **The cirrhotic symptoms**
   Cirrhotic symptoms are grouped under three stages:
   a. Stage I:
      - Slight fever
      - Liver is enlarged up to 3–5 cm, edges become sharp, giving a leafy boarder appearance
      - Children exhibit jaundice
      - Poor growth
      - Anorexia
      - Constipation/diarrhoea
      - Clay-coloured stools
      - Growth failure
   b. Stage II:
      - Diffuse hepatomegaly
      - Splenomegaly
      - Ascites
      - Oesophageal varices
      - Haemoptysis
      - Anaemia
      - Muscle weakness
      - Lethargy
      - Gastrointestinal bleeding
   c. Stage III:
      - It is the terminal stage of the disease
      - Restlessness
      - Confusion
      - Dyspnoea and cyanosis on exertion
      - Evidences of hepatocellular failure in the form of palmar erythema and spider nevus appearance on the upper torso
      - A peculiar garlic odour is present in patients with impending liver cell failure
      - Enlarged and hard spleen
      - Terminally, there is jaundice and hepatic coma and is often associated with gastrointestinal bleeding
      - The child may die at this stage either from hepatic failure or intercurrent infections

II. **Acute onset:** It is the sudden onset of disease and sometimes the child becomes symptomatic for a variable period and then shows the manifestations of the insidious onset. The symptoms include:
- Sudden onset of fever
- Jaundice
- Clay-coloured stools
- Hepatomegaly
- Maybe death as a result of hepatic coma

Diagnostic Evaluation

1) Perform history collection.
2) Complete physical examination: Liver can be palpable, very firm in consistency and its boarders will be sharp. On auscultation, hepatic bruit is present in severe cases. If there is ascites, fluid thrill test can be done.
3) Liver function test
   • Increased ALT (alanine transaminase, an enzyme present in hepatocytes)
   • Increased GGT (γ-glutamyl transpeptidase)
4) Prothrombin time (PT), clotting time and bleeding time should be assessed. PT will be prolonged.
5) Liver biopsy is done to find out the sclerosis of liver. It is a reliable method of arriving at a foolproof diagnosis.
6) Cupriuresis: It involves testing the presence of copper in urine after administration of D-penicillamine.

Multidisciplinary Management

If the condition is diagnosed in early stages, i.e. before the development of jaundice, ICC can be treated.

1. Initial stage:
   • An adequate diet with enough quantity of good-quality proteins, vitamins and minerals is desirable.
   • Antibiotics should be given to treat the intercurrent infections/infestations.
   • The drug of choice is D-penicillamine (which chelates copper) in a dose of 20–40 mg/kg per day for 12–18 months, which leads to marked improvement and even total reversal of the histopathological picture.
   • Symptomatic treatment should be given.
   • Immunomodulators such as levamisole can be used.
   • Corticosteroids and γ-globulins are also helpful.
   • Administer intravenous fluids if there is dehydration.
   • Prevention of infection: Follow aseptic techniques.
   • Prophylactic antibiotics can be given to prevent infection.

2. Terminal stage:
   If the patient has entered the precoma or coma stage, the protein intake should be reduced. Administration of neomycin by gavage and 20% i.v. glucose drip are helpful. Oxygen can be administered if necessary. Administer exchange transfusion to remove the circulating toxins.

Surgical Management

• No specific surgical correction is required. The only successful treatment of end-stage liver disease is liver transplantation.
• If there is portal hypertension with haematemesis, Sengstaken tube may help control the oesophageal bleed.
• A portocaval anastomosis may be done to relieve the portal hypertension and complications of hypersplenism.

Nursing Management

Nursing Diagnosis

1. Hyperthermia related to the inflammatory process in the liver
2. Impaired breathing pattern related to pressure on diaphragm secondary to ascites
3. Imbalanced nutrition less than body requirement related to anorexia
4. Diarrhoea or constipation related to acute abdominal condition
5. Parental anxiety related to management of the disease condition

Nursing Interventions

• Provide symptomatic treatment to the child.
• Provide adequate rest and place in a semi-Fowler's position.
• Check and record the abdominal girth every fourth hourly.
• Administer intravenous fluids if needed.
• Provide small and frequent meals.
• Provide protein-rich food and massive doses of vitamin B_6.
• Follow aseptic techniques to prevent infection.
• Intake and output (I&O) chart should be maintained.
• Provide parental education:
  • Explain the cause, symptoms and management of the disease.
  • Avoid food rich in copper such as dry nuts, chocolates, liver, etc.
  • Provide small and frequent meals to the child.
  • Advice the mother to breastfeed her baby for a longer period and not to introduce food supplements beyond the age of 6 months.
  • Milk used for the infant should not be boiled and stored in copper and copper alloy pots.
  • Reduce the use of brass and copper vessels.
  • Use aluminium and steel utensils.
  • Foods rich in tryptophan (milk, eggs, meat, nuts, beans, fish and cheese) should be reduced.
  • Provide more vitamin B_6 foods such as potato, banana, spinach, soya bean, fruits and vegetables. (Vitamin B_6 helps convert tryptophan to niacin.)

Malabsorption Syndrome

Definition/Description

Malabsorption syndromes are conditions that result in chronic diarrhoea, abdominal distension and failure to thrive. It is a disorder of the intestinal processes of digestion, transport, or both of carbohydrate, protein and fat across the intestinal mucosa into the systemic circulation. Congenital abnormality in the digestive or absorptive process or a secondarily acquired disorder of such a process may result in malabsorption.

Aetiology

Causes of malabsorption can be divided into congenital and acquired. It usually affects one or more steps of intestinal hydrolysis and subsequent transport of nutrients.

Genetically determined syndromes occur in 1% of the children, but the majority of cases are secondary to cow's milk or soy milk protein allergies, especially in infants and young children, with a prevalence of 3%. Cystic fibrosis is the second most common cause of acquired malabsorption syndrome. Another cause of malabsorption is related to acute-onset enteritis (rota virus) with transient malabsorption. Nonspecific diarrhoea in toddlers also causes malabsorption.

Other possible causes are as follows:
- Carbohydrate malabsorption results from deficiency of salivary and pancreatic amylase.
- Pancreatic insufficiency impedes the digestion of large starch molecules.
- Absence or reduction of the brush-border disaccharidases causes selective carbohydrate malabsorption.
- Glucoamylase and maltase are most resistant to the depleting effects of mucosal injury that result from infection, whereas lactase is the most sensitive because of its predominant distribution near the tips of the villi.
- Lack of sucrase and isomaltase is, by far, the most frequent congenital enzyme deficiency. This enzyme deficiency is inherited in an autosomal recessive manner.
- Small bowel bacterial overgrowth of normal flora alters the intraluminal metabolism of carbohydrates and results in their malabsorption.
- Fat malabsorption: Increased delivery of fat to the colon results in diarrhoea and soft, pasty, foul-smelling stools. It also alters absorption of fat-soluble vitamins (A, D, E and K).
- Exocrine pancreatic insufficiency is the principal condition that results in severe fat malabsorption in cystic fibrosis, Shwachman–Diamond syndrome and Johanson–Blizzard syndrome.
- Protein malabsorption: Malabsorption that results from congenital enterokinase deficiency is found in certain cases, but the incidence of such defect is rare.
- Creatorrhea, loss of protein in the stool (protein-losing enteropathy): It is caused by the leakage of protein from the serum as a result of inflammation of the mucosa (coeliac disease and protein sensitivity syndromes).
- Vitamin malabsorption: Malabsorption of vitamin B_{12} and folate may also result in this syndrome.

Factors that may cause malabsorption syndrome include:
- Damage to the intestine from infection, inflammation, trauma or surgery
- Prolonged use of antibiotics
- Other conditions such as coeliac disease, Crohn disease, chronic pancreatitis or cystic fibrosis
- Lactase deficiency or lactose intolerance
- Certain defects that are congenital (present at birth), such as biliary atresia (when the bile ducts do not develop normally and prevent the flow of bile from the liver)
- Diseases of the gallbladder, liver or pancreas
- Parasitic diseases
- Radiation therapy, which may injure the lining of the intestine
- Certain drugs that may injure the lining of the intestine, such as tetracycline, colchicine or cholestyramine

Risk Factors

- Mortality/Morbidity
  Mortality is rare except in cystic fibrosis, as it is the most lethal genetic disorder. Neonates and infants with severe malnutrition are at risk of dying. Associated comorbidity is also a threat.
- Race
  People of Canadian Eskimos and natives of Greenland are affected more. But adult-onset malabsorptions are seen in the people of Asians, Africans and Mediterranean origin.
- Sex
  All types of coeliac disease are more common in females, as autoimmune enteropathy is X-linked.
- Age
  Neonates and young infants are at a high risk as a result of milk protein allergies. The congenital malabsorption manifests early in life.

Pathophysiology

Carbohydrate, fat or protein malabsorption is caused by a disorder in the intestinal processes of digestion, transport, or both of carbohydrate, protein and fats across the intestinal mucosa into the systemic circulation as a result of congenital or acquired causes.

There are three characteristic phases in the digestion and absorption of major nutrients.
  Luminal phase: Dietary fats, proteins and carbohydrates are solubilized by digestive enzymes and bile. Deficiency of lipase and proteases leads to lipid and protein malabsorption.
  Mucosal phase: Brush-border hydrolase activity is more common in primary or secondary lactase deficiency.
  Postabsorptive phase: Hydrolysed nutrients are transported via lymphatic and portal circulation. Impairment of chylomicrons and lipoproteins may cause fat malabsorption or protein-losing enteropathy.

Absorption of Carbohydrates. The most common carbohydrates present in the diet are starches, sucrose and lactose. Out of these, only starches require preliminary luminal digestion by salivary and pancreatic amylases. The secretion of pancreatic amylase reaches the adult level in the first year. Starch malabsorption is rare in infants as a result of activity of the brush-border glucoamylase that develops in early life itself. The final hydrolysis of disaccharides and oligosaccharides occurs at the brush border of the enterocytes, where sucrase–isomaltase break down to maltose then to isomaltose (to glucose) and finally to sucrose (to glucose and fructose). The entry of these molecules (final monosaccharaides) into the enterocytes takes place through brush border via carrier molecules.

Malabsorption of carbohydrate can be a result of congenital disorders such as cystic fibrosis and Shwachman–Diamond syndrome, which cause amylase deficiency, the extremely rare congenital lactase deficiency, glucose–galactose malabsorption, sucrase–isomaltase deficiency and adult-type hypolactasia. The acquired ones are lactose intolerance, typically secondary to damage of the mucosa, such as viral enteritis, or conditions that cause mucosal atrophy, such as coeliac disease.

Absorption of Proteins. Proteins are first digested in the stomach, where pepsinogen, activated to pepsin by a pH of less than 4, hydrolyses them into large-molecular-weight peptides. Upon entering the duodenum, the pancreatic proteases (activated by trypsin) split large peptides into low-molecular-weight peptides (two to six amino acid residues) to 70% and free amino acids to 30%. Free amino acids are taken up by enterocytes through specific Na-linked carrier systems.

Disorders of Protein Digestion. Lipase is responsible for the first partial hydrolysis of triglycerides; this enzyme becomes active in persons with low gastric pH levels and is active even in premature infants. The largest part of triglyceride digestion is accomplished in the duodenojejunal lumen because of a complex of pan-*congenital disorders* of protein digestion (cystic fibrosis, Shwachman–Diamond syndrome and enterokinase deficiency) causes inadequate intraluminal digestion. No congenital defects have been described in any of the brush-border-bound peptidases or in the peptide carrier. *Acquired disorders* of protein digestion and/or absorption are nonspecific (they also affect the absorption of carbohydrates and lipids) and result from damage of the absorptive intestinal surface, such as extensive viral enteritis, milk protein allergy enteropathy and coeliac disease.

Absorption of Fats. Like amylase, lingual creatic enzymes – lipase–colipase complex, also develop slowly, and this results in a low capacity of babies to absorb lipids, termed 'physiological steatorrhoea' of the newborn. Additionally, adequate concentrations of intraluminal conjugated bile salts are needed to form micelles, and the secretion of bile acids may also be partially inadequate in very young patients.

Clinical Features

Gastrointestinal tract symptoms
- Abdominal distension and watery diarrhoea, with or without mild abdominal pain, associated with skin irritation in the perianal area as a result of acidic stools are characteristic of carbohydrate malabsorption syndromes.
- Periodic nausea, abdominal distension and pain, and diarrhoea are common in patients with chronic *Giardia* infections.
- Vomiting, with moderate-to-severe abdominal pain and bloody stools, is characteristic of protein sensitivity syndromes or other causes of intestinal injury (e.g. inflammatory bowel disease).
- Poor appetite is common in food sensitivity syndromes. The child becomes conditioned to refuse foods that cause inflammatory reactions of the intestine (this is typical in coeliac disease).
- Malabsorption syndromes not associated with inflammatory reactions typically cause an increase in appetite (e.g. cystic fibrosis).

Stool characteristics
- Patients with toddler's diarrhoea often have loose stools with undigested food particles. This should not be taken to imply the presence of true malabsorption.
- Frequent loose watery stools may indicate carbohydrate intolerance.
- Pasty or loose foul-smelling stools indicate fat malabsorption, also termed steatorrhoea (hepatic and pancreatic dysfunction and protein sensitivity syndromes).
- Bloody stools are seen in patients with protein sensitivity syndromes.

Diagnosis

- History
  Diet history: Obtain complete history of diet including the amount, type, formula feeds and its constituents and how much is ingested each time. This history should be taken for a minimum of period of 1 week. The amount of fluids taken is also important, as the normal requirement is 100 mL/kg. If infants are given more than that amount, they will have loose stools. This will not cause malabsorption.
  Fat intake less than 3 g/kg also should be verified, as fat is important for slowing the movement of food through intestine. This low intake of fat is a cause for toddler diarrhoea.
  Find out whether children are fed with juice, especially purple grape juice. This can cause diarrhoea.
  Look for gastrointestinal symptoms such as mild abdominal gaseous distension to severe abdominal pain and vomiting. Abdominal pain and vomiting also can be seen.
  Periodic nausea, abdominal distension and watery diarrhoea are the characteristic features that help in diagnosis along with history.
  Stool characteristics: Loose stools indicate carbohydrate indigestion; frequent loose stools indicate lactose intolerance. Differentiate it with viral and protozoal causes of diarrhoea.
  Disaccharidases and pancreatic enzyme deficiencies need to be looked into. Systemic symptoms such as weakness, fatigue and failure to thrive.
  Infants with weight loss or little weight gain with chronic diarrhoea need investigation for malabsorption.
  Borborygmi (increased peristaltic movements) can be detected audibly and with tactile palpation as a result of decreased intestinal transient time.
- Laboratory findings
  The following laboratory studies are indicated in malabsorption syndromes:
  Stool analysis
  - The presence of reducing substances indicates that carbohydrates have not been properly absorbed. Acidic stool has a pH level of less than 5.5. This indicates carbohydrate malabsorption even in the absence of reducing substances.
  - Stool bile acids: Conjugated and unconjugated bile acids may be measured in the stool, and but it is not used in routine clinical practice.
  - Stool fat and the amount of fat intake should be measured and monitored for 3 days. Normal fat absorption depends on age (lower in the neonate) and 95% or higher by the end of 1 year. Moderate fat malabsorption ranges from 60%

to 80%. Fat absorption of less than 50% indicates severe malabsorption.

- The presence of serum proteins in the stool, such as α_1-antitrypsin, indicates leakage of serum protein and serves as a screening test for protein-losing enteropathy.
- Stool for the presence of ova and parasites or testing the stool antigen for the presence of *Giardia* species, a cause of acquired malabsorption syndromes in children older than 2 years, may be performed.
- Testing for other chronic intestinal infections that cause malabsorption, such as *Clostridium difficile* (assays for toxins A and B) or *Cryptosporidium* species (modified acid-fast examination of stool), may be performed.

Urinalysis

- Urine examination may reveal an unusually high concentration of the malabsorbed substance, as the kidney and gut use the same transporter.
- In glucose–galactose malabsorption, the urinary glucose level is elevated.

Other laboratory studies

- A complete blood cell (CBC) count may reveal megaloblastic anaemia in patients with folate and vitamin B_{12} malabsorptions.
- Neutropenia may be present in patients with Shwachman–Diamond syndrome (associated with pancreatic insufficiency).
- In patients with abetalipoproteinaemia, blood smears may reveal acanthocytosis.
- Total serum protein and albumin levels may be lower than the reference range in syndromes in which protein is lost or is not absorbed.
- Recently, a ^{13}C-sucrose breath test has been proposed as a noninvasive, easy-to-use, integrated marker of the absorptive capacity and integrity of the small intestine.
- These tests measure the level of specific nutrients in blood, such as vitamin B_{12}, vitamin D, folate, iron, calcium, carotene, phosphorus, albumin and protein.
- Breath tests: If hydrogen gas is detected in breath after ingesting a product containing lactose, lactose intolerance may be present.

Radio diagnosis

- Upper gastrointestinal radiography with small bowel follow-through shows thickened folds and increased fluid content in the jejunal loop.

Other tests are substance tolerance test, carbohydrate malabsorption tolerance test, D-xylose absorption test, mucosal biopsy, etc.

Histological findings of mucosal biopsy are villous atrophy, infiltration of the epithelium by cytotoxic intraepithelial T lymphocytes and crypt hyperplasia. However, the spectrum can range from a simple intraepithelial lymphocytosis without villous blunting or crypt hyperplasia to total villous atrophy with severe crypt hyperplasia. Biopsy of the small intestine remains the criterion standard for the diagnosis of coeliac disease.

Multidisciplinary Management

- Treatment is based on specific entity and hence varies widely. If malabsorption results from carbohydrate malabsorption, the treatment is based on that and if it is a protein problem, then the treatment is based on that.
- Chronic diarrhoea as a result of proximal small bowel bacterial overgrowth is treated with oral, broad-spectrum antibiotics, particularly those with anaerobic coverage (e.g. metronidazole).
- Malabsorption secondary to short gut needs to be aggressively treated, and pharmacological options are now available.
- In children with chronic diarrhoea secondary to bile acid malabsorption, the use of cholestyramine (Questran) to bind bile acids may help reduce the duration and severity of the diarrhoea.
- Pancreatic enzyme deficiency is treated with oral supplements.
- Immunosuppressive medications can be used to control autoimmune enteropathy and should only be prescribed by a specialist.
- Children with malabsorption secondary to food allergic enteropathy need to be on an elimination diet, avoiding offending food antigens.
- So, identification of exact aetiology is very important in managing malabsorption.

Surgical care: Usually, surgical care is not required. But children who are on parenteral nutrition for a prolonged period may require multivisceral organ transplantation.

Nursing Management

- Provide supportive management and reassurance to parents.
- Diet management: Children with carbohydrate intolerance should be advised to take diet that is devoid of carbohydrate until diarrhoea resolves.
- For infants, use a glucose polymer (polycose)-based formula.
- Children with severe carbohydrate intolerance should be given a casein-based formula that contains essential amino acids and medium-chain triglyceride (MCT) oil and no carbohydrate.
- Usual practice is to begin with 14 g of fructose/L of formula and gradually advance in 14-g increments to a maximum of 56 g of fructose/L of formula. Once this goal is reached, slowly replace fructose with Polycose until 56 g of Polycose/L of formula is tolerated. Once 56 g of Polycose/L of formula is tolerated, begin introducing Pregestimil, a lactose-free formula.
- For older children, eliminate simple carbohydrates and lactose from the diet until the diarrhoea is resolved. Simple sugars, including fruit juices, should be avoided for several weeks.
- If after several weeks of a relatively carbohydrate-free diet symptoms return when carbohydrates are reintroduced, one must understand that the child has a congenital defect in carbohydrate transport or digestion.

Fat intolerance should be managed as follows:

- MCT oil is used to treat patients with poor weight gain that results from fat malabsorption. MCT oil does not require traditional fat metabolism and thus is more easily absorbed into the enterocyte and transported through the portal vein to the liver.

- Fat-soluble vitamin supplements are required for patients with fat malabsorption or short gut syndrome.
- Supplements in patients with fat malabsorption should also include linoleic and linoleic fatty acids.
- For children with short gut, appropriate parenteral nutrition may be given.

  Alternative formulas
  - Soy formulas can be effectively replaced with hydrolysed protein formulas.
  - High-degree protein hydrolysate formulas can be replaced with crystalline amino acids (e.g. Neocate, EleCare, EO28) as the protein source to reduce allergic reactions.

  Digestive enzymes
  - Pancreatic enzyme deficiency may occur because of steatorrhoea secondary to malabsorption. Pancrelipase (Ultrase, Pancrease, Creon) assists in the digestion of protein, starch and fat. It contains lipase, protease and amylase.

Coeliac Disease

Definition

It is an autoimmune disorder occurring in genetically predisposed individuals when they eat foods containing gluten that leads to damage of small intestine.

Incidence

It affects one in 100 people worldwide. It is hereditary. The risk of developing this disease is as high as 1:10 in first-degree relatives (parents, siblings and children) if they have coeliac disease.

Gluten is a protein found in wheat, barley, rye and other certain grains. This protein gives the chewy texture to breads. This disease has about 200 symptoms and varies among individuals and hence it is difficult to diagnose.

Pathophysiology

If children predisposed to gluten deficiency eat foods containing gluten, their body overreacts and produces damage to the small intestine and the villi get injured. Once the villi get injured, they will not be able to absorb nutrients. This leads to malnourishment and loss of bone mass.

Clinical Features

Two types of symptoms, namely gastrointestinal (typical) and nongastrointestinal (atypical), are present. Children have more of gastrointestinal symptoms. The common ones are as follows:

- Abdominal bloating and pain
- Chronic diarrhoea
- Vomiting
- Constipation
- Pale, foul-smelling or fatty stool
- Weight loss
- Fatigue

- Irritability and behavioural issues
- Dental enamel defects of the permanent teeth
- Delayed growth and puberty
- Short stature
- Failure to thrive
- Attention-deficit/hyperactivity disorder (ADHD)

Diagnosis

- Anti-gliadin antibodies testing: Antibodies (IgG and IgA) to the gluten protein in wheat, rye and barley. This test is relatively cheap and easy to perform, but it has poor sensitivity and specificity.
- Endomysial antibody (EMA) IgA-based antibody against reticular connective tissue around smooth muscle fibres. The test has high sensitivity and specificity but can be false-negative in young children; it is operator dependent, expensive and time consuming, and false-negative in IgA deficiency.
- Tissue transglutaminase (TTG): IgA-based antibody against TTG (coeliac disease auto-antigen). It has high sensitivity and specificity (human TTG) and nonoperator dependent (ELISA/RIA). It is relatively cheap but is false-negative in young children.

Multidisciplinary Management

- Only treatment of coeliac disease is a gluten-free diet (GFD)
- Strict, lifelong diet
- Avoid: Wheat, rye and barley

Lactose Intolerance

Lactose intolerance is most common of all the syndromes of carbohydrate malabsorption. The primary cause is lactase deficiency. It is a clinical syndrome with symptoms such as abdominal pain, diarrhoea, nausea, flatulence and/or bloating after ingestion of lactose or lactose-containing food substances.

Types

There are many types of lactose intolerance.
They are:
- Congenital – Very rare
- Primary – Develops after 2 years of age
- Secondary – Usually resolves in 1–2 weeks
- Developmental lactase deficiency

Aetiology

Lactase deficiency is either primary or secondary. Primary deficiency is caused by the relative absence of lactase, and secondary deficiency results from small bowel injury such as in gastroenteritis, persistent diarrhoea and hereditary lactase deficiency.

Clinical Features

Symptoms vary from individual to individual, depending on the amount of lactose ingested. Symptoms are a result of imbalance between the amount of ingested lactose and the capacity for lactase to hydrolyse the disaccharide. Other features are:

- Abdominal distension, flatulence
- Abdominal cramping
- Diarrhoea

Diagnosis

- History
- Stool test for pH
- Hydrogen breath test

Multidisciplinary Management

- Lactose-free and lactose-reduced milks (and lactose-free whole milk for children younger than 2 years)
- Lacto-free, NAN lactose-free
- Administration of lactase enzyme
- Vitamin (A, D, E and K) and mineral supplements (calcium, zinc and iron)

ACUTE ABDOMINAL PAIN

There are multiple causes for acute abdominal pain in children. These can be classified as intra-abdominal and extra-abdominal causes.

Intra-abdominal causes are either medical or surgical.

Medical Causes	Surgical Causes	Extra-abdominal Causes
• Gastroenteritis • Mesenteric adenitis • Urinary tract problems • Urinary tract infection • Pyelonephritis • Hydronephrosis • Renal calculi • Henoch–Schonlein purpura • Diabetic ketoacidosis • Sickle cell anaemia • Hepatitis • Inflammatory bowel diseases • Constipation • Recurrent abdominal pain of childhood • Gynaecological problems in puberty • Psychological • Lead poisoning • Unknown	• Acute appendicitis • Intestinal obstructions such as intussusception • Inguinal hernia • Peritonitis • Meckel diverticulum • Pancreatitis • Trauma	• Upper respiratory tract infections • Lower lobe pneumonia • Torsion of testis • Hip and spine problems

The exact cause must be identified to provide management of acute abdominal pain. Management depends on the cause. If it is a surgical cause, surgical management will be provided. Other causes are treated as per the cause. Nursing management is, too, dependent on the cause and the type of multidisciplinary management.

TRACHEOESOPHAGEAL FISTULA AND OESOPHAGEAL ATRESIA

These are malformations that results from failure of the oesophagus to develop as a continuous passage, and a failure of the trachea and the oesophagus to separate into distinct structures and an abnormal connection between the two exist. This can occur as two defects or sometimes occur in combination.

Aetiology and Incidence

Aetiology is like any other congenital malformations/anomalies as a defect in the development. Incidence is estimated to be from one in 3000 to one in 3500 live births. Both sexes are equally affected. The birth weight of the affected babies is lower than average. A high incidence of prematurity is also common. Approximately 50% of the infants with oesophageal atresia and TEF have associated anomalies (VACTERL syndrome – vertebral, anorectal, cardiovascular, tracheoesophogeal, renal and limb abnormalities) and CHARGE association (coloboma, heart defects, atresia choanae, retarded development, genital hypoplasia and ear abnormality). Prenatal karyotyping is advised in such conditions.

In total, 50% of children with TEF have associated anomalies that worsen prognosis. Duodenal atresia is also common along with TEF. The risk of subsequent pregnancies with TEF is less than 1%.

Pathophysiology

Oesophagus develops from the segment of the embryonic gut. During fourth to fifth weeks of intrauterine life (IUL), the foregut lengthens and separates longitudinally and becomes two parallel channels (trachea and oesophagus) that join only at the larynx. Anomalies involving the trachea and the oesophagus develop from defective separation or incomplete fusion of tracheal folds following separation or altered cellular growth during embryonic development.

Clinical Manifestations

- Frothy saliva in the nose and mouth is present, with drooling accompanied by chocking and coughing.
- Swallowing produces cough, gag and chocking, and the fluid returns through the nose and mouth.
- The infant becomes cyanotic and stops breathing with aspiration of feeds.
- Crying may be associated with air gulping and results in distended stomach and causes thoracic compression.
- If the upper segment of the oesophagus opens into the trachea, the infant is in danger of aspiration of the swallowed material.
- Abdominal distension begins soon after birth because of the inspired air that enters the stomach.
- Respiratory distress (retractions, nasal flaring, expiratory grunt and seesaw respirations) is noted.

Types

First type: In total, 80%–95% are those in which the proximal oesophageal segment terminates in a blind pouch and the distal segment is connected to the trachea or primary bronchus by a short fistula at or near the bifurcation.

Second type: Pure oesophageal atresia (5%–8%) consists of a blind pouch at each end, which is widely separated and with no communication to the trachea.

Third type: The normal trachea and the oesophagus are connected by a fistula. It is an extremely rare anomaly that involves a fistula from the trachea to the upper oesophageal segment.

Both upper and lower segments with a fistula from the trachea can also occur. Different types of TEFs are shown in in the following figure.

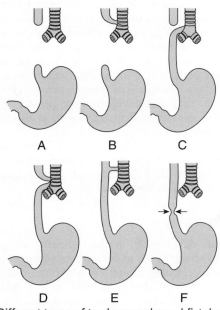

Different types of tracheoesophageal fistulas.

Clinical Signs and Symptoms

- Passage of a radiopaque catheter into the oesophagus will meet with resistance if the lumen is blocked but will pass unobstructed if the lumen is patent.
- Chest radiograph to ascertain:
- Oesophageal patency or the presence and level of a blind pouch.
- Presence of polyhydramnios prenatally is a clue to the diagnosis with signs and symptoms.

Multidisciplinary Management

Postnatal surgical management is dependent on the size and condition of the baby, length of the oesophageal gap and associated anomalies. Primary repair of the oesophagus is the treatment of choice; however, if not achieved, staged repair with upper oesophageal pouch care and gastrostomy or organ replacement with stomach or large bowel are other options. Associated anomalies require

evaluation and treatment. Advanced paediatric endosurgical centres may offer a minimally invasive thoracoscopic approach to the repair of TEF.

- Maintenance of patent airway
- Prevention of pneumonia
- Supportive therapy
- Surgical repair
- Surgical correction

Either one-stage operation or staging with two or more procedures according to the types of defects and associated defects is performed. The surgery consists of a thoracotomy with division and ligation of the TEF and end-to-end anastomosis of the oesophagus. Chest tube is inserted to drain chest fluid. In the staged procedure, gastrostomy is done for feeding to improve the condition of the baby; ligation of the TEF and drainage of the oesophageal pouch are done. Delayed oesophageal anastomosis is done after several weeks when the upper pouch elongates and the lower pouch hypertrophies. Sometimes, bougienage (the process whereby a blunt metal instrument is used to dilate fistula or lengthen membranous tissue) is performed. In unduly late anastomosis, a cervical oesophagostomy is done to drain the secretions. If the length of the segments is not enough for anastomosis, an oesophageal replacement procedure is used for correction.

Nursing Assessment

- Assess the infant's respiratory status (early recognition helps prevent aspiration).
- Assess for excessive amounts of mucus with drooling.
- Assess for coughing, chocking and cyanosis when fed.
- Check for expelled feeds through nose immediately following feeding (coughing, chocking, struggling and resultant cyanosis).
- Check for abdominal distension caused by inspired air.

Nursing Diagnoses

- Ineffective airway clearance
- High risk for injury
- Altered parental coping
- Parental anxiety
- Altered nutrition
  The expected outcome can be:
- The infant will maintain a patent airway and will have no signs of respiratory distress and infection.
- The infant will recover without any postoperative complications.

Interventions

- Maintain patent airway; observe for signs and symptoms of respiratory distress.
- Keep the neonate from crying because crying can cause air to pass through the fistula and distend the abdomen, causing greater respiratory distress.
- Administer oxygen as needed.
- Prevent aspiration pneumonia: Position the infant with at least 30° head elevation to decrease potential threat of aspiration and discontinue oral feeds immediately after diagnosis.

- Change position every 2 hours.
- Suction accumulated secretions.
- Elevate the head of the bed 20°–40° to prevent reflux of gastric contents.
- Place a nasogastric tube and connect to low intermittent suction.
- Initiate and monitor intravenous fluids as prescribed to prevent dehydration.
- Monitor I&O.
- Monitor electrolyte and glucose levels.
- Prepare for gastrostomy tube insertion, if indicated, and administer gastrostomy feedings.
- Observe for patency of all tubes. Do not clamp the gastrostomy tube.
- Use gentle suctioning of the upper pouch to minimize aspiration of saliva.
- Monitor the gastrostomy tube placement until total repair is performed.

Postoperative Care

- Maintain patency of airway by suctioning, positioning for comfortable ventilation and administration of oxygen and care of chest tubes.
- Prevent infection by meticulous care of the surgical site, observing for signs and symptoms of inflammation and infection, and maintain strict aseptic technique to prevent cross-infection.
- Maintain fluid–electrolyte balance by monitoring intravenous fluids, I&O records and weight recording and measuring urine specific gravity.
- Maintain the infant in an Isolette or radiant warmer with nebulized humidity.
- Provide adequate nutrition by gastrostomy feeding (usually the third postoperative day) and continue until the infant tolerates oral feeds (10–14 days postoperatively) according to his/her condition.
- Monitor gradual increase in feedings and elevation of the gastrostomy tube; feed slowly to allow swallowing and to provide infant rest; position upright to prevent aspiration; and burp frequently.
- Meet sucking needs of the infant by pacifiers, if policy permits.
- Prepare parents for discharge.
- Teach parents home care, care of tubing and suctioning.
- Educate parents to look for signs of complication, such as oesophageal constriction, chocking and breathing difficulty.

Treatment outcome: It is decided by improved perinatal management and inherent structural and functional defects in the trachea and the oesophagus. Quality of life is better in the isolated group with successful primary repair than in those with associated anomalies and delayed repair.

CONGENITAL DIAPHRAGMATIC HERNIA

It is the displacement of abdominal contents into the thoracic cavity through a defect in the diaphragm. It results from the failure of the transverse septum and pleuroperitoneal folds to completely develop and form the diaphragm.

The most common type of diaphragmatic hernia develops when the posterior part of the diaphragm fails to close and a triangular defect forms the foramen of Bochdalek. Often, if the diaphragm does not form completely, the intestines and other abdominal contents such as liver can enter thoracic cavity, compressing the lung. Lung growth may be arrested on the affected side and to a lesser degree on the contralateral side. Respiration is further compromised by hypoplasia and compression of the lung, including airways and blood vessels. In addition to the anatomic defect, pulmonary hypertension has also been noticed recently as an accompanying symptom. This is a very dangerous symptom which needs aggressive management.

Types

Hernia through the foramen of Bochdalek: This is the most common type of defect. The defect is always on the left side. It results from the failure of the pleuroperitoneal canal to close which normally occurs between 6 and 8 weeks of gestation.

Hernia through the foramen of Morgagni: It is rare and usually occurs on the right side. It occurs in the anterior portion of the diaphragm through the defects secondary to a developmental failure of the retrosternal segment of the septum transversum. Frequently, hernia contains only the omentum and the child will be asymptomatic.

Clinical Management

- Acute respiratory distress in newborn
- Entry of air into the intestine leads to further compression of lung, reducing thoracic space
- Dyspnoea
- Cyanosis
- Scaphoid abdomen
- Impaired cardiac output
- Severe cases of symptoms of shock

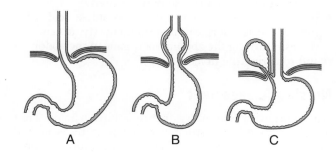

A   B   C

Diagnosis

Prenatal diagnosis by ultrasonography is possible as a result of three cardinal features such as polyhydramnios, mediastinal shift and absence of a stomach bubble in the fetus.

A majority of congenital diaphragmatic hernias (CDHs) are diagnosed on the 20-week anomaly scan, with a detection rate approaching 60%. Magnetic resonance imaging (MRI) accurately differentiating CDH from cystic lung lesions. Poor predictors of CDH are liver in the chest, polyhydramnios and fetal lung to head ratio (LHR) of less than 1.

After birth, diagnosis depends on the type of defect and presence of clinical manifestations that are confirmed by chest radiographs (fluid air-filled loops of the intestine on the affected side of the chest).

Multidisciplinary Approach

- Postnatal management is aimed at reducing barotrauma to the hypoplastic lung by introducing high-frequency oscillatory ventilation (HFOV) or permissive hypercapnia and treating severe pulmonary hypertension with nitric oxide.
- Surgery for CDH is not an emergency. Delayed repair following stabilization is employed in most paediatric surgical centres.
- Immediate respiratory assistance includes endotracheal intubation and gastrointestinal decompression with a double-lumen catheter to prevent further respiratory compromise.
- Maintain Fowler's position, which facilitates downward displacement of the abdominal content.
- In infants with mild respiratory distress, oxygen is administered by a hood.
- Maintain acid–base balance, which is vital in the management and prevention of pulmonary hypertension.
- Maintain low ventilation and least mean airway pressure combined with rapid ventilatory rates (80–120 breaths per minute) to reduce the incidence of pulmonary leaks from overinflation of the unaffected lung.
- Bag and mask ventilation is contraindicated (to prevent air entry into the stomach and intestine, which may further promote pulmonary function compensation).
- Administer intravenous fluids.
- Transcutaneous oxygen pressure monitor or pulse oximeter reading for oxygen saturation.
- Preoperative stabilization is achieved by opiates and paralyzing agents (such as pancuronium) and high-frequency ventilation. Also, extracorporeal membrane oxygenation (EMCO) is sometimes used.
- $NaHCO_3$ administration is done to combat acidosis.
- Perform early surgical management (treatment involves returning the abdominal organs to the abdomen and repairing the defect).

Nursing Assessment

A newborn with respiratory distress at birth who does not initially respond to resuscitation needs to be evaluated for CDH. Endotracheal intubation is the option for providing adequate oxygenation. A nurse in the neonatal unit should carefully watch and evaluate for CDH a neonate with scaphoid abdomen, respiratory distress and increased breath sounds, unilaterally with a positive history of hydramnios in the mother.

Preoperative Care

- Prompt recognition of resuscitation and stabilization assists in ventilatory support, blood gas measurement and administration of intravenous fluids. Position the infant on the affected side (to take advantage of gravity and also to aid in full expansion of the unaffected lung).

- Nurse the baby in incubator if it is a neonate.
- Assess respiratory status (use respiratory distress score).
- Watch for signs of impending shock.
- Place the baby in a Fowler's position.
- Prevent hypothermia.
- Follow strict aseptic technique for care to prevent infections.
- Insert a nasogastric tube and maintain gastric decompression.
- Monitor closely for acid–base balance.
- Watch for impending alkalosis and acidosis (see the chapter on fluid balance).
- Monitor vital signs.
- Monitor oxygen saturation (SaO_2) using noninvasive technique/methods as far as possible (use a pulse oximeter).
- Ascertain adequacy of oxygenation.
- Administer oxygen or provide care for ventilation.
- Administer medication as prescribed.

Postoperative Care

- Observe for respiratory distress.
- Maintain a calm environment to prevent any type of stimulation from any activities.
- Provide close attention to acid–base balance and ventilatory requirement.
- Maintain gastric decompression.
- Maintain thermoregulation.
- Maintain cardiac output and peripheral perfusion.
- Prevent infection.
- Administer prescribed medications.
- Provide appropriate pain management.
- Support parents by explaining the procedures and answering their queries because the management requires long hospitalization.
- Keep parents informed of their child's condition and make them prepare for acceptance of the child to the family environment.

  Treatment outcome: Lung hypoplasia and pulmonary hypertension account for most deaths in isolated CDH cases in newborns.

CLEFT LIP AND PALATE

Definition/Description

It is a birth defect that involves a fissure resulting from incomplete merging of embryonic processes that normally form the face or jaws. This condition is usually considered as a hereditary defect but may be familial, too.

Congenital anomaly involves one or more clefts on the upper lip ranging from a slight dimple to a large cleft involving nasal structures.

Aetiology and Incidence

Genetic, hereditary, environmental and teratogenic factors are the supposed causes of cleft lip and palate. The incidence of cleft lip is one in every 1000 live births; for palate defect, it is one in 2500 live births. Cleft lip is more common in male children and palate is more common in girls (double than that in male children).

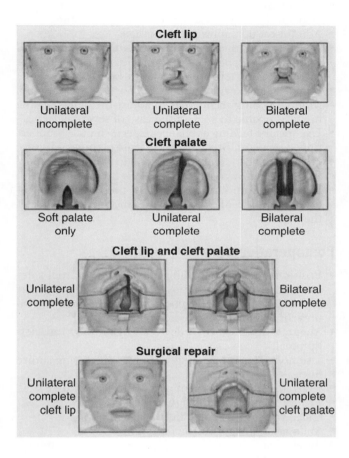

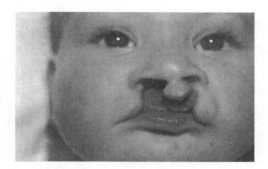

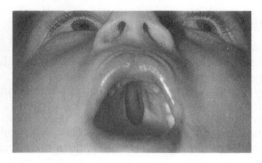

Pathophysiology

These defects occur during embryonic development. Cleft lip results from failure of fusion of lateral and medial tissues forming the upper lip. Cleft palate develops from the failure of fusion of tissues forming palate. Depending on the defects severity and the child's general health, surgical correction of cleft lip typically is done at the ages of 1–2 months and cleft palate repair is done between the ages of 6 and 18 months. Cleft palate repair requires several operations performed in stages.

Early correction of cleft palate enables development of more normal speech patterns. Delayed closure or large defects may require the use of orthodontic devices.

These defects may occur separately or in combination to provide complete unilateral or bilateral cleft from the lip through the soft palate.

Development of the primary and secondary palates takes place at different times and involves different developmental processes. Cleft lip with or without cleft palate results from failure of the maxillary processes to fuse with the nasal elevation on the frontal prominence at the sixth week of IUL. Merging of the upper lip at the midline is completed between the seventh and eighth weeks of gestation.

Fusion of secondary palate takes place later in development between the seventh and 12th weeks of gestation. At the time the primary palate is completed, two lateral palatine processes are situated in a vertical position at the side of the tongue. In the process of migrating to the horizontal position, they are, for a short time, separated by the tongue with the development of the neck and jaws, and the tongue moves downwards, allowing the palatine processes to fuse with each other and with the primary palate to form the roof of the mouth. If there is delay in this movement or if the tongue fails to descend soon enough, the remainder of the development proceeds but palate never fuses.

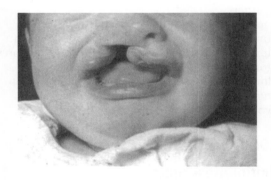

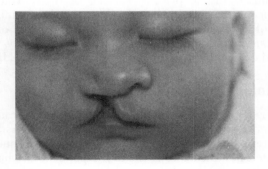

Clinical Manifestations

- Apparent at birth
- Determine whether the defect is isolated or a feature of a broader syndrome.
- Cleft of the lip may be unilateral or bilateral; extent of the defect and degree of nasal deformity are variable.
- Cleft palate alone can occur. Severity has an impact on feeding problems. The infant is unable to generate negative pressure and suction is created in the oral cavity. This impairs feeding.

Multidisciplinary Management

- Administer supportive therapy initially. Feed with special bottles (Haberman and squeezable bottles) at home.
- Surgical correction is the treatment of choice.
  Cleft lip: Closure of lip defects will be done during the first few weeks of life. Surgical correction is done when the infant is free of oral and respiratory infection or any systemic infection. Improved surgical techniques have minimized deformity related to scar retraction, but optimum cosmetic results are difficult with severe defects.
  Cleft palate: Surgery is done at a later stage, between 12 and 18 months of age, to take the advantage of normal growth. Clefts vary in size, shape and degree of deformity, and timing of repair is individualized. But it is preferable to correct before the baby develops faulty speech habits. Postpharyngeal flap procedure or palatal bone graft may be required later to treat persistent velopharyngeal insufficiency (nasal regurgitation and nasal speech).

Long-term problems may develop even with adequate anatomic closure. Children with cleft lip and palate have some degree of speech impairment and therefore require speech therapy.

Improper tooth alignment, varying degrees of hearing loss and improper drainage of the middle ear (as a result of inefficient function of the Eustachian tube) cause increased pressure in the middle ear, thereby leading to otitis media and hearing loss. These children also require orthodontics and prosthodontics during later stages.

Nursing Management

- Provide nursing assessment.
- Symptoms are readily visible at birth.
- Identify location and extent.
- Assess the emotional impact of birth of an infant with a cosmetic and functional disability to the parents.

Nursing Diagnoses

- Body image disturbances
- Ineffective parental coping
- Altered nutrition
- Altered growth and development
- High risk for injury/complication

Intervention

- Provide preoperative care.
- Prepare parents for surgical repair.

- Explain the impact of defect, how the surgery will help, etc.
- Consider different aspects of cleft lip and palate repair (explain the stage-wise treatment to the parents).
- Administer diet appropriate for age.
- Assist the mother with breastfeeding (position and stabilize the nipple well back in the oral cavity so that tongue action facilitates milk expression).
- Stimulate let-down reflex manually or by a breast pump.
- Modify feeding techniques to adjust the defect, as the infant is unable to suck in the case of severe defects.
- Use specific feeding appliances (special nipples, rubber-tipped syringes, Breck feeder, Asepto syringes, etc.).
- Hold the child in an upright position to prevent aspiration.
- Burp frequently to expel excessively swallowed air.
- Provide appropriate preoperative preparation: Physical preparation of the baby and emotional support to the parents.

Postoperative Care

- Position to allow for drainage of mucus (partial side-lying or semi-Fowler's position in cleft palate repair and back or side-lying position in cleft lip repair to prevent trauma to the operative site).
- Maintain lip protective device (Logan's bow) in cleft lip repair.
- Use nontraumatic feeding technique for caring suture lines.
- Restrain elbow to prevent access to the operative site.
- Prevent persistent and vigorous crying.
- Clean the suture gently after feeds.
- Maintain nonvigorous suctioning.
- Teach cleaning and restraining procedures to parents.
- Monitor intravenous fluids.
- Administer appropriate diet according to age and type of surgery.
- Teach feeding techniques to parents.
- Monitor behaviour and vital signs to assess pain.
- Administer appropriate pain medications to prevent vigorous crying as a result of pain.
- Administer antibiotics to prevent infection to the suture site.
- Involve parents in the care of child.

PYLORIC STENOSIS

Definition/Description

It is a condition that results from thickening of the circular muscle of the pylorus, causing obstruction at the gastric outlet. This is believed to be caused by a combination of muscular hypertrophy, spasm and oedema of the mucous membrane. When it occurs congenitally, it is called congenital hypertrophic pyloric stenosis (CHPS).

Aetiology and Incidence

It usually develops in the first few weeks of life (causing projectile vomiting). CHPS is more common in firstborn children, and males are affected five times more frequently than females. Incidence is one to five per 1000 live births.

Inheritance is polygenic with an increased risk in siblings and offspring of the affected persons. Pyloric stenosis can exist in twins, too. Hypertrophic pyloric stenosis is seen more in whites than in other populations.

It is more likely to affect full-term babies than premature infants.

Pathophysiology

Circular muscle of the pylorus is grossly enlarged as a result of both hypertrophy and hyperplasia. This produces severe narrowing of the pyloric canal between the stomach and the duodenum. In due course, inflammation and oedema develop that further reduce the size of the lumen, producing complete obstruction. The muscle is thickened, as much as twice its usual size (2–3 cm). The hypertrophied pylorus may be palpable as an olive-like mass in the upper quadrant of the abdomen.

Clinical Manifestations

- Persistent projectile vomiting (contains milk or formula and not bile-stained)
- Starts at the second or eighth week of age.
- Initially, the infant will be hungry and irritable
- Severe fluid loss and dehydration make the baby lethargic and malnourished.
- Visible peristalsis
- Palpable olive-shaped mass in the epigastrium just right of the umbilicus
- Dehydration
- Apathy
- Fails to thrive/weight loss
- Causes hypochloraemic metabolic alkalosis (serum bicarbonate level elevated 25–35 mEq/L)

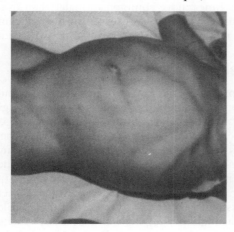

Diagnosis

- History and physical examination
- Presence of a palpable olive-shaped mass
- Laboratory findings show metabolic alterations with severe depletion of fluid and electrolyte
- Blood urea nitrogen (BUN) level elevated
- Multidisciplinary management
- Supportive therapy to combat dehydration
- Correction of metabolic alteration by parenteral fluids
- High Fowler's position
- Stomach decompression by a nasogastric tube
- Surgical correction by pyloromyotomy (Ramstedt operation)

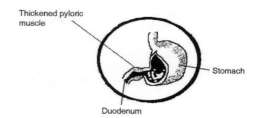

Nursing Management

- Observe for clinical features to establish diagnosis.
- Carefully take history.
- Provide intervention.
- Assess for vomiting that usually begins after 2 weeks and before 2 months of age.
- Vomiting progressively increases in frequency and force, and it is projectile in nature.
- Check for constant hunger.
- Evaluate stools for decrease in size.
- Observe for peristaltic waves.
- Assess for later symptoms.
- Monitor the infant for metabolic alkalosis from vomiting.
- Provide preoperative care.
- Ensure accurate regulation of intravenous fluid to prevent dehydration.
- Maintain an accurate I&O chart.
- Observe feeding behaviour.
- Support parents.
- Maintain proper insertion and observation of the gastric tube.
- Measure length of the tube externally on the infant from bridge of the nose to ear to stomach.
- Check position of the tube.
- Aspirate gastric content.
- Provide postoperative care for Fredet–Ramstedt operation.
- Maintain patent airway: Keep the baby in Fowler's position after anaesthesia has worn off.
- Observe for shock.
- Keep careful record of intravenous infusions and feeding behaviour to assist the surgeon in determining the progress of feeding.
- Begin feeds 4–6 hours after surgery to prevent adhesion formation.
- Do not handle the infant excessively after feeding.

INTUSSUSCEPTION

It is a condition in which a segment of the bowel telescope is inserted into the portion of bowel immediately distal to it.

Aetiology and Incidence

It probably results from hyperactive peristalsis in the proximal portion of the bowel, with inactive peristalsis in the distal segment. Boys are affected more than the girls.

Pathophysiology

- Intussusception is an invagination or telescoping of one portion of the intestine into another. The common sites of intussusception are:
- Ileocaecal valve (ileocolic) occurs when the ileum invaginates into the cecum.

- Ileoileal – One part of the ileum invaginates into another part of the ileum.
- Colocolic – One part of the colon invaginates into another part of the colon and usually occurs in the area of hepatic and splenic flexure.
- Invagination produces obstruction to the passage of intestinal contents beyond the defect. Moreover, the two walls of intestine pressing against each other cause inflammation and oedema and this leads to decreased blood flow. Ischaemia leads to necrosis, and perforation ultimately results in peritonitis and shock. These are serious complications of intussusception.

Clinical Features

- Sudden episodic attack of colicky pain in a well-thriving child between the ages of 3 and 12 months.
- Typical behaviours include screaming and drawing knees up to the chest.
- There will be normal intervals where the child will be comfortable.
- There may be vomiting, abdominal distension and infrequent stools with blood and mucus, called red currant jelly stool.
- The child may have fever and prostration and exhibits signs of shock.

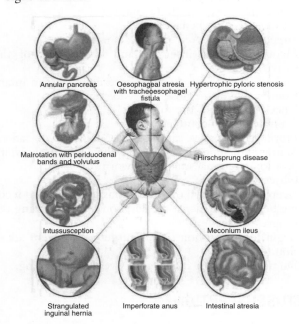

Annular pancreas

Oesophageal atresia with tracheoesophagel fistula

Hypertrophic pyloric stenosis

Malrotation with periduodenal bands and volvulus

Hirschsprung disease

Intussusception

Meconium ileus

Strangulated inguinal hernia

Imperforate anus

Intestinal atresia

Diagnosis

- Assess for signs and symptoms and provide definitive diagnosis by barium enema.
- Provide nursing assessment.
- Assess for sudden onset, with a detailed history.
- Evaluate for the clinical signs and symptoms of intussusception.

Multidisciplinary Management

- Initial management is nonsurgical hydrostatic/pneumostatic reduction, which is traditionally achieved by barium enema. In this case, the correction of invagination takes place at the same time as the diagnostic

testing. The force exerted by barium flow is enough to correct the invagination into the original position as is achieved by pushing an inverted finger out of a glove.
- At present, barium is replaced by water-soluble contrast and air pressure to reduce intussusception.
- Surgical correction involves manually reducing invagination and resecting necrotic intestine, if indicated.

Interventions

- Prepare the child for barium enema X-ray which frequently reduces the bowel obstruction.
- Observe and monitor for recurrence of symptoms, as surgery is indicated in recurrence.
- Observe and maintain intravenous fluids and electrolyte replacement.
- Perform nasogastric suction to deflate the stomach to prevent vomiting.
- Gradually reintroduce fluids and foods.
- Provide postoperative care to the child just as in any general surgery.

HIRSCHSPRUNG DISEASE

It is a congenital anomaly that results from mechanical obstruction from inadequate motility of a part of the intestine.

Aetiology and Incidence

It accounts for about one-fourth of all cases of intestinal obstructions. It may not be diagnosed until the late infancy or childhood. Incidence is one in 5000 live births. It is four times more common in males than in females, and a familial pattern is observed in a small number of cases. It is sometimes associated with Down syndrome.

Pathophysiology

Hirschsprung disease results from failure of craniocaudal migration of ganglion cell precursors along the gastrointestinal tract between the fifth and 12th weeks of gestation.

There is an absence of autonomic parasympathetic ganglion cells in the submucosal (Meissner) and myenteric (Auerbach) plexus of one or more segments of the colon. Lack of innervations produces functional defect (peristalsis) that causes accumulation of intestinal contents and bowel distension proximal to the defect (mega colon).

The aganglionic segment almost always includes the rectum and some part of the distal colon or entire colon or some part of the small intestine; intestinal distension may lead to ischaemia of the bowel wall leading to the development of enterocolitis.

Clinical Manifestations

- These vary according to the age of the child when symptoms are recognized, the length of affected bowel and the occurrence of complications.
- Neonate – Failure to pass meconium within 24–48 hours after birth, refusal of feeds and abdominal distension are the common features.
- Infants – Inadequate weight gain, constipation, abdominal distension, episodes of diarrhoea and vomiting.

Bloody diarrhoea, fever and severe lethargy and associated enterocolitis may also be seen.
- Children – Symptoms become chronic and include constipation, passage of ribbon-like foul-smelling stools and abdominal distension.
- Faecal mass may be palpable, and faecal impactions recur frequently.

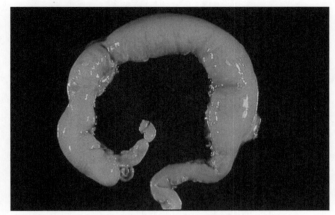

Hirschsprung's disease.

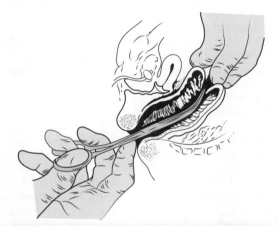

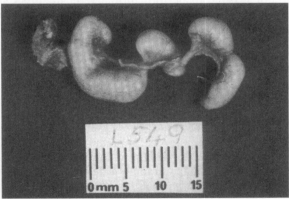

Diagnosis

In neonates, diagnosis is suggested on the basis of clinical signs and symptoms of intestinal obstruction. On examination, the rectum is empty, internal sphincter is tight, there is leakage of liquid stool and presence of accumulated gas. Barium enema demonstrates transition zone. The noninvasive procedure that may be used for diagnosis is anorectal manometry. The definitive diagnosis is done by rectal biopsy.

Multidisciplinary Management

Surgical correction aims at removal of aganglionic bowel to relieve obstruction, restore normal motility and preserve the function of external sphincter.

First, a temporary colostomy is created at least 10 cm proximal to the transition zone of the aganglionic segment to relieve obstruction and allow the normal, innervated, and dilated bowel to its normal size. The site is evaluated at the time of operation for the presence of ganglion cells on frozen section to avoid placing stoma in obstructed aganglionic bowel. If a colostomy is performed, a definitive pull-through procedure will be done later as corrective surgery.

Second, a complete corrective surgery is done when the child weighs approximately 10 kg (rule of 10). Definitive surgery may be one of the modified Duhamel (rectorectal) or Soave (endorectal) or Swenson (rectosigmoidectomy) procedure. The colostomy is also closed usually at this time. Overall, the survival rate is 90%. Most patients are continent. Soiling is a problem in 2%–3% of children after corrective surgery.

Nursing Assessment

- Assess the history regarding failure to pass meconium, symptoms of bile-stained vomiting and reluctance to feed.
- Evaluate for signs of intestinal obstruction.
- Assess for faecal odour of breath and stool.
- Note older children for symptoms of constipation, offensive odour, ribbon-like stools, etc.

Nursing Diagnoses

- Bowel elimination alteration
- High risk for injury
- Altered growth and development
- Risk for impaired peristomal skin integrity
- Impaired stomal tissue
- Body image disturbances

Intervention

- Prior to diagnosis, observe carefully for all gastrointestinal manifestations of the disease and report them accurately.
- Prior to colostomy procedure, clean the bowel and provide stool softeners, liquid diet and colonic irrigation with saline, if indicated.
- Apply pectin, methylcellulose-based solid skin barrier around the stoma to protect skin from contact with stool, which causes irritation.
- Zinc oxide cream (prepared by mixing zinc oxide powder with coconut oil) is used as a routine for this purpose in a majority of paediatric centres in India.
- Apply colostomy bag or pouch to collect faeces.
- In children, thoroughly cleaned cotton cloth pieces can be used as a good device by applying over the stoma to collect faeces and can be removed after soiling; it is also cheap for common people. This will not create any allergic reaction as well.
- Inspect stoma for redness, oedema and infection.

- Remove skin barrier every day to inspect the area for impairment and reapply the same to the skin around the stoma.
- Assess the stool quality and quantity.
- If colostomy is not eliminating the stool after return of bowel sounds, gently insert a nasogastric tube and irrigate the stoma with normal saline as prescribed.
- Prepare parents for the procedure.
- Clarify the surgical technique.
- Describe stoma care.
- Prepare for care of the stoma of the child with colostomy.
- Give parents opportunity to express their feelings about the procedure.

Postoperative Care

Provide general postoperative care. The special points to be remembered are the following:

- Maintain optimal nutrition.
- Closely observe for stools for re-establishment of normal elimination pattern.
- Maintain skin care of colostomy and anal areas.

OMPHALOCELE/EXOMPHALOS

It is the congenital herniation of bowel and solid viscera through the midline defect surrounded by the attachment of umbilical cord that occurs between 11th and 12th weeks of gestation when the alimentation tract should have been withdrawn back into the fetal abdomen.

Aetiology is unknown. Attention may be drawn to their presence during the second trimester because of raised maternal serum α-fetoprotein level or abnormal ultrasound scans. Exomphalos is characteristically a midline defect, at the insertion point of the umbilical cord, with a viable sac composed of amnion and peritoneum containing herniated abdominal contents.

Associated major abnormalities include trisomy 13, 18 and 21, Beckwith–Wiedemann syndrome (macroglossia, gigantism, exomphalos), pentalogy of Cantrell (sternal, pericardial, cardiac, abdominal wall and diaphragmatic defect), and cardiac, gastrointestinal and renal abnormalities and are noted in 60%–70% of cases.

Prenatal screening: Karyotyping, in addition to detailed sonographic review and fetal echocardiogram, is essential for complete prenatal screening.

If the defect is small and only a small bowel loop is herniated into the base of the cord, the defect is called as umbilical hernia. The size of omphalocele varies from 2 to 20 cm. In larger herniation, most of the abdominal contents lie outside the abdomen. At birth, the covering sac is a shiny, avascular transparent membrane consisting of amnion and Wharton's jelly and structures normally ensheath the umbilical cord. After 1 or 2 days, it becomes opaque and necrosed. If not treated properly, it may rupture and lead to evisceration and sepsis. In total, 40% of cases will not have associated anomalies such as EMG (exomphalos, macroglossia and gigantism), also called Beckwith–Wiedemann syndrome.

Smaller defects contain one or two loops of the intestine, whereas larger defects contain liver, spleen and a major portion of intestines. Cardiac anomalies are associated with 20% of cases.

Incidence is one in 10,000 live births.

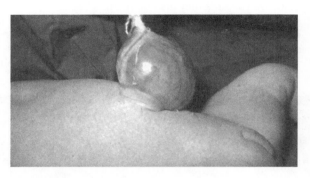

Multidisciplinary Management

Delivery by caesarean section is reserved only for infants with a large exomphalos with exteriorized liver to prevent damage. Surgical repair includes primary closure or a staged repair with a silo for giant defects.

Provide immediate management.

- Cover the defect with a moist, nonirritant antiseptic dressing (Betadine) to avoid rupture and infection. Withheld feeds and keep stomach empty by nasogastric aspiration.
- Prevent hypothermia.
- Aim of treatment is to provide a cover without increasing intra-abdominal pressure.
- Definitive treatment depends on the following:
  - Size of the hernial defect
  - Contents of the sac
  - Condition of the sac
  - Gestational age
  - General condition of the infant
  - Hypothermic problems and sepsis
  - Severity of additional malformations
- If the defect is less than 5 cm in diameter, it is possible to excise the sac, reduce the viscera and repair the defect in layers. When the defect is larger, it is not feasible to perform primary repair. First, skin flaps are mobilized and sutured and then hernial defect is repaired. Ruptured sac is resected and replaced with a Silastic silo (artificial sac).

Outcome: Postnatal morbidity occurs in 5%–10% of cases. Malrotation and adhesive bowel obstruction do contribute to mortality in isolated cases of exomphalos.

GASTROSCHISIS

Gastroschisis is protrusion of the abdominal viscera; usually, the entire midgut loops through a defect in the anterior abdominal wall at the level of umbilicus. Intrauterine rupture of a hernia of the umbilical cord produces gastroschisis.

It is an isolated lesion that usually occurs on the right side of the umbilical defect, with evisceration of the abdominal contents directly into the amniotic cavity. The incidence is increasing from 1.66 per 10,000 births to 4.6 per 10,000 births, affecting mainly young mothers typically younger than 20 years.

Associated anomalies are noted in only 5%–24% of cases, with bowel atresia being the most common coexisting abnormality. On prenatal scan with a detection rate of 100%, the bowel appears to be free floating and the loops may appear to be thickened because of damage by amniotic fluid exposure causing a 'peel' formation.

Clinical Manifestations

- Polyhydramnios
- Visualization by ultrasonography
- Elevated maternal serum α-fetoprotein level
- Preterm labour in the case of gastroschisis
- Visible defect over the abdominal area – Omphalocele is covered with a sac consisting of the peritoneum and the amniotic membrane; gastroschisis defect exposes viscera as a result of lack of any covering
- Intrauterine growth retardation in gastroschisis

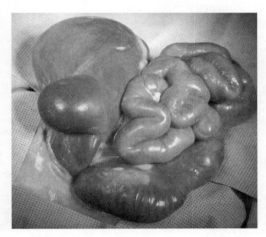

Gastroschisis.

Management

Delivery by caesarean section has no advantage over the normal vaginal route. Various methods of postnatal surgical repair include the traditional primary closure, reduction of bowel without anaesthesia and reduction by preformed silo or by means of a traditional silo. Coexisting intestinal atresia could be repaired by primary anastomosis or staged with stoma formation.

- Perform decompression of the upper gastrointestinal tract by nasogastric aspiration.
- Cover the exposed intestinal loops in a sterile polythene bag.
- Minimize fluid and heat loss.

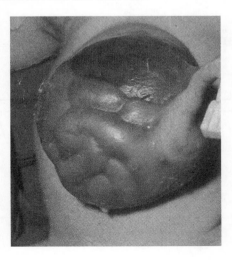

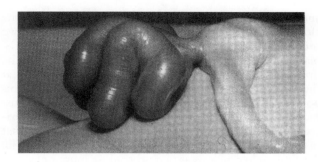

Nursing Interventions

- Provide immediate care.
- Cover the defect with a warm, normal saline-moistened sterile gauze and wrap over the dressing.
- Administer intravenous fluids and albumin.
- Keep nil per orally (NPO).
- Keep the dressing moist.
- Monitor glucose levels and electrolytes.
- Insert a nasogastric tube to decompress bowel.
- Maintain sterility of the dressing.
- Position the neonate to prevent any trauma or pressure on the defect.
- Administer antibiotics as prescribed.
- Place the infant in an Isolette and maintain a thermoneutral environment.
- Keep moistened dressings warm to prevent heat loss.
- Minimize the neonate's exposure to moist bedding.
- Support parents as they grieve for the loss of an 'idealized' perfect baby.
- Teach and explain possible treatment and other nursing care procedures to the parents.

Outcome of Treatment

The long-term outcome in gastroschisis is dependent on the condition of the bowel. In uncomplicated cases, the outcome is excellent in more than 90% of cases. The mortality of liveborn infants is 5%, with further 5% suffering short bowel syndrome and 10% requiring surgery for adhesive bowel obstruction. Health care professionals should be aware of third-trimester fetal loss, and this must be communicated while counselling parents.

ANORECTAL MALFORMATIONS

Anorectal malformations (ARMs) are congenital malformations caused by abnormal development of the rectum and anus.

Embryology

The major part of the anus and rectum develop during the fourth to sixth weeks of IUL. The common crown-to-rump length of the fetus is only 4–200 mm at this time. The upper rectum and the colon are derived from the cloaca. The division of the cloaca forms the portion of the rectum extending from the upper part of the anal canal to peritoneal reflection. Failure of division of the cloaca into the urogenital tract and the rectum results in the high- and intermediate-type anomalies. As the embryo develops, the cloacal membrane moves posteriorly and inferiorly. The urorectal fold or septum divides the cloaca into the rectum and the urogenital tract by two processes. First, there is a downward growth of mesoblastic tissue in a cranial-to-caudal direction. This is the Torneaux septum, which stops its downward growth at the level of verumontanum or Müllerian tubercle. This point is of great significance because it is here the most rectourethral fistulas occur in male. Below this, the urorectal septum has an outgrowth of mesenchyme that fuses laterally to the midline. This is called Rathke's fold. Anal tubercle develops as two protruding bumps of tissue beneath the fetal tail by 10th week of IUL. Partitioning of the anus from the uroanal tract is a process of growth of the urorectal and uroanal septum and ingrowth of genital folds. The genital tubercle becomes the phallus anteriorly. The inner and outer genital folds form between these structures. In males, the inner genital folds fuse, covering the posterior portion of the urogenital sinus to form bulbous and penile portion of urethra. In females, these folds form the labia minora. The outer genital folds fuse caudally to form scrotum and median perineal raphe in male, and it becomes labia majora in females. The junction of inner genital folds forms fourchette in females. Elongation of the genital folds and fusion of the anal tubercle above the anus and rectum form the genitourinary tract. The cloaca and the depressed anal pit, which is lined with the ectoderm, are finally joined by the atrophy and breakdown of the anal membrane. The junction makes the pectinate line. The low- and intermediate-type anomalies represent a failure of posterior migration of the anus away from urogenital sinus. There are various cloacal defects where rectum joins with the vagina and urethra to form a common channel. Failure of fusion of Müllerian ducts leads to bicornuate uterus, septate uterus or separate vagina in females

Aetiology and Incidence

Generally, any congenital malformations can cause ARMs. A family history of ARM is unusual. The risk of a family having subsequent infants with same anomaly is 1%. ARMs would appear to be autosomal recessive when genetically linked. The incidence is approximately one in 5000 live births.

Clinical Malformations

Clinical manifestations vary according to the type of anomalies present.

Imperforate anus – It encompasses several forms of malformation without an obvious anal opening, and many have a fistula from the distal rectum to the peritoneum or genitourinary system.

Cloacal exstrophy – It is a rare form that includes malformations of the urinary system, genital system and bowel with drain into a common channel that communicates with the peritoneum.

ARMs are also classified according to sex and the level of arrest of rectal descent. The level of rectal descent is determined by the relationship of the termination of bowel to the puborectalis sling of the levator ani muscle. Therapeutic intervention also depends on

the level of anomaly. According to the level of anomalies, they are classified as low-, intermediate- and high-type anomalies.

Low-type anomalies – The rectum descends normally through the puborectalis muscle, the internal and external sphincters are present and well developed with normal function and there is no connection to the genitourinary tract.

Intermediate-type anomalies – The rectum is at or below the level of puborectalis muscle, and the anal dimple and external sphincter are positioned normally.

High-type anomalies – The rectum ends above the puborectalis muscle, and there is an absence of internal sphincter; these are usually associated with a genitourinary fistula.

Wingspread Classification of Anorectal Anomalies

Level	Female	Male
High	Anorectal agenesis with rectovaginal fistula	Anorectal agenesis with rectal prostatitis, urethral fistula
	Rectal atresia	
Intermediate	Rectovestibular fistula	Rectal atresia
	Anal agenesis without fistula	Rectbulbar urethral fistula
		Anal agenesis without fistula
Low	Anovestibular fistula	Anocutaneous fistula
	Anocutaneous fistula	
	Anal stenosis	Anal stenosis
	Cloacal malformations	Rare malformations
	Rare malformations	

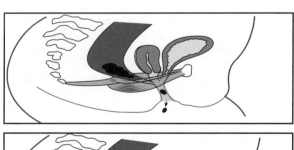

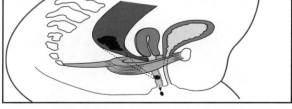

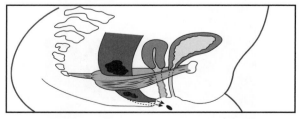

Pathophysiology

During embryonic development, the cloaca becomes the common channel for developing the urinary, genital and rectal systems. The cloaca is divided at the sixth week of gestation into an anterior urogenital sinus and a posterior intestinal channel by the urorectal septum. By the sixth week of IUL, the cloaca is divided into an anterior urogenital sinus and a posterior intestinal channel by the urorectal septum. After this, lateral fold joins the urorectal septum and separation of the urinary and rectal segments takes place. An interception in the development of the anterior genitourinary system and the posterior anorectal channel leads to incomplete migration of the rectum to its normal perineal position. Any description of pathology of ARMs should include the child's sex, level of lesion and presence or absence of fistula. The level of the rectal pouch must be related to the levator ani, specifically to the puborectalis muscle.

Lesion in the male – In low-grade lesions in males, the rectum penetrates the levator ani after leaving the internal sphincter intact. Anal stenosis presents a pinpoint opening at the normal site. A ring of fibrous tissue at the pectinate line causes constipation in mild anal stenosis. A completely covered anus consists of a heaped up mass of tissue covering the anus in the form of bucket handle. In intermediate-grade lesions, the rectum has penetrated through the puborectalis, which envelops the lower end of the bowel. There may be anal agenesis or the rectum may end in a fistula to the bulbar portion of the urethra. An invertogram or contrast study of distal colostomy shows that the bowel has penetrated well beyond the pubococcygeal line either at or just above the 'I' point (the inferior portion of the ischium). The internal sphincter is absent and external sphincter is variable.

In high-type anomalies, the blind rectal pouch lies above the levator sling. If the blind rectum has no communication with the urinary tract, it is called anorectal agenesis. Sometimes, there will be a fistula to the posterior urethra adjacent to the ejaculatory ducts. The fistula varies in size. The fistula is usually very short and is closely related to the urethra. The puborectalis sling encircles the urethra distal to the rectourethral fistula. X-ray shows the bowel to be present above the pubococcygeal line and is therefore completely supralevator. There is no internal sphincter and the external sphincter is variable.

Lesions in female – Simple anal or urorectal agenesis without a fistula is rare in females. The openings in all low or translevator lesions in females are easily visible on physical examination of the perineum. The simplest lesion is the anterior perineal anus. The perineal opening is normal in size or at most slightly stenotic, the orifice is skin linked and sphincter function is normal. From the anterior perineal anus, there is a continuing spectrum of lesions through which the anus is displaced forward to the vagina. The most anterior variety of the covered anus is an opening into the posterior margin of the vulva. The most common anal deformity in female children is anovestibular fistula.

Intermediate-type lesions consist of a rectovestibular fistula where the rectum has not penetrated the puborectalis

sling, but the long fistula connecting the rectum with vestibule is enveloped by the puborectalis. This need to be differentiated from an anovestibular fistula by a lateral roentgenogram obtained after injecting a contrast.

In high-type anomalies, the rectum may enter the back wall of the vagina at any point and is called rectovaginal fistula if the urethra is in the proper direction. There may be only one opening on the perineum. The rectum, vagina and urethra all join together creating a cloaca. Various types of defects are also associated with ARMs. A rectovesical fistula may occur in a female only in the presence of an absent or divided vagina and uterus.

Diagnosis

- Check for patency of the anus and rectum.
- Observe for passage of meconium.
- Perform digital and endoscopic examination.
- Invertogram is the classical method of determining the distance from the blind rectal pouch to a marker placed on or within the anal dimple. For male children, a 5-French gauge radiopaque catheter is placed in the urethra to determine relationship of the rectal pouch with the urethra.
- Obtain cross-table prone lateral X-rays.
- A voiding cystourethrogram and an intravenous pyelogram are indicated to find out associated anomalies.

Multidisciplinary Management

- Low anal stenosis – Perform manual dilatation.
- Imperforate anus – Perform excision, followed by daily anal dilatation.
- Intermediate-type anomaly – Reconstruction depends on the relationship of the anomaly to the puborectalis. Surgical correction is achieved by the abdominal pull-through procedure or anoplasty.
- High-type anomaly – It requires a diverting colostomy in the newborn period. After the condition improves, definitive surgery is performed (abdominal pull-through/ mid-sagittal anorectoplasty).

Intervention

- Assist in identifying the defect by newborn evaluation. (A newborn who does not pass stool within 24 hours requires further assessment.)
- General preoperative care as in any other general surgery.
- Prepare the baby for barium enema X-ray.

Postoperative Care

Provide general postoperative care along with the following:
- Observe and maintain intravenous fluids.
- Perform nasogastric suction to deflate the stomach to prevent vomiting.
- Withhold feedings.
- Check vital signs.
- Maintain temperature (thermoregulation).
- Prevent infection.

- Provide colostomy care.
- Check for return of peristalsis.
- Provide supportive care to parents before and after surgery.

STUDY QUESTIONS

- Why is it important for a paediatric nurse to know the fetal development of the gastrointestinal system?
- What are the consequences of abnormal embryonic development of the respiratory system?
- Prepare a nursing care plan using the nursing process approach for the following medical–surgical problems:
  a. A newborn with a tracheoesophageal fistula
  b. A neonate with congenital diaphragmatic hernia
  c. A 3-year-old baby admitted for Duhamel surgery
  d. A preschooler with acute abdomen
  e. A school-aged child with appendicitis
  f. A neonate with bilious vomiting
- Write short notes on:
  a. Omphalocele
  b. Gastroschisis
  c. Feeding problems of an infant with cleft lip and palate
  d. Management of respiratory problems in congenital diaphragmatic hernia
  e. Preoperative preparation of a toddler with intussusceptions
  f. Vomiting in children
  g. Common causes of acute abdomen

BIBLIOGRAPHY

1. Agarwal S, Mayer L. (2009). Pathogenesis and treatment of gastrointestinal disease in antibody deficiency syndromes. J Allergy Clin Immunol 124(4):658–664. PubMedCrossRef
2. Berni Canani R, Terrin G. et al. (2010). Congenital diarrheal disorders: improved understanding of gene defects is leading to advances in intestinal physiology and clinical management. J Pediatr Gastroenterol Nutr 50(4):360–366. PubMed
3. Braamskamp MJ, Dolman KM. et al. (2010). Clinical practice. Protein-losing enteropathy in children. Eur J Pediatr 169(10):1179–1185. PubMedCrossRef
4. Coran AG, eds. Pediatric Surgery. Vol 2. 5th ed. St Louis, Mo: Mosby-Year Book Inc, 1998:1925–1938. 15.
5. Heyman MB. (2006). Lactose intolerance in infants, children, and adolescents. Pediatrics 118(3):1279–1286. PubMedCrossRef
6. Hill ID, Dirks MH. et al. (2005). Guideline for the diagnosis and treatment of celiac disease in children: recommendations of the North American Society for Pediatric Gastroenterology, Hepatology and Nutrition. J Pediatr Gastroenterol Nutr 40(1):1–19. PubMedCrossRef
7. James J. Corrigan, Frank G. (Nov 2001). Boineau Pediatrics in Review. 22(11), 365–369. DOI: 10.1542/pir.22-11-365.
8. Yadav J, Sharma D, Yadav S, Shastri S. Indian Childhood Cirrhosis: Case Report and Pediatric Diagnostic Challenges. Pediatric liver study group of India. Metabolic liver disease in childhood. Int J Pediatr. 2015: Vol.3, N.5-1.
9. Marilyn J. Hockenberry, David Wilson. Wong's essentials of pediatric nursing. 8th edition, Elsevier publication. 2009.
10. Nayak NC. Indian childhood cirrhosis. In: MacSween RNM, Anthony PP, Scheuer PJ, eds. Pathology of the Liver. London: Churchill & Livingstone; 1979. pp. 268–9.
11. O P Ghai. Essential pediatrics. 5th edition. 2000; Naraina II, New Delhi.
12. Patra S, Vij M, Kancherala R, Samal SC. Is Indian Childhood Cirrhosis an Extinct Disease Now?—an Observational Study. Indian J Pediatr 2013;80(8):651–54.
13. Puri P, Höllwarth ME (eds) (2006). Pediatric Surgery. Springer, Berlin, Heidelberg.
14. Ramakrishna B, Date A, Kirubakaran C, Raghupathy P. Atypical copper cirrhosis in Indian children. Ann Trop Paediatr 1995;15(3):237–42.
15. Radhakrishna Rao MV. Histopathology of the liver in Infantile biliary cirrhosis. Indian J Med Res 1935;23:69-90.
16. Rao PS. (2007) Protein-losing enteropathy following the Fontan operation. J Invasive Cardiol 19(10):447–448. PubMed
17. Sampson HA, Anderson JA (2000) Summary and recommendations: classification of gastrointestinal manifestations due to immunologic reactions to foods in infants and young children. J Pediatr Gastroenterol Nutr 30(Suppl):S87–S94. PubMedCrossRef
18. Suraj Gupte. The short book of pediatrics. 10th edition. 2004; Jaypee publications, New Delhi.
19. Srivastava J. The genetic factor in infantile cirrhosis of liver: A preliminary report. Indian J Med Sci 1956;10:191-6.
20. Smith, E.D. (1998). The Bath Water Needs Changing But Don't Throw Out The Baby: An Overview of Anorectal Anomalies. Journal of Pediatric Surgery, 22, 335.
21. Sondheimer, J & Silverman, A. (1995). Gastrointestinal tract. In W. Hay. J. Groothuis, A Hayward & M. Levin (Eds). Current paediatric diagnosis and treatment 12th ed., 608-642, Norwalk, CT: Appleton & Lange.
22. Taylor SF, Sondheimer JM, Sokol RJ, Silverman A, Wilson H. Noninfectious colitis associated with short bowel syndrome. J Pediatr 1991;119:24-30 [CrossRef]
23. MedlineRoy CC, Silverman AS, Alagille D. (1995). Pediatric Clinical Gastroenterology. 4th ed. St Louis, Mosby.
24. Walkowiak J, Lisowska A. et al. (2010) Acid steatocrit determination is not helpful in cystic fibrosis patients without or with mild steatorrhea. Pediatr Pulmonol 45(3):249–254. PubMed

ALTERATION IN CARDIOVASCULAR FUNCTIONS

LEARNING OBJECTIVES

At the end of the chapter, the learner will be able to:

- Discuss the essential concepts related to cardiovascular system development.
- Describe the consequences of abnormal embryonic development.
- Describe the nursing management of children with congenital cyanotic and acyanotic heart diseases with other medical problems affecting the cardiovascular system, using the nursing process approach.
- Describe the nursing management of children with common infections affecting the cardiovascular system.
- Discuss the nursing management of children suffering from congestive cardiac failure.

THE CARDIOVASCULAR SYSTEM

Delivery of oxygenated blood and other nutrients to all body cells and removal of carbon dioxide and other metabolic waste products are the basic functions of the cardiovascular system. The cardiovascular system consists of a pumping unit (heart), a circuit (arteries, veins and capillaries) that transports blood through the body and numerous valves that regulate blood flow through the heart and vessels. The heart also has its own electrical system to maintain its rate and rhythm, but neural and hormonal systems complement the heart's intrinsic regulatory mechanism.

From conception through the postnatal period and childhood, the heart undergoes changes in size, structure and function. A basic understanding of fetal cardiogenesis and later development establishes a foundation for the understanding of normal cardiac findings as well as abnormal development. This chapter gives a basic understanding of the embryonic development of heart, consequences of abnormal heart development, developmental anomalies and certain pathological conditions that disrupt normal functioning of the heart and its nursing management.

Embryonic Development

Development of the cardiovascular system begins early in the fetal life, with cardiac structures formed during the third to eighth weeks of gestation. By the end of the eighth week, the heart beats and it is one of the first organ systems to function in utero. This early development permits the fetus to provide for nutritional, respiratory and excretory needs of developing cells and tissues. Embryonic design of the cardiovascular system is adapted to anticipate the shift that will occur in the metabolic centres in the later life. Functions managed by the placenta prenatally are transferred to the respiratory, digestive and renal systems after birth. The following section highlights the major events of the embryogenesis of the cardiovascular system. The development of each of the major structures is discussed separately, though they develop simultaneously.

Cardiac Tube

Early in pregnancy, the embryo relies on diffusion as a means of nutrient and waste exchange. But as the embryo grows, it requires its own transport system for servicing the developing structures. During the first 3 weeks of gestation, the mesoderm thickens and splits into two layers, the somatic and splanchnic mesoderm. The splanchnic mesoderm differentiates into a variety of cardiac structures within a fluid-filled space that becomes the pericardial cavity.

The splanchnic mesoderm initially forms a pair of tubes that soon fuse into a single endocardial tube. This primitive heart tube ultimately forms the endocardium, the inside layer of the heart. It is enveloped by a single fold of tissues that are formed by the rudiments of the myocardium, the muscular middle layer of the heart.

As the heart tube matures, sequential dilated areas appear to suggest the future structures of the heart. These regions are the sinoatrium (the sinus venosus joined with the common atrium), the ventricle, bulbus cordis and truncus arteriosus. In the mature heart, they become the atria, left ventricle, right ventricle and the aorta and pulmonary artery, respectively. Blood enters at the sinoatrium and leaves through the truncus arteriosus.

The heart tube, which is rapidly elongating within the pericardial cavity, is forced into a complex pattern of bends that enhance the formation of the cardiac chambers. Approximately 28 days after conception, the ebb and flow of blood cells begin through the heart.

Right and Left Atria

In the developing heart tube, endocardial cells proliferate and give rise to bulges of tissue within the canal; these thick pads are known as the endocardial cushions. From the top of atrium, the septum primum grows down and fuses with the endocardial cushions. From the superior and posterior walls of the atrium grows the septum secundum. As the partition develops, the septum secundum forms the flapped opening known as the foramen ovale. By the fifth week of gestation, the separation of atria is complete and blood flows from the right to left sides through the foramen ovale, which closes after birth.

Right and Left Ventricles

In early fetal development, the heart tube elongates and bends to bring the ventricle gradually at the posterior position of the atrium. Continued growth of the cardiac tube stimulates the absorption of the proximal end of the bulbus cordis into the right side of the common ventricle. About the same time, the ventral surface of the ventricle shows a distinct median, longitudinal groove that begins to divide the one ventricle into two chambers.

Between the fourth and eighth weeks of the fetal life, the muscular interventricular septum grows towards the endocardial cushions. Extension of the endocardial cushions and the swellings of other tissue fuse and form the membranous ventricular septum. This tissue merges with the muscular interventricular septum to complete the ventricular septum. By the eighth week of gestation, there is little trace of the foramen's existence.

Atrioventricular Valves

In the primitive heart, the atrioventricular (AV) communication is a single opening and the sinoatrium empties into a common ventricle. With division of the atrium and ventricles into the left and right sides, flaps of tissue arise from localized proliferations of endocardial tissue on the walls of the AV canal.

Each flap differentiates as a mass of fibrous tissue and becomes connected to special muscles of the ventricle (papillary muscles) by cords of the connective tissue (chordae tendineae). Three flaps or valvular cups are formed around the right AV canal, creating the tricuspid valve. The two flaps of tissue on the left side create the mitral (bicuspid) valve. These valves control blood flow from the upper chambers to the lower chambers.

Aorta and Pulmonary Artery

During the fifth week of gestation, the remainder of the bulbus cordis is divided into two channels by a spiral septum that appears as ridges of tissue. Similar ridges are found in the truncus arteriosus and are directly continuous with those of the bulbus cordis. The ridges enlarge and fuse to form the aorticopulmonary septum, creating the pulmonary trunk and a systemic trunk. These two trunks ultimately twist around one another and become the pulmonary artery and the ascending aorta, respectively. The semilunar valves (pulmonary and aortic valves) form inside the two vessels when truncal septation is almost completed and function to maintain blood flow in one direction, away from the heart.

Aortic Arch

The aortic arch pattern is laid within the first 4 weeks of gestation, but it is transformed into the familiar arrangements of arteries around the seventh week.

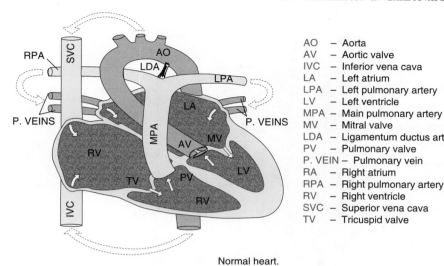

AO – Aorta
AV – Aortic valve
IVC – Inferior vena cava
LA – Left atrium
LPA – Left pulmonary artery
LV – Left ventricle
MPA – Main pulmonary artery
MV – Mitral valve
LDA – Ligamentum ductus arteriosus
PV – Pulmonary valve
P. VEIN – Pulmonary vein
RA – Right atrium
RPA – Right pulmonary artery
RV – Right ventricle
SVC – Superior vena cava
TV – Tricuspid valve

Normal heart.

Pulmonary Veins

The pulmonary veins begin to develop early in the third week of gestation. The primitive pulmonary vein arises as a sprout of the endothelium out of the left atrium and joins the pulmonary capillary plexus on the lung buds.

Consequences of Abnormal Development

The complex processes involved in the formation of the four-chambered heart and vascular pathways present many opportunities for malformations to occur. Most of the congenital defects of the heart are caused by the abnormal division or faulty separations of the heart tube and failure of specific vessels or tissues to grow during the time frame of normal development. Table 30.1 explains specific anomalies that develop during the intrauterine period.

FETAL CIRCULATION

Fetal circulation is well developed in utero to meet the demands of the growing fetus. The lungs are nonfunctional and the liver is only partially functional; most of the blood flows to the placenta and the brain. In fetus, the oxygenated blood from the placenta travels by way of the ductus venosus (it connects the umbilical vein to the inferior vena cava bypassing the liver) to the inferior vena cava. The blood that enters the inferior vena cava is shunted from the right atrium to the left atrium through the foramen ovale. From there, blood enters the left ventricle and the major part of this blood is routed to the brain and upper extremities. After circulating, blood from the head and upper extremities drains to the superior vena cava and blood from lower extremities empties into the inferior vena cava. Both vessels empty into the right atrium. Blood flows from the right atrium through the pulmonary artery and directly to the aorta by way of the ductus arteriosus. The shunt prevents most of the blood from entering the nonfunctioning lungs. Blood flow continues by way of umbilical arteries and returns to the placenta.

TABLE 30.1	**Anomalies Occurring in the Intrauterine Period**	
Fetal Age (in Weeks)	**Structure**	**Anomalies at Birth**
3	Pulmonary veins	Total anomalous pulmonary venous return (TAPVR)
		• Supracardiac
		• Cardiac
		• Infracardiac
		• Mixed
4–6	Atrial septum	Atrial septal defect (ASD)
		• Secundum ASD (centre)
		• Primum ASD (lower)
		• Sinus venosus ASD (high)
4–8	Ventricular septum	Ventricular septal defect (VSD)
		• Infracristal VSD
		• Supracristal VSD
		• Muscular VSD
		• Membranous VSD
4–8	Endocardial cushion region	Endocardial cushion defects – two major types
		• Partial AV canal
		• Complete AV canal
		VSDs
		ASDs
5–7	Pulmonary artery and aorta	Persistent truncus arteriosus
		Tetralogy of Fallot (TOF) – four defects
		• VSD
		• Pulmonary stenosis
		• Displacement or overriding of aorta
		• Right ventricular hypertrophy
		Pulmonary stenosis (PS)
		Trans position of great vessels (arteries) (TGA)
		Pulmonary atresia
5–7	Aortic arch	Coarctation of aorta (COTA)
		Interrupted aortic arch
		Aortic atresia
		Patent ductus arteriosus
		Vascular rings

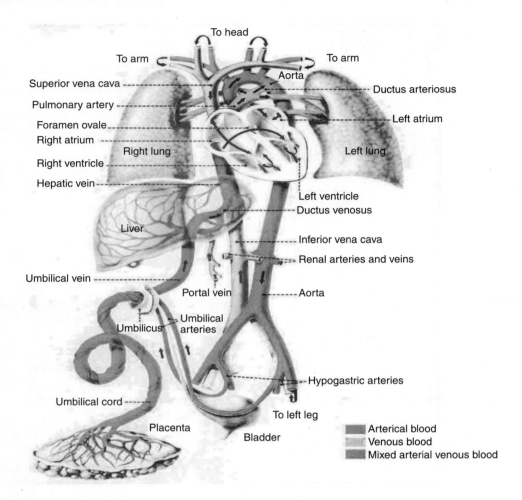

To head
To arm — To arm
Aorta
Superior vena cava -------- -------- Ductus arteriosus
Pulmonary artery -------- -------- Left atrium
Foramen ovale --------
Right atrium -------- Right lung   Left lung
Right ventricle --------
Hepatic vein -------- -------- Left ventricle
-------- Ductus venosus
Liver -------- Inferior vena cava
-------- Renal arteries and veins
Umbilical vein --------
Portal vein -------- Aorta
Umbilicus Umbilical arteries
-------- Hypogastric arteries
Umbilical cord --------
To left leg
Placenta   Bladder

Arterical blood
Venous blood
Mixed arterial venous blood

Fetal circulation.

POSTNATAL CIRCULATION

When the infant is born, two significant events immediately affect the change from fetal to neonatal circulation. The first event is the infant's initial breath of air and the second is the infant's separation from the placenta. After these events, the infant must rely on his/her own lungs for oxygen. Once the placental circulation is replaced by the pulmonary circulation, the following changes occur to the structure and function of the cardiovascular system:

- Pulmonary vascular resistance decreases and pulmonary blood flow increases; therefore, pulmonary artery pressure decreases.
- Foramen ovale closes as a result of pressure changes in the right and left atria.
- Ductus arteriosus closes as a result of increased oxygen tension in arterial blood.
- Ductus venosus closes as a result of the loss of blood flow from the placenta.
- Systemic vascular resistance increases as a result of removal of the low resistance from the placenta.
- The ductus constricts as blood flow is stopped with loss of the placenta. The smooth muscle of the ductus arteriosus responds to the oxygen, thus functionally closing the ductus arteriosus. The umbilical

arteries, vein and ductus venosus constrict within 3–7 days after birth and undergo infiltration.

Developmental Changes

The physical characteristics of the cardiovascular structures continue to change after birth. In infancy, the ratio of heart size to body size is higher and the heart requires a large space within the thoracic cavity. Growth and development of the child result in a reduction of that ratio. Yet, during the first year, the weight of the heart doubles; by 5 years, it quadruples; and by 9 years, the heart weighs six times as much as at birth.

At birth, the size of the ventricular walls is approximately equal, but with the demands of peripheral circulation after birth, the left ventricular wall becomes thicker than that of the right. The position of the heart also changes. At birth, it assumes a horizontal position but as the heart grows, it shifts to lie lower and more obliquely.

As the child's body lengthens, the heart increases in size to meet the growing demands of the circulatory system. Likewise, the walls of blood vessels become thicker to manage the increasing blood pressure (BP). Systolic BP quickly rises during the first 6 weeks after birth and then slows until puberty when it rises to adult levels.

CARDIOVASCULAR SYSTEM OVERVIEW

- A detailed health history that includes family history of congenital heart disease, feeding problems (fatigue, diaphoresis, poor weight gain, etc.), and respiratory difficulties (tachypnoea, dyspnoea, shortness of breath, cyanosis and frequent respiratory infections)
- Physical assessment – general appearance: Colour, position of comfort, facial expression, respiratory effort, level of activity and responsiveness to environment
- Baseline respiratory pattern, unusual rate, nasal flaring, grunting, retractions or other irregularities
- Tachypnoea, tachycardia, moist grunting respirations, orthopnoea, paroxysmal nocturnal dyspnoea
- Heart rate and rhythm or presence of murmurs
- All baseline vital signs including BP and pulses in all four limbs
- Chest deformities
- Location and depth of retractions
- Signs of venous engorgement – Periorbital oedema, hepatomegaly
  - Decreased urine output, diaphoresis
  - Abnormal heart sounds, rhythm; pulsus alternans
  - Feeding problems, tolerance of diet, growth pattern
  - Cool and clammy skin that is mottled, with poor capillary refill
  - Clubbing
  - Serum electrolytes
  - Hypotension or unequal BP in arms and legs
  - Murmurs, bruits and thrills
- Parental concerns and level of understanding of the child's condition, planned surgery, etc.

Laboratory Studies

Relevant laboratory findings may include the following:
- Compensatory increase in haematocrit (polycythaemia), haemoglobin and erythrocyte count
- Altered blood gas values
- Abnormalities in homeostasis such as thrombocytopenia; decreased platelet function, low prothrombin level, absent clotting factors, V, VIII or IX
- Important diagnostic tests include:
  - Electrocardiography (ECG)
  - Chest X-rays
  - Cardiac catheterization
  - Angiography
  - Echocardiography (Echo)

Cardiac dysfunctions include cardiac diseases and cardiac defects or lesions.

Cardiac defects or lesions are categorized as:
- Acyanotic, left-to-right shunts
- Cyanotic, right-to-left shunts

Cardiac lesions can be divided into four groups as follows:
- Lesions that increase pulmonary blood flow
- Lesions that decrease pulmonary blood flow
- Lesions that create obstruction
- Lesions that create directional shunts

Aetiology and Incidence of Congenital Heart Diseases

The aetiology of congenital heart disease in neonates is often unknown, with only 8% known to be associated with a single mutant gene or chromosomal abnormalities (Wolfe R R & Wiggins J W, 1991, p. 427). Most congenital cardiac anomalies are the result of a complex interaction of genetic and environmental factors.
- At least 90% are believed to be a result of multifactorial inheritance and a complex interaction between genetic and environmental factors.
- Teratogens are associated with a small percentage of congenital heart defects.
- Maternal rubella during the first trimester of pregnancy is associated with 50% cases of congenital heart defects (Hazinski, M F, 1984).
- Approximately 10% of infants of diabetic mothers who are insulin dependent may have congenital heart disease.
- Up to 50% of infants with fetal alcohol syndrome have associated congenital heart disease.
- Chromosomal anomalies or syndromes are associated with cardiac defects; approximately 30%–40% of neonates with trisomy 21 (Down syndrome) have cardiac anomalies.

The incidence of congenital heart disease is approximately 8–10 of every 1000 live births (Whaley L & Wong D, 1997).

Years ago, anatomic complexities of many cardiac defects were prohibitive of long survival and generally only supportive therapy was recommended. Nowadays, palliative and physiological repair of complex congenital heart anomalies is attempted in most centres with adequate facilities. Cardiac surgery pertains to both open and closed heart procedures for the palliation and correction of congenital disorders. Closed procedures may be accompanied through thoracotomy or modified thoracotomy. Open heart procedures include the use of cardiopulmonary bypass (i.e. use of heart–lung machine to divert the blood flow from the operative site and oxygenate the body while the heart is being repaired and deep hypothermia to reduce the body's oxygen needs).

Common complications of cardiac surgery include the following:
- Respiratory insufficiency following pulmonary artery binding
- Haemorrhage (more common in infants with preoperative cyanosis and compensatory polycythaemia)
- Cardiac tamponade
- Post-pericardectomy syndrome: Fever, leucocytosis, pericardial friction rub, pericardial or pleural effusion
- Conduction disturbances: Heart block, dysrhythmias
- Thoracotomy-associated syndromes such as chylothorax, phrenic nerve paralysis, etc.
- Leaks of baffle, conduit, anastomosis sites, valve malfunction, etc.
- Low cardiac output
- Congestive heart failure (CHF)
- Thromboembolus, cerebrovascular accident, etc.

NURSING MANAGEMENT OF CHILDREN WITH COMMON MEDICAL AND SURGICAL PROBLEMS AFFECTING CARDIOVASCULAR FUNCTIONS

Acyanotic Defects

Patent Ductus Arteriosus

Persistence of the fetal ductus arteriosus beyond the perinatal period with an anatomically and functionally open shunt exists between the pulmonary artery and the aorta.

Incidence
- Patent ductus arteriosus (PDA) occurs in 5%–10% of all congenital heart diseases in neonates, excluding preterm infants.
- In preterm infants, the incidence is 20%–60% among infants weighing less than 1500 g.
- PDA is common in neonates whose mothers had rubella in the first trimester of pregnancy (Wolfe R R & Wiggins J W, 1991).
- PDA is common in both females and males (Wolfe R R & Wiggins J W, 1991).

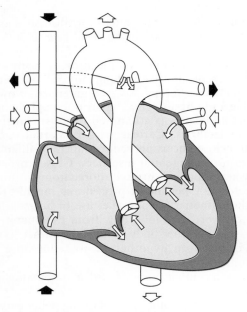

Patent ductus arteriosus.

Haemodynamics
- Large PDA
  Permits large aorta to pulmonary artery shunt under high pressure and CHF may occur
- Small PDA
  Less clinically significant and may be life-saving in infants with cyanotic heart disease and also in infants with compromised pulmonary blood flow.

Clinical Manifestations
- Harsh murmur heard at the second left intercostal space, at the left sternal border and inferior to the left clavicle.
- The murmur is systolic and then becomes continuous.
- Thrill over the supra sternal notch and along the upper left and right sternal borders; many a times the thrill can be visualized as active precordium.
- Bounding femoral pulses present.
- Pulse pressure is widened greater than half the systolic pressure.
- In preterm neonates, there will be respiratory distress with tachypnoea, retractions, hypoxaemia and hypercapnia.
- Presence of left-to-right shunt with CHF is demonstrated by increased dependency over oxygen respiratory support.
- Cardiomegaly: If the shunt is large, there is both left and right ventricular enlargement and if the shunt is small or moderate in size, the heart is not enlarged.

Diagnosis
- ECG may be normal or show left ventricular hypertrophy.
- Echo – Enlargement of left atrium indicates CHF.
- Chest X-ray shows cardiac enlargement.

Multidisciplinary Management
- Medical: Indomethacin (prostaglandin inhibitor) promotes ductus closure in neonates.
- Surgical: Ligation or division through a left thoracotomy is performed.

Atrial Septal Defect

Atrial septal defect (ASD) is an opening in the atrial septum that occurs as a result of improper septal formation in the early fetal cardiac development that permits shunting of blood between the two atria. An incompetent foramen ovale is the most common defect.

Incidence. This type of defect occurs in 10% of infants with congenital heart disease. Incidence is twice as common in females as in males and up to 40% spontaneously close within the first 5 years of life (Parks M K, 1996).

Types. There are three major types:
- Ostium primum – Positioned low in the atrial septum and results from incomplete fusion of the embryonic endocardial cushions which results from the lower portion of the atrial septum. This accounts for approximately 4% of all congenital heart diseases. The incidence is 20% in children with Down syndrome (Wolfe R R & Wiggins J W).
- Ostium secundum – It is the most common defect and occurs in the area of the foramen ovale or in an intermediate position on the atrial septum. This may be associated with mitral valve prolapse.
- Sinus venosus – It is located high in the septum and frequently associated with partial anomalous venous return (right pulmonary vein drains into the right atrium).

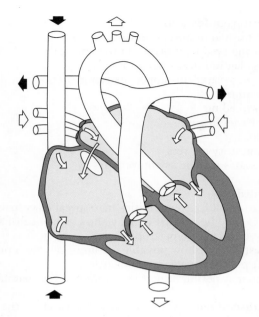

Atrial septal defect.

in size and may involve either the membranous or muscular portion of the ventricular septum.

Incidence. VSD is the most common among congenital heart diseases, with an incidence of 20%–25% among neonates with cardiac defects. It frequently occurs in association with other congenital heart disease. VSD is more common in males than in females.

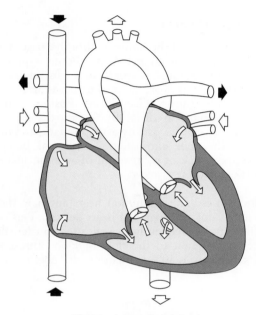

Ventricular septal defect.

Haemodynamics. Pressure in the left atrium is higher than that in the right atrium; therefore, blood is shunted from the left atrium through the defect to the right side of the heart. CHF is not common because the pressure increase on the pulmonary circulation is small.

Clinical Manifestations
- Many neonates with ASD are asymptomatic
- S2 widely split
- Grade I through III/IV ejection systolic murmur
- Diastolic flow murmur at the lower left sternal border in large shunts
- Widely radiating systolic murmur
- CHF

Diagnosis
- Chest X-ray shows cardiomegaly and the main pulmonary artery may show dilatation.
- Echo permits direct visualization of the defect and left-to-right shunt.
- ECG shows bundle branch block and right axis deviation.

Multidisciplinary Management. Treat CHF, if present. Primary or patch closure of the defect using cardiopulmonary bypass and atrial umbrella eliminates the need for corrective surgery of ostium secundum. Here, during cardiac catheterization, a catheter is advanced from the right atrium into the left atrium through the septal defect. A patch graft with claws that adhere to the atrial wall is carefully placed over the defect. The graft is held in place by high left atrial pressure.

Ventricular Septal Defect

Ventricular septal defect (VSD) is an opening between the right and left ventricles that results from imperfect ventricular formation during fetal development. It varies

Haemodynamics. A small defect may be asymptomatic and may close spontaneously. A shunting of blood from the left ventricle to the right ventricle occurs during systole because of a higher pressure in the left ventricle. In large defects, there will be increased pulmonary blood flow under high pressure resulting in pulmonary hypertension. If pulmonary hypertension is present, the blood shunts from the right ventricle to the left ventricle and cause cyanosis.

Clinical Manifestations
Small defects:
- Neonates usually show no signs other than a soft murmur.
- Normal growth patterns present.
- One-third of defects close spontaneously.

Large VSDs:
- Murmur is usually holosystolic and frequently accompanied by a thrill.
- They tend to become smaller with advancing age.
- Other signs of VSD are tachypnoea, poor feeding, diaphoresis and associated signs of CHF.

Diagnosis
- Chest X-ray shows cardiomegaly and left and right ventricular hypertrophy.
- Echo shows defects of 4 mm or larger.

Multidisciplinary Management
- Small defect – Asymptomatic children are treated conservatively, and a high incidence of spontaneous closure in the first 2 years of life exists.
- Large defect – Treatment of CHF and pulmonary artery banding (palliative procedure to reduce volume and pressure of pulmonary blood flow) are the main modes of management. Repair is accomplished through patch or suture closure using cardiopulmonary bypass.

Coarctation of Aorta

It is the narrowing of the lumen within the area of aortic arch. Three types of anomalies are noted – preductal, postductal and juxtaductal defects. In preductal defects, it can be a coarctation proximal to the ductus arteriosus or associated with other cardiac defects. Postductal defects may be a coarctation distal to the ductus arteriosus, wherein the neonate is usually asymptomatic and not associated with other anomalies. Juxtaductal being the most common type of coarctation of aorta in juxtaposition to the ductus arteriosus.

Incidence. It is a very common heart anomaly that accounts for 6% of all congenital heart defects. This occurs three times more frequently in males than in females. It produces obstruction to the flow of blood through the aorta. Its incidence is 30% in infants with Tuner syndrome.

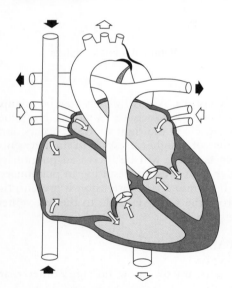

Coarctation of the aorta.

Haemodynamics. Constriction of the aorta reduces the amount of oxygenated blood to the descending aorta and sometimes produces cyanosis in the extremities. In preductal coarctation, severe CHF within hours or days of birth is reported if the aortic arch is small. If the narrowing is in the arch of aorta, there may be a difference of BP between the right and left arms. In postductal cases, there will be large resistance to blood flow; collateral vessels develop during the fetal life. BP in the upper extremities is increased, and left ventricular hypertrophy and CHF may also be present.

Clinical Manifestations
- Diminished or absent femoral pulses
- Blowing systolic murmur in the left axilla
- Pulse lag in lower extremities
- BP is greater in upper extremities than in lower extremities
- Poor feeding
- Poor weight gain
- Pallor
- Respiratory distress
- Neonates may be asymptomatic

Diagnosis
- BP from all four extremities may reveal discrepancies.
- ECG may be normal or may show evidence of slight left ventricular hypertrophy.
- Chest X-rays show possible cardiomegaly with prominent pulmonary venous congestion.
- Echo may permit direct visualization of the coarctation.

Multidisciplinary Management. Excision of the narrowed aortic area and reanastomosis of the resected area or closure with a patch with cardiopulmonary bypass assistance are the usual management.

Aortic Stenosis

It is an obstruction of the aorta interfering with left ventricular outflow.

Three types of aortic stenosis are seen. These are as follows:
1. Valvular stenosis (usually bicuspid) – The most common type where increased rigidity of the valve tissue and varying degrees of commissural fusion lead to obstruction to the flow of blood
2. Supravalvular obstruction
3. Subvalvular (subaortic) obstruction – As a result of fibrous ring or muscular obstruction

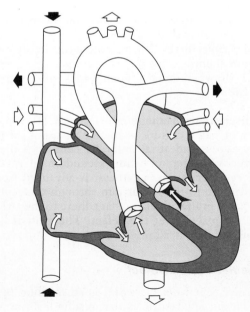

Subaortic stenosis.

Haemodynamics. It varies with the degree of obstruction. Increased left ventricular pressure causes left ventricular hypertrophy. Outflow into the aorta become extremely turbulent, producing loud murmurs and palpable thrills.

Clinical Manifestations

- Most aortic stenoses asymptomatic in infancy
- Systolic ejection murmur at the upper right sternal border
- Thrill on carotid arteries
- Systolic click at the apex of the heart
- CHF in aortic stenosis (peripheral pulses weak and thready, tachypnoea, increased respiratory effort, diaphoresis, poor feeding, poor weight gain)

Diagnosis

- Chest X-ray usually indicates that heart is not enlarged and the left ventricle is slightly prominent.
- Echo shows eccentric aortic valve closure and moderate to severe aortic obstruction.

Multidisciplinary Management

- Valvular stenosis – Aortic valvotomy and aortic valve replacement
- Subvalvular stenosis Excision of the membrane or fibromuscular ring
- May cause enlargement of the entire left ventricular outflow tract and annulus
- Supravalvular stenosis:
  - Excision of a discrete membrane, if present
  - Enlargement of the aorta with a prosthetic patch if the area is extensive.

Endocardial Cushion Defect

It is the improper fusion of the endocardial cushion during fetal development so that the right and left AV orifices are not correctly formed. Two types of defects are seen – ostium primum defect (defect low in the atrial septum) and complete AV canal defect where severe mitral insufficiency develops.

Haemodynamics. Ostium primum defect is similar to an ASD. In the complete AV canal, there will be left-to-right shunt of blood and increase in pulmonary blood flow. If the defect is large, CHF and right ventricular hypertrophy develop.

Multidisciplinary Management. Pulmonary artery banding is performed if CHF occurs. Definitive repair is patch closure of ASD and VSD on cardiopulmonary bypass, possible mitral valve replacement and division of common AV valves.

Cyanotic Defects

Tetralogy of Fallot

It is the lack of development of the subpulmonary conus during the fetal life producing pulmonary infundibular stenosis and malalignment of the conal septum

(Castaneda A R & Norwood W I, 1981). It includes four defects as follows:
- Pulmonary stenosis
- Overriding of aorta
- Ventricular septal defect
- Right ventricular hypertrophy

Aetiology and Incidence. It is the most common type of cyanotic heart lesion and accounts for 10%–15% of all congenital heart disease.

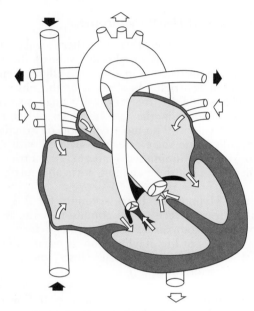

Tetralogy of Fallot.

Haemodynamics. The severity of symptoms depends on the degree of stenosis, the magnitude of VSD and the degree to which the aorta overrides the defect.

In mild stenosis, there will be minimal right-to-left shunting of blood and cyanosis. In severe stenosis, there will be decreased pulmonary blood flow, right-to-left shunting of blood, cyanosis and hypoxaemia.

Clinical Features

- Respiratory distress is present.
- Cyanosis – Degree is directly related to the extent of pulmonary stenosis (if the ductus arteriosus is patent, the neonate may have minimum cyanosis, and on constriction of the PDA, the infant will frequently have cyanosis upon exertion).
- Crying or feeding increases cyanosis and respiratory distress.
- Systolic ejection murmurs are located at the upper sternal border.

Diagnosis

- Chest X-rays may appear entirely normal, and right ventricular hypertrophy and boot-shaped appearance of the heart are secondary to the small pulmonary artery.
- Laboratory findings – Haemoglobin values are mildly to markedly elevated. Haematocrit and red blood cell

count are elevated depending on the extent of arterial oxygen desaturation.

- Echo shows right ventricular wall thickening and over-riding of the aorta and VSD.

Multidisciplinary Management
- Palliative – Aortopulmonary shunt
- Corrective surgery – Closure of VSD, resection of pulmonary stenosis and possible patch enlargement of the pulmonary outflow tract

Hypoplastic Left Heart Syndrome

It includes various defects that are either valvular or vascular obstructive lesions on the left side of the heart. There is severe obstruction in either the filling or emptying of the left ventricle. As a result of the obstruction during intrauterine life, there is a very small quantity of blood filling occurs in the left ventricle; subsequently, hypoplasia develops. The most common obstructive lesions include aortic valve atresia associated with mitral atresia or stenosis, diminutive or absent left ventricle, and severe hypoplasia of the ascending aorta and aortic arch.

Incidence. Hypoplastic heart accounts for 2% of all congenital heart defects. This condition is the leading cause of death from cardiovascular heart defects within the first 2 weeks of life. The neonate is usually duct dependent; as the ductus arteriosus closes, the neonate's condition deteriorates.

Haemodynamics. There will be resistance to flow to the aorta and inadequate perfusion of the systemic circulation. The flow of blood from the pulmonary artery through the ductus arteriosus supports life.

Clinical Manifestations
- Generalized cyanosis
- Soft, systolic murmur just left of the sternum
- Diminished pulses
- Tachycardia
- Tachypnoea
- Pulmonary rales
- Respiratory distress
- Pallor and mottling

Diagnosis
- Chest X-rays may appear normal at birth but later rapid and progressive cardiac enlargement and pulmonary venous congestion occur.
- ECG shows right atrial hypertrophy and right ventricular hypertrophy.
- Echo shows the diminished aorta and the left ventricle and the poorly defined mitral valve.

Multidisciplinary management
- Prostaglandin E$_1$ to keep the ductus arteriosus open.
- Surgical repair:
  - Stage I: Reconstruction of the diminutive ascending aorta and aortic arch, systemic artery to pulmonary shunt and creation of a large shunt.
  - Stage II: Removal of the systemic artery to pulmonary artery shunt, anastomosis of the right atrium to

the pulmonary arteries and insertion of an interatrial baffle to connect the left atrium to the right ventricle via the atrial septal defect.
- Other options: Heart transplantation is limited because of a small number of donor hearts.

Transposition of Great Vessels

It is a condition in which the aorta arises from the right ventricle and the pulmonary trunk from the left ventricle. Transposition is caused by an embryological abnormality in the spiral division of the truncus arteriosus. There is a straight division without the normal spiralling. As a result, the aorta originates from the right ventricle and the pulmonary artery originates from the left ventricle.

Haemodynamics. Unoxygenated systemic venous blood enters the right heart and the aorta and returns to the systemic circulation; oxygenated pulmonary venous blood enters the left heart and the pulmonary artery and returns to the lungs, resulting in severe systemic arterial hypoxaemia.

Clinical Manifestations
- Cyanosis: Most babies are cyanotic at birth.
- Usually, a large birth weight around 3.5–4 kg is reported.
- Possible pulmonic stenosis murmur is present, but some may not have murmurs.
- Signs of CHF: VSD is large and usually develops at approximately 3 weeks of age because of enormous pulmonary blood flow.
- Normal peripheral pulses are present.

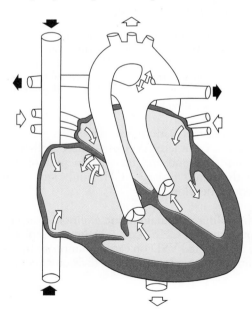

Transposition of great vessels.

Diagnosis
- Chest X-rays: Findings are usually nonspecific and indicate possible causes of cardiomegaly.

- Echo reveals abnormal relationship of the great vessels.
- Cardiac catheterization gives the definitive diagnosis and is used to perform a septotomy between the two ventricles.

Multidisciplinary Management
Palliative:
- Rashkind balloon atrioseptostomy via cardiac catheterization
- Pulmonary artery banding
- Blalock–Hanlon septectomy

Corrective surgery:
- Mustard procedure involves excision of the atrial septum and use of a pericardial baffle to redirect venous return.
- Senning repair is similar to the Mustard procedure; the atrial septum is preserved and utilized.
- In the atrial switch procedure, the pulmonary artery and the aorta are transected several millimetres above the semilunar valves and the pulmonary artery is sutured to the stump of the aorta; the aorta is sutured to the stump of pulmonary artery. Coronary arteries are detached from the aorta and reimplanted after the switch.
- In the Rastelli procedure, VSD is closed with a baffle; pulmonary valve is sewn closed, and the conduit connects the right ventricle to the main pulmonary artery.

Tricuspid Atresia

It is the absence of the tricuspid valve during fetal cardiac development which prevents blood flow between the right atrium and the right ventricle.

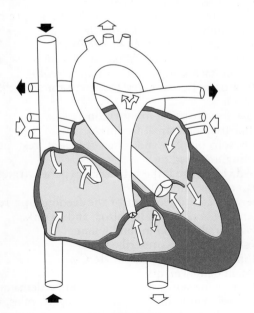

Tricuspid atresia.

Haemodynamics. The systemic venous blood must enter the left heart through a patent foramen ovale or an atrial septal defect. Pulmonary blood flow depends on the left-to-right shunt through a VSD, patent ductus arteriosus or surgical shunt. CHF may be present, and cyanosis is usually severe.

Multidisciplinary Management. If the foramen ovale is too small to allow adequate right-to-left atrial shunting, then Rashkind balloon septostomy or Blalock–Hanlon septectomy will be done. When CHF is unresponsive to medical management, pulmonary artery banding is done. If severe hypoxaemia is present, systemic to pulmonary artery shunt or Fontan's procedure is done (connection of the right atrium to the main pulmonary artery and closure of other existing shunts). This is ideally performed when the child of school-age to allow insertion of a large conduit.

Truncus Arteriosus

It is the inadequate division of the truncus arteriosus during the fetal life resulting in a single, large great vessel arising from the ventricles and giving rise to the pulmonary systemic and coronary circulations; a VSD is present because the truncal septum contributes to closure of the ventricular septum.

Classification
- Truncus arteriosus types I–III are direct branching of pulmonary arteries and aorta from the common trunk.
- Truncus arteriosus type IV or pseudotruncus is a single great vessel, and the aorta comes from the ventricles; blood enters this vessel through the VSD from both the right and left ventricles. The enlarged bronchial arteries and collateral vessels arising from the descending aorta carry unoxygenated blood to the lungs.

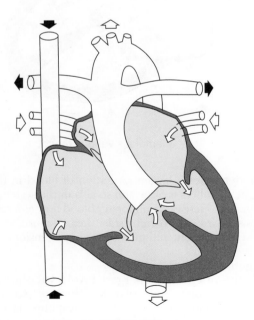

Truncus arteriosus.

Haemodynamics. In truncus arteriosus types I–III, both ventricles pump blood into a common trunk. There is an increased pulmonary blood flow unless pulmonary stenosis is present as well as right and left ventricular hypertrophy. In type IV, blood flow to the lungs is reduced and accomplished only through a patent ductus arteriosus or collateral circulation.

Management. For truncus arteriosus types I–III, pulmonary artery banding, closure of the VSD and insertion of a valved conduit are done by cardiopulmonary bypass. For type IV, an initial shunt procedure is done to increase pulmonary blood flow. Finally, closure of any associated septal defect and establishment of blood flow from the right ventricle to the pulmonary artery via the valved conduit are done.

Total Anomalous Pulmonary Venous Return

Drainage of the pulmonary veins into the right atrium occurs instead of the left atrium; pulmonary veins may be attached directly to the right atrium or to a systemic vein above or below the diaphragm.

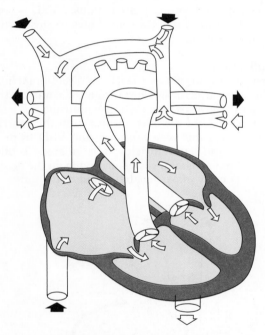

Total anomalous venous return.

Haemodynamics. Oxygen saturation of blood in the left and right chambers is same and so also in the systemic circulation. The increased pulmonary blood flow as a result of low resistance leads to right-sided heart failure, systemic venous engorgement and pulmonary hypertension.

Management
- Palliative or corrective surgery involves Rashkind balloon septostomy and corrective surgery. Corrective surgery includes anastomosis of the pulmonary veins to the left atrium, elimination of anomalous pulmonary venous connection and closure of ASD.
- Medications include digoxin, diuretics and antidysrhythmics, along with dietary management and social support.

GENERAL NURSING CARE

General nursing care for children with a congenital heart disease is same for all types of anomalies, with very little modification according to the condition of the child. Hence, a general care approach is followed in this chapter.

A general assessment is already described in this chapter along with a system overview. The reader is directed to review the same for nursing assessment.

The nursing interventions for infants and children with cyanotic and acyanotic heart defects are essentially the same, with an exception to education about specific defects and their management.

Major Nursing Diagnoses

- Alteration in tissue perfusion is related to decrease in circulating oxygen.
- High risk for alteration in nutrition: Less than body requirement is related to inadequate sucking, fatigue and dyspnoea.
- High risk for alteration in fluid volume: Excess is related to cardiac failure.
- Alteration in cardiac output: Decrease is related to cardiac failure.
- Alteration in respiratory function is related to decreased cardiac output.
- Activity intolerance is related to insufficient oxygenation secondary to cardiac defect.

Nursing Interventions

Alteration in tissue perfusion:
- Monitor BP and maintain within normal limits (the mean pressure should be 30).
- Administer vasopressor medications, as prescribed (dopamine, 5–20 mcg/kg per day).
- Assess capillary refill (1–4 seconds).
- Assess for signs of shock (pallor, thready pulse, hypotension, tachycardia, poor capillary refill).
- Monitor pulse oximetry (oxygen saturation 95 and above).

High risk for alteration in nutrition:
- Offer frequent, small feedings.
- Use soft nipples and offer frequent rest periods throughout feeding.
- Feed via gavage if the baby is tachypnoeic (rate more than 60 per minute).
- Increase calorie content of the feeding in a regular manner (24, 27, and 30 cal/oz, and so on).

High risk for alteration in fluid volume:
- Restrict fluids, as prescribed.
- Monitor intake and output (I&O).
- Obtain daily weights.
- Monitor for signs of fluid overload (oedema around the eyes, hands and feet; hepatomegaly, rales, rhonchi, cardiac enlargement and excessive weight gain).
- Offer high-calorie feedings to minimize fluid intake.
- Administer diuretics, as prescribed.
- Note time and response to diuretics.
- Have the child urinate prior to bedtime.

- Monitor electrolytes, especially potassium if Lasix is given, and supplement potassium, if indicated.

Alteration in cardiac output:
- Plan nursing care in such a way that minimum handling is needed.
- Maintain a neutral thermal environment to avoid cold stress.
- Minimize crying and agitation by using comfort measures.
- Feed by gavage if signs of respiratory distress are present.
- Administer medications according to prescription to increase cardiac output.

Alteration in respiratory function:
- Maintain bed rest in the semi-Fowler position.
- Avoid restrictive clothing or restraints around the abdomen and chest.
- Monitor blood gases, vital signs and pulse oximetry.
- Administer oxygen, as needed.
- Provide a humid atmosphere.
- Perform percussion, vibration, postural drainage and suction, as needed.
- Minimize agitation and crying by using comfort measures.
- Feed via gavage if signs of respiratory distress are present.

Activity intolerance:
- In non-duct-dependent lesions, increase oxygen concentration when the neonate is being suctioned or manipulated for a procedure.
- Avoid excessive stimulation; cluster interventions.
- Adapt feeding techniques to minimize energy expenditure.
- Organize nursing activities to allow for uninterrupted periods of sleep.

Preoperative interventions:
Provide preoperative education to parents and the child (age appropriate) including the followings:
- Tour to the intensive care unit and the operating room as per policy of the institution
- Anaesthesia, NPO (nil by mouth) orders and preoperative medications
- Postoperative pain management
- Type of incision
- Intubation, mechanical ventilation and the process of weaning to room air
- Pacer wires and pacemakers, if planned
- Use of cardiac/respiratory monitors
- Foley's catheter and its purpose
- Chest tubes
- Chest physiotherapy measures such as percussion, vibration, postural drainage, endotracheal saline and suctioning
- Arterial lines/intravenous/central venous lines
- Level of consciousness immediately following surgery
- Slow diet progression as the child recovers
- Encourage parents to stay with the child and to participate in the care as much as possible to decrease the child's anxiety and therefore decrease cardiac workload
- Counsel parents regarding the child's activity and possible activity restrictions; educate the child and parents the knee, chest or squatting position to facilitate breathing

- Allow for and provide therapeutic play opportunities appropriate to the child's age
- Provide parents opportunity to identify what is happening in the intraoperative period (messenger from intraoperative site will visit parents in waiting room to report about the child's condition to reduce the anxiety of parents.)

Postoperative care:
- Help maintain the optimal respiratory status by monitoring respirations and providing good pulmonary hygiene (monitor respiratory rate, breath sounds; monitor chest tubes, drainage and patency; monitor blood gases; provide chest physiotherapy; and observe for early signs of respiratory distress).
- Monitor cardiac status (heart rate and rhythm, BP, central venous pressure [CVP] and other haemodynamic parameters, heart sounds, peripheral pulses and perfusion and blood chemistry).
- Help prevent postoperative hypothermia.
- Closely monitor I&O.
- Help maintain skin integrity.
- Monitor for postoperative complications (hypoxia, acidosis, thromboembolism, electrolyte imbalance and poor systemic perfusion).
- Promote comfort measures.
- Help prevent problems of sensory overload by keeping the child oriented to time and place, prepare the child for all procedures and provide repeated age-appropriate explanations.
- During recovery, provide tactile stimulation for infants and distraction activities for older children.
- Provide emotional support to parents and children by addressing their concerns and answering their questions.
- Provide parent and patient education covering:
  - Activity restrictions
  - Incision site care
  - Dosage and administration of medications
  - Diet restrictions and fluid restrictions
  - Physiological complications to watch and report (fever, tachycardia, severe or persistent chest pain, tachypnoea, feeding difficulties, oedema over limbs and face)
  - Possible regressive behaviours

OTHER HEART DISEASES

Rheumatic Fever

Rheumatic fever is a condition that occurs as sequelae to streptococcal throat infection. It is an important cause of acquired heart disease in children. It is the post-streptococcal immune-mediated disorder related to cross-reaction between the connective tissue of the body and antibodies produced against streptococcal cell wall protein and sugars.

Incidence

The incidence of rheumatic fever is related to the incidence of group A streptococcal throat infection. More common in developing countries where overcrowding and poor sanitary conditions prevail. In crowded living conditions, the incidence is about 1%–3% such as in children's homes. The incidence is more common in fall, winter, early spring and autumn. It is more common in the age group of 5–15 years. Both sexes are equally affected. Rheumatic heart disease (RHD) is the sequelae of rheumatic fever.

Predisposing factors include poor socioeconomic status, overcrowding (orphanages, children's home, military recruits, etc.) and unhygienic living conditions.

It is believed to be following group A beta haemolytic streptococcal throat infection. The occurrence of rheumatic fever after the latent period following streptococcal throat infection gives credence to the immune-mediated mechanism. The presence of streptococcal M proteins in the human host after group A streptococcal throat infection is responsible for cross-reaction between the organism and the human host. The presence of common antibodies to the antigen found in the group A streptococcal cell membrane in the caudate nucleus of the brain in patients with Sydenham chorea also supports the abnormal autoimmune mechanism responsible for CNS manifestations of rheumatic fever. There is also a genetic predisposition for the development of rheumatic fever and RHD. The presence of specific alloantigen on the surface of non-T lymphocytes in 70%–90% of individuals with rheumatic fever compared with that in less than 30% of nonrheumatic individuals.

Assessment Findings

There is a set criterion for making the diagnosis as depicted by modified Jones criteria.

Modified Jones Criteria

Sl. No.	Major	Minor
1	Carditis	Clinical
2	Polyarthritis	1. Fever
3	Chorea	2. Arthralgia
4	Subcutaneous nodules	3. Previous rheumatic fever or RHD
5	Erythema marginatum	Investigation 1. Prolonged PR interval 2. Increased erythrocyte sedimentation rate (ESR) or the presence of C-reactive protein (CRP)

Essential Criteria

These include evidence of preceding group A streptococcal infection (culture, rapid antigen, antibody rise/elevation).

Typical Clinical Picture

A child suffers from streptococcal throat infection which alleviates spontaneously with or without treatment. One or few weeks later, the child develops fever with clinical features of rheumatic fever.

Major Criteria

Carditis is basically pancarditis with the involvement of endocardium, myocardium and pericardium. It occurs in 50%–60% of children with rheumatic fever. Though all the three layers are involved, the common manifestations of rheumatic fever result from the involvement of endocardium with valvular insufficiency. The most common affected valve is mitral valve. Sometimes, aortic valve is also affected along with it. Tricuspid and pulmonary valve involvement is not usual. Clinical feature of valvular insufficiency depends on the severity of involvement. This includes pansystolic murmurs of mitral insufficiency, apical mid-diastolic murmur or basal diastolic murmur. Tricuspid regurgitation is also seen. In severe cases, acute volume overload on the left ventricle results in left ventricular failure. Heart failure is the major cause of mortality in rheumatic fever. Myocarditis of acute rheumatic fever manifests with soft first heart sound, S_3 gallop, congestive cardiac failure (CCF), Carey Coombs murmur and cardiac enlargement.

Pericarditis of acute rheumatic fever presents with chest pain, pericardial rub and minimal effusion. Carditis is the only manifestation that leads to chronic conditions of RHD, which, in turn, leads to valvular stenosis.

Polyarthritis

This is the early manifestation that occurs in 70%–75% of cases. It is migratory in nature involving the large joints such as knees, ankles, elbows and wrists. It rarely involves small joints. The joints are swollen, red and severely tender and the movements are limited. Polyarthritis of rheumatic fever has no sequelae, and relief of the symptoms occurs with anti-inflammatory drugs. Prior anti-inflammatory therapy eliminates the migratory nature of polyarthritis of rheumatic fever. The saying that 'Rheumatic licks the joints and bites the heart' is 100% true.

Rheumatic Chorea (Sydenham Chorea)

It is a self-limiting late manifestation. It occurs usually after 3 months of acute rheumatic fever. The choreoathetoid type of movement makes diagnosis difficult. In school-going children, deterioration of handwriting is the best sign. The movements are purposeless and jerky resulting in deranged speech, muscular incoordination, awkward gait and weakness. This results in difficulty carrying out usual schoolwork.

Usual tests for confirmation of chorea are finger–nose test, buttoning the clothes test, dinner fork posturing of the outstretched hands, pronator test (pronation of the forearm when hands are raised above the head), dirtying tongue (tongue keeps moving like a bag of worms on protruding) and audible clicks during speech, clumsiness or inability in clear, organized writing.

Ataxia can be diagnosed by counting the digits test and sustained hung-up or double-knee jerk.

Subcutaneous Nodules

It is also a late manifestation, which is seen only in 3.5% of children with rheumatic fever. It is commonly seen in children with severe carditis. These are pea-sized, firm, nontender nodules usually seen on bony prominence such as knees, elbows, shines, over the spine and occiput. They usually disappear after few days or weeks.

Erythema Marginatum

It starts as nonspecific, pink macules over the trunk which spread and fuses together to form a serpiginous outline. It is a nonblanching, evanescent rash and difficult to be seen in children with dark complexion. It is a very rare finding as compared with other findings of rheumatic fever.

Minor criteria are less sensitive and only contributory findings in the diagnosis. Laboratory findings are increased ESR, positive CRP and prolonged PR interval that will be seen in all children with rheumatic fever. The 'gold standards' for diagnosis of rheumatic fever are positive throat swab culture and raised antistreptolysin O (ASO) titre.

Multidisciplinary Management

- Supportive medical management
- Treatment of associated clinical findings including anti-inflammatory therapy
- Treatment of group A streptococcal infections

Nursing Diagnoses

- Activity intolerance
- Comfort alteration in pain
- Potential for complications (RHD)
- Noncompliance
- Parental anxiety
- Alteration in nutrition
- Self-esteem disturbances

Nursing Interventions

- Provide complete/strict bed rest till the symptoms subside.
- Ideally, bed rest should be given for 6–8 weeks.
- Ambulate the patient only after the symptoms of carditis is not present.
- If CCF is present, bed rest need to be prolonged.
- Plan and provide a diet rich in protein, vitamin and micronutrients.
- If carditis/CCF is present, restrict salt intake.
- Administer medications, as prescribed.
  - Anti-inflammatory agents are the cornerstone of management.
  - Usual drugs are salicylates and steroids.
  - Aspirin is the drug of choice that causes decrease in fever, pain and swelling of the joints.
  - Joint symptoms disappear within 12–24 hours after administration of salicylates.
  - The usual dose is 90–120 mg/kg per day in four divided doses to maintain a blood level of 20–25 mcg/dL.
  - The total duration of therapy is about 12 weeks to suppress inflammation completely.

- Full dosage need to be administered for about 10 weeks and then dose needs to be tapered.
- Monitor for drug toxicity clinically as well as by estimation of blood levels.
- Observe for tinnitus as the early sign of salicylate toxicity.
- Report if there is any sign of toxicity.
- If toxicity is observed, dose needs to be reduced and continued with monitoring.
- Generally, steroids are not needed.
- The indication for steroid therapy is carditis with CCF or severe carditis.
- Steroid therapy is given for 4 weeks with prednisolone 2 mg/kg per day in divided doses.
- It should be slowly tapered, as instructed.
- Monitor the child for adverse effects of prolonged steroid therapy (infection, Cushing syndrome and osteoporosis).
- CCF related to acute rheumatic fever needs aggressive treatment with diuretics and digoxin.
- Chorea is self-limiting and does not require any treatment.
- If symptoms are severe, then administer phenobarbitone, diazepam or haloperidol, as prescribed.
- Reassure the parents and the child, especially with rheumatic chorea, to boost up self-esteem.
- Help children cope with anxiety.
- Institute stress reduction technique.
- Use storytelling modalities as a nursing intervention to build up self-esteem.
- Institute measures to prevent complications.
- Administer penicillin, as prescribed, after taking throat swab for culture to eradicate streptococcal infection.
- The usual dose is procaine penicillin 400,000 units i.m. b.d. × 10 days.
- Oral penicillin 4 lakh units (250 mg) can also be used.
- Provide prophylaxis every 21 days with benzathine penicillin 1–2 mg units.
- Administer erythromycin or tetracycline, as prescribed, for children who are sensitive to penicillin.
- Institute primary prophylaxis, if possible, to prevent rheumatic fever in all children with throat infection as prescribed by the acute respiratory infection (ARI) control programme or as per protocol.
- Educate the public on the dangers of untreated or poorly treated throat infections (common prophylactic treatment is with penicillin V, erythromycin, amoxicillin, cephalexin, clindamycin, nafcillin or oral penicillin G for 10 days).
- Secondary prophylaxis is by using long-acting penicillin, benzathine penicillin 1–2 mega units once in every 21 days.
- In smaller children, weighing less than 27 kg, the dose is 0.6 mg mega units.
- Parents should be informed about the consequences of rheumatic fever, the necessity for secondary prophylaxis and activity reduction.
- The nurse should be vigilant to prevent RHD in children with rheumatic fever, as the consequences are fatal in terms of morbidity and mortality along with treatment cost.

Rheumatic Heart Disease

It is the chronic sequelae of rheumatic fever and basically a valvular disease. Mitral valve is commonly affected and manifested with varying degrees of mitral regurgitation. The structural changes takes place are shortening and thickening of the chordae tendineae resulting in regurgitation. High volume of overload results in left ventricle enlargement and finally to left atrial enlargement. Persistent mitral insufficiency results in elevated pulmonary pressure, right ventricular enlargement and right-sided heart failure.

Assessment Findings

- Patients with mitral regurgitation may be symptomatic.
- Patients with moderate to severe mitral regurgitation develop easy fatigability and dyspnoea on exertion.
- Other symptoms are of CCF, palpitation and weakness.
- Cardiac enlargement is present.
- Apex displacement – Downward and outward displacement causes heaving apical impulse with apical thrill.
- First heart sound is normal, and the second sound is accentuated with augmentation of the pulmonary component.
- Pansystolic murmur is present at the apex with radiation to the left axilla, indicating increased early rapid filling of the left ventricle.
- Third heart sound is heard at the apex.
- In severe mitral regurgitation, diastolic murmur is heard at the apex as a result of large blood flow from the left atrium to the left ventricle.
- Diastolic murmur is of short duration and ends in mid-diastole.

Multidisciplinary Management

- Chest X-ray shows cardiomegaly, left ventricle and left atrial enlargement, and features of pulmonary venous hypertension.
- ECG is asymptomatic in mild cases. In moderate and severe cases, it shows left ventricular hypertrophy, left atrial hypertrophy and features of right ventricular hypertrophy.
- Echo shows enlarged left atrium and left ventricle.
- On Doppler Echo, severity of mitral regurgitation can be identified.
- Medical management includes treating mitral regurgitation and CCF, as well as prophylactic treatment of endocarditis.
- Surgical management involves prosthetic mitral valve replacement.
- Annuloplasty provides good results for older children, though valve replacement may be required later.

Nursing Diagnoses

- Activity intolerance
- Noncompliance
- Parental anxiety
- Health maintenance alteration

Nursing Interventions

- These are similar to that of a child with CCF till surgery is done.
- After surgery, the care is similar to that of any child undergoing cardiac surgery (refer to preoperative and postoperative care of child undergoing cardiac surgery).

Mitral Stenosis

It is less common in the paediatric population. It takes usually more than 10 years to develop after rheumatic fever. Juvenile mitral stenosis in children occurs rapidly within a few years after carditis.

Haemodynamics

Mitral stenosis results from fibrosis of the mitral ring commissural adhesions, contractures of the valve leaflets, chordae tendinea and papillary muscles. Reduction in valvular opening produces increased pressure and volume overload on the left atrium, resulting in its enlargement. Persistent high pressure leads to pulmonary venous hypertension, followed by pulmonary arterial hypertension, and right atrial and right ventricular enlargement that leads to right ventricular failure.

Assessment Findings

- Early presentation is tiredness and dyspnoea.
- Severe mitral stenosis leads to progressive exertional dyspnoea or even dyspnoea at rest, orthopnoea, paroxysmal nocturnal dyspnoea and palpitation.
- Blood-streaked sputum is seen in children with pulmonary oedema.
- Features of CCF (symptom develops when the size of the mitral opening reduces to 25%).

Multidisciplinary Management

- Management of CCF
- Surgery

Infective Endocarditis (Bacterial Endocarditis)

It is the infection of the endocardium of the heart along with that of the endocardium of the valves, mural endocardium and endothelium of the vessels. The commonest case is the infection with *Streptococcus viridans*. The other organisms responsible are flat *Streptococcus*, *Coxiella burnetii*, *Streptococcus pneumoniae*, *Haemophilus* species, *Staphylococcus epidermidis*, *Chlamydia* species, *Neisseria gonorrhoeae*, fungus, rickettsiae, etc. It is predominantly seen in children with acquired congenital heart disease but rarely seen in others as a part of septicaemia.

The most common risk factors are as follows:
- Underlying heart disease
- Valvular replacement surgery
- Drug abuse
- Cardiac surgery/catheterization
- Dental procedures
- Infective process anywhere in the body

- Genitourinary procedures
- Severity depending on the virulence of the organism
- The vegetation formed in any body part of the body may be carried to the endocardium, or vegetation formed at the site of endocardium through intimal erosion or from high velocity of blood ejection may be deposited on the endocardium. Or, the bacteraemia resulting from infection elsewhere in the body results in deposition of the bacteria on the endocardium, thus causing endocarditis. It can be either acute or subacute.

Assessment Findings

- Prolonged fever, high spiking fever with chills and rigors
- Night sweat and prostration
- Loss of weight
- Myalgia
- Arthralgia
- Headache
- Nausea and vomiting
- Signs and symptoms of CCF
- New murmurs or changing murmurs
- Splenomegaly
- Thromboembolic complications, brain abscess, etc.
- Embolism and mycotic aneurysms
- Vasculitis (Osler nodes – tender, pea-sized intradermal nodules in the pads of fingers and toes), Janeway lesions (painless erythematous or haemorrhagic lesion on the palms and soles), splinter haemorrhages below the nail bed, petechiae over the skin, mucous membrane and retina (Roth spot).

Multidisciplinary Management

- Blood culture
- Echo
- Considered as a medical emergency
- Hospitalization
- Prolonged antibiotics therapy for 4–6 weeks
- Penicillin G and aminoglycosides
- Supportive therapy
- Surgical treatment is an integral part of management and is needed for mitral and aortic regurgitation leading to severe CCF.
- Prophylactic and preventive treatments are advised by providing antibiotic coverage during dental, upper respiratory tract, gastrointestinal and genitourinary surgical procedures.

Pericarditis

It is the inflammation or noninflammational involvement of pericardium, causing accumulation of varying amount and nature of fluid in the pericardial cavity. The usual amount of fluid is 10–15 mL. This may be increased up to 1000 mL of serous or purulent or serosanguineous fluid, leading to cardiac tamponade causing shock.
   The common causes are as follows:
- **Bacterial**
   - Purulent – pneumonia/osteomyelitis/meningitis or tuberculosis
- **Viral**
   - Echovirus
   - Coxsackie virus
   - Epstein–Barr virus
   - Influenza
- **Fungal**
   - Histoplasmosis
   - Actinomycosis
- **Parasitic**
   - *Entamoeba histolytica*
   - Toxoplasmosis
- **Collagen disorders**
   - Rheumatic fever
   - Rheumatic arthritis
   - Systemic lupus erythematosus (SLE)
- **Neoplastic diseases**
   - Primary and metastatic malignancy
   - Haematological disorders
   - Thalassaemia
   - Leukaemia
- **Metabolic/Endocrinal disorders**
   - Uraemia
   - Hypothyroidism
- **Miscellaneous**
   - Radiation injury
   - Trauma
   - Chronic constrictive pericarditis

Assessment Findings

- Complaints of precordial pain
- Cough
- Fever
- Dyspnoea
- Arthritis
- Increased cardiac dullness
- Distant heart sounds (muffling)
- Pericardial friction rub
- Distended neck veins
- Pulses paradoxus (10–20 mm Hg inspiratory drop; over 20 mm Hg drop confirms cardiac tamponade)

Multidisciplinary Management

- Chest X-ray – Cardiomegaly
- ECG – Low voltage of the QRS complex, mild elevation of ST and generalized T-wave inversion
- Echo – Size and progression of effusion
- Medical treatment according to the cause – Steroids indicated in pericarditis associated with rheumatic fever, tuberculosis and collagen disorders
- Aspiration of pericardial effusion in the case of tamponade (up to 200 mL at a stretch)
- Surgical management includes radical pericardiectomy with decortication of pericardium)

Nursing Diagnoses

- Activity intolerance
- Altered breathing pattern
- Comfort alteration in pain
- Parental anxiety
- Ineffective parental coping
- Complication potential/high risk for injury/infection

Nursing Intervention

- Provide complete bed rest in a propped up position.
- Administer oxygen.
- Control temperature by administration of antipyretics.
- Monitor vital signs.
- Assist for laboratory investigations.
- Maintain fluid–electrolyte balance.
- Maintain adequate nutrition.
- Provide parental support.
- Reassure the child.
- Provide pain medication, as prescribed.

Myocarditis

It is the infection and inflammation of myocardium leading to myocardial damage as a result of a large number of conditions. The most common cause is viral infection with Coxsackie virus A, B, Echovirus, rubella virus, varicella zoster virus and influenza virus.

Assessment Findings

- Abrupt onset
- Unexplained dyspnoea
- Cardiovascular collapse
- CCF

Multidisciplinary Management

- Chest X-ray – Cardiomegaly
- ECG – Low-voltage and nonspecific ST-T abnormalities
- Medical treatment –Digoxin, steroid along with bed rest and antibiotics

Congestive Heart Failure

It is the failure on the part of the heart to maintain an output necessary for the needs of the body at rest or during stress following myocardial failure. It is a common paediatric medical emergency.

Left-sided heart failure occurs when the left ventricle is unable to maintain sufficient cardiac output to meet bodily needs. This is owing to inefficiency of the diseased left myocardium, leading to insufficient pumping of blood to systemic circulation. It can also occur because of increased afterload as in systemic hypertension and increased pulmonary vascular pressure (>30 mm Hg).

The common findings are nocturnal dyspnoea, dyspnoea on exertion, orthopnoea, cyanosis or pallor, palpitations, weakness, fatigue, anorexia, confusion, etc.

The right-sided heart failure results from increased pulmonary vascular resistance, which can be caused by left ventricular failure and pulmonary vascular congestion or certain lung diseases. Here, the right ventricular contractility is impaired resulting in increased right ventricular end-diastolic pressure and right ventricular preload increase, causing increased right atrial pressure and venous congestion. Increased venous pressure result in venous stasis, hepatic congestion, peripheral oedema and ascites.

The common findings include fluid retention, peripheral oedema, decreased urinary output, nausea, vomiting and anorexia.

Multidisciplinary Management

- Chest X-ray – To identify cardiac size, detect pulmonary congestion and detect congenital heart diseases and pulmonary aetiology
- ECG – Nonspecific T and ST segment changes; tall P wave and specific patterns of congenital and acquired heart disease
- Echo – To assess functional capacity and diagnosis of infective endocarditis
- Complete blood cell count, renal function, blood gas analysis, blood culture
- Medical management – Administration of digoxin, diuretics, potassium, oxygen and antibiotics, sedation and bed rest

Nursing Diagnoses (Left-sided Heart Failure)

- Impaired gas exchange
- Alteration in cardiac output
- Fluid volume excess
- Ineffective airway clearance
- Sensory perceptual alteration
- Parental anxiety

Nursing Interventions

- Monitor respiratory rate (↑ RR), rhythm and character every hourly. Be alert to increased respiratory rate; observe use of accessory muscles of respiration.
- Auscultate breath sounds, noting crackles, wheezes and other adventitious sounds.
- Provide supplemental oxygen to maintain SaO_2 to >95% by tent or nasal catheter.
- Assess arterial blood gases (ABGs); note changes in response to O_2 supplementation or treatment of altered haemodynamics.
- Suction secretions, as needed.
- Encourage deep breathing, coughing and turning every two hours (q2h).
- Place in the propped up position to maximize chest excursion (at an angle of 45°).
- Auscultate lung fields for crackles, rhonchi or other adventitious sounds.
- Monitor I&O. Report positive fluid state or decreased urine output.
- Check weight properly and daily and report changes.
- Observe for weight gain, pedal oedema and Jugular vein distention (JVD), S_3 gallop rhythm, murmurs, etc.
- Check heart sounds.
- Administer antibiotics, as prescribed, according to the cause.
- Monitor haemodynamic status hourly and report untoward symptoms.
- Administer diuretics (usual drug is furosemide in a dose of 1–3 mg/kg orally or 0.5–1.5 mg parenterally). Spironolactone is a potassium-sparing diuretic and the dose is 1–4 mg/kg.
- Observe for potassium deficiency.
- Limit oral fluids and provide sips of fluid to quench the thirst.
- Maintain prescribed activity level.

- Avoid strenuous activities of the chills that sedate the child, as prescribed.
- Administer digoxin, as prescribed.
- During digitalization, one-half of the total calculated doses should be given stat. Divide the remaining dose into two halves and administer at an 8-hour interval.
- Check the heart rate correctly to identify complications (remember the maintenance dose will be one-fourth to one-third of the total digitalizing dose, which is given as a single dose or in two divided doses).
- Organize nursing activities so that rest periods are provided properly.
- Assist in laboratory investigations and haemodynamic monitoring.

In right ventricular failure, administer positive inotropes (dobutamines, milrinone or amrinone) to support BP and to maintain cardiac output, if indicated.

Systemic Hypertension

It is defined as the BP of the 95th percentile or more with reference to the age and sex.

Normal Blood Pressure	
	Cuff Size
Infants	2.5 cm
1–2 month	5 cm
1–8 years	9 cm
Older children	12.5 cm

Systemic pressure is indicated by the appearance of Korotokoff sound, and diastolic pressure is ideally noted when the sounds are muffled. But usually, disappearance of sounds may be recorded as diastolic pressure. Both palpatory and auscultatory methods are used in children.

Aetiology

Ninety per cent of hypertension cases in children result from secondary causes.

- Renal causes   75%
- Essential hypertension 5%–10%
- Family history   ⎫
- Obesity   ⎬ Others
- Excess salt intake   ⎮
- Stress and other reasons ⎭

Assessment Findings

These depend on the underlying causes and severity of hypertension.
- BP is only slightly elevated with diastolic pressure at or slightly above the 95th percentile for age.
- Symptoms of hypertension include headache, nausea, vomiting, dizziness and irritability.
- Hypertension crisis and hypertensive encephalopathy in severe cases include convulsions, altered sensorium, visual disturbances, persistent vomiting, cranial nerve palsies and other neurological deficits.
- Secondary causes of hypertension as in renal causes are polyuria, oedema, decreased urine output, etc.
- Phaeochromocytoma will have palpitation, sweating and flushing.
- Cushing syndrome is characterized by obesity, buffalo hump, hirsutism and abdominal striae.

Classification

Hypertensive retinopathy is divided into following four grades:
- Grade I – Copper-wire appearance of arterioles, which assume the shape of broad yellow lines.
- Grade II – Thickened arterioles without a visible blood column hip vein.
- Grade III – Haemorrhages and exudates as well as considerably narrowed arterioles, with a diameter which is only one-fourth of that of veins and appear as broad white silver lines. Blood column is not visible. Dilatation of vein distal to the artery is apparent.
- Grade IV – Papilloedema on top of the changes seen in grade III retinopathy.

Multidisciplinary Management

- Proper recording of BP.
- Several recordings are important before labelling a child to be suffering from hypertension.
- Urine analysis – It is the most important screening test and should be done in all cases.

Nursing Diagnoses

- Altered cardiopulmonary, cerebral and renal tissue perfusions
- Pain
- Sensory perceptual alterations

Nursing Interventions

- Monitor BP and mean arterial pressure (MAP) every 1–5 (q1–5) minutes during titration of medications; as the condition stabilizes, q15–1h when oral medications begin to affect BP, wean nitroprusside and other potent antihypertensive to prevent hypotensive episodes. Continuous monitoring by arterial cannulation or automatic BP apparatus is recommended.
- Correlate cuff pressure with direct arterial pressure.
- Determine ideal range for BP control and maximal nitroprusside dose with the paediatrician.
- If hypotension develops, decrease or stop medications and inform the paediatrician.
- Assess for decreased renal perfusion by monitoring I&O and weighing the child twice daily. Also alert to azotaemia ($\uparrow$ BUN) $\downarrow$ creatinine clearance and $\uparrow$ serum creatinine.
- Assess for neurological deficit every hourly. Be alert to sensorimotor deficit if MAP > 130 mm Hg. As condition stabilizes, perform neurological assessment at least 4 hourly.

- Monitor for headache pain, rating discomfort using Age appropriate Pain Assessment Tool (APAT) or any other pain scales.
- Provide pain medications, as prescribed.
- Assess for effectiveness of pain medications.
- Maintain a quiet environment with minimum distractions.
- Assess for ↓ visual acuity by monitoring ability to read and recognize objects or people or use a hand-held Snellen chart. Evaluate coordination of movement to determine depth perception.
- If the child has decreased visual acuity, assist with activities of daily living.
- Reassure the child and parents.
- Involve parents in the care and clarify their queries to relieve anxiety.

Kawasaki Disease

Kawasaki disease (KD) is an acute inflammation of systemic blood vessels (systemic vasculitis) of unknown aetiology. It is the second most common vasculitic disorder of childhood. It is also known as mucocutaneous lymph node syndrome. It is one of the leading causes of heart diseases in children and can affect coronary arteries that supply blood to the heart.

Aetiology and Incidence

The exact aetiology of KD is unknown but thought to be a reaction of the immune system. KD is mainly seen in spring and early winter. It usually affects children younger than 5 years (80%–90%) and older than 6 months. In total, 20% of cases may lead to cardiac complications. Peak incidence is seen in children aged 1–2 years and is less common in children older than 8 years. It is noncommunicable in nature. Children who receive proper treatment recover without sequelae. KD is not preventable. Boys are affected 1.5 times more than girls. It is mostly seen in children of Asian origin.

One hypothesis is that KD is caused by a ubiquitous infectious agent that cause symptoms in certain genetically predisposed individuals (Asians). It is rare in the first few months of life (it will not be developed in the first six months of age) It is rare in adults. So adults are immune to KD and very young infants are protected by passive maternal antibodies. The genetic basis of susceptibility is still unknown.

Pathology

KD is a generalized systemic vasculitis involving blood vessels throughout the body with definite involvement of coronary arteries. Aneurysms may occur along with coronary arteries in other extraparenchymal muscular arteries such as the celiac, mesenteric, femoral, iliac, renal, axillary and brachial arteries. The affected blood vessels show oedematous dissociation of the smooth muscle cells. Swelling of the endothelial cells and subendothelial oedema are seen, with no change in internal elastic lamina. An influx of neutrophils is found in the early stages (7–9 days after onset), with a rapid transition to large mononuclear cells in concert with lymphocytes (predominantly CD8+ T cells) and IgA plasma cells. Eventual destruction of the internal elastic lamina with fibroblastic proliferation occurs at this stage. Active inflammation is replaced over several weeks to months by progressive fibrosis, with scar formation.

Pathological findings in lymph nodes include thrombotic arteriolitis and severe lymphadenitis with necrosis.

Clinical Features/Signs and Symptoms

The condition causes inflammation of the blood vessels and the symptoms can be severe. The specific symptoms are high temperatures that last more than 5 days, along with:

- Rash all over the body but more severe in the diaper area
- Red, bloodshot eyes without any pus, drainage or crusting
- Tender, swollen gland (lymph node) on one side of the neck
- Swollen hands and feet with redness on palms of the hands and soles of the feet
- Very red, swollen and cracked lips; strawberry-coloured tongue with rough, red spots
- Significant irritability and fussiness
- Effect on the function of the heart muscle or the heart valves, but with early treatment the child will recover without long-term complications
- Peeling fingers and toes (typically 2–3 weeks after the beginning of fever)

Risk factors:

There are three important risk factors:

- **Age.** Children younger than 5 years are most at risk of acquiring KD.
- **Sex.** Boys are slightly more likely than girls to develop KD.
- **Ethnicity.** Children of Asian or Pacific Island descent, such as Japanese or Korean, have higher rates of KD.
- KD is one of the leading causes of acquired heart disease in children.

Diagnosis

There is no specific single test to diagnose KD. If KD is suspected, cardiac monitoring with ECG, Echo, in addition to blood workup and urine analysis, is essential. The child may require a specialist consultation for rheumatology and cardiology for treatment assistance.

- **Urine tests** helps rule out other diseases.
- **Blood tests:** White blood cell (WBC) count will be elevated and there will be anaemia and inflammation. Presence of B-type natriuretic peptide (BNP), which is released when the heart is under stress, will be helpful in diagnosing KD.
- **Electrocardiogram shows rhythm changes.**
- **Echocardiogram** helps identify coronary artery abnormalities, if present.

KD must be differentiated from:

- Scarlet fever, which is caused by streptococcal bacteria and results in fever, rash, chills and sore throat
- Juvenile rheumatoid arthritis

- Stevens–Johnson syndrome, a disorder of the mucous membranes
- Toxic shock syndrome
- Measles
- Certain tick-borne illnesses, such as Rocky Mountain spotted fever
  Clinical criteria for diagnosis of KD include fever for 4 days or more, nonvesicular rash or nonpurulent conjunctivitis plus four of the following five criteria:
  Conjunctivitis
  Lymphadenopathy
  Rash (nonvesicular)
  Changes of lips or oral mucosa (red cracked lips, strawberry-coloured tongue)
  Changes of extremities (erythema, oedema, peeling of skin)

Complications

If not treated, it can lead to inflammation of the blood vessels. This situation is very dangerous as it affects coronary arteries. Aneurysms can also develop. But if treatment is initiated within 10 days, these dangers will not occur.

Heart complications include:
- Inflammation of blood vessels (vasculitis), usually the coronary arteries, that supply blood to the heart
- Inflammation of the heart muscle (myocarditis)
Heart valve problems

Multidisciplinary Management

- Admission to hospital is required for at least 24 hours till the dose of γ-globulin is completed.
- Administration of *intravenous γ-globulin* (IVIG). IVIG is given through an intravenous catheter as a single dose over 8–12 hours to lower the risk of coronary artery problems. Usual dose is 2 g/kg in a single dose. In **resistant cases**, the dose may be repeated. In infants and children with **fragile cardiac status**, the infusion may be divided to prevent cardiac compromise from the IVIG fluid volume.
- Administer high doses of aspirin to lower inflammation of heart muscles and to reduce joint pain and inflammation. It must be administered under supervision. Dosage: In **acute phase**, aspirin 30–50 mg/kg per day is advised and may be given up to 100 mg/kg per day. In **subacute phase**, aspirin may be decreased to 2–5 mg/kg per day and continued depending on results of cardiac Echo.
- Administration of steroids if inflammation does not subside. Sometimes, infliximab or etanercept is recommended.
- Once the fever goes down, lower the dose of aspirin. It may be given for at least 6 weeks and longer if the child develops a coronary artery aneurysm with its antiplatelet activity for preventing clotting.
- If the child develop flu-like symptoms or chicken pox, aspirin need to be stopped as it may lead to Reye syndrome, which can affect the blood, liver and brain after a viral infection.
- Monitor the child for heart symptoms regularly for quite some time.

Nursing Assessment

History/phase of illness (children tend to be very irritable during the course of KD)

The course of disease can be classified into three phases for providing excellent nursing care.

Acute Phase (lasts 7–14 days). This phase is characterized by the following symptoms:
- Progressive inflammation of small blood vessels (vasculitis)
- High fever
- Inflammation of the pharynx
- Conjunctivitis
- Rash
- Lethargic, irritable
- Strawberry-coloured tongue
- Red, cracked lips
- Swollen, reddened joints
- Hepatic dysfunction
- Aseptic meningitis
- Lymphadenopathy (Note: As internal lymph nodes swell, children may develop abdominal pain, anorexia, and diarrhoea)

Subacute Phase (10–24 days). In subacute phase, children manifest the following symptoms:
- Inflammation of larger vessels
- Thrombocytosis and hypercoagulability
- Aneurysms may develop, which may lead to sudden death from accumulating thrombi or rupture of the aneurysm
- Fever, rash and lymphadenopathy resolve
- Irritability, anorexia and conjunctivitis persist
- Desquamation (shedding of the epidermis) of palms and soles
- Arthralgia (pain in joints)
- Arthritis

Convalescent Phase (25–40 days)
Clinical signs of KD resolve in this phase.
- Laboratory results return to normal, usually 6–8 weeks from onset.
- Follow up with cardiology is important to monitor for new and/or resolving cardiac complications.
Other assessment parameters are as follows:
- Asses comfort.
- Assess for increased levels of anxiety (possibly as a result of cardiac complications or pain).
Neurological assessment includes:
- Neurological status per unit routine
- Extreme irritability or seizure activity as the child may develop aseptic meningitis
Respiratory status assessment includes:
- Assessment of respiratory distress (may be related to coronary abnormalities: CHF, coronary artery thrombosis, myocarditis, pericarditis, cardiogenic shock)
- Assessment for chest pain, type, location and severity

- Chest X rays to assess lung fields and cardiac silhouette
- Tachypnoea
- Nasal flaring
- Retractions
- Grunting
- Decreased oxygen saturations
- Diminished or abnormal breath sounds

Cardiovascular status assessment

- Provide continuous ECG monitoring while in bed.
- Assess and report chest pain.
- Observe and monitor and record V/S unit routine and clinical status of the patient.
- Assess perfusion.
- Check peripheral pulses.
- Monitor capillary refill.
- Monitor skin temperature, temperature line of demarcation.
- Check colour.
- Monitor urine output.
- Assess for cardiac arrhythmias, abnormal heart sounds as a result of coronary aneurysm, myocarditis, pericarditis, mitral regurgitation, etc.
- Assess for decreased ventricular function and valvular insufficiency.

Monitor laboratory values as ordered.
Integumentary system
Assess skin for signs and symptoms of rash and skin integrity.
Assess mouth for sores and fissures.
Assess eyes for conjunctivitis.
Renal
Assess for signs and symptoms of urethritis.
Maintain strict I&O per unit routine.
Daily weight
Gastrointestinal
Assess in every shift for abdominal pain, diarrhoea and vomiting.

Nursing Diagnoses

Comfort alteration related to pain/conjunctivitis/rash/swollen joints and extremities
Alteration in temperature (fever) related to disease process/vasculitis

Nursing Interventions

Decrease external stimulation (i.e. lights and noise) for extreme irritability.
Use nonpharmacological interventions to promote comfort to joints and swollen extremities:
Provide warm environment.
Apply warm compresses to joints.
Provide adequate hydration/mouth care.
Provide supportive positioning.
Provide distraction and apply relaxation techniques.
Maintain oxygen saturations ≥95%.
Administer O_2 as needed (prn) with chest pain, as ordered.
Prepare for and administer IVIG and aspirin treatment as ordered.

Perform ECG with any cardiac symptoms (e.g. abdominal/chest pain or onset of CHF).
Arrange cardiology consultation for the child.
Provide education on good personal hygiene for comfort and to promote skin integrity.
Provide skin care with lotions to alleviate itching that may occur with rash.
Provide mouth care at 2- to 4-hour intervals.
Ensure adequate hydration.
Strict I&O monitoring.
Take daily weight.
Administer medications, as prescribed.
Monitor for aspirin toxicity (tinnitus, headache, dizziness, confusion, etc.).
Administer Coumadin or heparin as ordered for treatment of severe coronary findings.
Apply soothing ointments to lips and provide gentle mouth care.
Provide soft, nonirritating foods as tolerated.
Provide cool liquids to maintain hydration and reduce mouth tenderness.

Outcomes: The child is free of fever, normal Echo and normal vital signs.
Family teaching
Instruct parents the need for follow-up, as well as the importance of looking for cardiac complications.

STUDY QUESTIONS

- What are the consequences of abnormal embryonic development of the cardiovascular system?
- What are the common acyanotic heart diseases?
- What is ASD? Describe its clinical features.
- What are the focus anomalies seen in tetralogy of Fallot?
- What is VSD? Describe haemodynamics in VSD.
- What are the common features seen in a child with congenital heart disease?
- What is rheumatic fever? Describe its clinical features.
- Describe the role of a nurse in preparing a child and his/her family for an open heart surgery that requires cardiopulmonary bypass.
- Describe the postoperative management of a child after tetralogy of Fallot repair.
- Explain the care of a child with congestive heart failure.
- What is Kawasaki disorder? How will you take care of a child with Kawasaki disorder?
- What are the nurse's responsibilities in the following situations:
    a. A 5-year-old child receiving digoxin
    b. A child with cyanotic spells
    c. A baby receiving potassium chloride and Lasix
    d. A baby with cyanotic heart disease receiving oxygen
    e. Discharge planning of a school-aged child with rheumatic fever
    f. A baby receiving antihypertensive for systematic hypertension

BIBLIOGRAPHY

1. Baas, L.S., Steuble, B.T. (1995). Cardiovascular Dysfunctions. In: Swearingen, P.L., Keen, J.H. (Editors): Manual of Critical Care Nursing, 3rd Edn. St. Louis. Elsevier.
2. Barron KS. (1998). Kawasaki disease in children. *Current Opinion In Rheumatology*, 10:29-37.
3. Belkengren R and Sapala S. (1997). Pediatric management problems. Kawasaki Disease. *Pediatric Nursing*, 23(4):404-405.
4. Brogan PA, Bose A, Burgner D, Shingadia D, Tulloh R, Michie C, Klein N, Booy R, Levin M, Dilon MJ. (2002). Kawasaki disease: an evidence based approach to diagnosis, treatment, and proposals for future research. *Arch Dis Child*. 86, 286-290.
5. Castaneda AR, Freed MD, Williams RG, & Norwood WI. (1977). Repair of tetralogy of Fallot in infancy: early and late results. *J Thorac Cardiovasc Surg*, 74:372–381.
6. Dracup, K., Dunbar, S.B., Baker, D.W. (1995). Rethinking Heart Failure, American Journal of Nursing, 95(7), pp 22–28.
7. Hazinski, M. (1984). Nursing care of the critically ill child. St. Louis. Mosby.
8. Hazinski, M. (1992). Nursing care of the critically ill child. 2nd edn. St. Louis, Mosby.
9. Jaffe, M. (1998). *Pediatric nursing, care plans*, (2nd edition). Englewood, Co: Skidmore-Roth.
10. Pahl E. (1997). Kawasaki disease: cardiac sequelae and management. Pediatric Annals, 26(2):112-115.
11. Norwood, W. I., Jr. Hypoplastic left heart syndrome. *Ann Thorac Surg*, 1991;52(3):688–695.
12. Payling, J. (1997). Kawasaki disease. *Professional Nurse*, 13(2): 108-109.
13. Pillitteri, A. (1995). *Maternal and Child Health Nursing: Care of the Childbearing and Childrearing Family*. (2nd ed). Philadelphia, PA: Lippincott.
14. Polacek TL and others (1992). Effect of positioning on arterial oxygenation in children with atelectasis following heart surgery. Heart Lung. 21(5): 457-462.
15. Pratt, N.G. (1995). Pathophysiology of Heart Failure. Critical Care in Nursing, Q18(1), pp 22–31.
16. Park M.K. (1996). Paediatric cardiology for practitioners. 3rd edn. St. Louis. Mosby.
17. Rubin B and Cotton DM. (1998). Kawasaki disease: a dangerous acute childhood illness. *Nurse Practitioner*, 23(2):34, 37-38, 44-48.
18. Shulman S, DeInocencio J, and Hirsch, R. (1995). Kawasaki Disease. *Pediatric Rheumatology*. 42(5):1205-1222.
19. Takahashi M. (1997). Kawasaki disease. *Current Opinion in Pediatrics*, 9(5):523-529.
20. Wright, J.M. (1995). Pharmacologic Management of Congestive Heart Failure. Critical Care in Nursing, Q18(1), pp 32–44.
21. Wacchter, E.H. Phillips J and Holaday, B. (1985). Nursing care of children. J. B. Lippincott, Philadelphia.
22. Waecher, E and Blake, R. (1976). Nursing of children. Lippincott. Philadelphia.
23. Whaley, L.F and Wong, D.L. (1991). Nursing care of infants and children. 4th edn. C.V. Mosby, St. Louis.
24. Wong, D.L and Wilson David. (1995). Whaley and Wong's Nursing care of Infants and children. 5th edn. C.V. Mosby, St. Louis.

ALTERATION IN GENITOURINARY FUNCTIONS

LEARNING OBJECTIVES

At the end of the chapter, the learner will be able to:

- Identify the essential concepts related to embryonic development of the genitourinary system.
- Discuss the consequences of abnormal embryonic development.
- Describe the nursing management of the common medical and surgical problems affecting genitourinary functions in children using the nursing process.

EMBRYOLOGY

Renal system development can be traced through three successive bilateral excretory systems in the embryo. These are the pronephros, the mesonephros and the metanephros (permanent kidney). These three systems are formed from the nephrogenic cord which is derived from mesoderm. Formation of pronephros begins around the end of the third week after conception, and approximately seven pronephric tubules are formed. These tubules degenerate as the mesonephric or metanephric tubules are formed. But one tubule is retained as a part of the mesonephros. Mesonephros develops in the middle of the fourth week after conception in a position caudal to the pronephros. Each mesonephric tubules has a glomerular structure and proximal and distal tubules.

Mesonephros is capable of urine formation unlike pronephros, which is nonfunctional in mammals.

In females, the mesonephric tubules begin to regress during the third month of gestation. In males, the mesonephric tubules remain and further develop to form parts of the male reproductive system (including vas deferens, epididymis and ejaculatory ducts).

The metanephros begins to appear 2 weeks after formation of the mesonephros. The meta-nephritic kidney is located in the pelvis and ascent to the abdominal cavity by the seventh to ninth weeks after conception. The metanephros is formed from the two different embryonic tissues. The excretory portion – collecting ducts, calyces, pelvis and ureter – develops ureteric bud. The metanephric blastema gives rise to Bowman's capsule, most of the glomerulus and the tubules of the nephrons. The collecting ducts and the tubules then make connections forming a functional system by 12–16 weeks. Nephron formation begins during the eighth week of gestation. At birth, a human kidney contains approximately 1 million nephrons at different stages of development. Most mature nephrons are seen in the medulla and the immature ones are seen in the cortex. Maturation of the renal system continues after birth, but no new nephrons are formed after birth.

Kidney development begins during the first few weeks of gestation but is not complete until the end of the first year of life. Glomerular filtration rate (GFR) at 28 weeks of gestation is only 25% of that of term. During the first 2 weeks of life, GFR doubles, increasing sixfolds from birth to 1 year of age. Infants are unable to excrete a water load at the same rate as older children and adults; GFR and absorption do not reach adult capabilities until the age of 1–2 years. Newborns are more prone to developing acidosis. Sodium excretion is also reduced during infancy and less adapted to sodium deficiency and excess.

The nephron (functioning unit) comprising glomeruli which filter water and solute from blood and tubules reabsorb the needed salts (water, protein, electrolyte, glucose and amino acids) and allow waste products to leave the body in urine. The functional kidney maintains body fluid volume and composition by responding appropriately to alteration in the internal environment caused by variations in dietary intake and external losses of water and solute. Secretion of hormone (erythropoietic stimulating factor – ESF), which stimulates production of red blood cells, and rennin, which stimulates production of angiotensin causing arteriolar construction and blood pressure elevation and aldosterone. Urine is formed in the nephron, which then passes into the renal pelvis through the ureter into the bladder and out of the body through the urethra. GFR in suspected renal failure can be rough estimate of GFR that can be obtained using the following formula:

$K \times$ length in (cm) ÷ serum creatinine in mg/dL = GFR in mL/min/1.73 m², where K is a constant. The value of K varies depending on the age of the child. It is 0.55 in children older than 2 years and is 0.33–0.45 in children younger than 2 years.

Relation between Specific Gravity and Osmolality

They are related but not the same. Normal urine osmolality has a very wide range 50–1200 Osm/kg. If specific gravity is known, we can calculate the approximate urine osmolality. This can be obtained by multiplying the last two digits of specific gravity by 33. If the specific gravity of urine is 1010, then urine osmolality is 10 × 33 = 330 m·Osm/kg. When the urine osmolality (normal 280–290 m·Osm/kg), then the concentration of urine is very high; if it is less than that of plasma, then urine is dilute.

Age-related normal creatinine values are as follows:

0–3 years	0.2
4–7 years	0.4
8–10 years	0.6
11–13 years	0.8

values increases by 0.2 every 3 years

CONSEQUENCES OF ABNORMAL DEVELOPMENT

It is not easy to pinpoint specifically the abnormal renal development because there is much overlapping of each stages.

Fetal Age in Weeks	Structure Formed	Anomalies at Birth
3–4 weeks	Pronephros	Renal agenesis
	Mesonephros	Patters syndrome
5 weeks	Beginning of metanephros	Renal agenesis

Fetal Age in Weeks	Structure Formed	Anomalies at Birth
8–9 weeks	Pelvis and ureter development	Posterior urethral valves
	Some functioning nephrons	Multicystic kidneys
		Dysplastic kidneys
20–22 weeks	Clearly demarcated medulla and cortex	Renal hypoplasia
		Polycystic disease
	One-third of nephrons formed	Medullary cystic disease

NURSING MANAGEMENT OF COMMON MEDICAL–SURGICAL PROBLEMS AFFECTING GENITOURINARY FUNCTIONS IN CHILDREN

Urinary Tract Infection in Children

Urinary tract infections (UTIs) are the most common infections faced by children. Infants have blood-borne UTIs, but urethral problems develop in older children. Girls have more frequent UTIs because of short urethras. The antibacterial properties of the prostate secretions also help prevent UTIs in boys. Most common agent is *Escherichia coli*. Symptoms of pain and bleeding in UTI are from irritation and inflammation of the urinary mucosa by bacteria.

If the infection is not treated by antibiotics early, backflow of urine through ureters to kidney (vesicourethral reflux [VUR]) causes infection and damage to renal parenchyma.

ACUTE GLOMERULONEPHRITIS

It is a self-limiting autoimmune disease that usually occurs as sequelae to group A beta haemolytic streptococcal infection (pharyngitis or impetigo) and is called post-streptococcal glomerulonephritis (PSGN).

Aetiology and Incidence

- Precipitating streptococcal infection (throat or skin)
- Commonly seen in children staying in hostels or after-care homes
- Primarily affects children of 5–12 years of age
- Incidence in boys is double that in girls
- Vasculitis, Henoch–Schönlein purpura (HSP), systemic lupus erythematosus (SLE), IgA nephropathy, polyarthritis nodosa

Pathophysiology

Onset commonly occurs within 7–14 days after the antecedent infection. After the streptococcal infection, there is release of membrane-like substance from the specific organism which is antigenic in nature. Antibody forms in response and an immune complex reaction occurs. Immune complex lodge in glomeruli, leading to inflammation and obstruction; subsequent decreased glomerulus filtration and tissue injury results in excretion of red blood cells (RBCs) and casts. Kidney gets enlarged and sodium and water retention occur leading to oedema. Protein is secreted in urine, and most children recover completely and some may experience chronic infection. The common complications are hypertensive encephalopathy, pulmonary oedema and acute renal failure (ARF).

Clinical Features/Assessment Findings

- Decreased urine output
- Hypertension
- Oedema – Periorbital
- Haematuria – Resembling tea-coloured urine
- Oliguria
- Weight gain
- Pallor
- Irritability and fatigue

Diagnostic Tests

- Complete blood studies – mild anaemia and leucocytosis, increased ESR
- Serum electrolytes, blood urea nitrogen (BUN) and serum creatinine
- Antistreptolysin O titre will be positive, indicating a recent streptococcal infection
- Renal biopsy

Multidisciplinary Management

- Administration of antibiotics, specifically penicillin
- Intravenous diazoxide and furosemide (Lasix) to treat severe hypertension
- Methyldopa or hydralazine along with reserpine or Lasix to treat hypertension
- Diuretic therapy such as hydrochlorothiazide or Lasix for treating severe oedema

Nursing Diagnoses

- Activity intolerance
- Nutrition alterations
- High risk for complications
- Fluid volume excess

Nursing Interventions

- Provide bed rest by providing quiet ambulatory play.
- Reassure parents.
- Administer medications as prescribed to control hypertension.
- Monitor blood pressure (BP) at regular intervals.
- Maintain adequate caloric intake and good nutrition by planning meals around the child's dietary preferences and serving meals in a pleasant atmosphere.
- Restrict sodium, potassium and fluid intake.
- Support the child and parents.
  Provide patient and family education – Follow-up, need for medical evaluation and culture of throat swab, home care measures, antibiotic prophylaxis for secondary prevention of bacterial endocarditis and renal damage, and watch for complications such as renal failure, chronic nephritis.

NEPHROTIC SYNDROME

It is a symptom complex characterized by increased glomerular permeability resulting in massive plasma protein loss via urine, leading to oedema, hypoalbuminaemia and hypercholesterolaemia. Nephritic syndrome occurs in two of 100,000 children per year and mainly seen in preschool children, with most common age being 1½–3 years. The prognosis of the condition shows that one-third of cases resolve directly, one-third of cases experience infrequent relapse and the other one-third have frequent relapse and are mainly steroid dependent.

Aetiology

- Congenital nephrotic syndrome is caused by a recessive gene.
- Secondary damage to glomeruli in conditions such as HSP, SLE, infections or allergens (e.g. bee sting), drug toxicity or chronic renal failure (CRF).
- Minimal change nephrotic syndrome (MCN) is idiopathic but often follows a nonspecific viral illness.

Clinical Features/Assessment Findings

- Periorbital oedema
- Scrotal, leg, and ankle oedema
- Ascites
- Breathlessness as a result of pleural effusions and abdominal distension
- Weight gain
- Anorexia and diarrhoea secondary to oedema of the intestinal mucosa
- Massive proteinuria
- Oliguria
- Pallor, irritability, fatigue and lethargy
- Increased susceptibility to infection

Pathophysiology

Disturbance in the glomerular basement membrane leads to increased glomerulus permeability to protein, resulting in leaking of protein through urine, especially albumin. This causes hypoalbuminaemia. Hypoalbuminaemia produces low colloid osmotic pressure in capillaries, leading to fluid shift to accumulate in interstitial spaces and body cavities, particularly in the abdomen, producing ascites. Massive fluid shift leads to hypovolaemia, which stimulates the rennin–angiotensin system to increase secretion of antidiuretic hormone (ADH) and aldosterone leading to sodium and water retention, causing oedema.

Investigations

- Urine protein
- Full blood count

- Serum electrolytes, urea, creatinine, albumin, complement – C3, C4
- Antistreptolysin O titre and throat swab culture
- Urine microscopy, protein, culture, urinary sodium concentration

Multidisciplinary Management

- Corticosteroid therapy
- Cytoxan (cyclophosphamide) for steroid resistant cases
- Diuretics (thiazides, otherwise spironolactone can be used with thiazides)
- Intravenous albumin
- Paracentesis for ascites
- Protein-rich diet

Nursing Diagnoses

- Fluid volume excess
- Disturbance in body image and self-concept
- Impaired skin integrity
- Ineffective breathing pattern

Nursing Interventions

- Perform detailed nursing assessment that includes nutritional assessment, weight, skin (oedema, breakdown), respiratory function, hydration, abdominal girth and urinalysis.
- Provide small frequent meals with increased protein.
- Assist in administration of plasma protein (intravenous albumin).
- Observe the intravenous site carefully for phlebitis.
- Administer corticosteroid as prescribed to resolve proteinuria (prednisolone at a dose of 2 mg/kg per day – average time for urine to be protein free is 10 days; after 4 weeks, the dose is reduced and given on alternate days).
- Administer cyclophosphamide as prescribed for steroid-resistant cases.
- Monitor side effects of steroids and cyclophosphamide (Cytoxan) (common features of steroid-resistant cases are age between 1 and 10 years; no macroscopic haematuria, normal complement levels; normal renal function).
- Administer spironolactone in combination with hydrochlorothiazide to treat severe oedema.
- Monitor intake and output (I&O).
- Monitor the effects of prescribed fluid and sodium limits.
- Monitor oedema by taking weight (weigh the child daily at a specific time).
- Examine urine for protein every 4 hourly and for specific gravity.
- Measure abdominal girth daily.
- Prevent skin breakdown by checking areas of oedema for skin breakdown, ensuring frequent position changes, using scrotal support in boys and good skin hygiene.
- Follow meticulous aseptic practices to prevent infection as they are susceptible to infection as a result of hypoproteinaemia and immunosuppressant therapy.

- Monitor vital signs and report alterations.
- Observe for signs of infection, especially opportunistic infections.
- Provide bed rest to conserve energy.
- Monitor for complications.
- Help improve the child's self-concept by providing positive feedback, emphasizing the strength.
- Support the family.
- Provide child and family education – Signs and symptoms of relapse to watch, urine testing, special dietary instructions, medication schedule and dosages, administration technique and special precautions, infection prevention, skin care, side effects of drug therapy and complications of the disease such as hypovolaemia, thrombosis (hypercoagulable state owing to losses of antithrombin, increased synthesis of clotting factors and increased blood viscosity from increased haematocrit).

ACUTE NEPHRITIC SYNDROME

Acute nephritic syndrome is a group of disorders that cause inflammation of the internal kidney structures (particularly the glomeruli) and is often caused by an immune response triggered by an infection or other disease.

Aetiology

The main causes in children and adolescents include:
- IgA nephropathy
- HSP
- Haemolytic uremic syndrome (HUS)
- PSGN

Other associated disease conditions include:
- SLE
- Infective endocarditis
- Vasculitis
- *Klebsiella* pneumonia
- Typhoid fever
- Hepatitis
- Measles, mumps, infectious mononucleosis
- Syphilis etc.

Pathophysiology

Inflammation of the glomeruli affects the function of the glomeruli in filtration and excretion. The inadequate functioning will lead to protein and RBC leaks to urine and accumulation of excess fluid in the body secondary to hypoproteinaemia. There will be high blood pressure and interstitial inflammation.

Clinical Features

- Blood in urine
- Decreased urine output
- Facial oedema, especially periorbital oedema
- Oedema on dependent parts of the body
- General body pain
- Headache and blurred vision

Late symptoms include the following:
- Convulsions
- Nausea and vomiting
- Cough
- Difficulty in breathing

Nursing Diagnoses

- Activity intolerance
- Alteration in cardiac output
- Alteration in nutrition less than body requirement
- Alteration in family process

Multidisciplinary Management

A large number of laboratory tests are required to differentiate it from glomerular nephritis, especially PSGN. It includes blood urea, creatinine, kidney biopsy, serum potassium, culture of throat swab, blood culture, Anti Nuclear Antibody (ANA), ANCA (antineutrophil cytoplasmic antibody for vasculitis), antiglomerular basement membrane antibody, etc.; hospitalization is required with strict bed rest. The aim of the treatment is to reduce glomerular inflammation. The diet restrictions include restriction of salt, fluids and potassium. Medications given are antihypertensive, corticosteroids and some other anti-inflammatory drugs to control inflammation. Other treatment options are according to the cause and symptoms.

Children have better prognosis and may recover completely. Adults often do not recover completely. Usually, the condition cannot be prevented, though treatment of illness and infection may help reduce the risk. Nursing management is somewhat similar to that for acute glomerulonephritis, as the nursing diagnoses and interventions seem to be similar.

ACUTE RENAL FAILURE

It is sudden and potentially reversible loss of kidney function.

Aetiology

It can be considered under the following three headings:
1. Prerenal causes (outside kidney)
   - Loss blood and body fluids
   - Circulatory inadequacy
   - Peripheral vasodilatation
2. Renal causes (damage to kidney)
   - Renal diseases
   - Tubular dysfunction
   - Vascular occlusion
   - Hypoxia
3. Postrenal causes (urinary tract obstructions)
   - Stones or crystals
   - Strictures
   - Tumours

Assessment

- Serum electrolyte (especially potassium) and BUN
- Weight

- Urine (volume, specific gravity)
- Vital signs (volume BP)

Multidisciplinary Management

- ARF can be prevented by adequate hydration of children at risk and cautious use of nephrotoxic drugs.
- Initiate fluid replacement.
- Perform Foley catheter drainage.
- Administer total parenteral nutrition (TPN), as necessary.
- Perform electrocardiographic monitoring.
- Reduce serum potassium.
- Administer calcium gluconate, sodium bicarbonate and Kayexalate (sodium polystyrene sulphate), phosphate binders (e.g. Amphojel [aluminium hydroxide]).
- Perform dialysis.

Nursing Diagnoses

- Activity intolerance
- Alteration in cardiac output
- Alteration in nutrition, less than body requirement
- Alteration in the family process

Nursing Interventions

- Monitor I&O, hourly heart rate and indications for electrolyte imbalances and peripheral oedema.
- Monitor weight daily.
- Provide education to the child and parent on the importance of eating limited amount of high-quality protein (e.g. egg, meat and milk).
- Decrease the child's tissue catabolism by decreasing stress (thermal, emotional).
- Provide low potassium foods and fluids (e.g. apple, banana, canned foods and refined cereals).
  Evaluation: The child gradually regains normal renal function as evidenced by stable weight, lack of oedema, and normal BUN and creatinine levels. The child and family can list the food items that need to be avoided and permitted in the child's diet (those with essential amino acids and low potassium).

CHRONIC RENAL FAILURE

It is a progressive, irreversible deterioration of kidney function over a prolonged time period in which more than 50% of nephrons have been destroyed. This results in fatal uraemia without dialysis or kidney transplant.

Now renal transplant has become a common therapeutic intervention for the treatment of **CRF**. Selection criteria for transplant in children are fairly liberal. Young children usually have the graft placed in their abdomen. In older children, it is placed in the extraperitoneal space. The child's own kidneys are usually left in place. Rejection of the transplanted kidney is the major complication. There are three types of rejection.

Hyperacute – It occurs immediately owing to an antibody antigen reaction and is reversible.

Acute – It occurs in the first few days through the first 6 months and usually responds to administration of Solu Medrol.

Chronic – occurs after the first 6 months but is an irreversible process.

Aetiology

- Urinary obstruction
- Congenital renal and urinary tract malformations (renal hypoplasia and dysplasia)
- Glomerular diseases Acute Glomerular Nephritis (AGN), Systemic Lupus Erythromatosis (SLE)
- Hereditary disorders (Alport syndrome, polycystic kidneys, congenital nephrotic syndrome)
- Renal and vascular disorders
- Metabolic diseases
- Nephrotoxic chemicals

Assessment Findings/Clinical Features

- Oedema
- Decreased urine output
- Altered level of consciousness
- Altered cardiac function
- Blood gas monitoring
- Nutritional status
- Loss of consciousness (LOC)
- I&O
- Vital signs
- Renal function
- Skin
- Serum electrolytes, especially BUN and creatinine
- Weight checking

Nursing Interventions

- Monitor diet – Restrict food high in phosphate (e.g. milk products), protein, sodium (e.g. crackers, sodas, instant cereals, smoked fish and meat) and potassium (e.g. nuts, bananas, orange, apple).
- Monitor the child for indications of impending seizures – BP, serum electrolyte imbalance and LOC.
- Regulate fluids as per amount prescribed.
- Monitor signs of cardiac compensation (e.g. tachycardia and shift of Point of Maximum Intensity (PMI)).

Evaluation: Maintain a normal fluid balance as evidenced by normal BUN and creatinine levels, stable weight, normal urine output (1 mL/kg per hour), no oedema, normal LOC, normal vital signs and normal serum electrolyte values.

Dialysis

It is used as a treatment option when renal function has been impaired, e.g. ARF and CRF.

Dialysis is the movement of fluid across a semipermeable membrane, resulting in the separation of molecules by osmosis, diffusion or ultra-filtration.

Osmosis is the passive movement of fluid from an area of low concentration to one of higher concentration.

Diffusion is the random movement from areas of greater concentration of substances to areas of lesser concentration.

Ultra-filtration – is the movement of fluid under pressure through a filtering medium with very small pores.

There are two types of dialysis, e.g. peritoneal and haemodialysis.

Peritoneal dialysis – Filtration of blood by the use of a dialysate administered through the abdominal cavity. The peritoneal membrane serves as the semipermeable membrane across which water and solutes move. This type of dialysis is used frequently for ARF or other acute conditions such as severe metabolic acidosis, accidental poisoning, intractable heart failure and hepatic coma.

Continuous ambulatory peritoneal dialysis (CAPD) can be performed in the homes of some children with CRF. Dialysate is introduced into the peritoneal cavity through a catheter that has been permanently sutured in place. The dialysate remains in the peritoneum for 4–6 hours. This makes children relatively active at home.

Haemodialysis is the filtration of blood across a dialyzer through an artificially constructed arteriovenous (AV) fistula or shunt or through a graft.

HAEMOLYTICA UREMIC SYNDROME

It is triad of ARF, microangiopathic haemolytic anaemia and thrombocytopenia. It is the most common renal cause of ARF in children.

Types

- Typical: Following a diarrhoeal infection
- Atypical: Because of other causes such as certain medications, genetic mutation, systemic infections, etc.

Pathophysiology

HUS typically occurs secondary to gastrointestinal infection with verocytotoxin producing *E. coli* or *Shigella*. It follows a prodrome of bloody diarrhoea. HUS develops from the activation of neutrophils which damage vascular endothelium of kidneys. Platelet count is reduced, but the clotting is normal. Brain, pancreas and heart may also be involved. Familial HUS has no prodromal diarrhoea.

Clinical Features

- Fever
- Lethargy
- Irritability
- Vomiting
- Blood in stool
- Later may develop oliguria, which progresses to anuria
- Bruising, petechiae
- Pallor
- Rarely develops seizures

Multidisciplinary Management

Diagnosis: Complete blood cell count; peripheral smear shows schistocytes, elevated blood urea and creatinine levels, CRP

Stool culture to identify organism

Monitoring of vital signs, especially blood pressure, neurological status, oedema

Fluid therapy

Dialysis

Packed red blood cell (PRBC) and platelet transfusion

Management of hypertension with antihypertensive

Nutritional support

Nursing Management

Nursing management is similar to that of ARF.

ENURESIS

It can be daytime enuresis or nocturnal enuresis. In daytime enuresis, the child will have lack of bladder control during the day. The child will be old enough to be continent as per age.

The common causes are as follows:

- Detrusor instability
- Bladder neck weakness
- Neurogenic bladder
- UTI
- Constipation
- An ectopic ureter

Secondary enuresis is the one in which the child has lost previously obtained bladder control. The common causes are emotional upset, UTI, polyuria from osmotic diuresis in diabetes mellitus, renal concentrating disease, etc. Examples are sickle cell disease or CRF.

Assessment

- Urine must be checked for microscopy examination, culture and sensitivity, glycosuria and proteinuria. Assessment of urinary concentration by measuring the osmolality of an early morning urine sample. These are specifically done for secondary enuresis. For day time enuresis, ultrasonography (USG) to identify bladder anomalies, urodynamic studies – X-ray of spine may reveal a vertebral anomaly. MRI to identify teething of spinal nerve roots.

Management

Management is according to the cause of enuresis and nursing management depends on the type of enuresis and its management.

UNDESCENDED TESTIS (CRYPTORCHIDISM)

Embryology

The testis is formed from the urogenital ridge on the posterior abdominal wall close to the developing kidney.

Gonadal induction to form a testis is regulated by genes on Y chromosomes. During gestation, the testis migrates down towards the inguinal canal guided by mesenchymal tissue known as gubernaculums under the influence of anti-Müllerian hormone.

Inguinoscrotal descent of the testis takes place with the help of testosterone from the fetal testis. The processus vaginalis (an extension of peritoneum) precedes the migrating testis through the inguinal canal and obliterates after birth. Failure of obliteration of the processus vaginalis may lead to inguinal hernia and sometimes hydrocoele.

Definition

In the undescended testis, there is an arrest in the normal descent of the testis. In total, 5% of full-term male infants may have unilateral or bilateral undescended testes. Incidence in preterm infants is higher than that in term babies. There are three varieties.

Retractile – The testis can be manipulated into the bottom of the scrotum without tension but subsequently retracts back to the inguinal canal, pulled up the cremasteric reflux. Follow up is essential to see that there is no problem.

Palpable – The testis can be palpated inside the groin.

Impalpable – No testis can be felt on careful examination and may be intra-abdominal.

Assessment

- USG is used to identify inguinal testis in obese boys.
- Administration of human chorionic gonadotropin (HCG) and serum testosterone response are monitored.
- Laparoscopy is used to identify impalpable testis.

Management

Surgical placement of testis in the scrotum (orchidopexy) is done for various reasons.

Fertility – Testes need to be in the scrotum below body temperature to optimize spermatogenesis. Timing is controversial. Preferred time is the second year of life. Fertility after orchidopexy for the unilateral undescended testis is close to normal. But bilateral undescended testes (impalpable) are usually sterile. The risk of malignancy is very high if the undescended testis is not treated surgically, especially in the intra-abdominal testis. Surgery is also advised for cosmetic and psychological reasons.

Orchidopexy is done via inguinal incision. Testis is mobilized by preserving the vas deferens and testicular vessels; the associated patent processus vaginalis is ligated and divided, and the testis is placed inside the scrotum. Orchidopexy in the intra-abdominal testis is done to reduce the risk of developing malignancy.

Nursing Management

Provide psychological support. Surgery is usually done as a day case; after the surgery, the child is observed for side effects of anaesthesia and is discharged by evening.

HYPOSPADIAS

Definition/Description

In the male fetus, tabularization occurs in the proximal-to-distal direction under the influence of fetal testosterone. Failure to complete this process leaves the urethral opening proximal to the normal meatus on the glans. This abnormality is called hypospadias.

It consists of the following:

- A ventral urethral meatus – In most cases, the urethra opens on or adjacent to the glans penis, but in severe cases, the opening may be on the penile shaft or in the perineum.
- A hooded dorsal foreskin – The foreskin has failed to fuse ventrally.
- Chordee – A ventral curvature of the shaft of penis owing to the presence of fibrous band of tissue most apparent on erection and is associated with a severe form of hypospadias.

Various types of hypospadias are as follows:

- Glandular – May be of cosmetic concern
- Coronal
- Anterior penile
- Mid-shaft
- Posterior penile
- Penoscrotal – All these may cause major functional problems
- Scrotal
- Perineal
- Additional genitourinary anomalies may be present that need to be excluded.

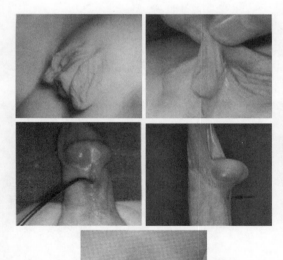

Signs and Symptoms

- Dribbling of urine – the stream
- Improper and painful excretion owing to chordee

Diagnosis

- Prenatal USG
- Physical examination at birth
- Urethroscopy and cystoscopy
- Excretory urogram

Management

Surgery is usually done before 2 years of age to prevent possible psychological problems in preschool children. Aim of management includes a terminal urethral meatus so that the boy can stand and micturate, straight erection and normal looking penis.

Preoperative hormonal stimulation performed with HCG and testosterone administration.

Common surgical procedures performed are meatal advancement glanuloplasty (MAGPI), tubularized incised urethral plate repair (TIP), etc.

Nursing Management

- Before surgery, nurses need to manage anxiety of parents with proper explanation regarding diagnosis, usual treatment options, prognosis and need for not doing circumcision.
- Postoperative care:
  Management of pain: Assess location, characteristics and intensity.
  Change position.
  Provide diversional therapy.
  Administer analgesics.
  Maintain skin integrity: protect incision.
  Monitor urinary elimination.
  Maintain strict I&O chart.
  Note the colour of urine
  Provide parental education regarding care of the site and monitoring of stream of urine.

EPISPADIASIS

A congenital malformation in which urethra opens into the dorsum of the penis in boys. Generally, girls are not affected. It is a rare condition.

Aetiology

Exact aetiology is unknown. Commonly related to development of the pubic bone and also associated with bladder extrophy.

Clinical Features

- Males:
  - Urethra opens on the dorsal aspect
  - Short wide penis
  - Abnormal curvature
- Female:
  - Opening is usually between clitoris and labia
  - Sometimes abnormal clitoris and labia

- Other common features are:
- Urinary incontinence
- UTI
- Retrograde flow of urine

Types

- Glanular
- Penile
- Penopubic

Multidisciplinary Management

Diagnosis: Physical examination
    To identify associated anomalies – intravenous pyelography (IVP), MRI, CT pelvic X-rays, USG of urinary system and genitals.
Surgery:
    Males: Modified Cantwell–Ransley technique
    Mitchell technique
    Females: Genital reconstruction

Nursing Management

- Assist in the identification of defects.
- Prevent potential complications.
- Promote parental understanding and attachment.
- Promote normal voiding pattern.
- Postoperatively – Manage pain, keep the area clean, assess for postsurgical complications and enable the parents.
- Discharge advise should include care of the area, dressing, activity restriction and monitoring of signs and symptoms of complication.

ECTOPIA VESICA (EXSTROPHY BLADDER)

It is the commonest of the exstrophic lesions that arise in the hind end of the embryo. Other exstrophic anomalies are epispadias, superior vesical fissure and covered exstrophy and cloacal exstrophy (vesicointestinal fissure). There is diastasis of the pubic bones. The extent of diastasis is proportional to the severity of the visceral lesion, as the two halves of the pelvis are separated anteriorly, the acetabula with the femoral heads are rotated externally.

Incidence

Incidence rate is one in 10,000 live births, and the male to female ratio is 2.3:1. Epispadias and cloacal exstrophy are extremely rare. Usually, siblings are also affected including those of different sexes.

Embryology

It is because of the failure of primitive streak mesoderm to invade the allantoic extension of the cloacal membrane (infraumbilical membrane). This results in the ectoderm and endoderm to remain in contact with the developing abdominal wall, without intervening the mesoderm. This produces an unstable state that results into disintegration of the cloacal membrane leading the pelvic viscera to be laid open onto the surface of the abdomen. The abdominal musculature derived from an ingrowth of thoracic somite mesoderm is normal on each side of the ventral defect. The abnormally extensive cloacal membrane produces a wedge effect holding apart the developing structure resulting in the deficiency of the abdominal wall, the pubic diastasis and, in severe cases, exomphalos. Double phallus or duplication of the female genital tract results from the same effect, causing failure of fusion of the originally paired genital tubercles or of the Müllerian ducts.

The type of defects depends upon the extent of the allantoic expansion of the cloacal membrane and upon the stage of embryonic development when the membrane dehisces. Vesical exstrophy with epispadias results from breakdown of an extensive membrane after completion of the urorectal septum at about the 16-mm stage so that the primitive urogenital sinus is exteriorized. Epispadias results without exstrophy bladder from the less extensive cloacal membrane that is limited to pubic area. If the cranial portion of the cloacal membrane (infraumbilical membrane) is not invaded by the mesoderm, it leads to superior vesical fissure.

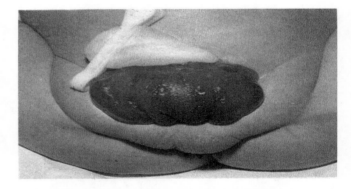

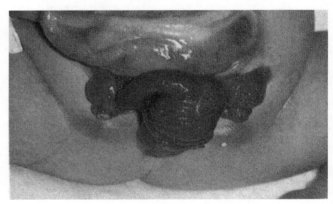

Management

Management includes staged reconstruction with primary closure of the bladder in the neonatal period. Initial operation is not intended to produce a continent bladder. Secondary operation is intended to produce competent bladder neck, enlargement of the bladder or both, which is delayed until the child is older. Neonatal closure is contraindicated in neonates with other anomalies. Small bladder is now treated by way of augmentation or substitution cystoplasty.

Pubic diastasis is treated by pelvic osteotomy to get satisfactory repair and cosmetic effect to the closure of abdominal wall.

Complications of bladder reconstruction include breakdown of the distal urethral repair, secondary changes in the upper renal tract, VUR and renal calculi.

Nursing Interventions

- Educate parents to prevent irritation.
- Provide support to the family by answering questions and providing information about diagnosis, tests and treatments. As appropriate, explain the surgical treatment, its stages and the parents' role in the case of children.
- Provide patients and family education covering measures to help prevent UTIs, such as good perineal hygiene (e.g. cleaning a girl from the urethra back towards the anus), avoid tight-fitting clothing, wearing cotton clothes and maintaining acidic urine by providing apple juice or giving ascorbic acid.
- After surgery, provide pre- and postoperative care. Provide routine postoperative care (dressing change, vital signs).
- Prevent skin excoriation, and use barrier cream.

POSTERIOR URETHRAL VALVE

It is the most common type of obstructive uropathy in male newborns leading to renal failure. Valve exhibits in a wide spectrum of clinical presentations and pathological manifestations that can be detected radiographically and endoscopically. Prenatal USG will help in diagnosing the condition, but few may escape detection and present later in life as voiding dysfunction with urinary urgency and frequency, daytime wetting and enuresis. Three types of valves are seen. Most common one is type I valve. The accentuation of normal folds that emanate from the distal aspect of verumontanum is seen in type I valve. These valves vary in thickness and the extent with which they course in an anterolateral direction. In more severe cases, they diffuse with the opposite valves in the anterior midline and result in a higher degree of outlet obstruction.

Type II valves are very rare and can be seen along with type I valve. Type III valves are diaphragmatic in configuration and arise from the verumontanum or from a more distal direction in the proximal anterior urethra. In some children, a combination of the three types of valve can occur.

Diagnosis

In older infants and children, renal and bladder USG, followed by VCUG, is used as a diagnostic measure. This helps in identifying dilated urethra and abrupt distal narrowing. Bladder may be narrowed and VUR may be present, especially on the left side.

Management

Primary treatment is ablation of the valve or fulguration of the valve which is done by using a cutting electrode with a low current. Placement is done very carefully to avoid damage to verumontanum, external urethral sphincter and normal urethra. If VUR is present, a urethral catheter is placed for complete urethral emptying to assess urethral drainage in the presence of a reflux. Most patients' symptoms improve after relief of urethral obstruction. Renal function of the left kidney is usually decreased. Reflux or urethral obstruction is corrected by reimplantation. Patients with posterior urethral valve (PUV) have long-term problems, and urodynamic studies are indicated in such patients. Some children may suffer from renal failure and need renal transplantation.

Complications are polyuria, infertility, incontinence, inadequate growth and hypertension.

VESICOURETHRAL REFLUX

Retrograde flow of bladder urine occurs up to the ureters during voiding.

Aetiology

Primary VUR results from congenital abnormalities on insertion of ureters into the bladder. Secondary VUR results from infection and ureterovesical junction incompetency related to oedema, neurogenic bladder and progressive dilation of ureters following surgical urinary diversion.

There is a positive history for the development of VUR. The incidence is about 10 times greater in girls than in boys.

Pathophysiology

VUR results when there is pressure of a full bladder that forces urine into the upper urethra and when the pressure is decreased, urine refluxes back to the bladder causing UTI in children. There are different grades of VUR:

Grade I – Reflux only into the lower ureter
Grade II – Ureteral and pelvic filling without calyceal dilation
Grade III – Ureteral and pelvic filling with mild calyceal blunting
Grade IV – Marked distension of pelvis, calyces and ureter
Grade V – Massive reflux associated with severe hydronephrosis. It is an important cause of renal damage as a result of infection brought to the kidney by the ascending urine. Large amount of refluxed urine produces urge to void even shortly after voiding and a small amount of refluxed urine leads to stasis of urine in the bladder to result into calculi.

Assessment Findings/Clinical Features

- Dysuria
- Urinary frequency, urgency and hesitancy
- Urine retention

- Cloudy, dark or blood-tinged urine
- Urinalysis showing RBCs or pus cells.
- Structural abnormalities can be determined on IVP, voiding cystourethrography and cystoscopy

Management

- Administration of continuous low-dose antibiotics, usually nitrofurantoin, trimethoprim or sulfisoxazole
- Correction of structural anomalies

Nursing Diagnoses

- Altered family process
- Potential for infection
- Potential for complications
- Pain
- Knowledge deficit
- Altered patterns of urinary elimination
- Urinary retention

Nursing Interventions

- Administer the prescribed medications and educate parents and the child if possible the precautions to be taken during drug administration.
- Teach a double voiding technique to the understanding of children.
- Provide support to the family by clarifying their doubts and by giving adequate information about the clinical course of the disease.
- Provide pre- and postoperative care, as indicated.
  - Monitor quantity and quality of urine.
  - Observe and protect the drainage tubes from kinking, clogging and ascending infection.
  - Administer drugs as prescribed (analgesics, antibiotics and antispasmodics).
  - Provide routine postoperative care.
  - Provide parental education.
  - Measures to prevent UTIs; keep good perineal hygiene, e.g. cleaning a girl from the urethra back towards the anus, avoiding irritants such as tub baths or swimming in ponds, tight-fitting clothes, wearing cotton underpants, scheduled voiding, preventing overfilling of bladder and taking apple juice or vitamin C to keep urine acidic to prevent growth of bacteria.

SPECIAL PROCEDURE

Bladder Training

Children with neurological, neuromuscular or physical disability need bladder training. At home, the child's individualized pattern of bladder training is given importance. At the hospital, nurses observe this to prevent nosocomial infection. Occasionally, children will be on a Foley catheter but it has risk of infections. Other types of diversion include urostomy and cystostomy. Transurethral emptying is done by the Credè procedure.

- Position the child on back in the bed or on toilet (if developmentally appropriate).
- Check for bladder level; if unable to palpate, begin the Credè procedure below umbilicus.
- Place the hand in semi-fist (fingers flexed to second knuckle but not to palm of the hand) and place the hand on abdomen, pressing toward the spine and downward toward feet; continue to hold pressure while urine is being evacuated.
- Remove the hand and wait for 1 minute.
- Reposition the hand slightly below the initial starting point and repeat the cycle.
- Replace the hand just above the symphysis pubis and repeat this cycle; if a moderate amount of urine is expressed, repeat this cycle.
- Record output.
- Do not perform the Credè procedure on males if they have erection, as they have voided at this time.
- Delay the Credè procedure if the child is crying and the abdomen is tense.

For the child with unimpaired myelomeningocoele:
- Relax for 1 minute after each cycle and repeat the cycle, beginning at the symphysis pubis.
- Repeat the cycle if a large amount of urine is expressed at the level of symphysis pubis.

Intermittent Catheterization

If intermittent catheterization is followed, catheterization schedule will be every 3–4 hours. At night, it can be extended up to 6–8 hours if the child is old enough. Clean procedure can be used at home, but at the hospital, strict aseptic precautions should be followed to prevent nosocomial infection.

A child with urinary surface stoma presents several challenges. If there is no collecting appliance, the problems of ammoniacal dermatitis or *Candida albicans* infections may occur. When a collecting bag is used, breakdown around the stoma site may be a problem. Application of barrier cream such as zinc oxide is essential to prevent skin breakdown.

Kock pouch is a collection reservoir of urine created from a portion of small intestine. Here, two nipple valves are created from portions of the ileum. The ureters are implanted near the inlet nipple valve. The urine leaves the pouch through the outlet nipple valve and stoma. A catheter can be inserted through stoma into the pouch. This is done four to six times a day. (This is a urinary diversion procedure like that of the ileal conduit.)

STUDY QUESTIONS

- What are the consequences of abnormal development of the genitourinary system?
- What is posterior urethral value? What is its surgical management?
- What advice will you provide to mother of a girl baby with ectopia vesica?
- What are the major protocols used in ectopia vesica management?

- Prepare a nursing care plan for a preschooler admitted with nephritic syndrome.
- Differentiate between nephritic syndrome and acute glomerular nephritis.
- Describe the nursing management of a child with post-streptococcal glomerulonephritis.
  a. Haemolytic uraemic syndrome
  b. Cryptorchidism
  c. Hypospadias
  d. Epispadias
  e. CRF
  f. ARF
  g. Peritoneal dialysis
  h. Bladder wash
  i. Bladder training.
  j. Urinary incontinence
  k. Pyelourethroplasty

BIBLIOGRAPHY

1. Edelmann, C.M., Jr. (1988). Urinary Tract Infection and Vesicourethral Reflex. Paediatric Annals, 17, pp 568–582.
2. Foreman, J.W., Chan, J.C.M. (1988). Chronic Renal Failure in Infants and Children. Journal of Paediatrics, 113, pp 793–8000.
3. Gaudio, K.M.; Siegel, N.J. (1987). Pathogenesis And Treatment of Acute Renal Failure. Paediatric Clinics of North America, 34, pp 771–787.
4. Gray, M.L. (1992). Genitourinary Disorders. St. Louis: Mosby.
5. Jordan, S.C., Lemire, J.M. (1982). Acute Glomerulonephritis. Paediatric Clinics of North America, 29, pp 857–873.
6. Haws, R.M., Baum, M. (1988). Efficacy of Albumin And Diuretic Therapy in Children With Nephritic Syndrome. Paediatrics, 91(6), pp 1142–1146.
7. Lerner, G.R., Flesischmann, L.E., Perlmutter, A.D. (1988). Reflex Uropathy. Paediatric Clinics of North America, 34, pp 747–770.
8. McFarland, K. (1988). Paediatric Peritoneal Dialysis. Paediatric Nursing, 14, pp 426–429.
9. Sheldon, C.A.; McLorie, G.A.; Churchill, B.M. (1987). Renal Transplantation in Children. Paediatric Clinics of North America, 34, pp 1209–1232.
10. Seigler, R.L. (1988). Management of Haemolytic Uraemic Syndrome. Journal of Paediatrics, 112, pp 1014–1020.

CHAPTER 32

ALTERATION IN CENTRAL NERVOUS SYSTEM FUNCTION

LEARNING OBJECTIVES

At the end of the chapter, the learner will be able to:

- Describe the essential concepts related to central nervous system development.
- Identify the consequences of abnormal development.
- Describes nursing management of various medical and surgical conditions affecting the central nervous system using the nursing process.

During the third week of embryonic life, the differentiation of the three primitive germ layers – the ectoderm, endoderm and mesoderm layers – occurs. The ectoderm layers give rise to the central nervous system (CNS), consisting of the brain and spinal cord and other structures (e.g. skin).

A cellular rod (notochord) develops during the third week of gestation, defining the primitive axis of the embryo that gives some rigidity. The embryonic ectoderm over the notochord (neuroectoderm) thickens to form the neural plate. At about 18th day, the neural plate invaginates to form the longitudinal neural groove with two adjacent neural folds. The neural folds move together and fuse to form the neural tube by the end of the third week. The fusion of the neural folds begins centrally and expands to form the future brain (rostrally) and the sacral area. The rostral end closes first and the caudal end closes later after 2 days. Cranial two-thirds of the neural tube forms the brain, and the caudal one-third gives rise to spinal cord. The neural tube canal becomes the ventricles of the brain and the central canal of the spinal cord. The process of the development of the

neural tube that forms the neural plate is called neurulation and is completed by the fourth week.

The brain continues to grow and develop after birth. The most of the brain growth takes place during the first year of life. At birth, the brain reaches 25% of its adult weight; by 6 months, it reaches 50%; and by 1 year, it is 90% of the adult size. The brain grows by hyperplasia during the prenatal period, by hyperplasia and hypertrophy from birth to 6 months, and by hypertrophy until puberty. Genetic, environmental and nutritional factors are the major influences on development of the CNS.

Neural tube gets separated from the surface ectoderm as the neural folds fuse. Neuroectoderm cells lying on the crest of each neural fold are collectively called the neural crest that forms a mass between the surface ectoderm and neuroectoderm. The neural crest cells differentiate into the peripheral nervous system, autonomic nervous system, cranial nerves, skeletal nerves and muscular components of the head.

During the fourth week before closure of the caudal and rostral neuropores, three primary brain vesicles begin to appear and later develop as the brain. The most rostral vesicle is the forebrain (proencephalon), the middle one is the midbrain (mesencephalon) and the caudal one is the hindbrain (rhombencephalon). During the fifth week, two of the primary vesicles subdivide to the telencephalon and the diencephalons, and the rhombencephalon develops into the metencephalon and the myencephalon. The mesencephalon does not undergo any change.

During the fourth week, a longitudinal groove called sulcus limitans forms along the lateral surface of the neural tube. This groove subdivides the dorsal part (alar plate) of the spinal cord from the ventral part (basal plate). The alar plate is associated with efferent function.

Failure of closure of the neural tube during the fourth week leads to neural tube defects. Caudal defects lead to the varying degrees of spina bifida. Defective closure of the rostral opening of the neural tube results in anencephaly or exencephaly. Other CNS malformations results from faulty histogenesis of the cerebral cortex, interference with cerebrospinal fluid (CSF) circulation and absorption and defective formation of the cranium.

MYELINATION

In the late fetal period, formation of myelin sheaths in the spinal cord begins and most nerve tracts are not fully functioning until myelination occurs. This process continues throughout the childhood and possibly to the adulthood. Complete myelination of fibre tracts is associated with full function of those tracts.

At birth, myelination of the peripheral nervous system, optic pathways and bulbar structures accounts for crying, sucking and primitive reflexes in the newborn. Myelination occurs in a cephalocaudal direction. As a result, children are able to sit before standing and stand before walking. This is followed by the ability to control bowel and bladder functions. When there is a delay or impairment in myelination, attainment of developmental milestones at anticipated intervals may be negatively affected.

REFLEXES

By the time the fetus reaches 28 weeks, the nervous system is able to control some of the body functions and some weak reflexes are present. This has implications for assessment of the gestational age and viability of preterm infants. At 40 weeks of gestation, the newborn possess numerous vital reflex functions. As the CNS matures, some of these primitive reflexes disappear and actions become intentional.

CONSEQUENCES OF ABNORMAL DEVELOPMENT

A number of CNS anomalies are associated with defects in neural tube closure. A defect in closure with the rostral or cranial end of the neural tube can inhibit development of the brain. When cerebral tissue is missing and remaining brain tissue is exposed because of lack of cranium, the condition is termed as anencephaly. If the defect is in the spinal column, the meninges or the spinal cord may protrude through the vertebral opening, exposing neural tissue. This is called as spina bifida. Hydrocephalus is caused by an abnormal accumulation of CSF. The normal structure and function of the CSF pathway can be affected by an obstruction of flow of CSF in the ventricles often in the aqueduct, impaired absorption of CSF or excessive production of CSF as a result of tumour of villi similar to the choroid plexus.

Arnold–Chiari malformation is a congenital herniation of the cerebellum and medulla through the foramen magnum into the vertebral column. This herniation causes an obstruction in the flow of CSF through the fourth ventricles.

Microcephalus occurs when the brain is small and underdeveloped. In this condition, the forebrain is most affected. Because of genetic or environmental causes, the cranium remains small and the head circumference falls below average because the growth of the cranium is partially caused by the pressure of the growing brain.

Fetal Age in Weeks	Structure Formed	Anomalies
Fourth week of the intra-uterine life	Closure of caudal neuropore	Spina bifida – occulta, meningocoele, meningomyelocoele
fourth week of the intra-uterine life	Closure of rostral neuropore	Cranial meningocoele, anencephaly

NURSING MANAGEMENT OF CHILDREN WITH ALTERATION IN CENTRAL NERVOUS SYSTEM FUNCTION

Head Injury

It is a pathological injury resulting from a mechanical force involving the scalp, skull, meninges or brain.

Aetiology

Brain damage occurs from falls, motor vehicle injuries, bicycle injuries, physical abuse, etc. Boys are twice as often prone to suffer head injury as girls. Young children are involved in head injury as passengers or pedestrians in motor vehicle accidents or as cyclists.

Infants left unattended on beds, high chairs and other places may fall. The head is proportionally large for infants and toddlers and is heavy compared with other parts of the body. It is most likely to be injured. Incomplete motor development contributes to falls at young ages, and natural curiosity and exuberance of children increase their risk of a head injury.

Pathophysiology

- Head injury is directly related to the force of impact. Intracranial contents (brain, blood, CSF) are damaged because the force is too great to be absorbed by the skull and musculoligamentous support of the head.
- The skull of infants and young children is pliable and absorbs much of the direct energy of physical impact to the head and offers protection to intracranial structures. Though nervous tissue is delicate, it requires a severe blow to cause significant damage.
- The larger head size and insufficient musculoskeletal support render the very young child particularly vulnerable to acceleration and deceleration injuries.
- The surface area of the child's scalp is large with remarkable vascularity; therefore, the child can bleed to death from a severe scalp laceration.
- Common head injuries are skull fractures, contusions, intracranial haematomas and diffuse injuries.

- Complications are hypoxic brain damage, increased intracranial pressure (ICP), infection and cerebral oedema.
- Hypoxia and hypercapnia threaten the energy requirements of brain and increase cerebral blood–brain barrier, plus the loss of autoregulation exacerbates cerebral oedema.
- Pressure inside the skull is greater than the arterial pressure which results in inadequate perfusion.
- Infants and young children tolerate increased ICP better than older children and adults (ability to expand and their skull is more compliant).

Impact of head injury produces acceleration or deceleration/deformation. Acceleration usually occurs when a stationary head receives a blow and causes deformation of the skull and mass movement of the brain. Continued movements of the intracranial contents allow the brain to strike parts of the skull or edges of the tentorium. Brain changes shape in response to the force of impact to the skull. This movement can cause bruising at the point of impact (coup) or at a distance as the brain collides with the unyielding surfaces far removed from the point of impact (counter-coup); e.g. an injury to the occipital bone/region can cause a severe injury to frontal or temporal areas of the brain.

Acceleration/deceleration – Children with an acceleration/deceleration injury demonstrate diffuse generalized cerebral swelling produced by increased blood volume or redistribution of cerebral blood volume (cerebral hyperaemia) rather than by increased water content (oedema) as seen in adults.

Brain movement or shearing stresses may tear small arteries and cause subdural haemorrhage. Severe compression of the skull causes the brain to be forced through tentorial opening.

Concussion – It is a transient and reversible neuronal dysfunction with instantaneous loss of awareness and responsiveness that results from trauma to the head and persists for a relatively short time, usually minutes or hours. It is generally followed by amnesia for the moment of the injury. Concussions are traumatically induced alteration in the mental status. Confusion and amnesia following head injury are the hallmarks of concussion.

Contusion and laceration – These are used to describe visible bruising injury and tearing of the cerebral tissue. Contusions represent petechial haemorrhages along the superficial aspects of the brain at the site of impact. Major areas susceptible to contusions or lacerations are the occipital, frontal and temporal lobes. Irregular surfaces of the anterior and middle fossae at the base of the skull are capable of producing bruises or lacerations on a forceful impact.

Fractures – There are mainly five types of fractures:
1. Linear fractures – These are those fractures in which the lines of the fracture are predetermined by the site and velocity of the impact as well as strength of the bone. It is the most common type of fractures. It presents with swelling or tenderness. Usually, they heal spontaneously. Management is treating the underlying cause, haemorrhage and brain injury.
2. Depressed fractures – Usually, the bone is locally broken into several irregular fragments that are pushed inward and a tear in the dura is seen. It is uncommon in children younger than 3 years because of soft, malleable skull bones.
3. Compound fractures – These consist of lacerations to skin that extend to the site of bony fracture which can be linear, depressed or comminuted. It requires immediate surgical intervention. These concern damage to the underlying tissue, especially depression >5 mm of the thickness of the skull.
4. Basilar fractures – These involve basilar portion of the frontal, ethmoid, sphenoid, temporal or occipital bone. Proximity to the brainstem produces seriousness. These are most common in children younger than 4 years and the cause is seizable blunt trauma. No specific treatment is available. Monitoring for epidural haemorrhage is advised.
5. Diastatic fractures – There involve traumatic separations of cranial sutures, mostly at the lambdoid suture. These are most common in children younger than years and the cause is seizable blunt trauma.

For any type of head injury, antibiotics and tetanus prophylaxis are advocated.

Complications

- Haemorrhage
- Infection
- Oedema
- Herniation.
- Subdural haemorrhage
- Cerebral oedema
- Posttraumatic meningitis should be suspected in children with increased drowsiness and fever.
- Subdural haematoma and retinal haemorrhage are seen in children with shaken baby syndrome and hence need to be assessed for child abuse.

Diagnostic Evaluation

A detailed health history, both past and present, needs to be taken to differentiate craniocerebral trauma from drug allergies, haemophilia, diabetes mellitus and epilepsy.

Initial assessment includes assessment of airway, breathing, circulation (ABC), evaluation of shock, a neurological examination, especially level of consciousness (LOC), pupillary symmetry and response to light and sound and seizures.

Look for signs of increased ICP:
- Deep, rapid, periodic or intermittent and grasping respirations, wide fluctuations or noticeable slowing or fluctuations in blood pressure (BP) are signs of brainstem injury.
- Ocular signs such as fixed and dilated pupils, fixed and constricted pupils and pupils that are poorly reactive to light and accommodation indicate increased ICP.
- Observation of asymmetric pupils or one dilated unreactive pupil in a comatose child is neurological emergency.

- Bleeding nose and ears need future evaluation.
- Watery discharge from nostrils needs to be evaluated for CSF rhinorrhoea.

Clinical indications for radiological studies in paediatric head injuries are as follows:

- Altered LOC
- Seizures
- Focal neurological deficits
- Depressed skull fractures
- Compound skull fractures
- Progressive worsening
- Full fontanel

Special Tests

- Computed tomographic (CT) scan
- Magnetic resonance imaging (MRI)

Diagnosis

Diagnosis involves preclinical signs.

- Raccoon eyes (periorbital bruising)
- Haemotympanum, cranial nerve palsies, battle sign
- Bloody rhinorrhoea and CSF rhinorrhoea
- Neurobehavioural assessment and assessment of posttraumatic syndrome

Emergency Management

- Assess the child's ABC.
- Stabilize neck and spine.
- Clean abrasion with soap and water.
- Apply clean dressing.
- Apply ice at the site of severe bleeding for an hour to relieve pain and swelling.
- If there is no vomiting, clear fluids can be given.
- Check pupillary reaction every 4 hours for the first 48 hours.
- Awaken the child during the night to check LOC.
- Seek medical help for any untoward symptom.
- Manage increased ICP by head-end elevation and administer osmotic diuretics (mannitol).
- Provide seizure prophylaxis.

Surgical therapy is needed for lacerations, depressed fractures, haematoma, etc.

Nursing Management

- Perform careful neurological assessment including vital signs and epiphenomena.
- Watch for increased ICP and LOC.
- Provide bed rest with adequate safety measures.
- Observe for complications such as bleeding from ear, nose and CSF rhinorrhoea.
- Apply no suctioning through nares or nasogastric tubes because there is a high risk of infection and probability of the tube entering the brain substances through the fracture.
- Provide family support.
- Provide rehabilitation.
- Provide prevention through education of parents and children.

Intracranial Pressure Monitoring

Indications

- Glasgow Coma Scale (GCS) score less than 7
- GCS score below 8 with respiratory assistance
- Deterioration of condition
- Subjective judgement regarding clinical appearance

Four Major ICP Monitors

- Intraventricular catheter with fibroscopic sensor attached to a monitoring system
- Subarachnoid bolt (Richmond screw)
- Epidural sensor
- Anterior fontanel pressure monitor

Catheter Method

Introduction of a catheter into the lateral ventricles or placed into the subdural space. Catheter use permits drainage of CSF to decrease the pressure.

Bolt Method

The end of the bolt is placed into the subarachnoid space. The bolt cannot be adequately secured in a small child's pliant skull, although special modification has been developed for children younger than 6 years. The bolt should be adjusted by the neurosurgeon alone.

Epidural Sensor

It is placed between the dura and the skull through a bur hole and connected to a stopcock. ICP measurement from the anterior fontanel is noninvasive but may prove to be accurate.

Nursing Intervention

- Apply proper and prompt suctioning as indicated.
- Maintain proper nutrition and hydration.
- Administer medications as prescribed.
- Maintain body temperature (thermoregulation).
- Meet the elimination needs and prevent constipation.
- Maintain skin hygiene.
- Provide passive and range-of-motion (ROM) exercises.
- Give adequate stimulation.
- Provide family support.

SEIZURES

A seizure is an excessive, disorderly discharge of electrical impulses by neuronal tissue causing sudden, transient alteration in CNS function. It characteristically consists of transient involuntary alterations in consciousness or abnormalities in motor activity, behaviour, sensation or autonomic function. Epilepsy traditionally refers to recurrent seizure activities but has fallen out of common usage for more acceptable seizure disorder. Most of the childhood seizure tendencies do not persist into the adulthood may be because of the brain's increasing functional maturity with age.

Aetiology

- Simple febrile seizures
- Traumatic head injury
- Nontraumatic increased ICP
- CNS infection, congenital disorders and tumours of the brain
- Ingestion of toxins or exposure
- Anoxia
- Fluid–electrolyte imbalances
- Metabolic disorders
- Idiopathic epilepsy

Risk Factors of Paediatric Seizures

- Neurological/developmental abnormality before seizure
- Initial febrile seizure is focal/multiple or greater than 15 minutes.
- History of nonfebrile seizure in one or both parents.

Classification

Correct classification of seizure activity is essential for correct management of the disorder.

Generalized seizures arise from neuronal hypersynchronized discharges from groups of cerebral neurons in both hemispheres.

- *Partial*: Local focus of abnormal electrical discharge, usually in the cerebral cortex.
  It includes simple partial and complex partial types.
- *Generalized*: Multifocal arising in the reticular formation and involving both hemispheres of the brain. Types include tonic–clonic (grand mal), absence (petit mal), atonic, akinetic and myoclonic (including infant myoclonic seizures).
- *Status epilepticus*: Continuation of grand mal seizures with no recovery period or regaining of consciousness between attacks; a medical emergency.

Multidisciplinary Management

Emergency management of seizures:
- Administer oxygen.
- Put intravenous line.
- Start anticonvulsant therapy (refer ABCs of paediatric emergencies).
- Intubate if the condition worsens.

Nursing Diagnoses

- High risk for injury/complications
- Ineffective airway clearance
- Altered parenting
- Ineffective coping
- Altered self-concept
- Impaired social interaction
- Alteration in bowel elimination: incontinence

Nursing Intervention

- Ensure a patent airway:
  - Position on the side, if possible, for airway protection.
  - Prepare suction, if necessary.
  - Insert oropharyngeal airway, if possible, but avoid placing potentially occlusive objects into the mouth (padded tongue blade).
- Provide supplemental oxygen.
- Protect from physical injury:
  - Do not restrain.
  - Remove the child from the immediately dangerous environment.
  - Loosen restrictive clothing.
- Maintain continuous monitoring during seizure and postictal phase:
  - Observe for seizure activity.
  - Examine the mental status.
  - Monitor vital signs.
  - Watch injuries secondary to seizure.
- Prepare to administer anticonvulsant drugs as prescribed
  - -Prepare to start intravenous line
  - Determine accurate paediatric doses of anticonvulsants (see the Appendix)
  - Administer anticonvulsants as prescribed.
- Provide parental support.
- Help the child and family to cope with difficulties to prevent social isolation.

Febrile Seizure Characteristics

- Seizures usually occur between 3 months and 6 years of age.
- Seizures are associated with acute fever of less than 24 hours of duration.
- There is no history of neurological problems or nonfebrile seizures.
- There is no evidence of intracranial injury or CNS disease.
- The seizures are usually nonfocal in nature.
- The seizures activity is typically less than 15 minutes of duration.
- A positive family history is present but negative for nonfebrile seizures.

MENINGITIS

Meningitis is the inflammation of the meninges caused by the invasion of microorganisms. There are many causative agents responsible for the development of meningitis in children. These are as follows:
- Bacterial
- Viral
- Protozoa

Organisms responsible for bacterial meningitis are as follows:

Neonate–3 months	Group B *Streptococcus*
	Escherichia coli and other coliforms
	Listeria monocytegenes
1 month–6 years	*Neisseria meningitidis*
	Streptococcus pneumoniae
	Haemophilus influenzae
>6 years	*Neisseria meningitidis*
	Streptococcus pneumoniae

Pathophysiology

Bacterial infection of meninges follows bacteraemia from the foci of infection anywhere in the body. Damage from meningeal infection results from the host response to infection and not from the organism itself. The release of inflammatory mediators and activated leucocytes together with the endothelial damage leads to cerebral oedema, increased ICP and decreased cerebral flow.

Signs and Symptoms

The child will present with a history of fever, headache, photophobia, lethargy, irritability, poor feeding, vomiting, hypotonia, drowsiness, loss of consciousness and seizures. On examination, the child will have neck rigidity associated with Brudzinski's sign (flexion of the neck with the child in the supine position causes flexion of the knees and hips). This may not be seen in all children. Other signs include Kernig's sign (with the child in the supine position and with the hips and knees flexed, there is back pain on extension of the knee), signs of shock, focal neurological signs, altered LOC and papilloedema.

Diagnosis

- Full blood cell count and differential count
- Blood glucose
- Coagulation studies
- Lumbar puncture (LP) for CSF studies
- CSF and blood cultures and biochemical analysis
- Culture of urine, stool and throat swabs for bacteria and viruses

Difference in CSF Findings in Bacterial and Viral Meningitis

Bacterial meningitis – CSF is cloudy in appearance, with decreased glucose level, markedly increased protein level and a slightly increased or normal lymphocyte count.

Viral meningitis – Clear CSF, normal glucose level, slightly increased or normal protein level and a markedly increased lymphocyte count.

Contraindications for Lumbar Puncture

- Cardiorespiratory instability
- Focal neurological signs
- Signs of increased ICP (coma, increased BP, decreased heart rate and papilloedema)
- Coagulopathy
- Thrombocytopenia
- Local infection at the site of LP

Multidisciplinary Management

- Administration of appropriate antibiotics (third-generation cephalosporins)
- Supportive therapy – antipyretics, anticonvulsants
- Dexamethasone to reduce cerebral oedema and long-term complications

Common Types of Meningitis

Meningococcal Meningitis

Neisseria meningitidis is the causative agent for meningococcal meningitis. Incidence is increased over last 5 years. It remains as endemic and leads to large outbreaks. It is a disease that strikes fear into the public, parents, doctors and other health care professionals as a result of its virulent nature, as it can kill previously healthy children within hours. Meningococcal septicaemia carries a worse prognosis but has the lowest risk of long-term sequelae among bacterial meningitis. Septicaemia is accompanied by purpuric rash that may arise anywhere on the body and then spreads. The rash is irregular in size and outline, with a necrotic centre. The extensive rash is called purpura fulminans. Any child who develops fever and purpuric rash needs to be treated immediately with antibiotics.

Vaccination is available for groups A and C but not for group B.

Haemophilus influenzae type B is the second most common meningitis seen. Vaccination against *H. influenzae* has reduced the risk of this infection in Western countries, but still it is a problem in countries such as India.

Pneumococcal Meningitis

About 10% of meningitis in Kerala is caused by pneumococci. In total, 30% of survivors suffer from neurological impairments.

Partially Treated Meningitis

It is also a problem usually faced by paediatric practitioners. It is owing to the fact that children with febrile illness in early stages may be treated with antibiotics without recognizing the exact aetiology and diagnosis. This results in difficulty for proper diagnosis and treatment.

Tuberculous Meningitis

It is caused by *Mycobacterium tuberculosis*. It usually results as a secondary infection or may have a positive contact with patients with tuberculosis (TB).

Diagnosis is confirmed by positive Mantoux test, abnormal chest X-rays and acid-fast bacilli that may be identified by Ziehl–Neelsen or auramine staining of CSF.

Treatment is by administration of three to four antituberculous drugs for 2 months (rifampicin, pyrazinamide, isoniazid ± amikacin or streptomycin). Total treatment duration is 1 year. Dexamethasone is given to reduce cerebral oedema and long-term sequelae.

Viral Meningitis

Two-thirds of all meningitis is caused by viruses. The common viruses are as follows:
- Epstein–Barr virus
- Adenovirus
- Mumps virus
- Enterovirus

The course of the disease is less severe than bacterial meningitis and can be identified by polymerase chain reaction (PCR) of CSF or culture of CSF, stool, urine and throat swab and serology.

Common Complications

- Hearing loss – Inflammatory damage to the cochlear hair cells may lead to deafness, especially after pneumococcal meningitis. Audio logical follow-up is indicated in such cases.
- Local vasculitis – This may lead to cranial nerve palsies.
- Local cerebral infraction – It may cause focal or multi-focal seizures that lead to epilepsy.
- Subdural effusion – It is common with *H. influenzae* and pneumococcal meningitis.
- Hydrocephalus – It may result from impaired resorption of CSF. A ventriculoperitoneal (VP) shunt may be required.
- Cerebral abscess – It can be seen as space-occupying lesions.

Nursing Diagnosis

- High risk for injury
- Ineffective airway clearance
- Altered thermoregulation
- Complication potential
- Altered family process

Nursing Interventions

- Provide care of seizure (see the nursing intervention of patients with seizure).
- Administer antibiotics and antiviral agents.
- Provide adequate rest and a calm and quite environment.
- Provide protection from injury.
- Follow universal precautions in caring the patient.
- Provide parental support.
- Monitor for complications, such as hydrocephalus, mastoiditis, brain abscess, focal neurological problems, etc.

ENCEPHALITIS

Encephalitis is an infection of the CNS mainly brain tissue. The major causative agent is virus. The best example for this is the Japanese encephalitis outbreak of Gorakhpur, Uttar Pradesh, in India in the year 2017. This disease causes strong lymphocytic infiltration in brain tissue and leptomeninges leading to cerebral oedema, brain ganglion cell degeneration and destruction of nerve cells diffusion (Anania P C, 2008). Encephalitis is an inflammation of the brain tissue that can be caused by bacteria, worms, protozoa, fungi or viruses.

The common viruses that cause encephalitis are herpes simplex virus, enteroviruses and measles, mumps, rubella and chickenpox viruses.

The signs and symptoms of encephalitis are same even if the causative agents are different.

Clinical Features

- Sudden rise of temperature
- Severe headache
- Sensitivity to light (photophobia)
- Stiffness of neck
- Seizures
- Skin rashes
- Loss of consciousness
- Difficulty in walking
- Paresis
- Nausea and vomiting

Diagnosis

Diagnosing encephalitis is difficult. The definitive diagnosis is by brain biopsy, which is very hard to do. So, usually a spinal tap to obtain CSF and a CSF study is conducted to find out the organism.

A detailed history is very important, and the clinical features are helpful in diagnosing the condition.

Multidisciplinary management
- Treatment is supportive and symptomatic
- The child may require ventilator support
- Treatment to reduce cerebral oedema, oxygen administration to maintain SpO_2 and SaO_2.
- Antibiotics/antiviral agents to treat infections
- Care of the child against hyperthermia

Nursing Interventions

This is essentially as that for children with meningitis.

Assess and monitor the child for LOC, monitor vitals and connect the child to cardiac monitors.

Give intravenous fluid as prescribed.

Meet the basic needs and activities of daily living (ADL).

Prevention of encephalitis is very important. Certain encephalitides such as Japanese encephalitis are transmitted through mosquito bites. So prevention against mosquito bites is very important. Advise children to wear long sleeve shirts, long pants and socks while outside, use bug spray and avoid areas of stagnated and dirty water as a preventive measure against breeding of mosquitoes. Instruct parents to wear light-coloured dresses as dark colours attract mosquitoes.

DISORDERS OF HEAD

Normal head is symmetrical at birth. Depending on the racial and familial characteristics, there is considerable variation in the general form. The size and shape of head may be altered by abnormality of the cranium or intracranial structures.

Abnormalities of Shape

1. *Cephalohaematoma*: An eccentric swelling over a part of the head as a result of subperiosteal haematoma resulting from birth trauma.
2. *Craniosynostosis*: A condition in which there is premature fusion (synostosis) of some or all of the cranial

sutures. Development of the skull is restricted in the region of fusion and compensatory growth occurs at the region of fusion and the remaining suture lines. If untreated, it will lead to severe cosmetic defect and mental retardation and optic atrophy as a result of raised ICP. In some cases, facial skeleton is also affected, producing craniofacial defect, e.g. Crouzon syndrome. Common defects are sagittal, coronal and metopic synostoses (metopic sutures help produce a broad and rounded forehead). When fusion of all sutures takes place, a tall or tower skull results, which is called oxycephaly or turricephaly.

Treatment is early surgical intervention with multiple craniectomies to restore the normal shape.

Abnormalities of Size

Hydrocephalus (Water in the Head)

It is a condition in which an increased volume of CSF is present in an enlarged ventricular system under pressure. The normal range of CSF volume in the intracranial and intraspinal space varies from 30 mL in infants to 150 mL in adults. The resting ventricular pressure is 80–100 cm of water. It is estimated that 200–300 mL of CSF is formed every day.

Aetiology and Incidence. In normal circumstances, there is a dynamic equilibrium between the amount of CSF produced and the amount absorbed. If there is overproduction or decreased absorption, this equilibrium is disturbed. In most cases, there is a pathological obstruction at some point on the pathway of CSF circulation to produce an obstruction in CSF absorption. Depending on the site of obstruction, hydrocephalus may be:

- Noncommunicating – The obstruction is somewhere in the ventricular system or the blockage occurs from the ventricular system to the subarachnoid space. So, the dilated ventricles do not communicate with the subarachnoid space.
- Communicating – The CSF can circulate unobstructed through the ventricular system and the subarachnoid space, which itself is the site of obstruction.

Obstructive factors are of three types:

- Congenital hydrocephalus– It is seen early in infancy. Common abnormalities are aqueductal stenosis, Arnold–Chiari malformations and Dandy–Walker syndrome.
- Acquired hydrocephalus – If pyogenic meningitis is not treated adequately, it leads to hydrocephalus. It is common in developing countries such as India, especially after tubercular meningitis. Head trauma at birth or later may lead to subdural haematoma producing CSF obstruction, which also causes hydrocephalus. Hydrocephalus can also develop as a complication after repair of spina bifida.
- Neoplasms – 3%–4% of cases are secondary to intracranial tumours, especially arising from the cranial fossa and pineal area.

The incidence of congenital hydrocephalus is one in 2000 live births, and the anomaly occurs at approximately the sixth week of gestation.

Pathophysiology. Production and circulation of CSF are necessary to understand the exact mechanism of the development of hydrocephalus. The two mechanisms by which CSF is formed include secretion by the choroid plexus and the lymphatic-like drainage by the extracellular fluid of the brain. CSF circulates throughout the ventricular system and then is absorbed within the subarachnoid space (entire mechanism is not clearly known).

CSF from the lateral ventricle flows to the third ventricle through the foramen of Monro, where it combines with the fluid secreted by the third ventricle. From there, CSF flows to the fourth ventricle through the aqueduct of Sylvius. The fourth ventricle produces more fluid. From the fourth ventricle, the fluid flows to lateral ventricle by way of the foramen of Luschka and the middle foramen of Magendie into the cisterna magna. From cisterna magna, the fluid passes to the subarachnoid space of the cerebrum and cerebellum. A large amount of fluid is absorbed here by arachnoid villi. The sinuses, veins, brain substances and dura mater also absorb some amount of fluid.

Although hydrocephalus develops from varied causes, the mechanism by which it develops results either from impaired absorption within the subarachnoid space (communicating hydrocephalus) or from obstruction to the flow of CSF through the ventricular system (noncommunicating hydrocephalus). Rarely, it can also develop from tumours of choroid plexus that cause increased production of CSF. Any imbalance between the production and absorption of CSF causes an increased accumulation of CSF in the ventricles. This accumulation results in enlargement of the ventricles, and it compresses the brain substances against the rigid bony wall of the cranium. When this occurs before the fusion of cranial sutures, it provides enlargement of the skull and dilation of the ventricles. Even previously closed suture lines may get opened (especially sagittal suture) in children younger than 10–12 years.

Noncommunicating hydrocephalus results from developmental malformations. This includes Arnold–Chiari malformation, aqueduct stenosis and gliosis, atresia of the foramen of Luschka and the foramen of Magendie.

Clinical Manifestations
- Head circumference greater than the 90th percentile for gestation
- Enlarged or full fontanels
- Wide or split suture lines
- Setting sun eyes
- Excessive rate of head growth
- Impaired extraocular movement
- Hypertonia of the lower extremities
- Generalized hyperreflexia
- Vomiting

Diagnosis
- X-ray of the skull with anteroposterior and lateral views to confirm sutural separation
- CT scan – Nature and severity of ventricular dilation
- MRI
- Ultrasound test
- Plotting of the head circumference

- Subdural or interventricular tap for culture and sensitivity
- Cerebral angiography

Multidisciplinary Management. Whatever may be the cause, treatment remains the same for all types of hydrocephalus. Ventriculoatrial (VA) or VP shunt is performed to divert the flow of CSF to one of the body cavity as atrium of the heart or peritoneal cavity.

Conservative Management
- Administration of glycerol and acetazolamide or other diuretics
- Anticonvulsants
- Intravenous antibiotics

N.B.: VP or VA shunt is placed to decrease the ICP by diverting CSF around the point of obstruction. The procedure consists of drilling a burr hole, inserting a ventricular catheter into the lateral ventricle and bringing the tubing through the skull to the subcutaneous space of the scalp where a right angle is made. The catheter is then connected to a selected valve and placed subcutaneously into the abdominal cavity or right atrium (through a vein) where CSF drains. VP shunts are the procedure of choice for infants and young children; VA shunts are used most frequently in older children and adults.

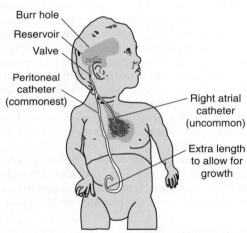

Positioning of Catheter in VP and VA Shunts.

Some shunts are equipped with flushing valves that can aid in assessing function and patency of both proximal and distal ends of the drainage system. Flushing devices work under the principle that CSF within the chamber can be forced out only if the distal catheter is patent and will refill only if the proximal catheter is patent. Once CSF drainage is stabilized, the child may be placed on and off shunt schedule. This prevents slit-like ventricles from forming and promotes normal head configuration.

Ventriculostomy. This procedure involves placement of a catheter via a burr hole in the skull and into the lateral ventricle; the catheter is attached to an external drainage system placed as an alternative to standard shunt placement and as a medication route to reduce ICP.

Nursing Diagnoses
- Ineffective thermoregulation related to hypothalamic injury or compression
- Impaired cerebral tissue integrity or risk for the same
- Impaired gas exchanges
- Alteration in the family process
- Potential/high risk for injury
- Decreased adaptive capacity related to damage of the brain
- Fluid volume excess related to imbalance between CSF production and absorption

Nursing Interventions
- Provide immediate preoperative care.
- Provide extra support of the neonate's head and neck while providing care and performing procedures.
- Maintain neck in the neutral position to prevent flexion and lateral movements that can significantly increase ICP. Stabilize the neck with towels or sand bags.
- Change head position frequently (every 2 hourly), maintaining proper alignment to ensure a patent airway.
- Clean and dry skin creases after feeding or vomiting.
- Monitor any reddened areas, and position the infant away from anything that may pose a skin breakdown.
- Feed small amounts frequently on a flexible schedule to accommodate diagnostic procedures (such as a CAT scan) which may induce an episode of vomiting.
- Restrict fluids to half of the daily maintenance level.
- Provide postoperative shunt care.
- Position the head so that the child will lie on the unoperated side or will not lie in the prone position if a VP shunt has been inserted.
- Determine what type of shunt has been inserted and plan care accordingly. (Some shunts require elevating the head of the bed 30° to facilitate drainage; some require positioning flat in bed to avoid rapid loss of intracranial fluid.)
- Assess neurological status (LOC, papillary reaction, motor function, reflexes, and vital signs) every hour.
- Assess respiratory rate, depth and rhythm.
- Auscultate lung fields for breath sounds.
- Deliver oxygen within prescribed limits.
- Maintain hydration; assess daily weights, intake and output (I&O).
- Assess tissue perfusion (temperature of extremities, peripheral pulses, capillary refill) every 2 hours.
- Prevent infection: Observe wound sites for redness, drainage, oedema, elevated temperature by monitoring vital signs.
- Monitor body temperature, as every 1°C increase in temperature there is 10%–13% increase in the metabolic rate. (Fever aetiology is important because it influences treatment. Increase in temperature may be a result of central fever or peripheral fever.
  - Central fever is directly attributed to brain damage, reflects derangement in hypothalamic function manifested by lack of sweating and there is no diurnal variation. Plateau-like elevation up to 41°C (105.8°F), absence of tachycardia and persistence for days/weeks. It can be controlled with external cooling rather than antipyretics. Hypothermia treatment increases metabolic demand and is not advisable.

- Peripheral fever is associated with CNS infection or other bacterial invasion. It is characterized by sweating, diurnal variation and tachycardia and responds to antipyretics.
- Provide comfort and medicate for pain.
- Flush shunts as ordered.
- Discuss signs of malfunction and infection with parents (infection: lethargy, nausea, vomiting, signs of meningeal irritation–obstruction: lethargy, vomiting, seizures, focal neurological signs, swelling around the shunt site [signs of increased ICP]).
- Instruct parents how to flush the shunt.
- If ventriculostomy is used as an interim therapy: Obtain specific written orders as to
  - Degree of elevation of the head of the bed
  - Height of inlet to the collection bag
  - Whether tubing is to be clamped, unclamped or on an alternating schedule
  - The characteristics of expected drainage
  - Need for intravenous fluids
- Continually assess the child for signs of increased ICP and amount of drainage from the system.
- Change the child's position carefully.
- Prevent infection by using aseptic technique when handling the drainage system.
- Secure all tubing with tape to prevent unnecessary breaks in the system.
- Note any changes in colour, consistency and amount of CSF.
- Monitor vital signs frequently.
- Use protective isolation if indicated.
- Clamp ventriculostomy tubing with a special label so that it is not mistaken.

SPINA BIFIDA

It is a major defect of the posterior body wall which is caused by the failure of development of the posterior vertebral arches with or without a neural tube defect where the posterior portion of the laminae of the vertebra fails to close during the fourth week of gestation.

Aetiology and Incidence

The exact aetiology is unknown. It is believed that interplay of genetic and environmental factors produces spina bifida. So, it is most commonly caused by multifactorial inheritance in which genes interact with environmental factors. The risk of neural tube defects increases in subsequent siblings. Consanguinity also increases the risk. Wide geographical variations are seen in incidence. Higher incidence is seen among Indians, especially north Indians (four to five in 1000 live births), whereas it is 0.6 in 1000 live births in Australians and one in 1000 live births in Americans. It occurs more frequently in females than in males (occurs more frequently in British Isles).

The incidence is decreasing globally as a result of prenatal screening and permitted medical termination of pregnancy.

Classification

Spina bifida is classified according to the severity and anatomical involvement into spina bifida occulta and spina bifida cystica. Spina bifida cystica is again divided into meningocoele and meningomyelocoele.

Meningomyelocoele (Myelomeningocoele)

It is the commonest form accounting for 95% of cases. The commonest site is lumbosacral. Defects are seen in the overlying muscles. Spinous process and posterior vertebral arches of several vertebrae are absent, producing a saucer-like bony defect lined on either side by malformed everted pedicles of the vertebral bodies.

The open myelomeningocoele is called myelocoele or rachischisis, where the bony defect is occupied by a pink, oval plaque with an ulcer-like appearance. In closed myelocoele, the bony defect is covered by a CSF-filled cavity which invariably contains neural tissue. The sac is usually irregular and the periphery is covered by the normal skin. Almost all infants with myelomeningocoele will have varying degrees of motor and sensory loss in the lower limbs and sphincter incompetence. The function distal to the lesion is usually absent or severely compromised. Hydrocephalus is associated with this type of lesion in 75% of cases. Only 60% of cases are operable (surgical correction). Other associated lesions are as follows:

- Arnold–Chiari malformation (there is an elongation and downward displacement of the cerebellar midline and midbrain deformity)
- Dislocation of hips
- Talipes equinovarus (clubfoot)
- Congenital scoliosis

Meningocoele

It is comparatively rare and constitutes only 4%–5% of all spina bifida cystica cases. Smooth, irregular and usually narrow-necked swelling covered with full-thickness skin and filled only with CSF is the characteristics. The spinal cord is anatomically and functionally normal, and there is no neurological deficit. Bony defect involve one or two vertebrae. Hydrocephalus is associated in 9% of the cases.

Another classification for spina bifida exists. It is divided into vertebral and dorsal defects. Vertebral defects are extremely rare and involve splitting of the vertebral body and the presence of a cyst that is neurenteric in origin. The lesion is usually seen in the lower cervical and upper thoracic vertebrae.

Dorsal defects are the most common types. These are subdivided into two categories: spina bifida occulta and spina bifida aperta.

Spina bifida occulta is limited to the vertebrae, with no visible external defect other than perhaps a tuft of hair. The spinal cord and meninges are normal; therefore, usually no symptoms are present. It is the most common type of spina bifida and occurs in 25% of all normal children. It is usually seen at the fifth lumbar and sacral vertebrae. It is usually associated with hydrocephalus. It is not obviously seen on inspection or examination, but there is a defective fusion of the posterior arches of L5 and S1 vertebrae. There are four groups of spina bifida occulta:

1. True spina bifida occulta is present in 10%–20% of normal individuals as asymptomatic, incidental radiological findings.
2. Spina bifida occulta present with an overlying superficial lesion such as tuft of hair or a capillary haemangioma.
3. Spina bifida occulta presenting as meningitis or overlying dermal sinus may end in a subarachnoid cyst or may go all the way to the spina theca providing a passage for bacteria which cause recurrent attacks of meningitis.
4. Occult spinal dysraphism (spina bifida with neurological symptoms). In addition to the superficial lesions described earlier, there is an underlying intraspinal lesion producing pressure or traction on the cord or the nerves of the cauda equina.

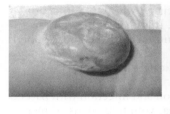
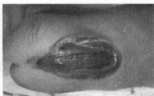
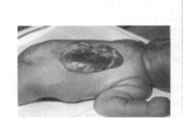
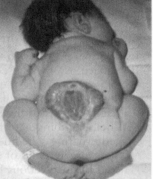

Various forms of spina bifida.

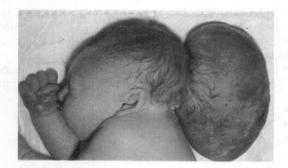
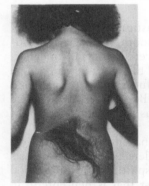
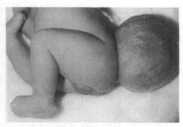
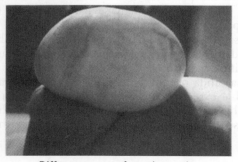

Different types of meningocele.

Clinical Manifestations

- α-Fetoprotein levels in maternal serum will be elevated in the antenatal period
- Ultrasound visualization of the defect possible
- A parent or sibling with spina bifida
- Hydrocephalic fetus
- Presence of a spinal lesion
- Tuft of hair over sinus tract in the lumbar area
- Enlarged head circumference – Hydrocephalus
- Lack of spontaneous movement of the lower extremities
- Hip clicks – Congenital hip dislocation
- Clubfoot
- Scoliosis
- Flaccid or spastic muscles in the lower extremities
- Sensory loss increasing the risk for burns and scalds
- Bladder and bowel dysfunction (the child dribbles urine: Important clinical signs are compressible urinary bladder, patulous anus and perianal anaesthesia)
- Additional malformations include genitourinary malformations (about 20% of cases) such as cystic kidneys, horseshoe kidneys, hypospadias, cryptorchidism, hydroureter and vesicourethral reflux. Along with these anomalies, there may be cardiac anomalies, exomphalos, ectopia vesica and Ano rectal anomalies (ARMs).

Diagnosis

- Radiographic studies of the spine, skull and hips
- Renal ultrasonography or intravenous pyelography (IVP)
- CT scan to identify ventricular dilation and subsequent treatment of hydrocephalus, as well as that of neuropathic bladder to preserve renal function and control urinary incompetence
- Routine urine examination, renal function tests (blood urea nitrogen [BUN], serum creatinine), voiding cystourethrogram, isotope renography, urodynamic studies, etc.

Multidisciplinary Management

- Main aim is to make an ambulant and continent baby with or without appliances.
- Active treatment is contraindicated in babies who have associated anomalies such as congenital cyanotic heart diseases, severe paralysis of lower limbs and sphincter incompetence, marked hydrocephalus at birth (2 cm above the 90th percentile), severe kyphosis and meningitis.
- In the absence of adverse factors, early surgery within 24 hours of birth is advised.
- Skeletal anomalies are corrected with orthopaedic management.
- Surgical correction of urinary incontinence.
- Teach the management of neuropathic bladder – Clean intermittent catheterization, bladder training and indwelling catheterization.
- Faecal incontinence presents as constipation or faecal soiling, which is managed by diet control, laxatives and suppositories and tap water washouts.
- The aim of operation is to cover the exposed neural plate with membranes and skin, thereby minimizing the chances of infection. Operation to close the defect can be conveniently done after 6 months.
- The most important part is the home care, education and rehabilitation.

Nursing Diagnosis

- High risk for injury
- Impaired skin integrity
- Ineffective family coping
- Altered family process
- Altered parenting
- Altered growth and development
- Complication potential

Nursing Interventions

- Place the neonate only in the prone or side-lying position.
- Cover the lesion with sterile, moist dressings.
- Keep meconium or urine away from the lesion.
- Administer antibiotics per the order.
- Institute nursing interventions to prevent hypothermia.
- Provide a sterile, warm, moist covering for the lesion and cover with a plastic wrap to prevent evaporative losses.
- Minimize the neonate's exposure to moist bedding.
- Support parents.
- Provide parental teaching to realistic goals, clarify the physician's explanations and reinforce the same.
- Instruct parents about ways in which they can be involved in the care of the baby.
  In the hospital:
- Encourage parents to ask questions and express their concerns.
- Support the grieving parents.
- Refer community resources, support groups and developmental and medical follow-up with rehabilitative measures.

CEREBRAL PALSY

Cerebral palsy (CP) is an upper motor neuron disease characterized by a group of disabilities caused by injury or insult to the brain sustained during the period of brain growth in the fetal life, infancy or childhood. This is the most common permanent disability of childhood. The term 'palsy' means disorder of movement. The affected part of the brain is the cerebrum. It also involves the connection between the cortex and other parts of the brain such as cerebellum. Causes of damage to brain in CP show that 75% of damage occurs during pregnancy, 5% during child birth and 15% after birth up to the age of 3 years. It is a nonprogressive (brain damage does not worsen) disorder, but secondary orthopaedic difficulties are common.

CP is a group of permanent disorders of the development of movement and posture, causing activity limitation (Hockenberry M J & Wilson C). In children with CP, there are disturbances of sensation, perception, communication, cognition and behaviour, secondary musculoskeletal problems and epilepsy

Aetiology

CP has prenatal, perinatal and postnatal causes.
Prenatal causes belong to maternal causes and fetal causes.

Maternal Causes

- Bleeding
- Cognitive impairment/seizures
- Diabetes/hyperthyroidism
- Exposure to radiation/toxins
- Genetic abnormalities
- Infections
- Incompetent cervix
- Malnutrition
- Medication use (e.g. thyroid, oestrogen, progesterone)
- Previous child with development disabilities
- Previous premature birth
- Polyhydramnios
- Severe proteinuria

Gestational Causes

- Chromosomes abnormalities
- Congenital malformations
- Fetal development abnormalities
- Genetic syndrome
- Inflammatory response
- Problems in placenta functioning
- Rh incompatibility infections
- Teratogen

Labour and Delivery

- Abnormal presentation
- Asphyxia
- Fetal heart rate depression
- Long labour
- Premature delivery
- Prolonged rupture of membranes
- Preeclampsia

Perinatal Causes

- Intraventricular haemorrhage
- Intrauterine growth retardation

- Low birth weight
- Meconium aspiration
- Mechanical ventilation for a prolonged period
- Prematurity and associated problems
- Periventricular haemorrhage
- Persistent pulmonary hypertension
- Sepsis and/or CNS infections
- Seizure

Postnatal Causes

- Brain injury
- Infections such as meningitis or encephalitis
- Traumatic brain injuries

- Toxin exposure
- Stroke

Classification

1. **Spastic cerebral palsy** (pyramidal)

   This type of CP is the most common one involving both sides of the body. Major features include hypertonicity with poor control of posture, balance and coordinated movement and impairment of gross and fine motor skills. The child may have persistent primitive reflexes, positive Babinski signs, ankle conus and eventual development of contractures. Common types of spastic CP are hemiparesis, quadriparesis and diplegia.

Patterns of cerebral palsy

Type of cerebral palsy	Aetiology	Clinical features
Unilateral cerebral palsy (hemiplegia) Spastic or dystonic	Often due to perinatal middle cerebral artery infarct	Spastic or dystonic tone, one side of body affected (oppositeto the side of the brain lesion) Arm often more affected than leg May have visual field defect on side of hemiplegia Risk of learning difficulties and seizures Often GMFCS level 1 and 2
Bilateral spastic cerebral palsy (diplegia)	Damage to the periventricular areas of developing brain often associated with prematurity. Leg motor fibres from the homunculus are closest to the ventricles, so legs more affected than arms.	Young child – pattern with walking on their toes with scissoring of the legs. Older child – crouch gait pattern is typical when the child gets heavier and can't remain on their toes.	Predominantly affects legs. Arms may be subtly affected (supination, fine motor control). Spasticity is main motor type. Usually no feeding or communication difficulties and good cognition. Often associated with squints. Frequently GMFCS level 1–3
Bilateral spastic cerebral palsy (quadriplegia, 4 limb pattern)	Extensive damage to the periventricular areas of the developing brain, including cortex.	Both arm and leg involvement – predominantly spastic but dystonia often also present. Associated with learning difficulty, feeding difficulties, problems with speech, vision and hearing. Seizures common. At increased risk of hip subluxation and dislocation and scoliosis. Usually dependent on others for activities of daily living Powered mobility a common requirement. Often GMFCS levels 4 and 5.
Dyskinetic cerebral palsy (dystonia, athetosis, chorea)	Perinatal asphyxia – particularly affecting the basal ganglia. Also kernicterus, but this is now rare.	Typical dystonic pattern with open mouth posture and internal rotation and extension of the arms.	Mixture of motor patterns including dystonia, athetosis and chorea. Cognition may be preserved but feeding difficulties are common. Risk of hip deformity and scoliosis. Many are dependent on others for activities of daily living due to their severe movement difficulties even if cognitively normal. Usually GMFCS level 4–5.

Source: Illustrated Textbook of Paediatrics, Fifth Edition by Tom Lissauer, Will Carroll. Elsevier Ltd; 2018. Figure 4.5, The different types of cerebral palsy.

2. **Dyskinetic or athetoid cerebral palsy**
   Children with this type of CP have abnormal movements that disappear during sleep and increase with stress. Major manifestations are wormlike movements called athetosis along with dyskinetic movement of mouth, drooling of saliva and dysarthria.

3. **Ataxic cerebral palsy**
   The child has wide based gait, and rapid repetitive movements are performed poorly. Disintegration of movements of the upper limb occurs when the child tries to reach objects.

4. **The mixed/dystonic cerebral palsy** is manifested by a combination of the characteristics of spastic and athetoid CPs.

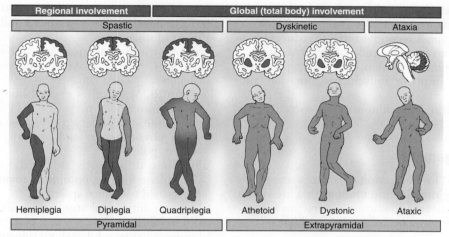

Source: Ferri's Clinical Advisor 2018: 5 Books in 1 by Fred F. Ferri. Elseveir Inc; 2018. Fig. E1, Classification of cerebral palsy. Although overlaps in terminology exist, cerebral palsy can be classified according to distribution (regional versus global involvement, hemiplegic, diplegic, quadriplegic), physiologic type (spastic, dyskinetic/dystonic, dyskinetic/athetoid, ataxic), or presumed neurologic substrate (pyramidal, extrapyramidal). Cerebral Palsy by Joseph S. Kass, Maitreyi Mazumdar (From Canale ST, Beaty JH: Campbell's operative orthopaedics, ed 11, Philadelphia, 2007, Mosby.)

Clinical Features

Physical Signs and Symptoms

- Clenched hands after 3 months
- Floppy or limp body posture
- Poor head control after 3 months of age
- Pushing away or arching back
- Persistent tongue thrusting after 6 months of age
- Uses only one side of the body or only the arms to crawl
- Stiff or rigid arms or legs
- Scissoring of legs
- Seizures
- Sensory impairment (hearing, vision)
- Cannot sit up without support by 8 months of age
  Other behavioural signs include:
- Irritability or crying
- Feeding difficulties
- Little or no interest in the surrounding
- Excessive stepping

Diagnosis

- Physical examination.
- History taking.
- Neurologic assessment.
- MRI to study the brain in more detail
- Ultrasonography to detect certain types of structural and anatomic abnormalities.
- CT scan to create a detailed three-dimensional model of the child's brain

- Electroencephalogram (EEG) to monitor brain activity
- Electromyogram (EMG) and nerve conduction studies (NCS) to test the electrical activity of muscles and to measure the conducting function of nerves.
- Laboratory studies to detect any blood clotting and screen for genetic or metabolic problems
- Tests to vision, speech and hearing impairments and intellectual disabilities
- Other developmental delays and movement disorders

Multidisciplinary Management

- Treatment is aimed at enhancing functional capacities and to develop self-help abilities.
- Treatment is mainly symptomatic and supportive.
- The main goals of treatment are to help the child develop integration of motor functions and obtain optimum appearance, to detect and correct associated anomalies and to promote socialization of the children and their parents within the community.
- Treatment include **physiotherapy** to improve motor functions by reducing spasticity and control gait and involuntary movements. It improves mobility, child's strength and flexibility. Use of orthotic devices such as braces, casting and splints support the child during movements.
- **Occupational therapy** improves child's independence and is useful in training children to use alternative strategies and adaptive equipment for independent activities and to promote ADL. This will promote

children to have self-help at home, school or special schools or homes.
- **Speech and language therapy** is administered to improve communication. Sometimes, training in sign language is essential.
- **Recreational therapy** is administered to improve motor skills, speech and emotional well-being.
- **Pharmacological interventions include treatment to reduce the effects of CP and prevent complications.**
- **Analgesics are administered to reduce intense pain or muscle spasm.**
- Botulinum toxin type A is administered to reduce spasm after inhaled nitrous oxide or midazolam for sedation.
- Dantrolene sodium, baclofen, and diazepam are administered to improve muscle coordination and relaxation.
- Anticonvulsant drugs are administered to relieve or stop seizures.

Surgical Management

- Surgery is advised for correction of orthopaedic problems (lengthening muscles and tendons that are short) and orthopaedic surgery to correct contractures, spastic deformities and muscle and tendon problems.

Rhizotomy

- Selective dorsal rhizotomy (SDR) is a surgical procedure that can help children particularly with severe muscle stiffness in their legs to improve their walking. The operation involves cutting some of the nerves in the lower spinal column, which can help relieve leg stiffness.
- Gastrostomy is performed for feeding and correct associated gastroesophageal reflux (GER).
- Proper assessment of the infant for abnormal muscle tone and inability to achieve milestones at the desired age, and persistence of some of the neonatal reflexes such as Moro, Babinski, etc. needs to be checked.
- Parents must be given support and help them socialize themselves and their sick children.
- Encourage parents to express concerns, treat their concern as genuine, help them cope positively, etc. are very important along with other treatment protocols.
- Meeting nutrition through various means is also very important, e.g. special feeding techniques such as tube feeding, gastrostomy feeding.
- Provide all routine immunization as per the Universal Immunization Programme (UIP).
- Counsel parents.

Nursing Assessment

It involves a complete physical assessment and assessment of general condition, level of mobility, feeding problems and ADL.

Nursing Diagnoses

Impaired physical mobility/activity intolerance/self-care deficit

Alteration in nutrition less than body requirement
High risk for injury
Parental anxiety

Nursing Interventions

Assess the type of motor disorder.
Assess the orthopaedic, visual, auditory and intellectual deficits.
Assess abnormal reflexes seen in infants and children that may be persistent beyond the stipulated age.
Perform development assessment and note the development of milestones.
Plan activities to use gross and fine motor skills (holding toys, pen or spoon and encourage reaching for objects).
Perform ROM exercises every 4 hours for the child unable to move body parts.
Involve multidisciplinary team in the care of the child.
Provide physiotherapy and orthotic appliances such as walker, poles, etc.
Administer drugs such as benzodiazepines, baclofen, dantrolene sodium, botulinum toxin, tizanidine, etc. as prescribed to reduce spasticity.
Administer anticonvulsants such as diazepam and phenytoin sodium.
Administer haloperidol, sodium valproate, tetradiazepines, benzodiazepines, etc.
Assist in investigations such as EEG, CT, MRI, psychometric and evaluation of language and learning disabilities.
Assess the nutritional requirement and the present feeding schedule. Monitor weight and height.
Administer small frequent feeds.
Use appropriate utensils for feeding.
Teach family members techniques to promote adequate calorie, protein and other nutrients.
Position the child upright while feeding.
Place foods far back in the mouth to overcome tongue thrust.
Use soft and blended foods.
Allow extra time for chewing and swallowing.
Obtain adaptive handles for utensils and encourage self-feeding skills.
Prepare foods according to the nutritional needs of children.
Teach the signs and symptoms of food aspiration.
Administer strategies to prevent infection, especially respiratory tract infection.
Assist for surgical procedures such as tendon lengthening, tendon transfer, osteotomy, tendentomy, neurectomy and Selective Dorsal Rhizotomy (SDR).
Educate parents regarding care and preventive strategies such as skin care, different feedings techniques, etc.
Promote speech therapy, occupational therapy, cognitive therapy and behavioural therapy.
Administer medications as prescribed such as anticonvulsants, skeletal muscle relaxants and antacids.
Botulinum toxin injection to muscles is a recent therapy used to control muscle spasm.
Provide time for parents to verbalize the impact of sickness on the family.

Assess family's ability to adapt and cope with the child's health problems.

Explore community services for rehabilitation, respite care, child care and other needs and refer family as appropriate.

Teach the family skills required to manage the child's care – medication administration, ROM exercises, physical rehabilitation, seizure management, etc.

Involve siblings and other relatives also in the care of the child.

Expected outcome: The parents and the child will adapt to the medical condition, socialize with the community and perform ADL within limits.

ENCEPHALOCOELE

It is a condition resulting from bony defects in the cranial vault, which leads to herniation of the meninges with or without differentiated brain tissue. If there is herniation of dura and brain tissue, then it is called meningoencephalocoele and if the ventricular system also herniates then it is called meningohydroencephalocoele. In encephalocoeles, the defect is usually covered with skin and it is seen in the occiput region. It can also affect the frontal bone, and this defect is common in Asia. The condition has variable outcome and shunt may be required. This condition may be associated with Dandy–Walker cyst formation, hydrocephalus and dysplasia of cerebellum and optic pathways.

Surgical correction is attempted if it is correctable.

STUDY QUESTIONS

- What are the consequences of abnormal embryonic development of CNS?
- What are the types of head injury?
- How will you assess the level of consciousness in a child with head injury?
- Describe the modified Glasgow Coma Scale used in children.
- How will you monitor ICP?
- What is a seizure? How will you protect a child during a fix?
- What is a febrile seizure? How will you differentiate a febrile seizure from an epileptic seizure?
- What are common causes of meningitis?
- Define tuberculosis meningitis. Differentiate it from viral meningitis.
- What is hydrocephalous? State its clinical features.
- Prepare nursing care plan for children with the following medical and surgical problems using the nursing process approach:
  a. An adolescent with head injury
  b. A neonate with meningomyelocoele
  c. An infant with hydrocephalus
  d. A preschooler with meningococcal meningitis
  e. A toddler with epilepsy
- Write short notes on the following:
  a. Care of a child during a fit
  b. Discharge planning for a child with febrile convulsions
  c. Care of an infant after spina bifida repair
  d. Maintenance of patent airway in a child with head injury
  e. Complications of hydrocephalus
  f. Care of bladder and bowel in children with meningomyelocoele repair
- What is encephalocoele?
- What are the causes of cerebral palsy?
  a. State five physical features of spastic CP.
  b. Prepare a nursing care plan for a 3-year-old child with athetoid CP.

BIBLIOGRAPHY

1. American Academy of Pediatrics & American College of Emergency Physicians. (1981). Pediatric Advanced Life Support. Elk Grove Village, IL & Dallas, TX.
2. Anania, et al. 2008. Nursing: *Memahami Berbagai Macam Penyakit*: Jakarta: Indeks.
3. Bruce, D.A., Schat, L., Sutton, L.N. (1988). Neurosurgical Emergencies. In: Fleisher, G., Ludwig, S. (Editors): Textbook of Pediatric Emergency Medicine. 2nd Edn. Baltimore: Williams & Wilkins, pp. 1112–1126.
4. Gill, F.T. (1989). Pediatric Trauma Nursing. Willkins: Ave Rockville.
5. Honkenberry, Marilyn, J & Wilson, David. (2011) Wongs – Nursing care of infants and children. (9th ed.) Elsevier Mosby: Canada.
6. Jones MW, Morgan E, Shelton JE. Primary care of the child with cerebral palsy: a review of systems (part II). J Pediatr Health Care. 2007 Jul-Aug; 21(4):226-37.
7. Kliegam, Robert M & Berbman, Richard E. (2009). Nelson text book of paediatrics. (18th ed) Sauder Elsevier: United States.
8. Kitt, S., Kaiser, J. (1990). Emergency Nursing – A Physiologic and Clinical Perspective. Philadelphia, pp. 534–535.
9. Weller F. B. (ed). Bailliere's Nurses' Dictionary: for nurses and health care workers (24th ed.). United Kingdom.
10. Whaley, L., Wong, D. (1987). Nursing Care of Infants and Children. 3rd Edn. St. Louis: Mosby, pp. 9-669–681.

WEBSITES

1. http://www.nlm.nih.gov/medlineplus/cerebralpalsy.html
2. http://www.ninds.nih.gov/disorders/cerebral_palsy/cerebral_palsy.htm
3. nursingcrib.com/nursing-notes-reviewer/maternal-child.../what-is-cerebral-palsy
4. https://www.slideshare.net/drlibinthomas/cerebral-palsy-etiology-and-classification
5. www.hindustantimes.com/...encephalitis...children/story-E1dFf1KGTDeAprdt9N7wg
6. kidshealth.org/en/parents/encephalitis.html

ALTERATIONS IN HAEMATOLOGICAL FUNCTIONS: NURSING CARE OF CHILDREN WITH HAEMATOLOGICAL DISORDERS

CHAPTER OUTLINE

- Essential Concepts: Embryonic Development of Blood and Blood Components
- Anaemia
- Thalassaemia
- Aplastic Anaemia

- Haemophilia
- von Willebrand disease
- Idiopathic/Immune Thrombocytopenic Purpura (ITP)
- Haemopoietic Stem Cell Transplantation

LEARNING OBJECTIVES

At the end of the chapter, the learner will be able to:
- Identify the essential concepts related to blood formation and consequences of abnormal development.
- Describe nursing management of children with various haematological disorders using nursing procedures.

INTRODUCTION

This chapter describes haematological functions by examining various formed elements of the blood, transport of oxygen and carbon dioxide between lungs and other organs of the body, phagocytosis and other defence mechanisms, and homeostasis along with nursing management of children suffering from various haematological disorders.

EMBRYONIC DEVELOPMENT

Blood formation begins early in human embryonic life in specialized centres called blood islands. Haematopoiesis begins in these blood islands of the yolk sac in the second week of life from stem cells called haemocytoblasts, which were formerly undifferentiated mesenchyme cells. Haemopoietic cells are transferred from the yolk sac to embryo proper by the sixth week of embryonic life. Initially, liver is established as the major haemopoietic centre (about 1 month of the intrauterine life) for the

production of white blood cells (WBCs). The spleen also functions as an erythropoietic organ from the third to fifth fetal months. In the last half of gestation, there is a shift in haematopoiesis to the bone marrow. By birth, most blood formation takes place in the bone marrow. In human beings, bone marrow produces erythrocytes, granulocytes, monocytes and platelets and supplies precursors of lymphocytic tissues. Although liver is haematologically inactive in human after birth, it reserves its potential for haematopoiesis, which can be resumed in cases of bone marrow failure.

After birth, there is further change in the sites of haematopoiesis. In infancy, most of medullary spaces in bones are filled with 'red bone marrow' (a term given to the haemopoietic bone marrow). Gradually, during childhood, fatty tissue or yellow marrow replaces the red marrow of long bones. In older children and adults, active blood formation occurs in the marrow of selected bones, ribs, sternum, vertebrae, pelvis, skull, clavicles and scapulae. In circumstances of severe haematological stress (bleeding), the yellow marrow of the long bones of the extremities can resume active haematopoiesis.

CONSEQUENCES OF ABNORMAL DEVELOPMENT

Abnormal development in the embryo leads to death, arrested development or congenital problems as indicated in Table 33.1. Also, a number of genetically linked blood disorders may lead to haematological dysfunction in newborns and children. For example, sickle cell anaemia, glucose-6-phosphate dehydrogenase deficiency (G-6-PD), pyruvate kinase deficiency, hereditary spherocytosis, Wiskott–Aldrich syndrome, haemophilia and thalassaemia syndrome are genetically linked or transmitted.

TABLE 33.1	**Consequences of Abnormal Development**	
Fetal Age	**Structure**	**Abnormalities at Birth**
2 weeks	Blood islands of the yolk sac	Termination of growth
	1	2
6 weeks	Haemopoietic cells are transferred to the embryo	
	Development arrested from the yolk sac	
	Liver is the major haemopoietic centre	
3–5 months	Spleen also functions as an erythropoietic organ	
6–9 months	Shift of haemopoiesis to the congenital aplastic anaemia, bone marrow	Blackfan–Diamond syndrome, Fanconi anaemia

- Haemopoiesis is defined as the formation and development of blood cells.
- Haematopoiesis activity occurs by the second week of embryonic life; blood islands arise from the yolk sac and liver.
- From the second to fifth months of gestation, liver is the most active site of haematopoiesis.
- Bone marrow becomes active around the fourth month within 2–3 weeks after birth; the bone marrow is the main site of haemopoietic activity.

Primary Functions of Blood Cells and Cellular Elements

- Blood consists of liquid plasma and formed elements, erythrocytes, leucocytes and thrombocytes.
- Plasma transports formed elements and helps maintain homeostasis.
- Erythrocytes transport oxygen to and carbon dioxide away from body tissues; this activity relies on haemoglobin (Hb), an erythrocyte component. Erythrocytes also give blood its red colour. Their life span is 120 days.
- The primary function of leucocytes is to protect the body against infection. Two types of leucocytes exist: granulocytes and agranulocytes.
- Thrombocytes, the smallest blood cells, contain coagulation factors and help regulate haemostasis through a sequence of events known as the coagulation process.

Haematological System Overview

Health history should focus on bleeding or bruising tendencies, medication use and a family history of bleeding problems.

Main points should include the following:
- Skin colour, flushing, jaundice, purpura, petechiae, ecchymosis, pruritus, cyanosis, brownish discolouration, decreased capillary refill time
- Eyes jaundiced sclera, conjunctival pallor, retinal haemorrhage, blurred vision
- Mouth gingival and mucosal pallor
- Lymph nodes, lymphadenopathy, tenderness
- Cardiac tachycardia, murmurs, signs and symptoms of congestive heart failure
- Pulmonary tachypnoea, orthopnoea, dyspnoea
- Neurological headache, vertigo, irritability, depression, impaired thought processes, lethargy and cold sensitivity
- Gastrointestinal (GI) anorexia, hepatomegaly, splenomegaly
- Musculoskeletal weight loss, decreased muscle mass, bone pain, joint swelling and pain

Laboratory Studies and Diagnostic Tests

Complete blood cell count includes the following:
- Red blood cell (RBC) count
- WBC count
- Differential count
- Haemoglobin
- Haematocrit
- Mean corpuscular volume
- Mean corpuscular Hb
- Mean corpuscular Hb concentration
- Platelet count
- Bleeding time and clotting time

Other diagnostic tests include the following:
- Bone marrow aspiration that helps in the diagnosis of aplastic anaemia, pernicious anaemia, agranulocytosis, thrombocytopenia and leukaemia.
- Reticulocyte count helps differentiate between types of anaemias.
- Coagulation and homeostasis studies aid in differential diagnosis of haemorrhagic disorders.

Remember – Children with haemorrhagic disorders usually undergo a multitude of invasive procedures and treatments, which lead to anxiety and stress.

NURSING MANAGEMENT OF COMMON HAEMATOLOGICAL PROBLEMS OF CHILDREN

Red Blood Cell Disorders

The most common disorders affecting blood are those that in some way alter the function or production of erythrocytes or RBCs. Such common disorders are described as follows:

Anaemia

The term 'anaemia' describes a condition in which the number of RBCs and/or the Hb concentration is reduced to below normal. Anaemia is caused by inadequate supply of iron for normal RBC formation, resulting in smaller cells, depleted RBC mass, decreased Hb concentration and decreased oxygen-carrying capacity of the blood.

Anaemia is the most common haematological disorder of infancy and childhood. It is not a disease itself but an indication or manifestation of an underlying pathological process.

Aetiology and Incidence
- Excessive blood loss
- Destruction of erythrocytes
- Decreased or impaired production of erythrocytes (e.g. sickle cell anaemia)
- Decreased or impaired production of erythrocytes or their components
- Morphology

Sickle Cell Anaemia

Sickle cell anaemia is a chronic disease characterized by production of abnormal haemoglobin S and periods of crisis. It is most common in the people of African origin; in India, it is seen in the tribal population. (In Kerala, it is commonly seen in the tribals of Wayanadu.) In sickle cell anaemia, amino acid sequence in the β-peptide chain is abnormal. When only one mutant gene is inherited, it leads to sickle cell trait. Homozygous state causes sickle cell disease. Under conditions of anoxia and acidosis/dehydration, RBC changes its shape to sickle. These sickled RBCs cause anoxaemia locally. This, in turn, leads to further sickling causing infraction. Infraction to vital organs such as liver, spleen, muscles, bones, etc. leads to sickle cell crisis.

The common precipitating factors are as follows:
- Dehydration as a result of vomiting/diarrhoea/increased sweating or exposure to heat
- Exposure to extreme climates/travelling to high altitude
- Excessive physical exertion
- Infections

Vaso-occlusive crisis (thrombocytic crisis): Here, the malformed RBCs occlude small and peripheral blood vessels, leading to infraction of a given area.

Sequestration crisis: Blood pools in liver or spleen produce circulatory collapse (more common in infants and frequently fatal).

Aplastic crisis: This results from lack of production of RBCs.

Hyperhaemolytic crisis: This results from increased destruction of RBCs.

Crisis periods can be precipitated by dehydration, trauma, infection and extreme fatigue, exposure to cold, respiratory distress or unusual physical exertion (Hazinsky M F).

Multidisciplinary Management
- Administer intravenous fluids or oral fluids depending on the condition of the child.
- Temperature and pain control: Narcotic analgesics are most effective in relieving pain; non-narcotic analgesics are most effective for musculoskeletal pain.
- Provide treatment of the precipitating factor, if known.
- Administer antibiotics to prevent infection.
- Provide blood transfusion.
- Administer oxygen therapy.

- Prevention of further attack of crisis is achieved by proper health education and prophylactic therapy.
- The crisis is managed by analgesics, sedation and intravenous fluids.
- Agents stimulating fetal Hb (hydroxyurea, azacytidine, butyrates, etc.) are usually prescribed.
- Red cell haemoglobin S concentration reducing agents (DDAVP and calcium channel blockers, etc.) are also administered.
- Membrane active agents and bone marrow transplantation are other modes of treatment that are prescribed for sickle cell disease.

Nursing Diagnoses
- Comfort alteration in pain related to ischaemia
- Complication potential related to ischaemia and necrosis
- Parental anxiety
- Alteration in growth and development
- Self-esteem disturbance
- Noncompliance related to knowledge deficit and economic crisis
- High risk for injury

Interventions. Emergency management includes establishing intravenous line for fluids and pain medications and sending blood samples for laboratory studies. No time should be wasted in managing the crisis, as it may cause irreversible damage and even death.
- Record intake and output chart.
- Administer intravenous fluids, as indicated.
- Encourage child to drink more fluids (approximately 1½–2 maintenance fluids).
- Be alert to urine output <0.5 mL/kg per hour for two consecutive hours, which could signal onset of acute tubular necrosis (ATN) secondary to decreased renal perfusion.
- Evaluate efficacy of fluid administration.
- Assess for signs and symptoms of volume depletion (signs of dehydration).
- Observe laboratory values for Hb, haematocrit and electrolyte imbalance.
- Note the presence of anorexia, irritability, weakness, fever and pallor.
- Help parents/child to identify precipitating factors and plan to prevent further attacks.
- Maintain bed rest.
- Provide oxygen, as ordered.
- Monitor for decreased oxygen saturation. Be alert to sustained decrease in oxygen.
- Provide passive range-of-motion exercises when not in crisis.
- Apply warmth to painful areas; avoid use of cold application (exacerbates crisis).
- Monitor effectiveness of analgesics.
- Monitor for signs of discomfort. Use a pain scale.
- Reassure that pain will decrease as crisis subsides.
- Discuss home management with parents and the child as follows:
  - Prevent tissue deoxygenation by avoidance of strenuous physical activity, contact sports,

emotional stress, low oxygen environments, infections (even mild ones)
- When to seek medical help – Temperature greater than 38.5°C
- Pain controlled by oral medications
- Inability to drink sufficient fluids
- Refer genetic counselling to parents, if desired

Thalassaemia

Thalassaemia is a disease characterized by deficiency in the rate of production of specific globulin chain in the Hb. The term 'thalassaemia' originated from the Greek word *thalassa* meaning sea. It is more common among people living near the Mediterranean Sea (e.g. Italians, Greeks and Syrians). In India, it came with Alexander during his invasion with Greeks and Egyptians who eventually settled in India. It is more common among north Indians. Wide geographical distribution, probably as result of genetic migration through intermarriage, made thalassaemia to spread to south India. It is classified depending on the Hb chain affected and the amount of globin chain that is synthesized; e.g. α-thalassaemia.

β-Thalassaemia is the most common type and has three forms:
- Thalassaemia minor or trait thalassaemia (heterogeneous form)
- Thalassaemia intermedia – manifested as splenomegaly and severe anaemia
- Thalassaemia major – A homozygous form that results in anaemia of variable severity that is not compatible with life without transfusion

Mode of Transmission. It is an autosomal recessive disorder with varying expressivity.

	Heterozygous parent A/a		
	Gametes	**A**	**A**
Heterozygous parent A/a	A	AA Normal	Aa Carrier
	A	Aa Carrier	aa Affected

Pathophysiology. Normal postnatal haemoglobin (HbA) is composed of two α chains and two β-chains. In β-thalassaemia, there is partial or complete deficiency in the synthesis of the β-chain of Hb molecule. Hence, there is a compensatory increase in the synthesis of α-chains, and γ-chain production remains activated in defective Hb formation. This unbalanced polypeptide unit is very unstable when it disintegrate. It impairs RBCs causing severe anaemia. As a compensatory mechanism to haemolysis, a large amount of erythrocytes are formed unless there is bone marrow suppression by transfusion therapy. Excess iron will be formed by the rapid haemolytic process that will get deposited in various organs causing haemosiderosis.

Clinical Features. Thalassaemia major:
- Defective syntheses of HbA
- Structurally impaired RBCs
- Shortened life span of RBCs
- Major consequences from pathological condition, resultant hypoxia and multiple blood transfusions as a supportive measure
- Other features include anaemia (haemolysis exceeds erythrocyte production) and chronic hypoxia, which produces bone pain and decreased exercise tolerance
- Haemosiderosis in spleen, liver, lymph glands, heart and pancreas
- Haemochromatosis (excess iron storage, with resultant cellular damage)
- Haemosiderin deposits under the skin, which leads to bronze appearance of the skin
- Retarded growth
- Bone changes – Frontal bossing, dental malocclusion
- Vision problems

Diagnostic Studies. Blood investigation (peripheral smear) shows changes in RBCs – microcytosis, hypochromia, anisocytosis, poikilocytosis, target cells, basophilic stippling of immature RBCs and Hb electrophoresis for distinguishing type and severity.

Multidisciplinary Management
- Maintain sufficient Hb levels to prevent hypoxia.
- Transfusions are the foundation of medical management.
- Chelation therapy (iron removal) using Desferal (deferoxamine). Usually, it is given with vitamin C. Preferred route is intravenous or subcutaneous (subcutaneous administration by a portable infusion pump or syringe pump over 8–10 hours and intravenous over 8 hours at the time of blood transfusion).
- Provide folic acid supplementation.
- In children with severe splenomegaly, splenectomy may be performed. Major complication after splenectomy is severe infection.
- Children should be protected from pneumococcal or meningococcal infection by immunizations.

Nursing Diagnoses
- Complication potential related to anaemia and haemosiderosis
- High risk for injury/infection related to low resistance and blood transfusions
- Parental anxiety related to disease condition
- Noncompliance related to lack of knowledge
- Self-esteem disturbances/body image disturbances related to disease condition

Nursing Interventions
- Provide care of the child during blood transfusions.
- Assist in investigation.
- Administer chelating agent (deferiprone [DFP] is an effective oral iron-chelating agent with minimal toxicity. It is given at a dose of 75–100 mg/kg per day in

divided doses as prescribed). Side effects are arthropathy and agranulocytosis.

- Teach parents and the child the use of syringe pump and administration of deferoxamine at home for chelation.
- Explain the need for frequent blood transfusions and chelation.
- Inform them the need of continuation of treatment.
- Refer the parents for genetic counselling, if desired.
- Explain after-effects of the disease.
- Prevent infection.
- Pre- and postoperative care of splenectomy, if advised. If splenectomy is advised, they must be instructed for the possible complications and the need for protection from infections, especially vaccination against pneumococcal and *Haemophilus influenzae* infections.
- Support family.
- Engage them with thalassaemia associations.
- Assist coping with effects of disorder.
- Care for growth and self-concept.
- Assist in orthopaedic appliance arrangement and use, if needed, for bone pain and deformity.

Aplastic Anaemia

It refers to condition in which all formed elements of the blood are simultaneously depressed. Peripheral blood smear demonstrates pancytopenia or the triad of profound anaemia, leucopoenia and thrombocytopenia. Hypoplastic anaemia is pure red cell aplasia, marked by complete or almost complete absence of all cells of the erythroid series with normal production of other myeloid cells. Aplastic anaemia can be primary (congenital) and secondary (acquired). Congenital aplastic anaemia is an outstanding feature of Fanconi syndrome (a rare hereditary disease) manifested with pancytopenia, hypoplasia of bone marrow and patchy brown discolouration of the skin as a result of the deposition of melanin along with multiple congenital anomalies.

Acquired aplastic anaemia may result from multiple factors such as the following:

- Multiple transfusions
- Haemolytic syndrome (as in sickle cell anaemia or thalassaemia)
- Autoimmune or allergic states
- Infections
- Hepatitis
- Radiation
- Drugs
- Exposure to household chemicals

Manifestation of anaemia will be as leucopoenia and decreased platelet count.

Multidisciplinary Management. It is aimed at restoring bone marrow function. Mainly two approaches are used. They are immunosuppressive therapy to remove presumed immunological function and replacement of marrow through transplantation. Principal drugs used are antilymphocytic globulin (ALG) or antithymocytic globulins (ATGs).

Nursing Interventions. It is similar to the care of patients with leukaemia.

Important – ATG administration should be done carefully to prevent extravasations, as it produces subcutaneous necrosis of tissues. Administration of chemotherapy also requires this precaution. For other nursing interventions, refer to nursing intervention of children with leukaemia.

Haemophilia

It is a bleeding disorder resulting from the deficiency of one of the factors necessary for coagulation of blood. It is an inherited disorder and is X-linked recessive. Two most common forms are factor VIII deficiency (haemophilia A) or classical haemophilia and factor IX deficiency (haemophilia B) or Christmas disease.

Mode of Transmission. Even though it is X-linked recessive, one-third cases of haemophilia may be caused by gene mutation. Usual pattern is a cross between an unaffected male and a trait carrier female. The chances of its occurrence are 25% or 1:4.

Pathophysiology. The basic defect of haemophilia A is a deficiency of factor VIII (antihaemophilic factor – AHF). AHF is produced by liver and is essential for thromboplastic formation on phase I of blood coagulation. Haemophilia is generally classified into three groups according to its severity: severe, moderate and mild. The effect of haemophilia is prolonged bleeding.

Clinical Features
- Prolonged bleeding
- Subcutaneous and intramuscular haemorrhage
- Haemarthrosis – Bleeding into the joints and cavities, especially knees, elbows and ankles, resulting in bone changes to affected joints
- Epistaxis and bleeding anywhere from injury is common

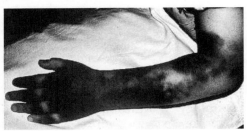

Diagnosis. Various tests of haemostasis are helpful to recall.

Multidisciplinary Management
- Administration of factor VIII concentrate to be reconstructed with sterile water immediately before use, DAVP (1-deamino-8-D-arginine vasopressin) – a synthetic vasopressin.
- Cryoprecipitate is no longer recommended.
- Aggressive factor concentrate replacement therapy is initiated to prevent crippling effect from joint bleeding.

- Corticosteroids are used judiciously to treat inflammation of the joints.
- Nonsteroidal anti-inflammatory drugs (NSAIDs) such as aspirin should not be administered, as it promotes bleeding.
- Provide a regular programme of exercise.
- Avoid contact sports.
- Provide treatment without delay in case of injury.

Prognosis. Home infusion and the concept of comprehensive haemophilia treatment have helped improve the prognosis.

Nursing Diagnoses
- Altered protection
- Risk for fluid volume deficit
- High risk for injury

Nursing Interventions
- Prevent bleeding.
- Recognize and control bleeding.
- Discuss bleeding history with the patient and parents.
- Monitor coagulation/clotting tests.
- Support tissue oxygenation via oxygen administration; monitor arterial oxygen saturation with continuous SpO_2.
- Monitor closely for increased bleeding, bruising, petechiae and purpura.
- Decrease risk of further bleeding by using alcohol-free mouthwash with swab sticks for oral hygiene, avoiding unnecessary venipuncture and intramuscular injections, applying pressure over invasive sites for 3–5 minutes and 10–15 minutes for arterial punctures.
- Prevent crippling effect of bleeding.
- Administer blood, as prescribed.
- Check blood to be transfused.
- Observe for allergic reactions.
- Provide family support and prepare for home care.
- Identify associations involved in the welfare of haemophiliac patients and introduce the patient and family members to the same (Hemophilia Foundation).
- Identify persons at risk.
- Promote genetic counselling.

von Willebrand Disease

von Willebrand disease (**vWD**) is a hereditary bleeding disorder characterized by factor VIII deficiency and low levels of factor VIII-related antigen (FVIII R:Ag). In addition, the functional component of factor VIII molecule that is required for platelet adhesion to vascular subendothelium (known as von Willebrand factor) is reduced. So, platelets fail to adhere to the walls. There will be prolonged bleeding time, and severe bleeding from the mucous membrane will be the characteristic feature, especially from gum, nose (epistaxis), easy bruising and menorrhagia in females. This affects both males and females, as the inheritance is autosomal dominant.

Multidisciplinary Management. Primary treatment is with DDAVP or a special clotting factor called Humate-P.

Nursing Interventions. Nursing interventions are similar to those of haemophilia.

Idiopathic Thrombocytopenic Purpura/ Immune Thrombocytic Purpura (ITP)

It is also known as Werlhof disease and purpura haemorrhagica. It is characterized by spontaneous small haemorrhages/bleeding from the skin, mucous membrane and internal organs. There will be petechiae and purpura on the skin and the mucous membrane.

Incidence. Three-fourth of all cases of ITP are seen in children. Both sexes are equally affected. About 85%–90% of children with ITP may have spontaneous remission. Antiplatelet autoagglutinins have been infrequently seen in ITP. The bleeding in ITP is caused by increased vascular permeability and thrombocytopenia.

Assessment Findings. The age of onset is 3 years, with a peak incidence at 5 years. Two stages are noted as acute and chronic. Acute cases are followed by an infection, especially upper respiratory tract infection. Onset is sudden, and the child presents with bruising, petechiae and bleeding from the nose, gums and urinary tract; spleen may be just palpable in 25% of the cases.

In chronic type, ITP exists for more than 6 months even after steroid therapy. It accounts for 10%–15% of the cases.

Multidisciplinary Management
- Tourniquet or Hess test is positive.
- Complete haemogram is obtained to find out the Hb status and any abnormal cells.
- Platelet count is usually less than $20,000/mm^3$.
- Bleeding, clotting and clot retraction times are abnormal.
- Capillary fragility test ≥1+ signals that >11 petechiae are present in the radial area on the skin after prolonged application of the blood pressure (BP) cuff.
- Obtain bone marrow to ascertain the adequacy of megakaryocytes and to rule out leukaemia and aplastic anaemia.
- Medical treatment is with corticosteroids, prednisolone or methylprednisolone and other drugs such as anti-Rh globulin (anti-D).
- Provide intravenous immunoglobulin transfusion.

Nursing Diagnosis
- Altered protection related to decreased platelet count, increased bleeding
- Decreased adaptive capacity or risk for the same
- Pain to joint inflammation

Nursing Interventions
- Monitor for signs of bleeding; ↑ heart rate and respiratory rate, ↓ BP, oozing from the invasive site, petechiae

purpura, bruising, haematoma, GI bleeding (i.e. vomitus, stool, gastric aspirate, melena, etc.).

- Monitor central venous pressure (CVP) (↓).
- Assess for abdominal pain, tenderness, guarding or back pain (to find out intra-abdominal bleeding).
- Avoid intramuscular injections, all venous punctures/arterial punctures.
- Monitor platelet count. Be alert for sustained low values.
- Avoid administration of NSAIDs.
- Assess signs of ↑ intracranial pressure (ICP) or ↓ level of consciousness (LOC). Monitor for headache, visual disturbances and motor dysfunctions which are symptoms of ↑ ICP.
- Head end of the bed to be elevated to 30°–40°, and the neck is placed in a neutral position to decrease ICP.
- Use stool softeners.
- Use a pain assessment scale to assess pain.
- Elevate legs to decrease joint pain.
- Monitor fatigue and malaise.
- Avoid knee flexion if haemarthrosis is present.
- Decrease stress on joints.
- Evaluate anxiety level.
- Provide emotional support.

HAEMOPOIETIC STEM CELL TRANSPLANTATION

It is the transplantation of haemopoietic progenitor cells to reestablish normal haemopoiesis in subjects with serious haematological and malignant diseases.

Indications

- Leukaemias, especially acute myeloid leukaemia (AML) and acute lymphocytic leukaemia (ALL)
- Congenital haemolytic anaemias (e.g. thalassaemia, sickle cell anaemia)
- Bone marrow failure (e.g. aplastic anaemia)
- Blackfan–Diamond syndrome, Fanconi anaemia
- Lymphoproliferative disorders, especially Hodgkin lymphoma, non-Hodgkin lymphoma and multiple myeloma
- Solid tumours such as Wilms tumour, neuroblastomas and Ewing sarcoma
- Immunodeficiencies, especially severe combined immunodeficiency (SCID), chronic granulomatous disease (CGD), Wiskott–Aldrich syndrome and Chediak–Higashi syndrome
- Miscellaneous: Mucopolysaccharidosis, leucodystrophies

Types

- In syngeneic haemopoietic stem cell transplantation (HSCT), stem cells are obtained from identical twins.
- In allogenic HSCT, normal appearing marrow is obtained from the patient taking cytotoxic drugs. This

marrow is preserved and subsequently transfused back into the patient.

- Alternative for obtaining stem cell is blood, including umbilical cord blood.

Complications

- Graft versus host disease (GVHD) of both acute and chronic types
- Superimposed infections, e.g. *Mycoplasma pneumoniae* infection
- Protozoal infections, especially as a result of *Pneumocystis carinii* infection

STUDY QUESTIONS

- Describe blood formation.
- What are common types of anaemia seen in children?
- What are the characteristics of nutritional anaemia? Describe its basic management.
- What is sickle cell anaemia? Describe its mode of inheritance.
- What is sickling? How will you manage a child in a sickling crisis?
- Describe the fluid and pair management in sickling crisis.
- What is thalassaemia? Describe its types and mode of inheritance.
- What is chelation therapy?
- What are the uses of deferoxamine?
- How will you administer deferoxamine to children with thalassaemia?
- What are the roles of a paediatric nurse in administering blood to a thalassaemic child?
- Describe the nursing management of a child with a plastic anaemia.
- What is haemophilia? Describe its mode of inheritance.
- Write short notes on the following:
  a. Nurses responsibility in genetic counselling in parents of haemophilic children, sickle cell disease and von Willebrand disease.
  b. Alteration in the family process related to disease condition in haemophilia.
  c. Haemopoietic stem cell transplantation.
  d. Idiopathic thrombocytopenic purpura.
  e. Aplastic anaemia.

BIBLIOGRAPHY

1. Angostiniotin, M., Model, B., et al. (1995). Prevention and Control of Hemoglobinopathies. Bull WHO, 77, p 375.
2. Baird, M.S. (1995). Hematologic Dysfunctions. In: Swearingen, P.C., Keen, J.H. (Editors): Manual of Critical Care Nursing. 3rd Edn. St. Louis: Mosby.
3. Balgir, R.S. (1989). Ethnic and Regional Variations in the Red Cell Glucose 6 Phosphate Dehydrogenase Deficiency in India. Journal of Hematology, 7, p 101.ss.
4. Beutlar, E. (1991). Glucose 6 Phosphate Dehydrogenase Deficiency. New England Journal of Medicine, 324, p 169.
5. Choudhry, V.P. (1997). Oral Deferiprone: Controversies on Its Efficacy and Safety. Indian Pediatrics, 64, p 395.

6. Choudhry, V.P., Desai, N., et al. (1991). Current Management of Homozygous Beta Thalassemia. Indian Pediatrics, 28, p 1221.

7. Coffland, F.L., Shelton, D.M. (1993). Blood Component Replacement Therapy. Critical Care Nursing Clinics of North America, 5(3), pp. 543–556.

8. Kimbrell, J.D. (1993). Acquired Coagulopathies. Critical Care Nursing Clinics of North America, 5(3), pp 453–458.

9. Rogers, G.P. (1997). Overview of Pathophysiology and Rational For Treatment of Sickle Cell Anemia. Seminars in Hematology, 34, p 2.

10. Rogers, Z.R. (1997). Hydroxyurea Therapy for Diverse Paediatric Population with Sickle Cell Disease. Seminars in Hematology, 34, p 2.

11. Saxena, R., Jain, P.K., et al. (1998). Prenatal Diagnosis of β Thalassemia Experience in a Developing Country. Prenatal Diagnosis, 18, p 1.

12. Williams, W.J. (1995). Approach to the Patient. In: Bentler, E., et al. (Editors): Williams' Hematology. New York: McGraw-Hill.

CHAPTER 34

ALTERATION IN ENDOCRINE FUNCTIONS: NURSING MANAGEMENT OF CHILDREN WITH ENDOCRINE DISORDERS

LEARNING OBJECTIVES

At the end of the chapter, the learner will be able to:

- Identify the essential concepts related to endocrine functions.
- Describe the nursing management of children with various endocrine functions using the nursing process.

EMBRYOLOGY

Most endocrine glands develop during the first trimester of pregnancy. The thyroid gland develops in three stages, between 7 and 14 weeks of gestation. The parathyroid gland can be identified at 5–7 weeks of gestation. The pancreas forms two different cells which fuse to form a single organ at 7 weeks of gestation. Insulin can be detected in β cells several weeks later. Pituitary originates from the fusion of two ectodermal processes. The primordial of anterior and posterior segments can be seen by the fourth week of gestation. The gland takes its permanent shape and location in the sella turcica between the third and fourth months of gestation. The adrenal gland reaches its maximum size by the fourth month of gestation. The medulla arises from the ectoderm via the neural crest, the cortex, from the lateral plate of the embryonic mesoderm. Both corticosterone and aldosterone are secreted in utero.

The endocrine system includes cells or glands that transmit chemical signals via hormones, target cells or end organs that receive chemical signals, an environment or medium through which the chemical signals travel,

lymph, blood and extracellular fluid. This system regulates energy production, growth, sexual reproduction, response to stress and various metabolic processes.

The endocrine and autonomic nervous systems function collectively to maintain homeostasis and called the neuroendocrine system. Signals of the endocrine system are primarily transmitted through blood, the autonomic system via neural impulses. Systemic responses to the endocrine system are usually slow but long-lasting, affecting multiple cells and organs unlike the autonomic system which are immediate.

NURSING MANAGEMENT OF CHILDREN WITH ENDOCRINE DYSFUNCTIONS

Juvenile Diabetes Mellitus, Type 1

Juvenile diabetes mellitus (JDM) a metabolic disease in which carbohydrate utilization is reduced and that of lipid and protein is enhanced. Nutritional deficiency of insulin causes diabetes. This condition is on the increase. About two out of 1000 children suffer from diabetes mellitus (DM). Almost all children with diabetes are insulin dependent (type 1). Only children with severe obesity may suffer from type 2 diabetes that occurs as a result of insulin resistance.

Aetiology

- Genetic predisposition
- Environmental precipitants
- Inherited susceptibility is demonstrated by an identical twin of a diabetic mother has 30%–50% chance of developing DM. The risk of a child developing diabetes increases if one of the parents has insulin-dependent

diabetes (one in 20–40 if the father is affected and one in 40–80 if the mother is affected). Increased risk of DM exists among those who are HLA-DR3 or -DR4 and decreased risk in children with HLA-DR2 and -DR5.

- Molecular mimicry occurs between environmental triggers (viral infection, diet – cow's milk protein) and antigen on the surface of β cells of pancreas. This results in an autoimmune process which impairs the pancreatic β cells and leads to an absolute insulin deficiency.
- There is an association with other autoimmune disorders such as hypothyroidism.

Assessment Findings/Clinical Features

- Age at presentation – Uncommon before the age of 1 year. Incidence rises steadily from the early school age to a maximum at 12–13 years of age. The symptoms can be categorized as early and late manifestations.
- The early most common classical triad of symptoms include polydipsia, polyurea and weight loss (present only for few weeks) and develop secondary symptoms such as enuresis, skin sepsis and *Candida* and other infections.
- The late symptoms are mainly of ketoacidosis – As smell of acetone on breath (fruity smell), vomiting, dehydration, abdominal pain, hyperventilation as a result of acidosis (Kussmaul breathing), hypovolaemic shock, drowsiness and coma.

Diagnosis

Diagnosis is confirmed by raised random blood sugar level in a symptomatic child (>11.1 mmol/L by the WHO definition), glycosuria and ketonuria. In doubt, fasting blood sugar (>7.8 mmol/L) is also performed. Glucose tolerance test (GTT) is rarely required in children.

Management

Initial management depends on the child's condition. Those with diabetic ketoacidosis need urgent hospitalization. Children who are not in coma and are alert can eat, drink and be managed with insulin alone. If there is vomiting, intravenous fluids may be required to correct dehydration. Others can be cared at home with parental education by the diabetes team. Synthetic insulin which is chemically identical to human insulin has been synthesized by recombinant DNA technology or chemical modification of pork insulin. Pork (porcine) and cow's (bovine) pancreas-derived insulin is still available. Insulin is available as short-acting (Actrapid and Humulin S), medium-acting (Insulatard and Humulin I) and long-acting (Ultratard) formulations.

A number of mixed preparations are also available. Most available insulin is human insulin and is available in concentration of 100 U/mL. (Insulin types or species without prior consultation with diabetes team should not be interchanged.) Insulin may be injected into the subcutaneous tissues of the upper arm, lateral aspect of the thigh, abdomen and buttocks. Rotation of the injection site is essential to prevent lipohypertrophy or lipoatrophy (rare). Intradermal injection should be avoided as it produces scaring. In young children, insulin is given twice daily before breakfast and evening meals with a mixture of short-acting (30%) and medium-/long-acting insulin (70%). Older children and teenagers increasingly use three to four injections a day (basal bolus).

Diet – Insulin and diet regimen need to match to optimize metabolic control in order to maintain growth and development in growing children.

Blood glucose monitoring – Regular blood glucose profiles and blood glucose measurements are required when a low or high level is suspected. The aim is to maintain blood glucose level as close to normal (4–6 mmol/L) as possible. Urine ketone and glucose testing is to be regularly undertaken.

Nursing Diagnoses

- Activity intolerance
- Alteration in nutrition
- Alteration in the family process
- Fluid volume deficit
- Impairment of skin integrity
- Knowledge deficit
- Noncompliance sensory–perceptual alteration
- Self-concept disturbances
- Social isolation

Nursing Interventions

- Use exchange lists for meats, vegetables, fruits, breads, milk and fats to plan three meals and two snacks (midafternoon and evening) per day.
- Distribute calories throughout the day to avoid hyperglycaemic peaks and hypoglycaemic episodes.
- Teach JDM children to include some of their favourite foods into the exchange system.
- Use sugar-free substitutes.
- Educate parents/child as soon as possible the following:
  - Basic understanding of the pathophysiology of DM
  - Three pronged approach to management: Insulin, diet and exercise
  - Concept of chronicity: Controllable but not curable
  - Glucose testing and blood glucose monitoring: Why, how and when?
  - Recording and reporting results
  - Urine testing for sugar and ketones: How and when?
  - Injection of insulin: What kind/s, how to administer, when to give, what it does, action (onset, peak and duration), sites and need of site rotation
  - Hypoglycaemia: Signs and symptoms, treatment and prevention
  - Hyperglycaemia and ketonuria: Signs and symptoms, management, aetiologies and prevention
- After 3–4 weeks of initial education, review and reinforce the previous education with additional points as follows:
  - Diet: Matching food intake with insulin and exercise
  - Normal nutrition incorporating cultural preferences and adjustments for growth changes, exercises, guideline for illness, eating away from home

- Adolescent need to be warned about crash diets
- Importance of exercise on insulin demand and blood sugar
- Hygiene: Treatment of cuts and injuries and scratches, importance of regular eye and dental examinations; this is not so frequent like adults but need to be every 3–5 years), correct nail trimming, foot care and preventing injuries to extremities
- Complications of diabetes need to emphasized and teach about precautions to be followed.
- Discussion of effects of diabetes on future plans:
  - Sexuality
  - Marriage and childbearing
  - Career
  - Regular review of growth and pubertal development, as there is some delay in the onset of puberty.
  - Obesity is also a problem, especially in females if their insulin dose is not adjusted.
  - Blood pressure (BP) must be checked for evidence of hypertension.
  - In renal disease, detection of microalbuminuria is an early sign of nephropathy.
  - Eyes: Retinopathy or cataract is rare, but check-ups must be conducted every 5 years.
  - Feet: Encourage to take good care of feet.
  - Other associated illnesses: Thyroid diseases and coeliac diseases are easily missed.
- Self-management and problem solving:
  - Evaluation should be done with follow-up, as the child has no hypoglycaemic attack and hyperglycaemic episodes.
  - Consistently perform basic survival skills: Blood sugar monitoring, urine testing, taking insulin self, identify the signs and symptoms of hyper- and hypoglycaemia, seek assistance as and when required.

Adolescent Diabetes

Diabetes in children has many after-effects.
- Delayed physical and sexual maturation
- Invasion of privacy with frequent medical examinations
- Difficulty in conformity with the peer group, as they have fixed meal
- Problems of self-image and self-esteem related to parental overprotection and reluctance to allow their child to be away from home and they battle over diabetes

Hypoglycaemia

The blood glucose level is lower than normal and occurs relatively quickly in diabetes.

It results from decreased caloric intake, increased exercise, overdosage of insulin or gastroenteritis.

It is a common problem in neonates and is rare after this period in normal infants. The common causes of hypoglycaemia in infants and children beyond neonatal period are as follows:
- Insulin excess
- B-cell tumours
- Drug induced
- Beckwith syndrome

- Liver diseases and hormonal deficiency
- Fasting

Other causes are galactosaemia, fructose intolerance, maternal diabetes, etc.

Sign and Symptoms

Sweating, pallor, central nervous system (CNS) signs of irritability, headache, seizures and coma

Multidisciplinary Management

- Administration of intravenous dextrose 2–4 mL/kg of 10% to prevent permanent damage to the brain.
- Care must be taken to avoid excess volume. Corticosteroids may also be given if there is a possibility of hypopituitarism.

Nursing Diagnosis

- Activity intolerance
- Alteration in comfort: Pain
- Potential for injury
- Sensory–perceptual alteration

Goal

The child's blood sugar will remain within normal limits.

Nursing Interventions

- For mild attacks, give food that increases the glucose level (e.g. sugar, honey, orange juice, milk).
- For moderate attacks, give concentrated sugar solution.
- Educate parents and other close relatives to detect early signs and symptoms of hypoglycaemia.
- Instruct them to keep easily available glucose or sugar preparations to manage hypoglycaemia.

Diabetic Ketoacidosis

It is a possible complication of DM in which there is low pH and reduced bicarbonate concentration in the blood as a result of accumulation of ketone bodies.

Signs and symptoms are already described along with DM.

Management

- Intravenous fluids: In shock, initial resuscitation is with normal saline to correct dehydration over 48 hours. Rapid rehydration should be avoided, as it may lead to cerebral oedema. Monitor fluid intake and output, electrolytes, creatinine and acid–base status regularly, as well as central venous pressure (CVP).
- Insulin either bolus (half intravenous, half subcutaneous) or continuous infusion adjusted according to blood sugar level.
- Potassium (when urine output is established) level is adjusted according to blood levels and ECG changes.
- Bicarbonate is administered to correct acidosis if necessary, as acidosis will be self-corrected with fluids and insulin therapy.

- Re-establish oral fluids or nasogastric tube feedings but do not stop intravenous insulin until subcutaneous insulin has been given.
- Insert Foley catheter, if necessary.
- Treatment of the underlying causes, such as infection or trauma or noncompliance to treatment that triggers the episode.

Nursing Diagnoses

- Alteration in cardiac output
- Fluid volume deficit
- Ineffective breathing pattern
- Potential for injury
- Sensory–perceptual alteration

Nursing Intervention

- Record changes in laboratory values and report significant deviation.
- Monitor intravenous infusion rates and adjust rates as ordered to maintain blood sugar within normal limits.
- Monitor cardiac rhythm, serum potassium and regulate intravenous potassium, as ordered.

Evaluation

The child's blood sugar and serum potassium are within normal limits, and ECG is normal; no vomiting and abdominal pain; and the child is alert and oriented.

Hypothyroidism

Severe maternal hypothyroidism can affect the developing brain of the fetus as in the normal case; there is only minimum transfer of thyroxin from the mother to the fetus. Fetal thyroid predominantly produce reverse T3, which is largely inactive.

Congenital hypothyroidism needs to be detected as early as possible to prevent cretinism. The prevalence is high – one in 4000 live births. This is a preventable cause of mental retardation, too. The causes are as follows:

- Maldescent of thyroid or athyrosis
- Dyshormonogenesis – Inborn errors of thyroid hormone synthesis
- Iodine deficiency
- Hypothyroidism as a result of TSH deficiency

Assessment Findings

Congenital	Acquired
FTT	Short stature
Feeding problem	Cold intolerance
Prolonged jaundice	Dry skin
Constipation	Cold peripheries
Pale, cold and mottled dry skin	Thin, dry hair
Coarse facies	Pale, puffy eyes with loss of eyebrows
Large tongue	Goitre
Hoarse cry	Slow relaxing reflexes
Goitre	Constipation
Umbilical hernia	Learning difficulties

Diabetes Insipidus

It is characterized by profound ADH (antidiuretic hormone) deficiency or is related to decreased renal responsiveness to ADH. Deficiency of ADH synthesis in the hypothalamus or decreased release from the posterior pituitary may be nephrogenic in origin, resulting from decreased water permeability of collecting tubules as a result of decreased ADH effect. The after-effect of the same may produce dehydration, hypotension, hypovolaemic shock and increased blood viscosity with risks of thromboembolism.

Assessment Findings

- Increased excretion of large qualities (5–10 L per day) of hypotonic urine
- Extreme thirst
- Altered level of consciousness (LOC), orthostatic hypotension
- Poor skin turgor, dry mucous membrane
- Vital signs: respiratory rate will be abnormal if ICP is increased
- Heart rate is increased; BP is decreased; temperature may be increased if the ICP is increased
- CVP decreases
- Urine osmolality decreases to 200 mOsm/kg
- Serum osmolality increases to 300 mOsm/kg
- Increased serum Na >147 mEq/L
- Plasma ADH is decreased

Multidisciplinary Management

- Water deprivation test: Monitor and asses the baseline weight, serum/urine osmolality, urine specific gravity, etc.
- Measure every hourly the aforementioned variables.
- Prohibit fluid intake.
- Assess for negative results:
  - Urine specific gravity >1.020
  - Urine osmolality >800 mOsm/kg
- Assess for positive results:
  - ≥5% of body weight loss
  - Urine specific gravity not to increase for three consecutive hourly measurements
- Vasopressin test:
  - Administer vasopressin subcutaneously.
  - Urine specimens are collected every 30 minutes for 2 hours and evaluated for quantity and osmolality. Urine osmolality generally increases significantly in response to ADH unless diabetes insipidus is nephrogenic in origin.
- Medical treatment includes rehydration with hypotonic solutions to replace fluid/weight loss.
- Rapid rehydration is advised until the child is stabilized and then administer as per urine output.
- Administer exogenous vasopressin.
- Administer thiazide diuretics; low Na, low-protein diets are advised in nephrogenic diabetes insipidus.

Nursing Diagnoses

- Fluid volume deficit
- Risk for injury

- Altered peripheral tissue perfusion
- Altered cerebral perfusion/altered sensorium
- Parental anxiety
- Knowledge deficit

Nursing Interventions

- Keep careful intake and output records.
- Be alert for urine output more than 200 mL per hour for two consecutive hours.
- Additional fluid therapy may be required for such a child.
- Provide adequate fluids.
- Administer hyperosmolar tube feedings or solutions with extra caution (as it can cause osmotic diarrhoea).
- Administer intravenous fluids as prescribed.
- Administer vasopressin: Document its effects/side effects.
- Weigh the child daily at the same time and using the same scale and garments to prevent errors in recordings.
- Monitor for continued fluid deficit, poor skin turgor, dry mucous membrane, rapid and thready pulse and CVP.
- Monitor serum Na, serum urine osmolality and urine specific gravity to evaluate response to therapy.
- Monitor orientation, LOC and respiratory status.
- Keep oral airway, manual resuscitator and mask and supplemental oxygen at the bedside for intervening emergency.
- Reduce the likelihood of injury caused by falls by keeping bed rails on.
- Place a gastric tube for intermittent suction in comatose children to decrease the likelihood of aspiration.
- Elevate head end of bed to 45° to minimize risk of aspiration.
- Initiate seizure precautions, if needed.
- Monitor haematocrit with proper fluid replacement. The values should return to normal limits.
- Assess peripheral pulses. Be alert for decreased amplitude or absence of pulses.

- Be alert to signs and symptoms of deep vein thrombosis, erythema, pain and tenderness, warmth, swelling, bluish discolouration, prominence of superficial veins, especially in lower extremities.
- Assist in range-of-motion (ROM) exercises to all extremities 4 hourly to increase blood flow to tissues.
- Provide proper parental and child education to prevent complications of injury, altered LOC, decreased peripheral tissue perfusion, etc. along with treatment protocols.

STUDY QUESTIONS

- What is juvenile diabetes?
- How will you manage a child with juvenile diabetes mellitus?
- What are the features of ketoacidosis?
- How will you manage a child with hyperglycaemia?
- Differentiate between hypoglycaemia and hyperglycaemia.
- Write short notes on the following:
  a. Diabetic insipidus
  b. Hypothyroidism
  c. Insulin administration

BIBLIOGRAPHY

1. Ansley- Green A, Polack JAM, Bloom SR. et al (1981). Nesidioblastosis of the Pancreas. Definition of the syndrome and the management of the severe neonatal hyperinsulinemic hypoglycemia. Arch. Dis. Child 54:496.
2. Pilliteri A. (2007). Maternal and Child Health Nursing Care of the Child bearing and rearing family. 5th edn. Philadelphia: Lippincott Williams & Wilkins, 1506-1538.
3. Pollack ES, Pollack CV Jr. (1993). Ketotic hypoglycemia: A case report. J Emerg Med. 11:531.
4. Tyrala EE, Chen X, Boden G. (1994). Glucose metabolism in the infant weighing less than 1100 gms. J Paediatr 125:283.
5. Wong DL and Hockenberry MJ. (2003). Wong's Nursing care of Infants and children. 7th edn, Mosby. 1703-1756.

CHAPTER 35

ALTERATION IN MUSCULOSKELETAL FUNCTIONS: NURSING MANAGEMENT OF CHILDREN WITH MUSCULOSKELETAL DISORDERS

LEARNING OBJECTIVES

At the end of the chapter, the learner will be able to:

- Identify the essential concepts and consequences of abnormal embryonic development of the musculoskeletal system.
- Describe nursing management of children suffering from various musculoskeletal disorders.

The musculoskeletal system includes bones, joints, muscles and connective tissue. These components work in harmony to produce the actions that allow a child's independence in exploration and discovery. The skeleton is the framework of the human body, but the muscles produce movement by exerting a force on the bones to which they are attached. This unit describes the essential concepts related to development of the musculoskeletal system and the consequences of abnormal development.

EMBRYONIC DEVELOPMENT

Development of the musculoskeletal system is controlled by genetic make-up. However, environmental factors in utero can also affect the developing fetus. During the third week after conception, three germ layers (ectoderm, mesoderm and endoderm) are formed from the inner cell mass of the embryo and give rise to all the tissues and organs of the developing fetus. The musculoskeletal system is derived from the mesoderm layer.

Skeleton

Bone formation begins during the eighth week of gestation and involves the delivery of bone cell precursors to the sites of bone formation and aggregation of these cells at the primary centre of ossification. During the early fetal life, the fetal skeleton mainly consists of hyaline cartilage that eventually undergoes ossification and bone formation. Intramembranous ossification occurs when osteoblasts are in the flat form and secrete a matrix that calcifies and acts as a precursor to osteocytes. This network of matrix and osteocytes forms the basis of the spongy bone. Endochondral ossification is the means by which cartilage develops into bone in the long bones. This ossification begins in the shaft (diaphysis) and the ends (epiphysis) of the long bones. The formation of bones from cartilage continues until two thin strips remain at the ends of the bones (epiphyseal plates). Any teratogenic insult to these plates may result in abnormal growth patterns for the child during prenatal and postnatal growth and development. During the fourth week of gestation, the upper buds appear and are followed by the lower limbs around the seventh week. The cephalocaudal growth pattern is retained throughout embryonic development.

Joints

Joints begin to develop during the sixth week of intrauterine life (IUL) and by the end of the eighth week, they closely resemble adult joints. Synovial joints (e.g. knee and elbow) are formed when mesoderm between the bones forms a capsule and differentiates into articular cartilage and synovial membranes. The resulting space forms the joint cavity. Fibrocartilaginous joints are formed when the mesoderm between the developing bones differentiates into hyaline cartilage (e.g. costo-chondral joints) and fibrocartilage (e.g. symphysis pubis). Fibrous joints are formed when the mesoderm in the joint differentiates into dense fibrous connective tissue (e.g. sutures of the skull).

Vertebral Column and Ribs

During the fourth week of gestation, mesodermal cells from the somites migrate and form the vertebral column dorsally and the ribs ventrally. Ossification becomes evident in the vertebral column around the eighth week. By the 40th week of gestation, the vertebral column consists of three bony parts – the centrum and two halves of the vertebral arch – which are all connected by cartilage. The ribs form from the meso-dermal costal processes of the thoracic vertebrae. Initially, the ribs are cartilaginous, but by the 13th to 14th weeks, they begin to ossify.

Skull

The fetal skull develops from the mesoderm surround-ing the developing brain. The fetal skull separates into the parietal, frontal, temporal and occipital bones by weeks 20–24. These bones are separated by dense con-nective tissue membranes that form fibrous joints called sutures. The fibrous areas where the sutures meet are called fontanels. These sutures and fontanels enable the fetal skull to accommodate brain growth and to change shape during the birth process. This accommodation of the fetal cranial vault is called moulding.

Muscles

All muscles except those of the ribs are formed from myoblasts that are derived from the mesoderm. The skeletal muscles show their classic cross-striations and multinucleations by the 12th week. Smooth muscles evolve from myoblasts that elongate and develop con-tractile characteristics. Cardiac muscles are formed from the splanchnic mesoderm that surrounds the heart tubes during the third week. The first heartbeat occurs around the fourth week of gestation.

Ultrasonography can detect fetal muscle movement in the neck, trunk and limbs by the seventh week. By the 11th week, the fetus demonstrates sucking and swallow-ing reflexes. The 12th week brings about fetal responses to skin stimulation. By the end of the 12th week, the fetus can bend, flux and turn its body all around the uterus. However, these movements are so minute and weak that they cannot be felt by the mother. The fetal movements can usually be felt by the 20th week, and this initial motion of the fetus in the uterus is called quickening.

CONSEQUENCES OF ABNORMAL DEVELOPMENT

The period during which limb development is critical is from 24 to 42 days after fertilization. Consequently, any environmental or teratogenic agent which a pregnant woman is exposed to or ingests during this crucial time may result in congenital anomalies or musculoskeletal deformities. Genetic factors over which the parents have no control may also cause these abnormalities. Interruption in the normal development of the musculoskeletal system during the prenatal period can have deleterious effects on the spinal column, hips and limbs, creating serious problems with ambulation and activities of daily living. Prenatal detection of fetal abnormalities can be done through the maternal history and physical examination, ultrasonography, radiological studies, fetoscopy and blood tests.

Fetal Age	Structure	Anomalies
4 weeks	Neural tube, spinal column	Spina bifida
4 weeks	Limbs	Amelia (absence of limbs)
5–6 weeks	Limbs	Meromelia (partial absence of limbs)
5–6 weeks	Maxilla, palate	Cleft palate
6 weeks	Upper lip	Cleft lip
6–7 weeks	Ankles, feet	Talipes equinovarus (congenital clubfoot)
Through out	Limbs	Amniotic band deformi-ties, constriction bands and amputations
Through out	Acetabulum	Congenital hip dysplasia

NURSING MANAGEMENT OF CHILDREN WITH ALTERATION IN MUSCULOSKELETAL FUNCTIONS

Bone Tumours

A vast majority of bone tumours in children are benign. But there are few aggressive and malignant tumours. The common benign tumours are desmoid tumours, haeman-giomas, neurofibromatosis, vascular malformations, an-eurismal bone cyst, Baker cyst, chondroblastomas, etc.

Osteogenic Sarcoma

Definition – It is the malignant tumour originating from osteoblasts (bone-forming cells). The incidence is more common in boys than in girls (2:1 ratio).

Assessment Findings

- Usually located at the end of long bones (metaphysis)
- Mostly seen at the distal end of the femur or proximal end of the tibia

- Presenting symptoms are pain at site, swelling and limitation of movement
- Common site of metastasis is lung

Multidisciplinary Management

- Diagnosis by X-rays and bone scan along with clinical features
- Nursing diagnoses
- Comfort alteration in pain
- Impaired physical mobility
- High risk for injury
- Parental anxiety
- Body image disturbances

Nursing Interventions

- Provide care for amputation, followed by chemotherapy.
- Administer chemotherapeutics and monitor frequently used drugs:
  - Vincristine
  - Cytoxan
  - Actinomycin D
- Provide parental support.
- Involve parents in care.

Ewing Sarcoma

Definition – It is the malignant tumour of the bone originating from myeloblasts, with early metastasis to lung lymph node and other bones.

Assessment Findings

- Usually located on the shaft of the long bones – femur, tibia and humerus
- Pain at site, swelling and tenderness
- Increased temperature
- Multidisciplinary management
- Diagnosis is by X-rays, signs and symptoms and bone scan
- Amputation
- Radiotherapy
- Chemotherapy
- Treatment of side effects and symptomatic management

Nursing Diagnoses

- Comfort alteration in pain
- Parental anxiety
- Body image

Nursing Interventions

- Prepare and assist for amputation.
- Provide postoperative care.
- Prepare for chemotherapy and radiation.
- Administer chemotherapy.
- Watch for side effects of chemotherapy and radiation.
- Treat the side effects of chemotherapy and radiation.

- Encourage inclusion of parents and children in the care.
- Listen to parents, child and siblings as they express denial, anger and acceptance and allow them their grieving process.
- Promote age-appropriate activities and group discussion with peers.
- Assist parents in avoiding overprotection.

Congenital Dislocation of the Hip

Definition – It is the malrotation of the hip at birth. The exact cause is unknown.

Assessment Findings

- Unequal major gluteal folds
- Presence of a hip click on abduction
- Femur may appear shortened

Multidisciplinary Management

- Complete history, case finding and referral
- Application of splint with good alignment
- Protection of skin under splint
- Bryant's traction

Nursing Diagnoses

- Impaired mobility
- High risk for impaired skin integrity
- Parental anxiety

Nursing Interventions

- Educate parents how to apply splint and maintain splint alignment.
- Protect skin under the splint.
- Provide age-appropriate adequate play materials/toys and avoid boredom.
- Maintain hip flexion and abduction.
- Provide double diapering.
- Monitor Bryant's traction.
- Provide parents support.

Congenital Clubfoot (Talipes Equinovarus)

Definition – It is a congenital deformity in which the foot has a club-like appearance, whereby the inner area of the foot is turned up, anterior half of the foot is adducted and the foot is in plantar flexion.

Assessment Findings

- Foot deformity is usually accompanied by other problems such as neurological defects or spina bifida.
- Assess general health status to provide treatment.

Multidisciplinary Management

Three stages of treatment are exercise, manipulation, casting and splint.

1. Provide passive exercises (manipulation) of the foot.
2. Demonstrate the same to parents.
3. Apply the cast and Denis–Browne splint.

Nursing Diagnoses

- Parental anxiety
- Impaired mobility
- Nursing interventions
- Assist in passive exercise
- Demonstrate it to parents (hold in position to the count of 10 and continue for 10 minutes several times a day).
- Provide cast care (change frequently).
- Assist in care of the infant with a splint.
- Instruct parents in cast care/splint care.

Osteomyelitis

Definition – It is an infection of the long bones caused mainly by *Staphylococcus aureus*. It is most common in boys between 5 and 15 years of age.

Assessment Findings

- Abrupt onset
- Fever, malaise and pain, localized tenderness in the bone at the metaphysis
- Swelling and redness over the affected bone

Multidisciplinary Management

- Antibacterial therapy
- Control of pain by nonsteroidal anti-inflammatory drugs (NSAIDs)
- Immobilization

Nursing Diagnoses

- Comfort alteration in pain
- Impaired mobility
- Diversional activity deficit

Nursing Interventions

- Administer antibiotics, as prescribed.
- Increase the fluid intake.
- Administer analgesics (NSAIDs).
- Immobilize the affected limb.
- Control movements.
- Provide diversional activities such as painting and crafts, passive games (snake and ladder, chess) and interaction with peers.

Scoliosis

It is the lateral curvature of the spine. There are two types of scoliosis: 'C'-shaped and 'S'-shaped. A young child has a greater chance of developing deformity. Deformity increases during growth periods and is not noticed until adolescence. Girls are more affected than boys.

Types of Spine Deformities

Kyphosis – It is a flexion deformity at the thoracic spine.
Lordosis – It is a fixed extension deformity that usually occurs to compensate for other abnormalities.
Scoliosis – It is the lateral curvature of the spine and can be nonstructural. Scoliosis is caused by changes outside the spine and treated with exercises. In *structural scoliosis*, the spine itself is rotated and is treated by bracing, exercises and insertion of the Harrington rod or the Luque procedure.

Assessment Findings

- Fatigue, dyspnoea and backache
- History of breathing difficulty
- On examination, difference in shoulder height, elbow level and height of iliac crests.
- Associated deviation of hips, rib cage, shoulders and iliac crest
- Mild pain and discomfort

Multidisciplinary Management

- Application of the Milwaukee brace
- Strict skin care under the brace

Operative Management

- Harrington rod is used in decortication of the bone over the laminar and spinous processes.
- Bone graft from the iliac crest is inserted to achieve fusion of the vertebrae.
- Rods are inserted along the vertebrae and attached by Harrington hooks.
- Postoperative casting is achieved.

Luque Procedure

- Wire loops are placed under the lamina at the vertebral level.
- Steel rods are aligned along the curvature of the spine and fixed to the spine with wires.

Nursing Diagnoses

- Body image disturbances
- Comfort alteration in pain
- Parental anxiety
- Complication potential

Nursing Interventions

- Assist in laboratory investigations.
- Provide age-appropriate preoperative preparation to the child and the family.
- Assess the pulmonary function.
- Teach postoperative exercise, deep breathing, coughing, etc. preoperatively.
- Provide parental support.
- Provide postoperative care.

- Check vital signs every 15 minutes until stable and thereafter hourly for 12 hours, 2 hourly for 24 hours and 4 hourly for 48 hours.
- Watch for hypovolaemia, tachycardia, blood pressure, etc.
- Assess respiratory function postoperatively, breath sounds, respiratory rate, chest excursion, colour, grunting, flaring and retractions.
- Check arterial blood gases (ABGs).
- Maintain strict intake and output (I&O) chart and monitor urine output hourly.
- Check colour, movement and sensation (CMS) of lower extremities hourly for 8 hours, every 2 hours for 24 hours and then 4 hourly.
- Turn the child only by logrolling.
- Maintain spine alignment.
- Provide pain medications for respiratory depression from narcotics.
- Maintain nothing by mouth (NPO) until bowel sounds return.
- Start diet with sips of clear fluid.
- Watch for paralytic ileus.
- Provide skin care and prevent skin breakdown and bedsores.
- Provide patient education.
- Children with a Harrington rod can get up in 1–2 weeks after the cast has been applied.
- Cast stays for 6 months.
- After removal of the cast, the Milwaukee brace is worn for support for approximately 3 months and can be removed at night.
- In the Luque procedure, the child can get up 3–5 days postoperatively.
- No immobilization is required.
- Follow-up is essential and must be emphasized.

Fracture

Definition – Any break in the continuity of bone is called fracture. A child's bone can be bent up to 45° before breaking.

Types

Greenstick – It is a crack and bending of the bone with an incomplete fracture and affects one side of the periosteum.

Comminuted fracture – It is a bone broken completely in a transverse, spiral or oblique direction or may be broken into pieces.

Open or compound fracture – The bone is exposed to air through a break in the skin.

Closed or simple fracture – The bone is broken, but the skin remains intact.

Compression – The fractured bone is compressed by other bones.

Complete – The bone is broken with disruption of both sides of the periosteum.

Impacted fracture – One part of the fractured bone is driven into another.

Depressed fracture – Fragmented bone are driven inward.

Assessment Findings

- Cardinal signs
- Pain or tenderness over the involved area
- Loss of function of extremity
- Deformity – Overriding, angulations (limb in an unnatural position)
- Crepitation – Sound of grafting bone fragments
- Ecchymosis or erythema
- Oedema
- Muscle spasm
- Patients may present with signs of anxiety and readiness for treatment

Multidisciplinary Management

- Diagnosis is made by signs and symptoms; X-rays are obtained to find out the exact location and type of fracture.
- Treatment is by traction and reduction.
- Reduction can be either open reduction or closed reduction.
- Closed reduction – Manual manipulation is usually done under anaesthesia to control pain and muscle relaxation to prevent complications.
- Apply cast after closed reduction.
- Open reduction – It is the surgical intervention with internal fixation devices such as screws, plates, wires, etc.
- Cast is applied after wound care.

Nursing Diagnoses

- Pain anxiety
- Complication potential for hypovolaemic shock
- High risk for injury/infection

Nursing Interventions

- Provide emergency care of fracture.
- Immobilize the affected extremity to prevent further damage to soft tissue and nerves.
- Institute triage by primary initial assessment.
- In compound fracture, do not attempt to reduce the fracture.
- Apply splint (an external support is applied around the fracture to immobilize the broken ends).
- Any hard materials can be used as splints (wood, magazines, plastics, etc.).
- Splinting helps prevent additional trauma, reduces pain, limits movement and prevents complications such as fat embolism in long bone fractures.
- Monitor traction as the treatment of fracture.
  Traction can be either skeletal traction or skin traction.
  Skeletal tractions – Mechanical tractions are applied to bone using pins (Steinmann), wires (Kirschner) or tongs (Crutchfield). It is used in fractures of femur, tibia and humerus.
  Balanced suspension tractions – These are used along with skeletal or skin traction (e.g. Thomas splint with Pearson attachment) and help in producing a counterforce.

*Skin traction*s – These are applied with the help of elastic bandages, Mole skin strips or adhesives.

Common types are Russell's traction, Buck's traction, cervical traction or temporary cervical immobilization and pelvic traction.

- Maintain alignment through proper care of traction.
- Ensure that weights hang freely and do not touch the floor.
- Ensure that pulleys are not obstructed.
- Check the ropes in the pulley to see they move freely.
- Secure a knot in the rope to prevent slipping.
- Maintain proper body alignment.
- Do not remove or lift weights without specific order.
- Cover sharp edges of the traction to prevent injury.
- Provide proper cast care.
- Allow 24–48 hours for drying for plaster of Paris (for synthetic cast, 30 minutes is enough).
- Do not handle cast during the drying process, as it creates indentation from finger marks and can cause skin breakdown.
- Keep extremity elevated to prevent oedema.
- Observe the casted extremity for signs of circulatory atrophy.
- Provide and teach isometric exercise to prevent muscle atrophy.
- Provide a comfortable position with pillows to prevent strain on the unaffected extremity or areas.
- Provide passive exercises, as required.
- Observe skin and traction frequently to prevent skin breakdown.

STUDY QUESTIONS

- What are the common types of bone tumours?
- What is congenital dislocation of hip? How will you provide nursing care to a baby with congenital dislocation of hip?
- What are the nurse's responsibilities while providing care to a child with a compound fracture?
- What are the responsibilities of a nurse in caring a child with hip spica?
- Write short notes on the following:
  a. Talipes equinovarus
  b. Osteomyelitis
  c. Scoliosis
  d. Ewing sarcoma

BIBLIOGRAPHY

1. Brosnan, H. (1991). Nursing Management of the Adolescents with Idiopathic Scoliosis. Nursing Clinics of North America, 26(1), pp 17–31.
2. Butler, A.B., Salmond, S.W., Pellino, T.A. (1994). Orthopaedic Nursing. Philadelphia: W.B. Saunders.
3. Hansell, M.J. (1988). Fracture and Healing Process. Orthopaedic Nursing, 7(1), pp 43–49.
4. Rose, C.D. (1992). Pharmacological Management of Juvenile Rheumatoid Arthritis. Drugs, 43(6), pp 849–863.
5. Voznak, L. (1988). My Life with Scoliosis. Orthopaedic Nursing, 7(1), pp 22–26.

CHAPTER 36

NURSING MANAGEMENT OF CHILDREN WITH EYE, EAR, NOSE AND THROAT DISORDERS

CHAPTER OUTLINE

- Amblyopia
- Conjunctivitis (Pink Eye)
- Chalazion
- Stye
- Preseptal or Orbital Cellulitis
- Cortical Visual Impairment (CVI)
- Developmental Abnormalities
  - Double Vision or Diplopia
  - Genetic Eye Disease

- Congenital Glaucoma
- Refractive Errors
- Paediatric Cataract
- Paediatric Glaucoma
- Prevention of Eye Injuries
- Tonsillitis
- Peritonsillar Abscess (PTA)
- Otitis Media

LEARNING OBJECTIVES

At the end of the chapter, the learner will be able to:
- Discuss various infections affecting the eye.
- Explain the refractive errors.
- Describe the nursing management of children with paediatric cataract.
- Describe the nursing management of children with paediatric glaucoma.
- Discuss various measures to prevent eye injuries in children.
- Describe the nursing management of a child with tonsillitis.
- Explain the medical and nursing management of a child undergoing myringotomy.

There are many eye conditions and disorders that affect children and their vision. The common focus and alignment disorders and infections are discussed in this section. Early diagnosis and treatment are very essential to maintain vision and eye health in children.

AMBLYOPIA

Amblyopia is a term used to describe poor vision in one of the eyes of a child who has not developed complete normal vision. It is seen in early childhood and is otherwise called 'lazy eye'. It occurs when visual acuity is much better in one eye than in the other. Amblyopia is common and affects 2%–3% of children.

Aetiology

Usual causes are as follows:
- Strabismus (misaligned eyes)
- Refractive error
- Disruption of light passing through the eye (e.g. paediatric cataract)

Clinical Features

- Signs and symptoms to watch for include misaligned eyes
- Squinting in one eye
- Bumping into objects or other signs of poor depth perception
- Head tilting
- Double vision

Diagnosis and Treatment

- Amblyopia therapy includes glasses, patching, eye drops and sometimes surgery.
- If recognized early (in preschool years), amblyopia generally responds well to treatment.
- If recognized later (after 9–10 years of age), amblyopia is much more difficult to treat and the child may have permanent vision loss.

ASTIGMATISM

It is a blurred vision. Objects both at near and far are seen blurred. This causes uneven curvature of the cornea and lens, preventing light rays to focus on a single point on the retina. Astigmatism usually occurs along with myopia (nearsightedness) or hyperopia (farsightedness).

PTOSIS

It is the drooping of upper eyelid that covers the eye either somewhat or entirely, thus blocking the vision.

CHILDHOOD TEARING

It is called epiphora. It is often noted soon after birth and can develop later, too. This causes chronic irritation and infection of the eye. In infancy, it results from blockage of the tear drainage system. It usually heals itself by 6–12 months. Management is massage of the tear sac and eye drops. It requires detailed examination to find out whether the cause is paediatric glaucoma.

CONJUNCTIVITIS (PINK EYE)

Conjunctivitis is the inflammation of the conjunctiva as a result of bacterial or viral infection. It is very contagious. It can also result from allergic reactions.

Clinical Features

Red or pink eyes result from inflammation of the conjunctiva.
A thin filmy membrane covers the inside of eyelids or sclera of the eye.
Tearing with discharge is present.
Itchy eyes may also be present.
It can be uncomfortable.
If it is a result of viral infection, the child may have runny nose, sore throat and fever.
If conjunctivitis is contagious, the child should be kept at home to prevent the spread and instruct the child to take care of the eyes if the child can comprehend.
It will take 3–7 days to resolve conjunctivitis.

CHALAZION

It is a small lump on the eyelid and may occur when a Meibomian gland is clogged. It is not related to infection.

STYE

It is a red sore lump near the edge of the eyelid and is caused by an infected eyelash follicle.

PRESEPTAL OR ORBITAL CELLULITIS

It is an infection related to trauma or upper respiratory tract infection. The tissue around the eye appears red and is swollen. It is painful, and the child will have fever. It requires medical treatment.

CORTICAL VISUAL IMPAIRMENT

Cortical visual impairment (CVI) is the vision loss as a result of abnormality of the visual centre in the brain. The eyes are normal, but the visual interpretation centre in the brain does not function properly and prevents normal vision.

DEVELOPMENTAL ABNORMALITIES

During development of the fetus, certain abnormalities in the visual system can occur. These are coloboma, microphthalmia (small eye) and optic nerve hypoplasia. These abnormalities cause vision loss in children.

Double Vision or Diplopia

This is caused by misalignment of the eyes (strabismus), which make one to see an object in two different places at the same time. The object can be displaced in a horizontal, vertical or diagonal fashion. Double vision can result from many conditions and should be evaluated at the time of onset. Usual treatment is strabismus correction surgery, prism glass and Botox injection.

Genetic Eye Disease

Many eye diseases have a known genetic abnormality. These diseases are often inherited and frequently there are other family members who have had the disease. In cases of known inherited eye disease in the family, early evaluation is important along with genetic counselling.

Congenital Glaucoma

It is a disease that results from damage of the optic nerve. Elevated eye pressure is the most common risk factor. This pressure can damage the optic nerve. Optic nerve is very critical in proper vision. Congenital glaucoma is seen at birth and can also be seen in childhood.

Signs and symptoms of paediatric glaucoma are cloudy cornea, tearing, frequent blinking, light sensitivity and redness of the eye.

REFRACTIVE ERRORS

Hyperopia (Farsightedness)

It is a condition in which a person can see distant objects more clearly than near objects. Typically, the farsighted eye is smaller than the normal eye. As a result, light rays do not focus properly on the retina at the back of the eye and causes blurring.

Aetiology

It can be inherited. Infants and young children are typically somewhat farsighted, but this lessens as the eye grows. Certain children have a higher amount of hyperopia, leading to constant blurring of images in one or both eyes and prevent normal eye development (amblyopia). If it is not recognized in time, then it will lead to permanent eye damage and visual loss. Hyperopia in children can cause inward crossing of the eyes (usually seen in children between 2 and 7 years of age).

Treatment

Appropriate eye glasses can be used to correct strabismus.

Myopia (Nearsightedness)

It is a condition in which children can see near objects more clearly than distant objects. In myopia, the light from distance objects focuses before it reaches the retina, causing blurred vision. Excessive myopia causes amblyopia or lazy eye. Children will hold objects very close to the eye. This is an indication for adults to suspect myopia in children.

Treatment is correction according to the cause, e.g. glasses or corrective surgery.

Nystagmus

Nystagmus is an involuntary, rhythmic oscillation of the eyes. The eye movements can be side-to-side, up and down or rotary. It may result from abnormal binocular fixation early in life. It may be present at birth or acquired later in life. A number of eye disorders and neurological disorders can be seen along with nystagmus.

PAEDIATRIC CATARACT

Description: Cataract is the opacity or cloudiness of the lens. The lens appears grey or milky. According to the World Health Organization, cataract is the leading cause of blindness worldwide. Paediatric cataract is one of the most treatable causes of childhood blindness. The management of paediatric cataract is more challenging and demanding than adult cataract management.

The prevalence of childhood cataract has been reported as 1–15 cases in 10,000 children in the developing countries. It is estimated that, globally, there are 200,000 blind children as a result of bilateral cataract.

Aetiology of Childhood Cataract

The main causes of infantile cataract are genetic, metabolic disorders, prematurity and intrauterine infections (TORCH infections). Other causes of cataract in older children include trauma, drug-induced causes, radiation and laser therapy for retinopathy of prematurity (ROP). Trauma is one of the commonest causes of unilateral cataract in the developing countries. Bilateral cataracts occur commonly as a result of the long-term use of topical or systemic steroid, ergot alkaloids, dinitrophenol, naphthalene or extended exposure to ultraviolet rays (toxic cataract). Inherited cataracts contribute significantly in the aetiology of childhood cataract. Zonular cataract is the commonest type of congenital cataract.

Clinical Features

First symptom is a white or partially white reflex noted by the parents. In unilateral cataract, strabismus may be the initial manifestation, and nystagmus or poor visual fixation may be seen in bilateral lens opacities during infancy.

Children who can verbalize may complain of **blurred vision** and may be frequently rubbing their eyes in an attempt to clear the vision. They may complain of glare (pain felt when looking directly to light).

Halos and double vision may be present.

Diagnosis

It includes ocular examination for visual acuity assessment, pupillary response and ocular motility.

The slit lamp biomicroscopic examination is performed to evaluate the size, density and location of cataract. It is essential to plan the surgical procedure.

Fundus examination is performed after pupillary dilatation.

A-scan helps measure the axial length for calculating intraoccular lens (IOL) power and monitoring the globe elongation postoperatively.

B-scan is an important tool to rule out posterior segment pathology.

Paediatric system-wise examination is performed to rule out systemic association of cataract, anomalies and congenital rubella.

Leucocoria is a usual finding among family members.

In children with bilateral cataract, membranous morphology, lenticonus, inflammatory pathology or any history of maternal illness during pregnancy need to be elicited.

Blood workup includes fasting blood sugar, urine for reducing substance for galactosaemia after milk feeding and urine amino acids for Lowe syndrome.

Plasma phosphorus, red blood cell transferase, galactokinase levels and calcium evaluation for hypothyroidism are important. The titres for toxoplasma, rubella, cytomegalovirus and herpes simplex (TORCH titres) should be carried out to rule out these disorders.

It is essential to screen parents and siblings to rule out familial causes. History to be taken from parents to ascertain the cause of cataract. It is important to quantify the visual acuity of the child with cataract as precisely as possible. The grade of visual fixation is also important.

Multidisciplinary Management

Management of childhood cataract is very complex. The physiology and anatomy of the growing eyes of children are so different from those of adults. Low scleral rigidity, increased elasticity of the anterior capsule and high vitreous pressure are among the major problems. Cataract surgery in children is complicated, with increased postoperative inflammation, a changing refractive state, higher re-surgery rate and an inherent risk of amblyopia. Unilateral cataract is operated within the first 6 weeks of life to prevent development of deprivation amblyopia.

Polar opacities (those involving only the anterior capsule), smaller nuclear cataracts and lamellar cortical opacities that transmit light centrally are left alone till a reliable assessment of visual potential is possible.

Pharmacological management include four doses of dilating drops every 10 minutes at least 1 hour before surgery. Antibiotic drugs to prevent postoperative infection and inflammation are required.

Cataract Removal

The lens material may be removed using either phacoaspiration or automated irrigation and aspiration. However, membranous or calcified cataract may need phacoemulsification. **In phacoemulsification,** a portion of the anterior capsule is removed, allowing extraction of the lens nucleus and cortex whereas the posterior capsule and zonular support are left intact.

Extracapsular cataract extraction (ECCE). ECCE removes the anterior lens and cortex, leaving the posterior capsule intact.

Intracapsular cataract extraction. This procedure removes the entire lens within the intact capsule.

Hydrodissection: Hydrodissection is essential to ensure maximum removal of lens cortex and lens epithelial cells from the equatorial region. It may be a single-site or multiple-site hydrodissection. It is performed by injecting Ringer's lactate or balanced salt solution using a 2-mL disposable syringe with 27- to 30-G cannula under the capsulorhexis margin. It should be avoided in posterior lenticonus cataract or posterior polar cataract.

Intraocular lens implantation: Capsular bag implantation of IOL is the best choice to reduce the contact of IOL with uveal tissue and to achieve IOL centration.

The single-piece hydrophobic acrylic IOLs are ideal for implantation into the small capsular bag of children.

Aphakic glasses are used for magnification of objects. Aphakic glasses provide 25% magnification, making objects appear closer.

Contact lens provides almost normal vision and is usually used in teens and young adults.

Postoperative Management

Postoperatively, there will be more tissue reaction. This inflammatory response is managed with topical steroid application every 4 hours. The steroids are tapered over a period of 6–8 weeks.

Topical antibiotics thrice daily are also used for 10–14 days.

Homatropine eye drops (2%) twice a day or atropine eye ointment once a day is used for about 4 weeks to prevent posterior synechia formation. Check refraction as soon as inflammation subsides, and appropriate correction should be provided according to the age of the child.

Preschool-aged children may be provided with a near addition incorporated into the bifocals during retinoscopy. Older children should be given bifocal glasses.

Postoperative amblyopia therapy is essential.

Occlusion therapy for unilateral cataract after surgery is instituted for children considered to be at high risk of developing amblyopia.

Complications

Postoperative complications after paediatric intraocular surgery are high as a result of a greater inflammatory response.

Uveitis results from increased tissue reactivity in children. Intensive topical steroids and cycloplegic agents in the postoperative period have reduced the incidence of uveitis after cataract surgery.

Posterior capsular opacification (PCO) is the most common complication after cataract surgery with or without IOL surgery in children. In a thick PCO, surgical posterior capsulotomy is required to prevent amblyopia.

Visual axis opacification (VAO) is the most common complication after a successful cataract surgery in children.

Pupillary capture occurs when a portion of the optic nerve passes anterior to the iris. The incidence of pupillary capture is very high. Fixation of posterior chamber IOL in the capsular bag decreases the incidence of this complication.

Decentration of IOL – Capsular bag placement of IOL is mandatory to reduce this complication.

Retrobulbar haemorrhage can develop as a result of retrobulbar infiltration of anaesthetic agents when the ciliary artery is involved.

Acute bacterial endophthalmitis. It is a devastating complication that occurs in about one in 1000 cases.

Toxic anterior segment syndrome. It is a noninfection inflammation as a result of anterior chamber inflammation.

GLAUCOMA

The incidence of glaucoma following paediatric cataract surgery varies. Glaucoma occurring soon after surgery is usually a result of pupillary block or peripheral anterior synechia formation, whereas open-angle glaucoma may occur late. This implies a lifelong follow-up of children after cataract surgery.

Intraocular pressure (IOP) should be periodically recorded to detect and treat this vision-threatening complication.

Secondary membranes are common after infantile cataract surgery and traumatic cataract.

Retinal detachment after cataract surgery is also noticed, but it is usually a late complication.

Amblyopia is one of the most important vision-threatening complications. Suitable optical correction after surgery is essential in an aphakic or pseudophakic child. Postoperative patching of the normal eye in cases of unilateral congenital or developmental or traumatic cataract is done to achieve binocular vision and stereopsis.

Visual outcome after cataract surgery is good provided the surgery is successful, followed by prevention of complications.

Nursing Management

Nursing assessment includes the following:
Preoperatively, assess the history of medications such as anticoagulants, as they may increase the possibility of retrobulbar haemorrhage.
Assist in preoperative tests, as there is a standard battery of tests such as blood count, urinalysis, etc.

Monitor vital signs, as it is important to stabilize vital signs.
Assist in assessing visual acuity tests.

Nursing Diagnoses

- **Disturbed visual sensory perception** related to altered sensory reception or status of sense organs
- **Risk for trauma** related to poor vision and reduces hand–eye coordination
- **Anxiety of parents related to child's vision, as there is a threat of permanent loss of vision**
- Deficient knowledge related to disease condition and prognosis
  The major goals for the child and parent are as follows:
  - Regaining of usual acuity and vision
  - Recognizing awareness of sensory needs
  - Be free of injury
  - Identifying potential risk factors in the environment
  - Relieving anxiety or reducing it to a manageable level and verbalize it

Nursing Interventions

- Preoperatively, taking the history of medications, stabilizing the vitals, alleviating anxiety of parents and children and preparing them for surgery including preoperative medications should be undertaken.
- Postoperatively, parents and children must be given exact information about how to care children at home without injury, explain need of eye patching, how to administer eye drops and also teach them how to recognize complications and obtain emergency care.
- Document all plan of care including the assistive devices given to the child.
  Evaluate the child's progress before discharge. This includes regained level of vision, awareness of sensory needs, being free of injury, identification of potential risks in the environment and being free from anxiety.

Patient Education/Family Education

This includes the permitted activities and the activities to be avoided to keep the IOP normal:
Protective eye patch to prevent accidental rubbing or poking of the eyes for 24 hours.
Eye glasses worn during day and night.
Expected side effects such as slight morning discharge, scratchy feelings and how to remove eye discharge using clean wet clothes.
Inform the surgeon or report to the surgeon if the child has new floaters in vision, flashing lights or decreased vision, as it may be warning of retinal detachment.
Increased redness also needs to be reported, as it may be a sign of infection.

PAEDIATRIC GLAUCOMA

Description: Glaucoma in children is characterized by improper development of the eye's aqueous outflow system which results in an increased IOP leading to damage to the optic nerve resulting in loss of vision.

When the pressure is too high, there will be difficulty in draining the aqueous fluid. Early identification and treatment of paediatric glaucoma are very important to restore vision.

Types

There are different types of glaucoma. One way to classify glaucoma is based on age.
1. Congenital glaucoma is present at birth.
2. Infantile glaucoma develops between 1 and 24 months of age.
3. Juvenile glaucoma has an onset after the age of 3 years.

Glaucoma can be primary or secondary. Primary glaucoma is congenital, and developmental glaucoma is associated with syndromes and systemic abnormalities. The two categories of primary childhood glaucoma are as follows:

Primary congenital glaucoma (PCG). Children with PCG have enlarged eyes and frequently have corneal clouding. It consists of three subtypes based on the age of the child at onset.
  1. Neonatal onset develops before 1 month of age.
  2. Infantile onset develops between 1 and 24 months of age.
  3. Late onset develops after 24 months of age.
Juvenile open-angle glaucoma (JOAG). This type of glaucoma develops after the age of 3 years and is associated with normal sized eyes and the absence of corneal clouding.

Secondary glaucoma is related to disease conditions such as uveitis, congenital cataract surgery, neurofibromatosis and aniridia, which are dominantly inherited and are passed on to 50% of children.

There are four categories of secondary childhood glaucoma:

Glaucoma following cataract surgery. It is also called aphakic glaucoma. This refers to the type of glaucoma that can occur in children who have had cataract surgery.
Glaucoma associated with acquired conditions. This type of glaucoma occurs as a result of conditions such as ocular injury, inflammation or infection of the eye or medication use (corticosteroids).
Glaucoma associated with nonacquired systemic disease or syndrome. This type of glaucoma is associated with systemic conditions that are present at birth such as Down syndrome, Marfan syndrome, and Sturge–Weber syndrome.
Glaucoma associated with nonacquired ocular anomalies. These types of conditions are usually associated with structural abnormalities or systemic conditions. Some of these are associated with certain ocular conditions present at birth such as aniridia, Axenfeld–Rieger anomaly or Peters anomaly. But some other conditions are chronic steroid use, trauma or previous eye surgery such as childhood cataract removal. Neurofibromatosis is another disease condition that causes this type of glaucoma.

Incidence

Primary congenital glaucoma occurs in one of every 10,000 births in the United States
- Primary congenital glaucoma accounts for approximately 50%–70% of all cases of congenital glaucoma.
- In diagnosed cases, about two-thirds of the patients are male. In about three-fourths of all cases, glaucoma affects both eyes (bilateral).

The incidence of childhood glaucoma is estimated to be 2.29 per 100,000 patients younger than 20 years. Primary congenital glaucoma is the most common form of childhood glaucoma. Paediatric glaucoma is also associated with an elevated IOP and progressive optic nerve damage.

Causes

The exact aetiology of childhood primary glaucoma is unknown. It is sporadic in occurrence. But there is evidence suggesting an autosomal recessive pattern of transmission. The incidence of glaucoma is higher after cataract surgery or other ophthalmic problems. In total, 50% of patients with aniridia will develop glaucoma during their lifetime. Incidence is higher when there is a genetic reason. Higher mortality is observed in the case of bilateral glaucoma (about 75%). Congenital glaucoma occurs in all races. Male (65%) children are more affected than female children. Primary glaucoma is diagnosed immediately after birth or within the first year of life.

Pathophysiology

Primary congenital glaucoma is related to a developmental abnormality and affects the trabecular meshwork. This helps distinguish it from other childhood glaucoma cases. Secondary glaucoma develops as a result of other ocular disorders such as inflammation, trauma and tumours.

Clinical Features

The classic triad of manifestations includes epiphora (excessive tearing), photophobia and blepharospasm. Other symptoms are cloudy dull eyes and signs of optic nerve cupping (enlargement of the centre 'cup' portion of the optic nerve). Juvenile glaucoma develops without any obvious symptoms such as that in adult glaucoma. Patients with juvenile glaucoma often have a family history. On examination, the eye pressure will be elevated and there may be optic nerve cupping.

Complete Ophthalmological Examination

A child suspected of having glaucoma must be examined under anaesthesia to get an accurate finding of the structure and IOP.

The average horizontal corneal diameter at birth is less than 10.5 mm. Increased IOP causes distension of the globe (buphthalmos), which leads to enlargement of the cornea. If the corneoscleral junction is more than 12 mm in diameter in the first year of life, it is suggestive of glaucoma. Corneal oedema may be a direct result of the elevated IOP, producing a corneal haze. Haab striae represent tears in the Descemet membrane as a result of the elevated IOP. In advanced cases, a dense opacification of the corneal stroma occurs. Tonometry often can be accomplished in a child's eye with a hand-held instrument such as Perkins' tonometer or a Tono-Pen.

Diagnosis

Measurement of IOP (best under anaesthesia; straining increases IOP), cornea diameter (for increased size), cornea clarity (for cloudiness and Haab striae, which are breaks in the back surface of the cornea), axial length (for elongation of the eye – caused by stretching from increased pressure), refractive error (for myopia – also caused by stretching) and the optic nerve (for abnormal cupping which infers optic nerve damage). Diagnostic visual field examination is done to look for peripheral vision. Paediatric glaucoma needs to be differentiated from birth trauma, congenital anomalies of the nasolacrimal duct, congenital clouding of the cornea, infections of the eye, megalocornea, Peters anomaly and sclerocornea.

Laboratory Studies

Laboratory methods of diagnosing primary congenital glaucoma include hybridization analysis, direct mutation analysis and hybridization of an allele-specific oligonucleotide with amplified genomic DNA.

Imaging studies include high-resolution anterior segment optical coherence tomography.

Other Tests

In addition to tonometry, corneal measurements, gonioscopy and ophthalmoscopy should be performed in the operating room. In the operating room, pachymetry to quantify corneal oedema and A-scan ultrasound study to determine axial distention often are useful.

Multidisciplinary Management

Paediatric glaucoma is treated by lowering the IOP via medical and/or surgical means.

Primary paediatric glaucoma cases are treated with surgery. Trabeculotomy and goniotomy, which open the drainage canals, are performed. Other procedures create a bypass for the aqueous humour (fluid made by the eye) to drain out of the eye.

Trabeculectomy creates a guarded opening from the front of the eye to a space underneath the conjunctiva. A tube shunt is a device which is inserted into the front of the eye or into the vitreous cavity (back part of the eye). Fluid from the eye then drains to a reservoir that is located underneath the conjunctiva.

Laser procedures can also be beneficial in some cases.

Control of the glaucoma usually requires multiple procedures and examinations under anaesthesia.

Eye drops and oral medications are the primary treatments of secondary and juvenile glaucoma.

Eye drops and oral medications are used as adjuvant therapy after surgery for primary paediatric glaucoma.

Many children with paediatric glaucoma develop myopia (nearsightedness), which requires glasses, amblyopia (decreased vision) and strabismus (crossing or wandering eye), which may require treatment with patching or surgery.

The Follow-up

In the early postoperative period, close observation is required to attain the success of the procedure and may require multiple examinations under anaesthesia.

Complications

Serious complications of surgical intervention include misdirection into the suprachoroidal space hyphaema, infection, lens damage, cyclodialysis cleft, iris tear and uveitis.

Prognosis

Corneal oedema may persist for weeks after successful reduction of the IOP. Changes in the optic nerve head provide the most important indicator of the course of the disease. Cupping can reverse in successfully treated cases.

IOP is also a significant factor in postoperative visual capacity, with substantially better vision among those patients whose eye pressure remains no higher than 19.

Even when the IOP is well controlled, approximately 50% of children do not achieve vision better than 20/50.

Reduced visual acuity may result from persistent corneal oedema, nystagmus, amblyopia or large refractive errors.

Nursing Management

Nursing assessment includes a detailed history and looking for signs and symptoms.

Nursing Diagnoses

Preoperative nursing diagnoses are as follows:
1. Disturbed sensory perception (visual) related to reception of sensory disturbances
2. Pain (acute/chronic) related to increased IOP
3. Anxiety related to disease condition
4. Deficient knowledge (learning needs) related to the disease process

Postoperative nursing diagnoses include the following:
1. Pain (acute/chronic) related to the invasive procedure, increased IOP and vitreous loss
2. Risk for injury/infection related to surgical intervention

Nursing Interventions

Administer cycloplegic eye drops in the affected eye. The nurse must be very careful, and the drug should be administered only in the affected eye, as it will precipitate angle closure glaucoma in the unaffected eye, too.

After trabeculectomy, administer pupil-dilating drugs, as ordered.

Apply steroid as ordered to rest the pupil.

Protect the affected eye by applying an eye patch and eye shield.

Position the patient on his/her back or the unaffected side and do not allow making hasty movements or activities that increase IOP.

Encourage ambulation as early as possible.

Stress the importance of compliance to medications after surgery.

Inform parents and children to look for visual changes and report untoward symptoms immediately to the concerned surgeon.

Monitor IOP.

Instruct how to modify the child's environment to adapt to the situations and to ensure safety.

Patient/Family Education

The patient and family must understand that IOP elevation can recur at any age in individuals with primary congenital glaucoma, and these patients must receive follow-up care throughout their lives.

PREVENTION OF EYE INJURIES

It is essential to maintain safety of eyes, and adults should help them use protective goggles as and when needed.

In India, every year thousands of children sustain eye injuries during play and festival seasons when firecrackers are used. These injuries can lead to blindness in children.

All chemicals and sprays must be kept out of reach of small children.

Parents and others who provide care and supervision to children need to practice safe use of common items that can cause serious eye injury, such as paper clips, pencils, scissors, bungee cords, wire coat hangers and rubber bands.

Avoid projectile toys such as darts, bows and arrows, and missile-firing toys. Teach children to be EyeSmart by safeguarding their own sight.
- Use safety gates at the top and bottom of stairs. Pad or cushion sharp corners.
- Put locks on all cabinets and drawers that kids can reach.

Avoid projectile toys such as darts, bows and arrows, and missile-firing toys.

Protect young children from bites of dogs and cats, as there is always a chance for eye injuries.

Road safety is also important. Keep children always in the back seat with protective seat belts.

Pad sharp items so that they will not cause injuries.

First Aid

While seeking medical help, provide care to the child as follows:

- DO NOT touch, rub or apply pressure to the eye.
- DO NOT try to remove any object stuck in the eye. For small debris, lift eyelid and ask child to blink rapidly to see if tears will flush out the particle. If not, close the eye and seek treatment.
- Do not apply ointment or medication to the eye.
- A cut or puncture wound should be gently covered.
- In the event of chemical exposure, flush the eye with plenty of water.

TONSILLITIS

Tonsillitis is inflammation of the pharyngeal tonsils mainly caused by group A β-haemolytic *Streptococcus pyogenes* (GABHS). The inflammation usually extends to the adenoid and the lingual tonsils. It can be acute, recurrent or chronic tonsillitis and peritonsillar abscess (PTA). Tonsillitis had gained a lot of medical attention after quinsy as the differential diagnosis in George Washington's death.

Tonsillitis rarely occurs in children younger than 2 years. Tonsillitis caused by *Streptococcus* species typically occurs in children aged 5–15 years. Viral tonsillitis is more common in younger children. PTA usually occurs in teens or young adults but may present earlier, too.

Aetiology

Viral or bacterial infections and immunological factors lead to tonsillitis and its complications. Overcrowded conditions of living such as staying in dormitory, sharing common environment and malnourishment promote tonsillitis.

- The most common organism involved in tonsillitis is GABHS
- Respiratory viruses
- Herpes simplex virus
- Epstein–Barr virus (EBV)
- Cytomegalovirus
- Adenovirus
- Measles virus

Out of these organisms, EBV produces 19% of exudative tonsillitis cases in children.

Bacterial infection constitutes 15%–30% of cases of pharyngotonsillitis. Anaerobic bacteria also cause tonsillar disease.

Most common organisms that are isolated in recurrent tonsillitis are *Streptococcus pneumoniae*, *Staphylococcus aureus* and *Haemophilus influenzae*. The microbiology of recurrent tonsillitis in children shows more occurrences of GABHS.

Signs and Symptoms

Acute tonsillitis
- Fever
- Sore throat
- Foul breath
- Dysphagia (difficulty swallowing)
- Odynophagia (painful swallowing)
- Tender cervical lymph nodes

Airway obstruction may manifest as mouth breathing, snoring, nocturnal breathing pauses or sleep apnoea.

Diagnosis

Clinical features assist in diagnosis.

Multidisciplinary Management

Supportive management is indicated in acute cases that includes:

Analgesics
Antipyretics
Increased fluid intake
- Infection with GABHS requires antibiotics. This is mandatory if three out of four characteristic symptoms are presented and must be treated with antibiotics 'upfront' (before culture results are known): fever, discharge from the tonsils, no cough and tender lymph nodes.

Tonsillectomy may be required in children who develop frequent infections.

Tonsillectomy is advised if there are six episodes of infection in a year, five episodes of pharyngitis in two consecutive year and three or more episodes of tonsillitis or adenoiditis per year for 3 years in a row even after antibiotic treatment.

Nursing Diagnoses

Altered temperature
Pain
Altered nutrition
Fluid volume deficit

Nursing Management

- Pain management is the most important aspect, as the child will not be able to take food and fluid as a result of pain. The child may suffer from dysphagia and odynophagia as a result of pain. So, pain relief is very important. Administer pain medications as prescribed.
- Administer antipyretics as the child will have high fever related to infection. Care during fever such as tepid sponging, rest and medications on time is necessary.
- Monitor intake and output and document and inform the physician in this regard.
- If it is viral tonsillitis, aspirin should not be administered, as it may cause Rey syndrome in children which may affect the brain and liver.
- Administer antibiotics as prescribed. It is essential not only to treat current infection but also to protect from the dreaded sequel of rheumatic heart disease.
- Provide health education on prevention of further infection and prevention of sequelae.

- Look for PTA as another complication of tonsillitis.
- If the child is scheduled for surgery, then preoperative and postoperative care must be given as per protocol. The nurse should remember that the child will be coming from theatre with packs and haemorrhage is very common complication leading to respiratory problems. The nurse must observe for bleeding and further respiratory distress.
- Prevention of bleeding by administering cool drinks and ice cubes for chewing.
- Avoid hot drinks and foods until it is ordered.
- Teach parents how to look for bleeding and how to position the child to promote drooling of the saliva and discharges and not aspirating the same to the trachea.

Health education should be provided regarding healthy living conditions, care during acute illness, prophylactic antibiotic administration to prevent rheumatic heart disease and PTA. In the case of recurrent infection, family members may be advised to have check-up to see if they are asymptomatic (without symptoms) carriers of group A streptococci. If so, they may be given antibiotics to ensure that the whole family is *Streptococcus*-free and to protect the child from reinfection.

PERITONSILLAR ABSCESS

This occurs when a clump of bacteria are 'walled off' by new tissue growth. The abscess is not in the tonsil itself but on one side of it. Unlike simple tonsillitis, quinsy tends to be felt on only one side of the throat, and people with this condition can often be seen tilting their head to one side to reduce pain. Quinsy is more common in young adults with tonsillitis than in children. Multiple bacteria are isolated in PTA. Predominant organisms are the anaerobes *Prevotella*, *Porphyromonas*, *Fusobacterium* and *Peptostreptococcus* species. Major aerobic organisms are GABHS, *Staphylococcus aureus* and *H. influenzae*.

PTA presents with the following symptoms:
- Severe throat pain
- Fever
- Drooling
- Foul breath
- Trismus (difficulty opening the mouth)
- Altered voice quality (the hot-potato voice)

Prognosis

Because of improvements in medical and surgical treatments, complications associated with tonsillitis, including PTA, are rare in children. The incidence of rheumatic fever has declined significantly with administration of antibiotics and prophylactic treatment.

OTITIS MEDIA

'Otitis media' (OM) is an umbrella term used for a group of complex, infective and inflammatory conditions affecting the middle ear. It involves pathology of the middle ear and middle ear mucosa. OM is one of the leading causes of health care visits and is the major cause of preventable hearing loss in the developing world.

OM is a very common problem in childhood, especially among children who are bottlefed. There are two forms of OM, namely acute otitis media (AOM) and otitis media with effusion (OME). It is caused by bacterial or viral infection. Subtypes are acute otitis media, chronic suppurative otitis media, mastoiditis and cholesteatoma.

- AOM is acute inflammation of the middle ear and may be caused by bacteria or viruses. A subtype of AOM is acute suppurative OM, characterized by the presence of pus in the middle ear. The eardrum perforates in around 5% of cases.
- OME is a chronic inflammatory condition without acute inflammation, which often follows a slowly resolving AOM. There is an effusion of glue-like fluid behind an intact tympanic membrane in the absence of signs and symptoms of acute inflammation.
- Chronic Suppurative Otitis Media (CSOM) is long-standing suppurative middle ear inflammation, usually with a persistently perforated tympanic membrane.
- Mastoiditis is acute inflammation of the mastoid periosteum and air cells and occurs when AOM infection spreads out from the middle ear.
- Cholesteatoma occurs when keratinizing squamous epithelium (skin) is present in the middle ear as a result of tympanic membrane retraction.

AOM is a self-limiting illness, and a few episodes may become recurrent or chronic problems.

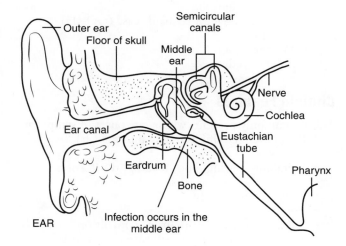

AOM is a very common childhood problem, and about two-thirds of young children suffer more than three episodes. The peak age of this disease is 6–15 months of age. About 75% of episodes occur below the age of 10 years and less common among school-aged children. It occurs more in winter than in summer and is usually associated with common cold. It is common issue of the developing world. Global incidence is about 10%, and about half of the cases occur in children younger than 5 years. Death occurs as a result of complications of OM, especially in developing countries.

Pathophysiology

The infecting organism reaches the middle ear from nasopharynx. Children are vulnerable to OM because of the fact that their Eustachian tube is straight and short. In small children, the less acute angle facilitates infected material to enter through the Eustachian tube to the middle ear.

- Most often, AOM is a complication of a preceding or concomitant upper respiratory tract infection.
- The most common bacterial pathogens are *H. influenzae*, *Streptococcus pneumoniae*, *Moraxella catarrhalis* and *Streptococcus pyogenes*.
- Culture of fluid obtained from the middle ear reveals pathogenic bacteria in up to 70% of cases. *Streptococcus pneumoniae* and *H. influenzae* together comprise 60%–80% of these cases.
- Since the introduction of the pneumococcal vaccine, the most common pathogen may be changing from *Streptococcus pneumoniae* to *H. influenzae*.
- The most common viral pathogens are respiratory syncytial virus (RSV) and rhinovirus.

Risk factors for AOM are as follows:
  - Younger age
  - Male sex
  - Smoking in the household
  - Day care/nursery attendance
  - Formula feeding – Breastfeeding for 3 months and above has a protective effect
  - Craniofacial abnormalities, e.g. Down syndrome, cleft palate

Associate factors are as follows:
  - Early first episode
  - Gastroesophageal reflux disease (GORD)
  - Dummy use
  - Winter season
  - Supine feeding

Clinical Features

AOM commonly presents with acute onset of symptoms:
- Pain (younger children may pull the ear)
- Malaise
- Irritability, crying, poor feeding, restlessness
- Fever
- Coryza/rhinorrhoea
- Vomiting
- High temperature (febrile convulsions may be associated with the temperature rise in AOM)
- A red, yellow or cloudy tympanic membrane
- Bulging of the tympanic membrane
- An air–fluid level behind the tympanic membrane
- Discharge in the auditory canal secondary to perforation of the tympanic membrane, which may obscure the view completely
- A red pinna

Very young children (younger than 6 months) show nonspecific symptoms. They may also have coexisting diseases such as bronchiolitis, and the tympanic membrane may be difficult to see: It often lies in an oblique position, and the ear canal tends to collapse closed.

Perforation of the eardrum often relieves pain. A child who is screaming and distressed may settle remarkably quickly and then the ear starts to discharge green pus.

Differential Diagnosis

There is long list of differential diagnosis.
  Otitis externa
  OME
  Respiratory infection
  Referred pain of toothache
  Foreign body in the external ear
  Temporomandibular joint pain
  Trauma
  Chronic suppurative otitis media
  Bullous myringitis (rare and caused by *Mycoplasma pneumoniae* manifested with bullous red blisters)

Investigations

- Usually, no investigation is required.
- Culture of discharge from the ear may be indicated in chronic or recurrent perforation or if grommets are present.
- Audiometry should be performed if chronic hearing loss is suspected but not during acute infection.
- CT or MRI may be appropriate if complications are suspected.

Multidisciplinary Management

A majority of cases usually resolve on their own.
Administer analgesics and antipyretics as required according to symptoms.
No antibiotics are required in mild to moderate cases.
- Antibiotics may be given immediately to children younger than 2 years with bilateral AOM and children of any age with perforation and/or discharge in the ear canal. Usual antibiotic given is a 5-day course of amoxicillin. For children who are allergic to penicillin, a 5-day course of erythromycin or clarithromycin is usually prescribed.
- For children with immunocompromised conditions, antibiotics are usually prescribed.
- Apply warm compress over the affected ear to reduce the pain.
- Antihistamines, decongestants and *Echinacea* are not found to be useful.

Artificial perforation of the tympanic membrane is required in certain cases, which promote drainage of pus.
If symptoms persist despite two courses of antibiotics, seek advice from an ENT specialist. In the case of recurrent AOM, the child may be referred to an ENT specialist, especially if the child has a craniofacial anomaly.
Some children require admission:
- Children younger than 3 months with a temperature of 38°C or more
- Children with suspected acute complications of AOM, such as meningitis, mastoiditis or facial nerve paralysis

- Children who are systemically very unwell
- Children younger than 3 months
- Children 3–6 months of age with a temperature of 39°C or more

Nursing Management

Reassure the parents.

- Tell them that usually this disease subsides by itself within 2–3 days. If treated properly, the risk of complications are less. Most cases of AOM will resolve spontaneously with no sequelae.
- Administer analgesics, antipyretics and antibiotics (if prescribed) properly.
- Provide care for fever.
- Provide warm compresses.
- Teach parents proper positioning while feeding, especially if the child is bottlefed.
- Instruct the importance of breastfeeding.
- Clean the ear if the discharge is present.
- Usually, there will not have any ear drops.
- Look for symptoms of AOM such as pulling the ear in infants, who cannot communicate, as a symptom of AOM.
- Educate parents not to expose children to passive smoking, and advise against using dummies and against flat, supine feeding. Advise them to have pneumococcal vaccine.

STUDY QUESTIONS

1. What is amblyopia?
2. What is coloboma?
3. What is stye?
4. List the common eye infections.
5. How will prevent the spread of conjunctivitis in children?
6. What are the common refractive errors seen in children?
7. What are the causes of paediatric cataract?
8. Describe the medical and surgical management of children with paediatric cataract.
9. What are the causes of paediatric glaucoma?
10. Describe the nursing care of children with paediatric glaucoma.
11. How will you prevent eye injuries in children?
12. What are the common causes of tonsillitis in children?
13. What is the medical management of tonsillitis in children?
14. How will you care a child after tonsillectomy?
15. What is peritonsillar abscess?
16. What are the consequences of a partially treated or untreated tonsillitis?
17. What are the causes of otitis media?
18. How will you care a child with otitis media?
19. What are the important modalities of treatment of otitis media?

BIBLIOGRAPHY

1. Aponte EP, Diehl N, Mohney BG. Incidence and clinical characteristics of childhood glaucoma: A population-based study. Arch Ophthalmol 2010; 128:478-82.
2. Beck AD, Freedman S, Kammer J, Jin J. Aqueous shunt devices compared with trabeculectomy with mitomycin C for children in the first two years of life. Am J Ophthalmol 2003; 136:994-1000.
3. Khitri MR, Mills MD, Ying GS, Davidson SL, & Quinn GE. (2012). Visual acuity outcomes in pediatric glaucomas. J AAPOS, 16(4):376–381.
4. Sippel KC. Ocular findings in neurofibromatosis type 1. Int Ophthalmol Clin 2001; 41(1):25-40. Review.
5. Biglan AW. Glaucoma in children: Are we making progress? J AAPOS. 2006 Feb;10(1):7-21.
6. Foster A, Gilbert C, Rahi J: Epidemiology of cataract in childhood. A global perspective. J Cataract Refract Surg 1997; 23:601-4.
7. World Health Organization. Global initiative for the elimination of avoidable blindness. WHO/PBL/97.61. Geneva.
8. Eckstein M, Vijayalakshmi P, Killedar M, Gilbert C, Foster A. Aetiology of childhood cataract in south India. Br J Ophthalmol. 1996; 80:628-32.
9. Jain IS, Pillai P, Gangwar DN, Gopal L, Dhir SP: Congenital cataract: Etiology and morphology. J Pediatr Ophthalmol Strabismus 1983; 20:238-42.
10. Scheie HG: Aspiration of congenital or soft cataracts. A new technique. Am J Ophthalmol 1960; 50:1048-56.
11. Wilson ME. Intraocular lens implantation: has it become the standard of care for children? Ophthalmology 1996; 103:1719-20.
12. Basti S, Ravishankar U, Gupta S: Results of a prospective evaluation of three methods of management of pediatric cataracts. Ophthalmology 1996; 103:713-20.
13. Vasavada A, Desai J: Primary posterior capsulorhexis with and without anterior vitrectomy in congenital cataracts. J Cataract Refract Surg 1997; 23(Suppl):645-51.
14. Holmes JM, Leske DA, Burke JP and Hodge DO. Birth prevalence of visually significant infantile cataract in a defined U.S. population. Ophthalmic Epidemiol 2003 Apr; 10:67-74.
15. Rahi JS, Dezateux C: British Congenital Cataract Interest Group. Measuring and interpreting the incidence of congenital ocular anomalies: lessons from a national study of congenital cataract in the UK. Invest Ophthalmol Vis Sci 2001 June; 42:1444-8.
16. Ashwin Reddy M, et al. (2004 May-June). Molecular Genetic Basis of Inherited Cataract and Associated Phenotypes. Survey of Ophthalmology, 49(3):300–315.
17. Pandey SK, Wilson ME, Trivedi RH, et al. Pediatric cataract surgery and intraocular lens implantation: current techniques, complications and management. Int Ophthalmol Clin. 2001; 41(3):175-96.
18. Vishwanath M, Cheong-Leen R, Taylor D, et al. Is early surgery for congenital cataract a risk factor for glaucoma? Br J Ophthalmol 2004; 88;905-910.
19. Gimbel HV, DeBroff BM. Posterior capsulorhexis with optic capture: maintaining a clear visual axis after pediatric cataract surgery. J Cataract Refract Surg. 1994 Nov; 20:658-64.
20. Infant Aphakia Treatment Study Group, Lambert SR, Buckley EG, Drews-Botsch C, Dubois L, Hartmann EE, Lynn MJ, Plager DA, Wilson ME. A randomized clinical trial comparing contact lens with intraocular lens correction of monocular aphakia during infancy: grating acuity and adverse events at age 1 year. Arch Ophthalmol. 2010 Jul; 128:810-8.
21. World Health Organization. (1997). Global initiative for the elimination of avoidable blindness. WHO/PBL/97.61. Geneva: WHO.
22. Lambert SR, Drack AV: Infantile cataracts. Surv Ophthalmol 1996; 40:427-58.
23. Eckstein M, Vijayalakshmi P, Killedar M, Gilbert C, Foster A. Aetiology of childhood cataract in south India. Br J Ophthalmol. 1996; 80:628-32.
24. Jain IS, Pillai P, Gangwar DN, Gopal L, Dhir SP: Congenital cataract: Etiology and morphology. J Pediatr Ophthalmol Strabismus 1983; 20:238-42.

CHAPTER 37

ALTERATION IN INTEGUMENTARY FUNCTIONS: NURSING CARE OF CHILDREN WITH DERMATOLOGICAL DISORDERS

CHAPTER OUTLINE

- Skin Problems in Children
- Bullous Impetigo
- Collodion Baby
- Epidermolysis Bullosa
- Melanocytic Naevi
- Napkin Rash
- Viral Infections – Viral Warts
- Molluscum Contagiosum
- Ringworm Infection
- Tinea Capitis (Scalp Ringworm)

- Parasitic Infestations – Scabies
- Pediculosis
- Psoriasis
- Pityriasis Rosea
- Acne Vulgaris
- Urticaria (Hives or Weals)
- Fever in Children
- Pyrexia of Unknown Origin or Fever of Unknown Origin
- Burns in Children

LEARNING OBJECTIVES

At the end of the chapter, the learner will be able to:
- State the common skin disorders, including viral infections in children, and their management.
- Identify the allergic skin disorders in children.
- Discuss the management of children with burns.
- Describe the causes and management of fever in children.

At birth, the skin of newborn is covered with vernix caseosa – a whitish greasy coat produced by epithelial cell breakdown. It protects the skin from amniotic fluid in utero. The common skin problems seen in children are briefly described. (For detailed information, the reader is advised to refer to dermatology textbooks.)

BULLOUS IMPETIGO

This is a blistering form of impetigo, seen particularly in newborns. It is most often caused by phage group, i.e. strain of *Staphylococcus aureus*.

Treatment of bullous impetigo is with systemic antibiotics.

COLLODION BABY

It is a rare manifestation of inherited ichthyosis.

EPIDERMOLYSIS BULLOSA

It is a condition with 20 subtypes. The main features are blistering of the skin and the mucous membrane. Autosomal dominant variants are milder than the autosomal recessive variants, which are very severe and fatal. Mucous membrane involvement leads to oral ulceration and stenosis from oesophageal erosions.

Management includes maintenance of adequate nutrition along with multidisciplinary team management with a dermatologist, a paediatrician, a plastic surgeon and a dietician.

MELANOCYTIC NAEVI

It occurs in up to 3% neonates and is usually small. It may become increasingly common as children get older, and the presence of a large number in an adult may be indicative of childhood sun exposure. Congenital moles carry a risk of developing as malignant melanomas. They need dermatological consultation and sometimes surgical removal by plastic surgery.

NAPKIN RASH

Napkin rashes are usually caused by the use of disposable napkin. Irritant dermatitis is the most common napkin rash that can occur even after regular cleaning. It results from the irritant effects of urine on the skin of susceptible infants. Common types are irritant dermatitis, seborrhoeic dermatitis, *Candida albicans* infection and atopic eczema.

Management includes avoiding irritants and precipitants such as soap, biological detergents, etc. Clothing next to the skin should be of pure cotton whenever possible, and avoiding nylon and pure woollen cloths. Emollients, as a mainstay of treatment, maintain moisture and soften the skin. Topical steroids are used, especially for eczema (1% hydrocortisone ointment). Antibiotics or antiviral agents, H_1 histamine antagonists, dietary elimination of allergens in eczema and psychological support to parents and children as appropriate are the mode of management.

VIRAL INFECTIONS

Viral Warts

Viral warts are caused by the human papilloma virus and are common in children. It is usually seen on fingers and soles (verrucae). Most warts disappear over few months or years. Treatment is needed only if there is superimposed infection and is painful or for cosmetic reasons.

Treatment is with application of salicylic acid or phenol or by cryotherapy with liquid nitrogen.

Molluscum Contagiosum

They are small, skin-coloured, pearly papules with central umbilication caused by a poxvirus. It can occur as single or multiple lesions. Lesions spread rapidly and disappear spontaneously. Secondary infection needs treatment with antibiotics.

RINGWORM INFECTION

It is caused by dermatophyte fungi that invade dead keratinous structure such as the horny layer of skin, nails and hair. The lesions are annular (ringed) and hence called ringworm infection. Severe inflammatory pustular patch of ringworm is called kerion.

Tinea Capitis (Scalp Ringworm)

It is usually acquired from pets. It can be identified by examination of skin scrapings for fungal hyphae.

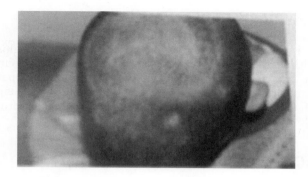

Treatment is with topical antifungals for several weeks.

PARASITIC INFESTATIONS

Scabies

Scabies is caused by an eight-legged parasitic arthropod called *Sarcoptes scabiei*. The mite burrows down the epidermis along the stratum corneum. Severe itching occurs 2–6 weeks after infestation (worse at night).

Complications are secondary bacterial infection.

Treatment includes application of permethrin cream (5%) applied below the neck and washed off after 8–12 hours, or benzyl benzoate emulsion (25%) applied below the neck all over the body for 12 hours and washed off thereafter, or malathion lotion (0.5%) applied below the neck for 12 hours and then washed off.

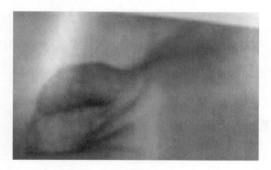

Pediculosis

Pediculosis capitis (head lice infestation) is the most common form of lice infestation in children. Treatment includes application of permethrin (1%) as a cream and rinsing after 10 minutes. Alternate treatment is malathion (0.5%) applied overnight and hair shampooed the next morning.

PSORIASIS

This is a familial disorder that rarely presents before the age of 2 years. Lesions are small, raindrop-like round or oval, erythematous, scaly patches on the trunk and upper limbs. The attack resolves over 3–4 months.

Treatment is with bland ointments; coal tar preparations are useful for plaque psoriasis. Chronic psoriasis may develop into arthritis.

PITYRIASIS ROSEA

It is a self-limiting condition of viral origin. It begins with a single, round or oval, scaly macule which is 2–5 cm in diameter. It is usually seen on the trunk and upper arms and thighs. The rash extends to follow the line of the ribs. Posteriorly, it shows the fir tree pattern. No treatment is required.

ACNE VULGARIS

It usually begins 1–2 years before puberty after androgenic stimulation of the sebaceous glands, causing increased secretion of sebum. There are different types of lesions. Initially, open comedones (blackheads) or closed comedones (whiteheads) are present that progress to form papules. Lesions occur mainly on the face, back, chest and shoulders. More severe lesions produce scaring. Menstruation and emotional stress cause exacerbation. Treatment includes topical application of keratolytic agents, such as benzyl peroxide, applied twice daily after washing. Secondary infections are treated with antibiotics.

URTICARIA (HIVES OR WEALS)

It results from a local increase in the permeability of capillaries and venules. These changes are dependent on activation of skin mast cells which contain a range of mediators including histamine. The cause may be allergy to substances such as cow's milk or drugs or anything under the sun. In children, the manifestations are severe and may develop angioneurotic oedema and anaphylaxis. Treatment is the same as that for anaphylaxis.

FEVER IN CHILDREN

It is an elevation of body temperature (rectal temperature of ≥38°C or 104.4°F in response to pathological stimuli/pyrogens; American College of Emergency Physicians – ACEP).

Bacteria, viruses, malignancies, connective tissue disorders, certain drugs or trauma may endogenously stimulate the production of pyrogens. Common endogenous pyrogens include interleukin (IL)-1, tumour necrosis factor and interferon. Other classes of endogenous pyrogens that cause fever include IL-6, IL-11, leukaemia inhibiting factor (LIF), ciliary neurotrophic factor (CNTF) and oncostatin-M. Exogenous pyrogens include lipopolysaccharides, entotoxins and exotoxins.

Advantages of fever include the following:
- Increased host defence mechanism
- Augmentation of immunological functions
- Suppression of growth of some microbes

Disadvantages of fever include the following:
- Increased incidence of febrile convulsions
- Increased temperature of above 41.5°C is hyperpyrexia and can cause irreversible organ damage

Fever may be of short or long duration. Short-duration fevers (<2 weeks' duration) are caused by infection as a result of viruses, bacteria or protozoa.

Common assessment findings include the following:
- Malaise
- Headache
- Nausea
- Vomiting, impaired appetite and flushed skin

Common causes of short-duration fever are as follows:
- Respiratory tract infection
- Urinary tract infection
- Exanthematous disorders
- Meningitis
- Pyogenic infections
- Malaria
- Typhoid fever
- Heatstroke

Common medical causes of prolonged fever (>2 weeks' duration) are as follows:
- Infections
- Hypersensitivity disorders
- Malignancy
- Rare causes include immunodeficiency disorders, haematological disorders such as hypothalamic and third ventricle lesions
- Genetic disorders
- Miscellaneous causes and metabolic causes

PYREXIA OF UNKNOWN ORIGIN OR FEVER OF UNKNOWN ORIGIN

Pyrexia of unknown origin (PUO) is a fever of more than 3 weeks' duration or fever above 101°F on multiple occasions and with a lack of specific diagnosis after 1 week.

Multidisciplinary Management

- Observe and document fever.
- Identify type, character and course of fever.
- Take a detailed history.
- Perform physical assessment with a special emphasis to identify foci of infection.
- Conduct laboratory investigation including total leucocyte count, peripheral smear (malaria and filariasis) and serological tests.
- Perform microscopic examination and culture of blood, urine, stool and throat swab for bacterial and fungal infections.
- Conduct polymerase chain reaction (PCR) test.
- Obtain X-rays of chest, barium studies of the gastrointestinal tract, ultrasonography and whole-body CT and MRI of various organs to identify the cause of fever.
- Medical management is administration of antipyretics, nonsteroidal anti-inflammatory drugs and steroids.
- Provide specific treatment of infection, if present.
- Rectal temperature between 38.2°C and 39°C needs no treatment.
- Temperature less than 41.2°C needs antipyretics (acetaminophen 45 mg/kg per day is a usual dose).

Nursing Diagnoses

- Alteration in body temperature (hyperpyrexia)
- Activity intolerance
- Parental anxiety
- Knowledge deficit

Nursing Interventions

- Closely monitor and record temperature to identify the type, course and duration of fever.
- Administer antipyretics as prescribed.
- Allow 30 minutes for the antipyretics to work before resorting to hydrotherapy.
- Use tepid water or lukewarm water if sponging is indicated.
- Massage body only gently so that the cutaneous vessels dilate and body heat is dissipated.
- Immerse or rinse all body areas for 20–30 minutes.
- Alternatively, wet towels or sheets can be placed around each extremity and trunk and replace as they become warm.
- Observe the child carefully for chilling or shivering; stop the bath if these occur.
- Recheck temperature 30 minutes after sponging.
- Use cooling blanket (hypothermia blanket), if available, when other methods fail for the child with prolonged hyperpyrexia greater than 102°F (39°C).
- See the blanket temperature at –41°C (5°C).
- Turn the blanket off when the child defervesces to temperature of 100.4°F (38°C).
- Set the blanket temperature to 104°F (40°C) if the child has problems with hypothermia such as in postoperative cardiothoracic surgery.
- Place the child directly on the blanket or have only one-sheet thickness between the child and the blanket.
- Place blanket rolls used for positioning under the blanket so that more of the child's skin surface is in contact with the blanket.
- Place one or more blankets on top of the child, if necessary.
- Monitor vital signs every 15 minutes for 1 hour; if stable, monitor every 30 minutes for 2 hours and then hourly.
- Turn off the cooling blanket if shivering occurs.
- Administer fluid for hydration, as fluid requirement increases by 10% for every 1°C rise in temperature above baseline.

BURNS

It is one of the most common causes of injury, disability and permanent disfigurement in children. Burns cause major physiological and psychological upset because every organ system of the body is affected.

Aetiology

Burns are caused from hot liquids, fire, electricity and chemicals. Children, especially toddlers, are inquisitive and get burned when they reach up to a stove and pull over a pot of hot liquid.

Classification of Burns

Burns are classified by aetiology as scalds, flame burns, electrical burns or chemical injuries. Severity of a burn is determined by its depth and the percentage of the body which is burned. Aetiology and the percentage of burn can easily be calculated, but the depth of the burn can only be estimated. A partial-thickness burn is one which spares the deeper skin appendages and heals spontaneously; full-thickness burn requires skin grafting.

First degree implies a superficial injury of the epidermis with basal layers left intact. The skin is red, oedematous and painful. Healing takes place by regeneration of the epithelium from the basal layers, with desquamation of the superficial corneum.

Second degree involves the epidermis and upper portion of the dermis but spares the dermal appendages. There is blistering and redness of the skin immediately after the burn. Healing normally takes place by regeneration of skin from deeper epidermal cells and the dermal appendages. It usually heals spontaneously within a reasonable period of time.

Full-thickness or **third-degree burn** is a burn in which the entire skin has been destroyed, sometimes with the underlying fat, tendon and other deeper structures. The tissues are dry, charred or dark brown after a flame burn. Thrombosed veins may be seen through the translucent skin and are clearly indicative of depth of the injury. This type of burn weep only very little fluid from its surface and is anaesthetic.

Classification of Burn Injuries

Degree	Structure Involved	Depth (Inches)	Clinical Appearance	Cause	Sensation
Superficial	Epidermis	0.002	Red, dry, erythematous	Sunburn, scald	Normal or sensitive to pain and temperature
Partial thickness (second degree)	Superficial dermis, deep dermis	0.02	Red, blisters, moist, erythematous; blanches with pressure	Scald, immersion, contact, grease, flash fire	Sensitive to pain and temperature
Full thickness (third degree)	Subcutaneous tissue and muscle	0.035–0.040	Dry, white, brown, black, or dark waxy yellow; skin surface cracked, avascular; if red, it does not blanch with pressure	Prolonged immersion, flame, contact, grease, oil	Anaesthetic to pain and temperature

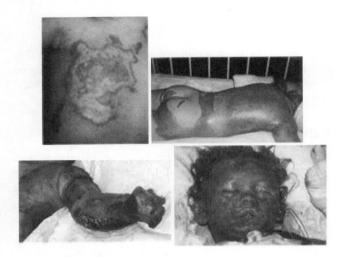

Severity is decided according to the extent of burn on the body. For overall severity of burn, the following factors need to be considered:
- The age of the child
- Depth of burns
- The percentage of burns
- The anatomic areas involved

Minor burns – less than 10% of the body surface – are of partial thickness and do not involve face, hands or perineum. A burn of 15%–30% is considered moderate, and if less than 10% of it is a full-thickness burn. Any burn of 30% or more is considered as severe. Any burn in a child younger than 2 years is more serious because of the thin skin and the difficulties with preventing infection and maintaining infant's nutrition.

A full-thickness burn of more than 30% of body surface area (BSA) is a real threat to life. But with optimum care and the patient's strong will to survive, a 70%–80% survival rate has been achieved.

Classification of Burn Severity

Minor	Moderate	Severe
<10% BSA covered with superficial burns	10%–20% BSA covered with partial-thickness burns <10% BSA covered with full-thickness burns	>20% BSA covered with partial-thickness burns >10% BSA covered with full-thickness burns Burns to hands, feet, face or perineum Electrical burns Inhalation injuries Burns complicated with other injuries

Methods to Determine the Extent of Burn Injury

Rule of Nines

In an adult, the Rule of Nine is used to estimate the relative percentage of a burn wound. In a child, the head

accounts for a larger percentage of total BSA and the legs account for a smaller percentage, so the Rule of Nine is not precisely applicable to children. However, a modified version of Rule of Nine is still used in some centres to calculate the percentage of BSA burned.

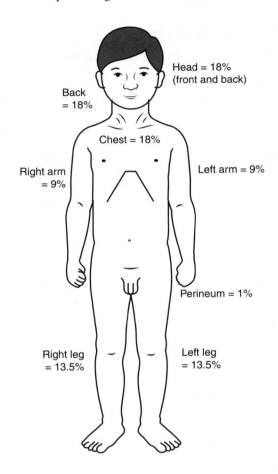

Rule of Palm

A child's palm area is considered as approximately measuring 1%. So, burn area can be approximated with the area of the child's palm and thus one gets an approximation of actual burns.

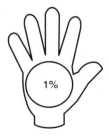

The Rule of Palm is probably the easiest method to use when determining the size of a child's burn. As a general rule, the surface of the child's palm is approximately 1% of the total BSA. By approximating the number of times the child's palm would fit into the burn area, one can estimate the percentage of BSA burned.

Lund and Browder Chart for Assessment of Burns

It is an accurate method of burn assessment and may be made into fill-in sheets for use in paediatric burn units.

The main disadvantage is that it consumes more time than any other burn assessment tool.

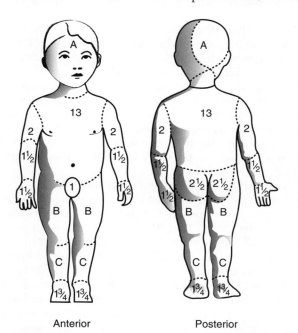

Anterior   Posterior

Relative percentage of body surface area (% BSA) affected by growth

Body part	Age (year)					
	0	**1**	**5**	**10**	**15**	**Adult**
A = Half of head	9.5	8.5	6.5	5.5	4.5	3.5
B = Half of thigh	2.75	3.25	4.0	4.25	4.5	4.75

Area	0–1 Year	1–4 Years	5–9 Years	10–15 Years	Adult	Second Degree	Third Degree	Total (%)
Head	19	17	13	10	7			
Neck	2	2	2	2	2			
Anterior trunk	13	13	13	13	13			
Posterior trunk	13	13	13	13	13			
Right buttock	2.5	2.5	2.5	2.5	2.5			
Left trunk	2.5	2.5	2.5	2.5	2.5			
Genitalia	1	1	1	1	1			
Right upper arm	4	4	4		4			
Left upper arm	4	4	4	4	4			
Right lower arm	3	3	3	3	3			
Left lower arm	3	3	3	3	3			
Right hand	2.5	2.5	2.5	2.5	2.5			
Left hand	2.5	2.5	2.5	2.5	2.5			
Right thigh	5.5	6.5	8	8.5	9.5			
Left thigh	5.5	6.5	8	8.5	9.5			
Right leg	5	5	5.5	6	7			
Left leg	5	5	5.5	6	7			
Right foot	3.5	3.5	3.5	3.5	3.5			
Left foot	3.5	3.5	3.5	3.5	3.5			
Total								

Relative percentage of body surface area (% BSA) is affected by growth.

Pathology

On contact with thermal or chemical energy, immediate coagulation necrosis of the superficial layer of the skin occurs. The depth of the tissue death depends on the temperature and duration of contact with the source of heat. Below the first layer of coagulation necrosis is the second zone that is damaged but still viable. There is reduction of capillary blood flow related to the damage to the microcirculation in the second zone. Venous thrombosis will lead to infraction in this area and convert the wound from a possible deep, second-degree burn to one of full-thickness tissue loss. In the third zone of injury, there is hyperaemia and vasodilatation. The necrotic tissue releases toxic materials into the bloodstream, causing red cell haemolysis, and this forms a culture medium until it is debrided or sloughed. The deeper, viable injured zone has importance in the first hours after injury. Here, capillary permeability increases and free loss of plasma proteins and electrolytes into the extravascular compartment takes place. The injury to the capillary membrane leads to lack of osmotic pressure to keep the plasma proteins within the blood vessels.

In extensive second-degree burns, half of the lost fluid and protein remain in the extravascular tissues, whereas the rest is lost through evaporation as superficial weeping and blister fluid. In severe burns, the fluid loss takes place primarily in the first 12 hours of burns. With burn shock, there is loss of endothelium. Vascular integrity in the unburned area leads to further exudation of fluid and proteins from the vascular space. In severe burns, reabsorption of fluid from the injured zone starts within 48 hours, but this may be delayed in burn areas of more than 50%. Other derangements in skin's normal function include the following:

- Loss of regular body temperature occurs (owing to injury to sweat glands as well as increase of evaporating water sources through the air–wound interphase).
- The loss of skin as a barrier against bacterial invasion is most important. The bacteriostatic properties of the normal skin are destroyed, and the dead tissues act as a perfect culture medium for proliferation of bacteria.
- The endogenous bacteria that remain deep in the patient's sweat glands and hair follicles may cause serious infections.

An extensive thermal injury exerts pathophysiological responses far beyond burns. Myocardial depressant is released from the burnt wound that decreases the cardiac output and reduces excess plasma loss. The hypovolaemic state is reflected or manifested as decreased urine output and increased circulatory norepinephrine, cortisol, aldosterone and antidiuretic hormone and rennin angiotensin. Hypermetabolism associated with burns is related to heat loss through evaporation of water from burn wound and through chronic catecholamine stimulation. The stress produced by a burn is prolonged till the burn wound is healed. During this period, the endogenous nutrition is depleted and the patient's needs for nutrition are tremendously increased. Fluid therapy helps maintain normal plasma volume. The diet should supply 25 cal/kg of body weight plus 40 kcal for each percent of the body burned to the patient to reduce nutritional deficiency and promote wound healing.

Initial Care

- Evaluate the child, his/her burn and his/her family.
- Burns involving less than 10% of body surface in children younger than 1 year can be managed on outpatient basis, but burns of the perineum and face need hospitalization.
- After the initial assessment, sterile, cold normal saline soak can be applied to the burn wound that relieves pain of first-degree burn and possibly reduces oedema.
- Wash the skin around the burned area with a bland soap.
- After washing the skin, gently wash the burned area with soap and water with new washed cloths or *gangi* pads. The wound should be irrigated with normal saline and dried with a sterile towel.
- Blisters are left untouched, as debridement of blisters remove excellent biological dressing and exposes the underlying epithelium to drying and mechanical irritation. Blister fluids help preserve capillary circulation in the second zone of injury. It is shown that the presence of blisters does not produce more infection.
- All attendants should wear a mask and gloves.
- Gloves need to be changed after burn wash and wear a new pair for dressing. Hospital practice is to apply silver sulfadiazine after drying the wound with sterile towel and follow open dressing pattern for burn care. In some hospitals, closed dressings are used for burn care. After drying the burn wound with a sterile towel, apply petroleum gauzes over the burn wound and bulky dressings are applied over the same and held securely in place by multiple layers of smoothly applied bandages (at some places, topical antibiotics are used instead of petroleum gauze). The initial dressing is left undisturbed for 5–7 days and then removed and reapply another bulky dressing which is removed after 10–14 days after soaking with normal saline. But if the child is febrile, then the dressings are removed and inspected for infection. If burn is infected, culture is taken for sensitivity to start appropriate antibiotics. The wound itself is treated with moist dressings, which are changed several times a day.
- The wound is washed again on the third day and topical antibiotics (silver sulfadiazine) are applied. This process is continued till the wound is ready for skin grafting.
- Evaluation and initial assessment:
  Evaluation of A, B, C and burn wound. The nurse must be vigilant to have all resuscitation equipment ready in the causality/emergency department. In addition to usual resuscitation equipment, sterile sheets must be available to cover the child. If the child has burns of airway, the child may be cyanotic and apnoeic. Initial treatment of any child suspected of having an airway burn consists of administration of humidified oxygen, postural drainage and tracheal suction.
- Resuscitation:
  Remove clothes completely and place the child on a sterile sheet (in Kerala, the child is placed on clean banana leaves). Venipuncture is performed or central line for fluid therapy is inserted for fluid administration. Blood is drawn for haematocrit and electrolytes and cross-match.
- Administer Ringer's lactate with an initial bolus of 20 mL/kg. If burn is more than 20%, a Foley catheter is introduced for urinary measurements.

- The percentage of body area burned is assessed using the Lund and Browder chart (see the figure) or by Rule of Palm or modified Rule of Nine. Estimation of relative areas of partial and full thickness along with the total percentage of body area burned needs to be done to provide adequate fluid management.
- Perform fluid calculation.

Essential Facts

- Accurate hourly urine output
- The sensorium   } Essential guide to fluid therapy
- The pulse

There are many formulas used for fluid calculation. According to Evans et al., 1 mL each of plasma and isotonic saline/kg per % of body surface area burned is required, as fluid loss is primarily plasma and extracellular fluid. In addition to plasma and saline calculated on the basis of the burned area, the child's usual maintenance is given as half of the first day's requirement in the first 8 hours after the burns and the other half of the formula is given during the rest of the 24 hours.

The Brooke Army formula provides only 0.5 mL plasma/kg per % of burn and includes 1.5% crystalloid plus maintenance fluids.

Current practice is an immediate bolus of 20 mL/kg in Ringer's lactate in 5% dextrose. If this provides an output of urine 1 mL/kg per hour, then 1 mL each of plasma and Ringer's lactate solution/kg per % of body burned are provided during the first 8 hours. During the second and third 8 hours, maintenance fluids are met with 0.2% saline in 10% glucose. Gastrointestinal losses are replaced and further lactate Ringer's solution is given by bolus if the urine output falls.

During the second 24-hour period, a minimum of 10 mL/kg plasma or 1 mL/kg per % of body burned is given. The hourly urine volume is continually monitored to observe the onset of diuresis, which heralds the resolution of the burn oedema.

Common formulas used for fluid calculation in burns are as follows:

1. Parkland's formula:
   4 mL of Ringer's lactate per kg of body weight per % of BSA burned given in the first 24 hours (4 mL × kg × % BSA).
   - Half the amount given in the first 8 hours
   - One-fourth of the amount given in the second 8 hours
   - Next one-fourth of the amount given in the third 8 hours
2. Duke's formula:
   3 mL of Ringer's lactate per kg of body weight per % of BSA burned, PLUS one-half ampoule of sodium bicarbonate per litre of the replacement fluid given in the first 24 hours.
   - One-half of the amount given in the first 8 hours
   - One-fourth of the amount given in the second 8 hours
   - One-fourth of the amount given in the third 8 hours

Summary of Initial Care

- Evaluate airway.
- Draw blood for haematocrit, type and cross-matching, electrolytes and blood urea nitrogen (BUN).
- Estimate the percentage of burned area.
- Start administration of intravenous Ringer's lactate solution and calculate the fluid needs.
- Insert a Foley catheter to all children with burns more than 30% of BSA or with burns to the perineum.
- Pass a nasogastric tube.
- Give prophylactic Tetanus Toxoid (TT).
- Give penicillin or appropriate antibiotics for the first 5–7 days to prevent β-haemolytic streptococcal cellulitis and septicaemia during this period.
- Give intravenous sedation if the child is in pain or restless and if the airway is not involved (usual dose for a child older than 1 year is 0.1 mg/kg morphine). It can be given by diluting it with saline.
- Start an intensive care flow sheet to record pulse, blood pressure, rest rate and urine output every half hourly.

Treatment of Burn Wound

Wounds must be protected from mechanical trauma and bacterial contamination in the case of partial-thickness burns. Slough of full-thickness burn may be removed so that the wound may be closed with skin graft. The occlusive dressing technique was formerly associated with a high incidence of wound infection and sepsis during the second and third post-burn weeks. Silver sulfadiazine is an effective agent against *Pseudomonas*, *Staphylococcus aureus* and a variety of other organism which colonize burn wounds. Primary excision and grafting of small non-life-threatening burns have always been a highly acceptable and desirable practice. Areas such as hands, face, etc. need early excision and grafting. The technique of primary excision has been further refined by the use of hypotensive anaesthesia, electrocoagulation of bleeding points and immediate coverage of the wound with both allografts and cadaver homograft. Burn less than 30% of BSA can usually be completely grafted with the patient's own skin at one sitting. The face, hands and flexion creases are grafted as first sheets of skin which provide uniform coverage to give a better functional and cosmetic result.

Nutrition

Nothing is more important than maintaining adequate nutrition in the total care of a child with burn injury. The common problem faced in maintaining adequate nutrition includes paralytic ileus and constant pain. Without intensive nutritional support in addition to what the child will eat him/herself, there is extensive weight loss, the burn wound is soggy and oedematous, grafts will not take and donor sites convert to third-degree wounds. The degree of catabolism is such that two to three times the usual maintenance requirements for calories, proteins and vitamins are necessary. Hence, an accurate daily calorie count with an estimation of protein intake is essential. As soon as the gastrointestinal tract commences to function, feeds must be given either through a nasogastric tube or orally according to the condition of the child. Parents must be encouraged to bring the favourite food of the child. Burns of more than 40%–50% of BSA require additional nutritional support. In some cases, intravenous hyperalimentation is practiced.

Sepsis

Delayed closure of the wound, poor nutrition and sepsis go hand in hand. During the first few days, patient him/herself will be the source. But as the time goes on, the hospital personnel, equipment and general hospital environment become the source. Suppurative thrombophlebitis is a significant cause for sepsis in burned patients. Prophylactic antibiotic therapy has reduced the incidence of sepsis. The most common fungal infections are caused by *Candida albicans* and *Aspergillus*.

Gastrointestinal Complications

During the first 24 hours after burns, there is a high incidence of acute gastric dilatation and paralytic ileus. Most serious complication is gastrointestinal bleeding. The so-called Curling ulcer occurs most commonly in the gastric antrum or duodenum. In children, duodenal ulcers are common. Haemorrhage occurs at any time but is more common during the third and fourth weeks. If the child develops melaena or haematemesis, a nasogastric tube is passed at once and the stomach is irrigated with 1% $NaHCO_3$. Vital signs and urine output are monitored and stabilized with transfusions.

Burn Wound Scars

Rehabilitation of a burned child requires many years. Scaring and contracture formation are quite common if adequate care is not taken. Areas which are of particular concern include axillae, neck, antecubital fossa, popliteal fossae and hands. As soon as possible after the initial injury, the knees and elbows are splinted in extension. Shoulders should be abducted with a bulky dressing or with a skin traction of the forearm if it is not burned.

Passive exercises of interphalangeal joints are advisable. The neck must be splinted with head extension. The child must be taught to do simple exercises of joints to prevent contraction.

STUDY QUESTIONS

- What are the common skin disorders seen in children?
- What are the common characteristics of allergic skin manifestations in children?
- How will you classify burns?
- What is the Parkland formula?
- What is the fluid management in burns?
- How will you prevent infection in a child with burns?
- What is pyrexia of unknown origin?
- Write short notes on the following:
  a. Impetigo
  b. Napkin rash
  c. Tinea capitis
  d. Parasitic infestation
  e. Urticaria
  f. Acne vulgaris
- What are the nurse's responsibilities while caring a child with PUO?

BIBLIOGRAPHY

1. Charles L. Fox., Jr. (1968). The role of alkaline sodium salt solutions in treatment of severe burns. Annals of the New York Academy of Sciences 150(3): 823-844.
2. Desai, M.H., et al. (1992). Candida Infection With and Without Nystatin Prophylaxis. Archives of Surgery, 127, pp 159–162.
3. Evans E.L., Purnell, O.J., Robinett P. W., Batchelor A., Martin M.: Fluid and electrolyte requirements in severe burns. Annals of Surgery, 804-17, 1952.
4. Kinner, M.A., Daly, W.L. (1992). Skin Transplantation. Critical Care Nursing Clinics of North America, 4, pp 173–178.
5. Martinez, S. (1992). Ambulatory Management of Burns in Children. Journal of Paediatric Health Care, 6, pp 32–37.
6. O'Neil, J.A. (1990). Inhalation Injury in Children. In: Happonik, E.F., Munster, A.M. (Editors). Respiratory Injury: Smoke Inhalation and Burns. New York: McGraw Hill.
7. Sorenesen B. Dextran solution in the treatment of burn shock. Scand. J. Plast.Reconstr.Surg, 1:68, 1967.
8. Zingg, B.M. (1993). Managing Burns in Children: An Intraoperative Nursing Care Plan. AORN Journal, 54, pp 568–575.

CHAPTER 38

NURSING MANAGEMENT OF CHILDREN WITH COMMUNICABLE DISEASES

LEARNING OBJECTIVES

At the end of the chapter, the learner will be able to:

- Describe the nursing management of children suffering from tuberculosis.
- Explain various communicable diseases and their medical and nursing management and preventive measures.
- Explain communicable diseases with viral aetiology.
- Explain care of children with HIV/AIDS.
- Discuss nursing management of children with chikungunya and dengue fever.

INTRODUCTION

In India, communicable diseases are still a threat to childhood morbidity and mortality. India being a signatory to WHO and UNICEF in implementing immunization programmes to control communicable diseases, the toll of deaths related to this remains a health care burden. In this chapter, nursing management of children with various communicable diseases that affect children is dealt with.

TUBERCULOSIS

Tuberculosis (TB) is still a public health problem in many parts of India, though there is a decline in the incidence and mortality related to TB. HIV infection has also added to the cause of TB. Re-emergence of multiresistant strains has also contributed to the increase in incidence of TB.

Pasteurization of milk has made a decline in the incidence of bovine TB, and the spread is usually by the respiratory route. Close proximity, infectious load and underlying immunodeficiency enhance the risk of transmission. Children usually get infected from adult contacts through direct droplet infection within the same household. Child-to-child transmission does not take place, as the primary complex is not infectious.

Signs and Symptoms

Primary infection can be asymptomatic or symptomatic. In about 90% of infants, the disease is asymptomatic and will show minimal sign and symptoms of infection. A local inflammatory reaction limits the progression of infection. The disease is latent and develops into active form at a later time. A positive Mantoux test (10 units) >10 mm of induration implies active infection (read after 48–72 hours). A dose of 10 units – 0.1 mL of 1:1000 of a purified protein derivative of tuberculin is given intradermally.

In symptomatic cases, the local inflammatory response fails to contain the inhaled tubercle bacilli, allowing lymphatic spread to the regional lymph node, leading to lymphadenopathy. The lung lesion and the lymph node constitute a primary complex (Ghon complex). When the host's cellular immune system responds to the infection (3–6 weeks), bacterial replication diminishes but systemic symptoms develop, such as:

- Fever
- Anorexia and weight loss

- Cough
- Chest X-ray changes

Primary complex usually heals and calcifies. The inflammatory reaction may lead to local enlargement of periorbital lymph nodes which may cause bronchial obstruction with collapse and consolidation of the affected lung. Local dissemination and pleural effusion may also develop. Primary infection usually develops in the lung. But it occurs in other regions, too.

Both asymptomatic and symptomatic infections may become dormant but can get reactivated and spread by lymphohaematological routes, leading to spread of infection to other organs such as central nervous system (CNS), kidney and pericardium.

Treatment is by DOTS.

Prevention is by BCG immunization.

DIPHTHERIA

It is an acute infectious disease caused by *Corynebacterium diphtheriae* and characterized by local inflammation of the epithelial surface, formation of pseudomembrane and severe toxaemia.

The bacteria (bacilli) proliferate and liberate a powerful exotoxin that causes the systemic and local lesions. Local lesions are the result of necrosis of the epithelial cells and liberate serous and fibrinous material which forms a greyish-white pseudomembrane and bleeds when an attempt is made to remove it. The surrounding tissues are inflamed and oedematous.

The systemic symptoms result from the effect of exotoxin that affects the heart, kidneys and nervous system. It causes myocardial fibre degeneration and enlargement of the heart, causing conduction disturbances. Nervous system involvement is manifested as polyneuritis. In the kidneys, it produces renal tubular degeneration with inflammation of the interstitial tissue.

Assessment Findings

- Incubation period is 2–5 days.
- In a nonimmunized child, the onset is acute with fever (usually 39°C).
- Malaise, headache and loss of appetite occur.
- The child looks sick, toxic, with clouded sensorium, and may be delirious.
- Circulatory collapse occurs owing to heart and renal involvement.

Types

- Nasal diphtheria
- Faucial diphtheria
- Laryngeal diphtheria

Nasal diphtheria

- It can be unilateral or bilateral.
- Serosanguineous discharge occurs from the nose and excoriation of the upper lip.
- Minimal toxaemia is present and the child looks ill.

Faucial Diphtheria

- Redness and swelling present over fauces.
- Exudates on tonsils coalesce to form a greyish-white pseudomembrane which may spread to the surrounding areas. Regional lymph node inflammation and enlargement are present.
- Sore throat, dysphagia and muffled voice are present.

Laryngeal Diphtheria

- Membrane over the larynx, brassy cough and hoarse voice
- Laboured and noisy breathing
- Chest retractions, both suprasternal and substernal retractions
- Increased respiratory effort and use of accessory muscles
- Respiratory distress leads to respiratory failure
- Unusual sites of involvement are conjunctiva and skin

Complications

- Myocarditis
- Palatal paralysis
- Loss of accommodation
- Polyneuritis
- Renal complications include oliguria and proteinuria

Multidisciplinary Management

- Diagnosis is by clinical findings

Medical Treatment

- Neutralization of circulating toxins is achieved by administration of antitoxin.
- Antitoxin is given intramuscularly or intravenously, but after the appearance of the symptom, it has no use. So, early administration is important.
- Dose for pharyngeal and laryngeal diphtheria of 48 hours' duration is 20,000–40,000 units.
- For nasopharyngeal diphtheria, it is 40,000–60,000 units.
- For swelling of neck, the dose is 80,000–120,000 units.
- Antibiotic penicillin or erythromycin is given.
- Procaine penicillin dose is 3-6 mL Intramuscular (IM) twice a day.
- Oral penicillin dose includes 125–250 mg q.i.d. or erythromycin 25–30 mg/kg.
- Total duration is for 14 days.
- Supportive management includes bed rest for 2–3 weeks to reduce heart complications.
- Symptomatic treatment is provided.
- Management of complications is essential.

Nursing Diagnoses

- Airway clearance ineffective
- Ineffective breathing pattern
- Activity intolerance
- Altered parenting

- Anxiety
- Decreased cardiac output
- Complication potential
- Altered renal, gastrointestinal/peripheral/cardiopulmonary/cerebral perfusion
- Nutrition alteration

Nursing Interventions

- Monitor vital signs every 1–2 hours; note pulsus paradoxus.
- Provide cool, moist environment.
- Administer aerosol or nebulizer treatment, as prescribed.
- Plan nursing tasks to allow for maximum rest.
- Administer sedatives, as ordered.
- Encourage anxious parents to take small amount of time away from the child to see if the child relaxes.
- Teach parents and the child signs and symptoms of the disease.
- Do not attempt to remove the pseudomembrane.
- Monitor vital signs closely and be alert for indications of airway obstruction and respiratory failure.
- Keep nothing by mouth (NPO).
- Maintain bed rest.
- Sedate the child, as needed.
- Observe for nervous system complications and for development of Guillain-Barré syndrome (GBS), as sudden death may occur as a result of renal failure, myocarditis and respiratory paralysis.
- Monitor cardiac/respiratory function for signs of respiratory arrest/failure.
- Establish airway.
- Control fever with cooling mattresses.
- Assess heart sounds every 4 hours.
- Change in the characteristics of heart sounds and murmur may be noticed to identify progression.
- Monitor heart sounds/rhythm continuously. Conduction defects may signal the spread of infection or atrial volume overload.
- Monitor for left ventricular failure – crackles, S3/S4 sounds, dyspnoea, tachypnoea, digital clubbing, increased pulse pressure and left ventricular end-diastolic pressure (LVEDP), decreased blood pressure (BP) and cardiac output.
- Monitor right ventricular failure – increased central venous pressure (CVP), jugular venous distension (JVD), positive hepatojugular reflux, oedema, jaundice and ascites.
- Monitor intake and output and measure weight daily.
- Decrease the preload by limiting fluid intake and by administering diuretics and venous dilators, as prescribed.
- If mean arterial pressure (MAP) is high, decrease the afterload with prescribed arterial dilators.
- If afterload decreases, increase it by administration of vasopressors.
- Increase contractility with positive inotropes.
- Limit child activities, schedule activities to level of tolerance.
- Provide sedation as needed to decrease oxygen consumption caused by anxiety and agitation.
- Monitor intake and output.

- Monitor peripheral pulses, colour and temperature of extremities.
- Monitor for convulsions, paralysis and dysphagia.
  Prevention: This dreadful disease can be prevented by vaccination.

WHOOPING COUGH

It is a highly contagious acute respiratory infection caused by *Bordetella pertussis*. It is also known as 100 days' cough. *Bordetella pertussis* is a nonmotile gram-negative bacillus. The infection is transmitted by droplets infection from infected persons. It commonly occurs in late winter and early spring. Peak age of incidence is seen in children 4 years of age. In developing countries, it occurs much earlier as a result of early exposure to infectious agents. Incubation period is 7–14 days. Clinical stages are divided into three stages:

- Catarrhal stage – It lasts for 7–10 days. It is the most infectious period. The initial manifestations are indistinguishable from upper respiratory tract infections. Children have cough and coryza with little nasopharyngeal secretion. The cough symptoms do not alleviate and become most severe and frequent with the passage of time. In the early stage, it is nonparoxysmal, but during the later part, it is paroxysmal in nature.
- Paroxysmal phase – It lasts for 2–4 weeks. This phase is characterized by rapid succession of cough in an explosive manner. The child may appear to be choking, unable to breathe, looks anxious and has a suffused face. The bout of cough terminates with a long drawn-out inspiratory crowning sound or whoop. The whoop is produced by air rushing in during inspiration through the half-open glottis. In infants, whoop may not be present; instead, cyanotic spells are seen. The paroxysms of cough are so frequent that it may occur even hourly or more frequently. Ulceration of frenulum as a result of frequent thrusting of the tongue is too common. After the paroxysms of cough, the child appears listless. Precipitating factors include food intake, cool liquids, inspiration of cool air, etc.
- Convalescent period – The interval between paroxysms of cough increases and severity of episodes decreases gradually. Vomiting episodes are less frequent. Appetite, general condition and health improve gradually. This stage lasts for 2–4 weeks but may also extend longer.

Complications

- Respiratory – *Bordetella pertussis* causes necrotizing inflammatory response, stasis, paralysis of cilia, inspiration of secretions causing patchy atelectasis and pneumonia. Interstitial pneumonia, bronchiectasis, subcutaneous emphysema and pneumothorax are other complications.
- Neurological – Convulsions and encephalopathy result from hypoxia and focal intracranial haemorrhages. Persistent seizures, hemiplegia, paraplegia, ataxia,

aphonia, blindness, deafness and decerebrate rigidity may occur.

- Gastrointestinal manifestations include hernias and rectal prolapse.
- Haemorrhage is subconjunctival in nature.
- Severe malnutrition may result from persistent vomiting and disinclination to eat the food because of fear of paroxysms of cough.

Multidisciplinary Management

The total leucocyte count is elevated, and there is absolute lymphocytosis. Quick diagnosis is possible by florescent antibody staining of the laryngeal swab. Other investigations include DNA probe, ELISA, etc.

- Medical treatment includes hospitalization in severe cases.
- Administration of erythromycin, especially estolate ester (40–50 mg/kg per day), is the preferred antibiotic.
- Small doses of bronchodilators are used to relieve bronchospasms.
- Nebulization is performed to control bouts of cough.
- Prevention is by active immunization with DPT vaccine.

Nursing Diagnosis

- Infective airway clearance related to bronchospasm
- Comfort alteration related to paroxysmal cough
- Nutrition alteration related to vomiting and feeding difficulty
- High risk for injury/complication potential related to the disease process
- Parental anxiety
- Ineffective parental coping
- Knowledge deficit

Nursing Interventions

- Assist in respiratory clearance/airway clearance.
- Administer bronchodilators.
- Do not allow the child to cry, as it stimulates paroxysms of cough.
- Administer antibiotics as prescribed.
- Give small, frequent, easily digestible feeds.
- Do not force food and fluids.
- Permit the child to have adequate rest.
- Protect the child from respiratory irritants.
- Allow the child to rest with head in an elevated position.
- Provide adequate rest.
- Do not provoke the child for any reason, as it stimulates paroxysms of cough.
  Prevention is through vaccination with DPT vaccine.

CHOLERA

It is a form of severe gastroenteritis characterized by the sudden onset of profuse rice water diarrhoea, followed by vomiting and dehydration. Severe type of cholera is called cholera gravis. It is caused by *Vibrio cholerae* 01 or *Vibrio cholerae* 0139 group 1.

Previously, it occurred as epidemics; now it is not common as epidemics. In Kerala, the epidemic outbreaks are common during rainy season and in tribal areas. Cholera is endemic in certain parts of India such as Maharashtra, Tamil Nadu, Madhya Pradesh, Andhra Pradesh and Assam. Transmission is by the faeco-oral route, and the channel of transmission is by contaminated water, food and direct person-to-person contact. The predisposing factor is poor environmental sanitation.

Assessment Findings

- Incubation period is 1–2 days and can extend up to 5 days.
- The disease has three stages:
- Stage 1 is characterized by profuse, effortless, watery diarrhoea with rice water stools, followed by vomiting and severe dehydration.
- Stage 2 is characterized by severe dehydration that ends up in shock.
- Stage 3 is the stage of recovery with alleviation of symptoms unless severe dehydration had not taken its turn.

Multidisciplinary Management

- Diagnosis is confirmed by direct microscopic examination of the stool, vomitus, water and food.
- Culture on peptone water tellurite medium (PWT) shows the growth of the organism.
- Biochemical tests are performed.
- Medical management consists of administering oral or intravenous rehydration therapy along with drugs to shorten the duration of diarrhoea to reduce the period of *Vibrio* excretion.
- Drug of choice is tetracycline.
- Other drugs include erythromycin, co-trimoxazole, furazolidone and ciprofloxacin.
- Usual duration of treatment is 3 days.
- Parental education is provided to improve sanitation.
- Environmental and food sanitation and disinfection of contact materials are strictly advised to follow.
  Prophylaxis – Chemoprophylaxis for household contacts is recommended as well as for a closed community outbreaks of cholera by using cholera vaccine (which kills 12,000 million *Vibrio*/mL) with a protective value of 50% for a period of 3–6 months. The dose is 0.3 mL for children older than 2 years and 0.2 mL for those between 6 months and 2 years of age. The route of administration is subcutaneous. The dose is repeated after 4–6 weeks.
  Reactions – These include local pain, swelling, erythema and abscess.
  Fever is seen only in a small proportion of children.

Nursing Diagnoses

- Fluid volume deficit
- Complication potential/high risk for injury/infection
- Parental anxiety
- Knowledge deficit

Nursing Interventions

- Assess the hydration status of children.
- Accurately monitor the type of diarrhoea and the amount of fluid loss.
- Monitor intake and output.
- Administer fluids as required.
- Administer prophylaxis to contacts.
- Activate public health measures to prevent the spread of cholera to other areas.
- Other nursing interventions are described in the chapter on fluid electrolyte imbalances.

Outbreak can be prevented through vaccination and chlorination of water sources.

SHIGELLOSIS (ACUTE BACILLARY DYSENTERY)

It is defined as passage of loose stools containing mucus, pus and blood. The accompanying features are fever, tenesmus and abdominal cramps.

There are four strains of *Shigella*. Invasive strains of *Shigella* enter through oral–faecal route after penetrating the epithelial cells of the intestine and multiply in the submucosa and lamina propria. It produces local inflammation and superficial ulcers that may bleed, causing blood in the stools. The infection results from a low level of personal and environmental sanitation that promotes breeding of flies.

Assessment Findings

- Incubation period is 1–3 days.
- Onset is sudden with fever.
- Prostration, vomiting, bloody diarrhoea, abdominal pain and tenesmus are present.
- Dehydration and electrolyte loss occur.
- Headache, drowsiness and convulsions follow and lead to coma in severe cases.
- Common complications include haemolytic uraemic syndrome (HUS), anaemia with hypoproteinaemia, rectal prolapse, arthritis, Reiter syndrome, vaginitis, etc.

Multidisciplinary Management

- Stool smear is obtained to find out red cells and leucocytes (pus cells).
- Blood culture reveals marked leucocytes with increased polymorphonuclear cells.
- Stool culture is collected to isolate organism.
- Medical management includes administration of antibiotics after culture and sensitivity tests.
- Common drugs used are ampicillin, co-trimoxazole, nalidixic acid and tetracycline.
- Supportive measures are correction of dehydration and electrolyte imbalances.

Nursing Diagnoses

- Fluid–electrolyte imbalances
- Knowledge deficit
- Complication potential

Nursing Interventions

- Assess dehydration.
- Administration of fluid and electrolytes should be done, as prescribed.
- Maintain intake and output.
- Assist in investigation, blood and stools culture and sensitivity and peripheral smear.
- Administration of antibiotics done as per prescription after culture and sensitivity tests.
- Observe for complication such as the dreaded HUS, which requires peritoneal dialysis.
- Provide parental education on the following:
  - Personal hygiene
  - Environmental sanitation
  - Provide anticipatory guidance

HIV INFECTION

HIV transmission occurs vertically from the mother to the child. Vertical transmission occurs during the intrapartum and intrauterine periods or via breast milk. Transmission of HIV to infants occurs from the mother who has a greater load of HIV and more advanced disease stage. In total, 25%–40% of infants get infected through breast milk. A majority of women are infected from their partners than by drug abuse or blood transfusions. The virus is rarely transmitted to children by infected blood products, and HIV transmission through blood products and contaminated needles is rare in children.

Diagnosis of HIV is reliable only in children older than 18 months. This is because infants born to infected mothers will have circulating maternal HIV antibodies and the test will be unreliable.

HIV-infected children (<18 months):
- Only if two tests are +ve, i.e. HIV culture, Ag or polymerase chain reaction (PCR) or clinical criteria.

HIV-infected children (>18 months):
- ELISA, Western blot +ve
- Perinatally exposed
- <18 months of age, ELISA, Western blot +ve
- HIV +ve mother, kid status unknown
- Seroverter
- <18 months, ELISA −ve twice
- >18 months, ELISA −ve once

Most important test is detection of viral genome by PCR. Other tests include HIV culture, P24 antigen, elevated immunoglobulins, low CD4 T cell count for age and clinical features.

- Paediatric AIDS in the West   1982
- Indian HIV-infected infant   1986
- Paediatric AIDS constitute   2%
- Mother-to-child transmission (MTCT)   15%–20%
- HIV-infected women and kids constitute   50%

Reduction of Vertical Transmission

- Avoidance of breastfeeding
- Use antenatal antiretroviral drugs to reduce perinatal and postnatal to reduce viral load, e.g. zidovudine or nevirapine

- Avoidance of labour and contact with the birth canal by elective caesarean section.

All these interventions reduce transmission of HIV/AIDS to a rate less than 2%.

HIV-infected children may remain asymptomatic for months or years before progressing to severe disease and immunodeficiency or to an AIDS diagnosis. Clinical presentation is according to the level of immunosuppression.

    Mild immunosuppression – Lymphadenopathy or parotitis

    Moderate – Recurrent bacterial infections, candidiasis, chronic diarrhoea and lymphocytic interstitial pneumonitis (LIP)

    Severe – Opportunistic infections, e.g. *Pneumocystis carinii* infection, severe failure to thrive (FTT), encephalopathy and malignancy (which is rare manifestation in children)

	Baby	Mother
Interstitial pneumonitis	Short	Longer
Bacterial infection	More	Fewer
Opportunistic infection	Less (Toxoplasmosis, Histoplasmosis and Cryptosporidiosis)	Common
LIP	Common	Rare
Kaposi sarcoma	Rare	Not common
Viral DNA	100%	60%–70%

Natural history of children with HIV with its difference from adults
- HIV antibody tests cannot be used to diagnose infection in infancy
- Faster rate of clinical disease progression in some children; 20–25% progress in the first year in the absence of antiretroviral therapy and PCP prophylaxis
- Primary disease with opportunistic infections more common than re-activation
- Lymphocytic interstitial pneumonitis (LIP) is common
- Bacterial infections are very common and occur at all stages of disease
- HIV encephalopathy presents differently
- Growth failure occurs as well as weight loss and wasting
- Kaposi's sarcoma is rare outside endemic areas

Adapted from Graham SM & Gibb DM. "HIV disease and respiratory infection in children" *British Medical Bulletin*, Volume 61, Issue 1, 1 March 2002, Pages 133–150

Treatment

Infants of indeterminate state should be immunized according to schedule except BCG. BCG should not be administered owing to the risk of dissemination. Infants born to HIV-infected mothers should be given BCG vaccine only if they are known to be HIV negative. A theoretical risk is postulated for immunocompromised caregivers if oral polio vaccine is given to a baby, so Salk polio vaccine is advised. Primary pneumocystis pneumonia (PCP) is prevented in HIV-infected children with administration of co-trimoxazole.

Factors that decide long-term morbidity and mortality are as follows:
- The plasma load of virus
- CD4 Count

Child with symptomatic HIV has a reduced CD4 count for age and a high viral load. Asymptomatic children or mildly symptomatic children require regular monitoring of viral load and CD4 count. These children require antiretroviral therapy if their count is low.

Stages

- **Asymptomatic stage:**
  - Progressive decline in CD4 and T cells
  - Immunosuppression
- **Early symptomatic stage AIDS Related Complex (ARC):**
  - CD4 <500/µL
  - Clinical illness — Lymph node enlargement (lymphadenopathy), thrush, Shingles (herpes zoster infection)

WHO Criteria	
Major Criteria	**Minor Criteria**
Weight loss/FTT	Generalized lymphnode Enlargement (GLE)
Chronic diarrhoea (>1 month)	Oropharyngeal candidiasis
Prolonged fever (>1 month)	Recurring common infections

- Severe/recurrent pneumonia
- Dermatitis
- Confirmed Mother HIV +ve

PAPULAR RASH

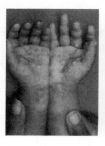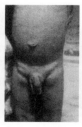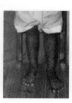

Antiretroviral therapy is most effective in suppressing viral replication and maintaining health status in children. The common antiretroviral agents used are:
- Nucleoside analogue reverse transcriptase inhibitors (NRTIs), e.g. zidovudine, didanosine, lamivudine
- Non-nucleoside analogue reverse transcriptase inhibitors (NNRTIs), e.g. nevirapine, efavirenz
- Protease inhibitors (PIs), e.g. ritonavir, indinavir, nelfinavir

The current regimen for antiretroviral therapy is two NRTIs with either an NNRTI or a PI. With this treatment, most children are living up to their teenage years which bring more problems.

The child and family need to be provided coordinated medical, psychological and social support which is a major aspect of HIV management. This is very important in Kerala, as many issues have developed recently in children with HIV-positive findings. This also helps in streamlining the treatment. Multidisciplinary team approach is essential in helping family cope with the social stigma associated with this condition. Children should be protected and confidentiality should be maintained as their schooling will be affected.

MEASLES

It is viral infection caused by rubella virus (RNA virus) characterized by fever, cough, coryza and Koplik spot in the pre-eruptive phase and maculopapular rash on the fourth to fifth days. Healing of the rash gives brown pigmentation of the skin. Infection occurs with invasion of the respiratory epithelium by the virus. Local multiplication produces viraemia and spreads to the reticuloendothelium.

Assessment Findings

- The incubation period is 14–21 days, and the period of infectivity is from the onset of coryza until 5 days of rash.
- Two distinctive phases are seen – prodromal phase and eruptive stage.
- The signs and symptoms usually start 10–14 days after cough.
- Exposure to droplets, which are highly infectious during viral shedding, causes symptoms.
- Other symptoms include conjunctivitis, coryza and Koplik spots, rash and increased temperature. Koplik spots are white spots on buccal mucosa, seen against the bright red background. It is the pathognomonic feature but difficult to visualize. These disappear by the end of second day of the rash.
- In the eruptive stage, rash appears by fourth to fifth days.
- Rash – It spreads downwards from behind the ears to the whole of the body. Discrete, maculopapular rash initially becomes blotchy and confluent and desquamate by the second week.
- Fever increases.

Complications

- Respiratory – pneumonia, secondary bacterial infection, otitis media, tracheitis, laryngitis
- Neurological – febrile convulsions, electroencephalographic (EEG) abnormalities, encephalitis and subacute sclerosing panencephalitis (SSPE)
- Others – diarrhoea, hepatitis, appendicitis, corneal ulceration, myocarditis, cervical lymphadenopathy
- Malnutrition can aggravate complications of measles, leading to a high mortality rate

Multidisciplinary Management

- Diagnosis is by clinical symptoms.
- ELISA and haemagglutination inhibition are also done.
- Medical management is supportive.
- Fever is controlled by antipyretics and hydration therapy.
- Mild to moderate cough need not be suppressed, as it brings out mucus.
- Prevention is by vaccination.

Nursing Diagnoses

- Activity intolerance
- Altered body temperature
- Complication potential/potential for injury/infection

Nursing Interventions

- Most of the interventions are same as that of chickenpox.
- But vitamin A 200000 Units (2 L units) given orally to children older than 1 year for two consecutive days decreases the severity, complication and mortality rate as a result of measles.
- Treatment of complications – Respiratory complications are treated with a combination of antibiotics, oxygen and other supportive measures. Convulsions are treated with anticonvulsants such as diazepam and phenobarbitone.

  Encephalitis occurs in only one in 5000 cases about 8 days after the onset of illness. Signs and symptoms include headache, lethargy and irritability proceeding to convulsions and ultimately coma. Mortality rate is 15%. Sequelae include seizure, deafness, hemiplegia and severe learning difficulties, affecting up to 40% survivors.

  SSPE usually develops 7 years after measles in one in 100,000 cases and develops in children who had measles before 2 years of age. Diagnosis is with clinical findings and a high level of antibody in blood and cerebrospinal fluid (CSF). With the use of immunization, SSPE has become extremely rare.

  Measles in malnourished children is very dangerous, especially in children with vitamin A deficiency. They develop severe complications. Giant cell pneumonia (a complication of measles, interstitial pneumonitis) develops in children with deficiency of effective T lymphocyte response in immunocompromised children. They are more prone to develop encephalitis.

MUMPS

It is a communicable disease caused by mumps virus. Its occurrence is worldwide. Period of infectivity is 7 days and the incubation period is 14–21 days similar to measles.

Signs and Symptoms

Onset is with fever, malaise and parotitis, but in up to 30% of cases, infection is subclinical. It starts with swelling of the parotid gland at one side, and bilateral involvement occurs over the next few days. Parotitis is associated with headache, earache and difficulty in swallowing food and water. On examination, the parotid gland will be swollen. Fever disappears within 3–4 days. Serum amylase levels are increased. Illness is usually mild and self-limiting.

Complications include viral meningitis and CNS involvement. Orchitis is the most dreaded complication, with the evidence of decreased sperm count and infertility in male children. In female children, rarely, oophoritis, mastitis and arthritis occur.

RUBELLA (GERMAN MEASLES)

It is a viral disease caused by rubella virus. Incubation period is 14–21 days. It spreads by droplets (respiratory route) from close contacts. The prodromal symptom includes mild low-grade fever or none at all. The maculopapular rash is often the first symptom that spreads centrifugally to cover the whole body and fades by 3–5 days. Suboccipital and postauricular node enlargement is also seen.

Complications are rare in childhood. Common ones are arthritis, encephalitis, thrombocytopenia and myocarditis. Rubella in pregnancy causes severe congenital anomalies in the fetus. Diagnosis is confirmed by serological examination.

Treatment is symptomatic. Prevention is by immunization. All adolescent females are advised to take immunization before they become pregnant to prevent congenital anomalies in the fetus.

CHICKENPOX

It is a highly contagious disease which presents with the sudden onset of low-grade fever, mild constitutional symptoms, a centripetal pleomorphic rash appearing on the first day of illness and a relatively short course of illness.

It is caused by varicella zoster virus which gives rise to vascular rash on the skin. The disease spreads through the respiratory route and is highly infectious during viral shedding. It progresses via blood and lymphatics to cause vesicular lesions on the skin. Its incubation period is 10–23 days.

Clinical manifestations are fever and rash, which comes in crops for 3–5 days. It starts as papules, progress as vesicles, pustules and crusts. The number of vesicles ranges from 200 to 500 lesions, starting on the head and trunk and progressing to peripheries.

The lesions begin as macules and quickly develop into papules and vesicles with scab and crust formation; the vessels are formed in prickle cell layer of the skin. The oesophagus, pancreas, liver, genitourinary tract and adrenal glands are affected with acidophilic inclusion bodies and foci of necrosis. It also causes disseminated interstitial pneumonia. The tissues of thymus, spleen, lymph nodes, liver, skin, conjunctiva and lungs are also infected with varicella. Latent infection is seen in dorsal root ganglia.

Assessment Findings

- Incubation period is 14–16 days.
- Prodromal symptoms are minimal with mild fever, malaise and anorexia.
- Rash appears on the first day.
- Macules quickly develop into papules and vesicles on erythematous base.
- New lesions appear in 1–7 days.
- The approximate number of lesions may be more than 250.
- Vesicles are not umbilicated and dry up to form scabs.
- Rashes are centripetal in distribution.
- Lesions are concentrated on the trunk, back and shoulders, with fewer lesions on the face, scalp and extremities.
- Vesicles may be seen on oral mucosa, pharynx, larynx, trachea, conjunctiva and genitals.
- Symptoms are more severe in immunocompromised patients or in children receiving steroid therapy.
- Common complications are of two types – cutaneous and systemic.
- Cutaneous complications are secondary bacterial infections of the skin and mucous membrane.
- Purpura fulminans and idiopathic thrombocytopenic purpura (ITP) also can occur a week after the onset of illness.
- Systemic complications are mainly neurological in nature such as acute cerebellar ataxia, GBS, transverse myelitis, optic neuritis, facial nerve palsy and postinfection encephalitis.

Multidisciplinary Management

- Diagnosis is done with clinical findings.
- It needs to be differentiated from impetigo, herpes simplex and coxsackievirus infection.
- Medical management is supportive and symptomatic.
- Antipyretics are used to relive fever, sedatives to provide rest and antipruritics to control itching.
- Oral acyclovir is given to healthy children within 24 hours of the onset but not used as a routine drug.
- The dose is 20 mg/kg four times a day.

Human varicella immunoglobulin (VZIG) is recommended in high-risk immunocompromised patients with deficient T-lymphocyte function after contact with chickenpox. (Recommended in bone marrow transplant patients, leukaemic children, HIV-infected patients, those who are taking steroids and neonates whose mother had chickenpox before or after delivery and who has been exposed to chickenpox. The dose is 125 U/kg to household contacts.)

Protection from infection with zoster immunoglobulin is not absolute and depends on how soon it is administered after contact with chickenpox. Intravenous acyclovir should be given in severe chickenpox.

Complications

Secondary bacterial infection occurs with *Staphylococcus* or *Streptococcus* species which leads to toxic shock syndrome or necrotizing fasciitis. Encephalitis occurs usually early within a week of the onset of rash. Purpura fulminous occur as a consequence of vasculitis on the skin and in subcutaneous tissues. Stroke is another very serious complication. Chickenpox in the immunocompromised children will cause progressive disseminated disease, leading to high mortality and Disseminated Intra-vascular Coagulation (DIC).

Nursing Diagnoses

- Activity intolerance
- Altered body temperature
- Altered nutrition less than body requirement
- Comfort alteration in pain and itching
- Knowledge deficit
- Infection potential
- Complication potential
- Social isolation
- Diversional activity deficit
- Altered parenting

Nursing Interventions

- Provide adequate rest.
- Provide administration of antipyretics.
- Increase fluid intake, especially energy-rich drinks.
- Administer easily digestible food.
- Provide administration of sedatives and antipyretics, as prescribed.
- If hospitalized, follow isolation precautions.
- Serve food on disposable dishes to all children with infectious diseases, if possible.
- Otherwise, autoclave the vessels after use.
- Wash toys that have come in contact with contaminants before use by another child.
- Double bag and label contaminated materials for disposal.
- Educate all individuals involved with care of the child to carry out isolation precautions.
- Be a role model to parents and others in providing care following isolation precautions.
- Institute protective measures as well as routine isolation precautions for children who may be in isolation because of overwhelming infection.
- Place children who are immunocompromised in private rooms.
- Discourage visitors as far as possible.

EPSTEIN–BARR VIRUS INFECTION

Epstein-Barr virus (EBV) infection is a major cause of the infectious mononucleosis syndrome. It is also involved in the pathogenesis of Burkitt lymphoma, lymphoproliferative disease in immunocompromised hosts and nasopharyngeal carcinoma. The virus has a particular tropism for B lymphocytes and epithelial cells of the pharynx. Transmission is oral contact.

INFECTIOUS MONONUCLEOSIS

This is a syndrome with features of fever, malaise, tonsillopharyngitis with often severe or limiting oral ingestion of fluids and rarely compromised breathing. Lymphadenopathy is a common feature, especially cervical lymphadenopathy. Petechiae on the soft palate, splenomegaly,

maculopapular rash and jaundice are also manifestations of this condition. Symptoms may persist for 1–3 months.

Treatment is symptomatic.

CYTOMEGALOVIRUS INFECTION

Cytomegalovirus (CMV) is usually transmitted through saliva, genital secretions or breast milk and rarely via blood products. As with EBV, CMV causes mononucleosis syndrome.

Treatment is with ganciclovir or other antiviral drugs.

KAWASAKI DISEASE (ACUTE FEBRILE MUCOCUTANEOUS SYNDROME)

It is mucocutaneous lymph node syndrome usually affecting children younger than 4 years, with its peak incidence from 6 months to at the end of the first year of age. It is more commonly seen in Japanese children than in other children. But incidence of this disease is not rare in Kerala. Aetiology is unknown. Clinical features are similar to streptococcal and staphylococcal shock syndrome that shows cervical lymphadenopathy, i.e. unilateral, nonpurulent bulbar conjunctivitis. It also causes vasculitis of small- and medium-sized vessels. In about one-third of cases, there will be coronary artery thrombosis or aneurysm, leading to ischaemia that can be visualized by echocardiography.

Treatment is with intravenous immunoglobulin which is given within the first 10 days. Aspirin is given in the anti-inflammatory dose till fever subsides and to continue the antiplatelet dose for coronary abnormalities. Intravenous immunoglobulin helps prevent coronary aneurysm, if given early. For further details, refer the chapter on cardiovascular disorders.

TOXIC SHOCK SYNDROME

It is caused by toxin-producing staphylococci and streptococci. The toxin is released from the infection site even from small abrasions. It causes systemic illness with high fever, diffuse maculopapular rashes, hypotension and shock. Desquamation of palms and soles is common after 1–2 weeks of onset.

Treatment is intensive care support to manage shock. Infected areas are surgically debrided. Intravenous immunoglobulin is given to neutralize the circulating toxin.

GUILLAIN–BARRÉ SYNDROME

GBS is acute or subacute postinfectious polyneuritis. It is considered as an autoimmune disorder owing to its occurrence with lymphoid tissue diseases and after infection. GBS mainly affects the Schwann's cells, which synthesize and maintain the peripheral nerve myelin sheath. Ventral root axons of anterior horn cells which innervate voluntary skeletal muscles are mainly involved. Dorsal root axons are also affected. Recovery is directly related to proliferation of Schwann's cells and axonal remyelination.

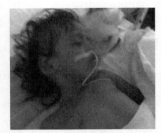

Baby with Guillain-Barre syndrome (GBS).

Assessment Findings

- Recent history of respiratory and gastrointestinal illnesses
- Recent vaccination
- Recent surgical procedure
- Rapidly developing muscle weakness
- Weakness is symmetrical and begins in distal muscle groups and ascends to more proximal muscles.
- Ascending flaccid motor paralysis is the most common presenting sign, associated with early loss of deep tendon reflexes (DTRs).
- Muscles of respiration (intercostals and diaphragm) are affected in 50% of all patients with GBS.
- Vital signs – respiratory rate ↑, weakness of muscles of respiration, heart rate within normal limits, BP often ↓ because of ↓ vascular tone.
- Temperature within normal limits. Hypoxaemia may be present. Expected recovery in 85%–90% of cases.

Multidisciplinary Management

- Lumbar puncture (LP) and CSF analysis, complete blood cell (CBC) count, arterial blood gases (ABGs), pulmonary function tests and electrocardiographic (ECG) studies
- Respiratory support, supplemental oxygen and if needed endotracheal (ET) intubation and tracheostomy with assisted mechanical ventilation
- Corticosteroids to ↓ inflammation
- Plasmapheresis – Complete exchange of plasma with removal of abnormal circulatory antibodies
- Maintenance of cardiovascular functions
- Management of bowel and bladder dysfunction
- Nutritional management and tube feeding
- Management of motor dysfunction

Nursing Diagnoses

- Impaired gas exchange
- Risk for disuse syndrome
- Dyslexia (or risk for the same related to noxious stimuli)
- Sensory/perceptual alterations (or risk for the same)

Nursing Interventions

- Assess neurological function every other hour and as often as needed. Ascending motor and sensory dysfunctions usually occur rapidly (over 24–72 hours) and can lead to life-threatening respiratory arrest.

- Monitor for respiratory distress: Adventitious (crackles or rhonchi) and ↓ or absent breath sounds.
- Following signs and symptoms are present: Temperature ≥37.8°C or 100°F; heart rate and BP ↑, tidal volume or vital capacity ↓ from baseline; ↓ in PaO_2 or ↑ in $PaCO_2$ ≥10–15 mm Hg or rhythm; ↑ restlessness or anxiety; confusions.
- If these signs and symptoms are present, be prepared to assist for intubation or tracheostomy.
- Suction airways as determined by auscultation findings. As paresis or paralysis subsides (after 2–4 weeks, usual time or dysfunction peak), cranial nerve functions will begin to return (i.e. gag, swallowing, coughing). Evaluate ability to cough.
- Deliver O_2 and humidification, as prescribed.
- Unless contraindicated, maintain adequate hydration (up to 2–3 L per day) to minimize thickening of pulmonary secretions.
- Turn and reposition patient for at least every 2 hours to prevent stasis of secretions.
- Assess neurological function starting with lower extremities and work upwards to determine level of deficit.
- Assess muscle symmetry by using side-to-side comparison.
- Assess muscle strength by having the child pull against resistance with each extremity.
- Assess DTRs of the Achilles tendon, patellae, biceps, triceps and brachioradialis (report ↓ (+1) or absent (0) responses).
- Asses for paraesthesias, presence/absence of vibratory sense, presence/absence of response to light, touch or pinprick to determine level of dysfunction and whether or not ascending.
- Turn the child in correct anatomic alignment every 2 hours or more often.
- Ensure that active or passive range-of-motion (ROM) exercises are performed, if appropriate.
- As indicated, apply splints to hands/arms and feet/legs to help prevent contractures; alternate splints so that they are on for 2 hours and off for 2 hours.
- Use pneumatic comparison device or other prescribed therapy to minimize risk of thrombophlebitis.
- Low air loss or fluidized bed beds may be used to manage respiratory, autonomic and musculoskeletal problems that can occur with GBS.
- Asses signs of Autonomic Dysfunction (AD): Cardiac dysrhythmias, heart rate <60 or >100 beats per minute (BPM), ↑ and sustained BP, facial flushing, ↑ sweating, extreme generalized warmth, profound weakness and complaints of severe headache or tightening in chest/abdomen.
- Place the patient on cardiac monitor during the first 10–14 days or if there are signs and symptoms of AD.
- Monitor carefully during activities known to precipitate AD Such as position changes, vigorous coughing straining with bowel movements, suctioning, etc.
- If indicators of AD are present, correct stimulating factors.
- Consult the paediatrician if symptoms do not subside within 15–30 minutes.
- If there is sustained increase in BP, administer antihypertensive agents.
- Evaluate cranial nerves III, IV and V by checking for extraocular eye movements, papillary light reflex, degree of ptosis and diplopia.

- If the patient exhibits a deficit, place objects where they can be seen.
- Assist with activities of daily living (ADL), as indicated.
- For diplopia, cover one eye with a patch; alternate patch every 2 hours or every 3 hours during waking hours.
- Use eyelid crutches for ptosis.
- Evaluate cranial nerves V and VII by checking facial sensation and movement, ability to masticate and correct reflex.
- If deficit is present, assess for corneal irritation or abrasion; apply artificial tear drops or ointments as prescribed. Secure eyelids in a closed position if corneal reflex is diminished or absent.
- Evaluate cranial nerves IX, X and XII by checking for pharyngeal sensation and movement (swallowing), absence of gag reflex and tongue control.
- If a deficit is present, suction during oral hygiene to be done. Do not feed the child orally until gag reflex returns.
- Assess cranial nerve XI by checking ability to shrug shoulders and turn head from side to side.
- If a deficit is present, place the head in a position of comfort and proper anatomic alignment.

CHIKUNGUNYA

Chikungunya is a viral infection from an alphavirus which is transmitted through the bite of an infected *Aedes* mosquito. The word 'chikungunya' originated from the Kimakonde language means '**to become contorted**' or 'to walk bent'. The virus exists in tropical regions of Asia and Africa. *Aedes* mosquitos breed in and around human habitations and feed on human blood during daytime and in the evening. The infected mosquitos cause fever and severe joint pain within 2–7 days after infection. Chikungunya spreads with the help of monkeys, birds and cattle unlike dengue virus, which spreads only with the help of mosquitos.

Aetiology

Chikungunya virus is an RNA virus and a member of the Togaviridae family. The disease was first described during an outbreak in Tanzania in 1952.

Clinical Features

Following are the symptoms:
 Fever
 Headache
 Retro-orbital pain
 Vomiting
 Diarrhoea
 Meningeal syndrome
 Muscle and joint pain and rash
 Symptoms usually begin 3–7 days after being bitten by an infected mosquito.
 Disease rarely causes death, and the symptoms are severe and disabling. High-risk groups are neonates infected around the time of birth and debilitated adults/older people with comorbidity such as diabetes and asthma. Children are highly vulnerable to the initial symptoms of body pain and fever.

Diagnosis

- Symptoms of chikungunya are similar to those of dengue fever and Zika virus disease.
- Dengue fever and Zika virus diseases are also transmitted by the same mosquito.
- Blood investigation is the definitive diagnostic tool. Tests include:
- Viral culture, serological tests and immunocapture PCR test
- Serum or plasma test to detect virus
- Viral culture can detect the virus in the first 3 days of illness.

 Serum or plasma test is done by examining the child's serum to detect the virus, viral nucleic acid or viral-specific immunoglobulin along with neutralizing antibodies. These antibodies can be identified in the first 8 days of disease.

Treatment

The major mode of treatment is symptom management.
- Provide rest.
- Maintain increased fluid intake to prevent dehydration.
- Administer acetaminophen or paracetamol to reduce fever and pain.
- Do not administer nonsteroidal anti-inflammatory drugs (NSAIDs) till differentiated from the diagnosis of dengue fever.

Complications

- **Uveitis**
- **Retinitis**
- **Myocarditis**
- **Hepatitis**
- **Nephritis**
- **Haemorrhage**
- **Meningoencephalitis**
- **Myelitis**
- **Guillain–Barré syndrome**
- **Cranial nerve palsy**

 These complications are seen in vulnerable populations such as neonates and debilitated children with other systemic diseases.

Nursing Management

- Assess the child's condition. Monitor vitals, especially temperature, frequently.
- Assess the pain.
- Provide supportive care for fever such as administration of paracetamol, tapid sponge and increased fluid intake.
- Protect the child from extreme weather.
- Administer energy-rich and easily digestible foods and fluids.
- Prevent further mosquito bites.
- Apply pain medications to joints if there are complaints of joint pain.
- Provide health education regarding prevention of chikungunya, as there is no vaccine available for this disease so far.

- Look and monitor for complications, as there is a chance for developing serious complications.
- Closely watch for the progress of the disease as well as the progress of the child.

Prevention

Chikungunya is spread in the first week, as the virus is seen in the blood during the first week of infection.

It passes from an infected person through mosquito bites. An infected mosquito spreads the virus to other people. So prevention is only by preventing mosquito bites.

Children should be protected from mosquito bites through various measures such as use of long-sleeved shirts and pants while outside of home.

Prevent mosquito growth by destroying mosquito breeding places, avoiding stagnant waters near human habitats and using mosquito repellents, preferably ones that contain DEET, picaridin, IR3535, oil of lemon, eucalyptus or *para*-menthane-3,8-diol (PMD), on exposed parts of the body.

- Keep the windows and doors duly locked. Use insecticide-treated mosquito nets, not only at night but also during daytime as these mosquitos bite maximum during daytime.
- Keep children indoors as much as possible, especially during early morning and late afternoon.
- Use air-conditioning. This deters mosquitos from entering rooms.
- Make children sleep under a mosquito net.
- Use mosquito coils and insecticide vaporizers.

DENGUE FEVER

Sudden outbreak of dengue fever is very common in certain parts of India. Kerala had witnessed this in the year 2017. Dengue fever is a vector-born disease caused by bites of infected *Aedes* mosquito that carries dengue virus. It is a fast emerging arboviral infection. The most common type of mosquito that spreads dengue fever is the female tiger mosquito. These mosquitos are found in the tropical and subtropical areas in South East Asia and are also known as Asian tiger mosquito. The fever occurs when an infected mosquito bites a person. Rashes are often developed. Dengue fever can also become severe and be fatal. The most severe complication of dengue fever is dengue haemorrhagic fever or DHF or dengue shock syndrome (DSS). It is a life-threatening condition that needs immediate medical attention.

Causes

The dengue viruses are members of the genus *Flavivirus* and family Flaviviridae *that* have an RNA strand as its genetic makeup. These small (50-nm) viruses contain a single-strand RNA as genome. Four types of viruses cause dengue fever (virus types 1–4, DENV1–4). All four types of viruses are closely related, but infection with one serotype will not provide immunity against other types. Infection with any one serotype confers lifelong immunity to that virus serotype. The viruses are transmitted from *Aedes aegypti* and *Aedes albopictus* mosquitos to humans in a viral life cycle that requires both humans and these mosquitos. There is no human-to-human transmission. Once a mosquito is infected, it remains infected for its lifetime. Secondary infection with another serotype or multiple infections with different serotypes lead to severe form of dengue (DHF/DSS). Both *Aedes aegypti* and *Aedes albopictus* carry high vectorial competency for dengue viruses. Vectorial competency denotes:

- High susceptibility to infecting virus
- Ability to replicate the virus
- Ability to transmit the virus to another host

The susceptibility of the human depends upon the immune status and genetic predisposition.

Clinical Features

In infants and toddlers, the following symptoms are present:

- A runny nose
- A small skin rash or a few skin rashes
- A slight cough
- A sudden temperature that can shoot up to a high fever very fast (105°F)
- Sore throat

Older children will have the following symptoms:

- A dull and continuous pain behind the eyes and in various joints of the body
- Very high fever up to 105°F
- Pain in the back
- Petechiae and bruises
- Muscle pain
- Flu-like cold and cough
- Headache and chills
- Nausea and vomiting
- A constant feeling of itching on the soles of the feet
- Rashes on the palms of the hands and the bottom of the feet
- Decrease in or complete loss of appetite
- Sudden bleeding from various parts of the body, such as the gums or the nose as a result of decreased platelet count (platelet levels are usually between 150,000 and 450,000/mL)
- Skin rash that may be itchy, usually seen after few days of fever

Clinical Features of Dengue Haemorrhagic Fever

A usual fever with dengue can turn into a serious condition called DHF and can subsequently move to DSS, a very serious problem in children. Both conditions are life-threatening. The symptoms of DHF and DSS are as follows:

- Children younger than 15 years are more prone to DHF and DSS
- Sudden and continuous bleeding from any part of the body, especially inside the abdomen
- A quick dip in the levels of blood pressure
- A sudden shock that is caused because of excessive and sudden bleeding or because of a leakage in the blood vessels
- Failure of different organs

Risk Factors

- Travelling to or living in endemic or outbreak areas, especially if no mosquito control is attempted by the people or government

- Mosquito bites
- A repeated infection with another serovar of dengue virus, with antibodies in the serum active against the first infecting virus type
- Not taking precautions to avoid mosquito bites and lack of mosquito control infrastructure
- Unplanned and uncontrolled urbanization leading to increased breeding places for mosquitos, introduction of nonbiodegradable plastic products, used tyres, etc.
- Microevolution of viruses
- Insufficient and inadequate water supply
- Improper solid waste management

Diagnosis

- Perform physical examination and check for the signs and symptoms.
- Take a recent history of travelling to find out whether the child had visited endemic areas.
- CBC and coagulation studies. Total white blood cell (WBC) count is usually normal. Mild thrombocytopenia (100,000–150,000 cells/mm^3) is common. Approximately, half of the children with dengue fever have decreased platelet count below 100,000 and may have severe thrombocytopenia. Mild rise in haematocrit values as a result of dehydration can also be seen.
- A MAC-ELISA assay (an immunoglobulin M-based test) is the most widely used test for dengue fever virus.
- Other tests are IgG-ELISA, dengue viral plaque reduction tests and PCR tests.
- Definitive diagnosis is made by isolation and identification of the dengue virus serovar from the child.
- Serum biochemistry is usually normal, but liver enzymes and aspartate amino transferase (AST) levels may be elevated.

Differential Diagnosis

Leptospirosis, typhoid fever, scarlet fever, Rocky Mountain spotted fever, meningococcemia, malaria, chikungunya and food poisoning

Multidisciplinary Management

- For mild fever: Increase fluid intake so as not to get dehydrated.
- Administer antipyretics and analgesics to control fever and headache and body pain.
- Do not administer aspirin compounds.
- In most cases, symptoms of fever subside within 1–2 weeks.
- If the symptoms are not getting resolved, there is a chance that it has converted to DHF, which can be life-threatening.
- DHF requires continuous monitoring, and platelet transfusions are required to improve platelet count and arrest bleeding.
- Fluid and electrolyte need to be replaced, and hydration level should be monitored carefully.
- Maintain rest, no work and no play.
- Provide nutritious food.
- If vomiting/diarrhoea persists, fluid therapy may be continued.

- Continuous monitoring of vitals, especially BP, to guard against DSS.

Prevention

- Remember that there is no specific treatment of dengue fever.
- Prevention is the best way to protect children.
- Prevent mosquito bites, use nets in bedroom, close windows and doors during peak hours at home to prevent the entry of mosquitos (early morning and evening hours).
- Prevent water logging near residential areas to check breeding of mosquitos.
- Keep home and courtyard clean and safe to prevent growth of mosquitos.
- Use anti-mosquito screens for doors and windows and keep closed them during afternoon or whole day if too much mosquitos are present.
- Make children wear proper leggings, soaks and other protective clothing with long sleeves when going out of the house.
- Make compulsory use of mosquito nets while sleeping.
- Use safe mosquito repellent at home.
- Make sure that children do not play in an area where the grass is tall and where there is stagnant water around.
- Use mosquito repellent cream on children when they step out of home.

Nursing Management

Administration of fluids, preferable orally, if tolerated. If oral fluids are not tolerated, intravenous administration is essential to maintain hydration.

Infants must be breastfed.

Administration of vitamin C, zinc, analgesics and antipyretics is performed.

No aspirin and ibuprofen are used.

Diets including papaya, kiwi and passion fruit are advised.

Continuously monitor for rashes, bruises and bleeding and check vitals.

Provide complete rest.

Provide supportive nursing care according to medical condition of the child.

H1N1

H1N1, otherwise known as swine flu, is an acute respiratory disease affecting nose, throat, trachea and bronchi. Swine flu was initially detected in people who had close contact with pigs. In 2009, WHO declared it as a pandemic owing to its rapid spread. In India, it was reported predominantly in the states of Andhra Pradesh, Telangana, Maharashtra, Karnataka and West Bengal.

Aetiology

H1N1 or swine flu is caused by virus. The virus mutates very fast, and the currently circulating strains in India as per WHO are predominantly H1N1, followed by A (H3N2) and B viruses. Some of these strains infect only animals and birds, whereas other strains infect only human.

Mode of Transmission

Mode of transmission is by droplets from cough and sneeze of an infected person. When an infected person sneezes or coughs, he/she releases multiple tiny droplets. Those who come in contact with these droplets get infected. Swine flu is NOT transmitted by eating pork.

Children at Risk

- Children suffering from chronic conditions such as asthma, diabetes, heart and other respiratory problems, sickle cell disease, kidney disease OR liver disease
- Children with cancer or weak immune system conditions
- Neuromuscular disease (such as muscular dystrophy)
- Young children
- Children with lethargy, low appetite, breathing difficulty are also at high risk
- Healthy children younger than 2 years are also considered HIGH-RISK (CDC: September 2009)
- Diseases requiring long-term aspirin therapy
- Adolescents with pregnancy

Clinical Manifestations

- High-grade fever with chills
- Headache
- Body ache
- Cough and cold
- Sore throat
- Runny nose
- Vomiting
- Severe tiredness
- Stuffy nose/runny nose
- Diarrhoea, vomiting

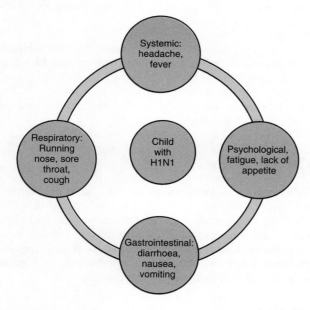

Diagnosis

- Culture of nasal and throat swabs. Theses swabs are then analysed using various laboratory techniques to identify the specific type of virus.

- Routine blood test is also done to differentiate between bacterial and viral infections.
  Multidisciplinary management.
  - Major line of medical treatment is with antiviral drugs. (Antiviral drugs such as Tamiflu should be started within 48 hours of flu symptoms). Tamiflu is used for prophylaxis if there is recent close contact with other children or adults with swine flu. It is indicated as a prophylaxis for those exposed to high-risk children.
  - For cough and respiratory symptom management, use antitussive agents.
  - For fever, antipyretics are prescribed. One should take caution not to administer aspirin to children younger than 18 years, as there is chance of developing Ryes syndrome.

Nursing Management

Nursing management is symptomatic similar to caring children with fever, runny nose, cough, dehydration and other symptoms.

Prevention advice and home care management are very important for nurses to implement.

Reassuring parents of children with swine flu is very important.

Teach preventive strategies:

Teach parents the importance of:

Washing hands often with soap and water or alcohol-based hand cleaners.

Avoid touching the eyes, nose or mouth. Germs on the hands can spread this way.

Try to avoid close contact with sick people.

Keep children at home when they are sick.

Cover the nose and mouth with a tissue when coughing or sneezing.

- Limit contact with others to avoid infecting them.

Face masks: Use disposable masks that may help avoid acquiring the disease as well as prevent the spread.

Vaccine:

- The best way to prevent swine (H1N1) flu is to get a yearly, seasonal influenza vaccine.
- Administration of Tamiflu can be used for prevention following close contact with a person who has swine flu.

Home care of children with swine flu involves the following:

- Isolate the child till symptoms subside.
- Keep the child at home.
- Give adequate fluid.
- Administer medications as prescribed.
- Avoid contact with others.
- Administer good nutrition, especially in the form of warm soups.
- Give plenty of rest as the child may have muscle pain.
- After the child recovers, give vaccination if possible so that the child may not get another attack, as there are different strains of swine flu.

Complications

If left untreated, H1N1 may lead to complications such as:

- Pneumonia: both viral and secondary bacterial (mainly in HIGH-RISK children)
- Bacterial infection
- Ear infections and sinus infections occur in 10% of children
- Influenza-induced flare-ups in those with asthma
- Muscle pains (viral myositis) in the legs can be severe and cause limping or refusal to walk
- Dehydration, often as a result of a severe sore throat that limits fluid intake
- Acute respiratory distress syndrome
- Multiorgan failure
- Death

STUDY QUESTIONS

- How will you prevent tuberculosis in children?
- What is BCG?
- How will you take care of a child with primary complex?
- Describe the nursing care of a child with tuberculosis.
- How is diphtheria transmitted?
- What are the types of diphtheria?
- Why diphtheria is considered a fatal disease?
- How will you manage a child with faucial diphtheria?
- What is the course of whooping cough?
- Why is pertussis called whooping cough?
- Prepare a nursing care plan for a child with whooping cough.
- How will you prevent outbreaks of cholera?
- Explain the fluid management of children with cholera.
- What medications are given to children with cholera?
- What is shigellosis? What are the common complications of shigellosis?
- How will prevent HIV transmission?
- What are the protocols for breastfeeding for a child if the mother is HIV-positive?
- What are the antivirals used for HIV/AIDS treatment in children?
- How will prevent HIV transmission from mother to child?
- What are the precautions to be taken during delivering a baby whose mother is HIV-positive?
- How will you care an infant after delivery if the mother is HIV-positive?
- What is chikungunya?
- How will you prevent chikungunya?
- What are the medical and nursing care of children with chikungunya?
- What is dengue fever? How will you prevent dengue fever?
- How will you identify haemorrhagic shock in dengue fever?
- What advise will you give to the mother of a child with dengue fever?
- What are the methods to compact platelet loss in children with dengue fever?
- What is H1N1? How is it transmitted?
- What advise will you give to parents in caring a child with swine flu at home?
- What are the complications of swine flu in children?
- What are the risk factors for developing swine flu?

BIBLIOGRAPHY

1. Anonymous. WHO Influenza A (H1N1)–update 55. *Morb Mortal Wkly Rep*. June 2009;58:1–4. PubMed
2. Anonymous. WHO weekly epidemiological record, No. 25. 2009; 84:249–260.
3. Barall-Inman, R.A. (1995). Question and Answer. Gullian–Barre Syndrome. J. Am Acad Nurs Pract. 7(4), pp 165–169.
4. Bhatia R, Narain JP. Re-emerging chikungunya fever: some lessons from Asia. Trop Med Int Health. 2009;14:940–6. Epub 2009 Jun 28. [PubMed]
5. Brooks, R., Joynson, D.H.M. (1990). Bacterial Diagnosis of Diphtheria. J Clin Pathol. 43, pp 576–580.
6. CDC. (1989). Measles Prevention: Recommendations of the Immunization Practices Advisory Committee (AcIp). MMWR, 38, pp 1–18.
7. CDC. (1996). Poliomyelitis Prevention. MMWR, 45, pp 8–10.
8. Chaudahari,A., S. Supriya., K Sashi., Rai, A., Rawat. D.S., Aggarwal R.K., and Chauhan L.S: Emergence of pandemic 2009 influenza AH1N1, India: Indian J Med Res. 2012 Apr;135(4) 534-537.
9. Chaturvedi U, Nagar R, Shrivastava R. Dengue and dengue haemorrhagic fever: Implications of host genetics. *FEMS Immunol Med Mic*. 2006; 47:155–166.
10. Centers for Disease Control and Prevention. (2010). Locally acquired dengue-Key West, Florida, 2009-2010. MMWR, 59(19): 577-581. Also available online: http://www.cdc.gov/mmwr/preview/mmwrhtml/mm5919a1.htm
11. Centers for Disease Control and Prevention. (2007). Dengue hemorrhagic fever-U.S.-Mexico border, 2005. MMWR, 56(31): 785-789. Also available online: http://www.cdc.gov/mmwr/preview/mmwrhtml/mm5631a1.htm. [Erratum in MMWR, 56(32):822. Also available online: http://www.cdc.gov/mmwr/preview/mmwrhtml/mm5632a5.htm.]
12. Cherry, J.D. (1980). The New Epidemiology of Measles and Rubella. Hosp. Prac., 115, pp 49–57.
13. Cherry, J.D., Brunell, P.A., et al. (1988). Report of Task Force on Pertussis and Pertussis Immunization. Paediatrics, 81, 939–984.
14. Friedman, R.L. (1988). Pertussis: The Disease and New Diagnostic Methods. Clin. Microbiol. Rev., 1, pp 335–336.
15. English, P.C. Diphtheria and Theories of Infectious Diseases. (1985). Paediatrics 76, pp 1–9.
16. Gregory, R.J. (1999). Understanding & Coping With Neurological Impairment. Rehabil Nurs, 20(2), pp 74–78, 130.
17. Hodder, S.L., Mortimer, E.A. (1992). Epidemiology of Pertussis And Reaction To Pertussis Vaccine. Epidemol Rev, 14, pp 243–268.
18. Mandell, G.L., Bennett, J.E., Dolin, R. (1995). Principles and Practices of Infectious Diseases. New York: Churchill Livingston.
19. Minor, P.D. (1992). The Molecular Biology of Polio Vaccines. J. Gen Virol, 73, pp 3065–3077.
20. Mohan A. Chikungunya fever: clinical manifestations & management. Indian J Med Res. 2006;124:471–4. [PubMed]
21. Mohan A, Sharma SK. Chikungunya fever. In: Singal RK, editor. Medicine update. Mumbai: Association of Physicians of India; 2007. pp. 634–8.
22. Mohan A. Chikungunya fever strikes in Andhra Pradesh. Natl Med J India. 2006;19:240.
23. Padbidri VS, Gnaneswar TT. Epidemiological investigations of chikungunya epidemic at Barsi, Maharashtra state, India. J Hyg Epidemiol Microbiol Immunol. 1979;23:445–51. [PubMed]
24. World Health Organization. Polio. The Beginning of The End. 1997. Geneva. pp 1–105.
25. Progress Towards Poliomyelitis Eradication in India, 2003. (2004 Mar 26). *Wkly Epidemiol Rec*, 79(13):121–125
26. Cherry, J. D., Brunell, P. A., Golden, G. S., & Darzon, D. T. (1988). Report of the task force on pertussis and pertussis immunization–1988. *Pediatrics, 81*(suppl), 939–984.
27. Rishnamoorthy K, Harichandrakumar KT, Krishna Kumari A, Das LK. Burden of chikungunya in India: estimates of disability

adjusted life years (DALY) lost in 2006 epidemic. J Vector Borne Dis. 2009;46:26–35. [PubMed]

28. Stowe, A.C. (1995). GBS. In: Swearingen, P.L., Keen, J.H. Manual of Critical Care Nursing. 3rd Edn. St. Louis: Mosby.

29. Suryawanshi SD, Dube AH, Khadse RK, Jalgaonkar SV, Sathe PS, Zawar SD, et al. Clinical profile of chikungunya fever in patients in a tertiary care centre in Maharashtra, India. Indian J Med Res. 2009;129:438–41. [PubMed]

30. World Health Organization, Regional Office for Southeast Asia. Chikungunya fever information sheet. http://www.searo.who.int/en/Section10/Section2246.htm (Accessed on 12 May 2010).

31. WHO South-East Asia Region: Reported Cases and Deaths of Dengue from 2003 to 2012. New Delhi: WHO-SEARO. http://www.searo.who.int/entity/vector_borne_tropical_diseases/data/graphs.pdf

32. World Health Organization. *International Health Regulations*. 2005. 2nd edn. Geneva: WHO, 2008.

33. World Health Organization, Special Programme for Research and Training in Tropical Diseases (TDR). Dengue: guidelines for diagnosis, treatment, prevention and control. New edition. 2009. http://www.cdc.gov/ (last accessed 12 August 2017).

34. WHO. Global strategy for dengue prevention and control. World Health Organization, Geneva; 2012.

35. World Health Organization, Regional Office for South-East Asia. Comprehensive guidelines for prevention and control of dengue and dengue haemorrhagic fever - revised and expanded edition. 2011. http://www.searo.who.int/ (last accessed 12 August 2017).

CHILDHOOD TUMOURS

LEARNING OBJECTIVES

At the end of the chapter, the learner will be able to:

- Identify the common tumours of childhood.
- Describe the nursing management of children with various childhood tumours using the nursing process approach.

Cancer of the blood-forming tissues is the most common form of childhood cancer. The annual incidence is 4.2 per 100,000 population in white children and 2.4 per 100,000 population in Indian children younger than 15 years. It occurs more frequently in males than in females after the age of 1 year, and the peak onset is between 2 and 6 years of age. This is the only cancer with good prognosis and prolonged survival rates.

LEUKAEMIAS IN CHILDREN

'Leukaemia' is a broad term that includes a group of malignant diseases of the bone marrow and lymphatic system. Classification is complex but essentially related to the identification of subtypes and therapeutic interventions.

Morphology

- Leukaemias are of different types according to predominant cell types and level of maturity:
  1. Lymphoid for leukaemias involving the lymphatic or lymphoid system
  2. Myeloid for those of myeloid (bone marrow) origin
  3. Blastic and acute for those involving immature cells
  4. Cystic and chronic for those involving mature cells
- In children, two forms are common. These are acute lymphoid leukaemia (ALL) and acute nonlymphoid

leukaemia (ANLL)/acute myelogenous leukaemia (AML).
  1. ALL (lymphatic/lymphocytic/lymphoblastic leukaemia)
  2. AML (granulocytic/myelocytic/monocytic/myelogenous/monoblastic and monocytic)
- According to cytochemical markers, leukaemias are of different types.
  1. Chromosomal studies – Trisomy of chromosome 21 has 15 times more risk than others. Hyperploid and translocation of chromosomes 4 and 10 have better prognosis (D.G. Poplack, 2002).
  2. Cell surface immunological markers – Cell surface antigens have permitted differentiation of ALL into three broad classes as follows: non-B-cell ALL and non-T-cell ALL (also called early pre-B cell); B-cell ALL and T-cell ALL (children with non-T-cell and non-B-cell ALL have best prognosis, especially if they have the common acute lymphocytic leukaemia antigen known as CALLA-positive antigen cell surface.

Pathophysiology

The unrestricted proliferation of immature white blood cells (WBCs) occurs in the bone marrow (blood-forming tissues). The clinical manifestations result from infiltration and replacement of the normal tissue with these immature nonfunctional leukaemic cells of the bone marrow and subsequently to other organs such as bones, liver, spleen, lymph nodes, brain, kidneys, ovaries, testis, gastrointestinal tract and lungs.

Essentially, the proliferating leukaemic cells depress the production of formed elements of the blood in the bone marrow by competing and depressing the normal cells of the essential nutrients for metabolism. Common presenting signs of leukaemia such as anaemia (pallor), infection and bleeding are the result of bone marrow infiltration. Infiltration of the bone marrow with leukaemic cells gradually weakens the bones, leading to pathological fractures. Periosteal invasion by leukaemic cells causes severe bone pain. Invasion of lymph node leads to lymphadenopathy.

Infiltration by leukaemic cells in the spleen, liver and lymph glands causes enlargement and eventual fibrosis. Invasion of leukaemic cells to central nervous system (CNS) produces meningeal irritation, increased intracranial pressure (ICP) and ventricular enlargement, leading to severe headache, vomiting, irritability, lethargy, papilloedema and eventual coma.

Leukaemic invasion of the testis/ovaries has become clinically more important as a result of long-term survivors. Proliferating leukaemic cells have greater metabolic needs that depress normal cells of nutrition, leading to metabolic starvation of normal cells.

Assessment Findings

It can be categorized into four main findings as follows:
- General:
  - Malaise
  - Anorexia
- Bone marrow infiltration:
  - Anaemia, pallor and lethargy
  - Neutropenia and infection
  - Thrombocytopenia, bruising, petechiae, nose bleeding
  - Bone pain
- Reticuloendothelial infiltration:
  - Hepatosplenomegaly
  - Lymphadenopathy
- Other organ infiltration:
  - CNS
    - Headache
    - Vomiting
    - Convulsions
    - Nerve palsy
- Testis: testicular enlargement

Diagnosis

- History
- Peripheral smear shows immature cells with a low blood count
- Bone marrow hypercellular with primarily blast cells
- FISH – fluorescent in situ hybridization

Multidisciplinary Management

There are following phases in the treatment:
- Induction therapy – This is to achieve a complete remission (disappearance of leukaemic cells).
- CNS prophylaxis – This is to prevent leukaemic invasion to the brain.
- Maintenance therapy with intensification (consolidation) – This serves to maintain the remission phase.

Remission Induction

Treatment is given immediately after establishing diagnosis. The principal drugs are as follows:
- Prednisolone (corticosteroids)
- Vincristine
- L-Asparaginase with or without doxorubicin or donorubicin
- Cystosine arabinoside

Common problems are as follows:
- Myelosuppression, especially the period after remission, is critical.
- Highly susceptible to infection and haemorrhage. Supportive therapy is essential in such cases.

CNS Prophylaxis

Treatment is intrathecal methotrexate, cytarabine and hydrocortisone. Some centres also provide CNS irradiation.

Maintenance Therapy

It is given after completion of successful induction and consolidation therapy to preserve the remission and decrease the number of leukaemic cells. Also, combined drug regimens are used.

Reinduction following relapse

When the leukaemic cells are observed in bone marrow, CNS or testis, there is relapse. Treatment includes administration of prednisolone and vincristine along with a combination of other drugs which are not used before. CNS prevention by intrathecal drugs and irradiation and maintenance therapy is again followed.

Bone Marrow Replacement Therapy

Bone marrow replacement therapy (BMT) is successful in children with ALL and AML. BMT is not used for children with ALL during first remission because of the excellent results with chemotherapy. BMT is used with first remission for children suffering from AML as a result of poor prognosis. Peripheral blood stem cell (PBSC) transplantation is also used as an alternative or in conjunction with BMT.

Prognosis

Factors deciding prognosis are as follows:
- Initial WBC count – Children with normal or low WBC count, non-T, non-B ALL and presence of CALLA-positive antigen have better prognosis.
- Age of the child at diagnosis – Children between the ages of 2 and 9 years have better prognosis.
- Type of the cell
- Sex of the child
- Karyotyping and analysis – Children with DNA index >1.6 and translocation of chromosomes 4 and 10 have better prognosis.

Late effects of treatment lead to increased survival. No organ is exempt from infiltration, and almost all antineoplastic drugs are used including radiation therapy, leading to adverse effects and secondary carcinomas. This causes many problems in children, parents and their family members.

Clinical Manifestations

Assessment is routine physical examination. Usually, children will have vague complaints. Fatigue, pain in a limb, night sweating, lack of appetite, headache and general malaise are the earliest clues that need to be taken seriously.

- Signs and symptoms of anaemia, pallor, fatigue and cardiac murmurs
- Poor wound healing, fever, anorexia and lymphadenopathy related to neutropenia.
- Petechiae, ecchymosis, purpura, epistaxis, easy bruising and blood in urine or emesis related to decreased platelet production
- Bone and joint pain related to leukaemic invasion into the periosteum
- Headache, vomiting, papilloedema and other signs and symptoms of increased ICP related to leukaemic cell invasion of the CNS.

Nursing Management

- Nursing care of leukaemic children is directly related to the regimen of therapy.
- Nurse needs to set realistic goals depending on the type of therapy prescribed.
- Curative treatment is given with a goal of disease eradication.
- Adjuvant therapy is given for eradication of disease and subclinical micrometastases with systemic adjuvant modalities.
- Palliative therapy is aimed to provide quality survival with symptom control.
- Provide supportive role and help them understand various therapies to prevent and manage expected side effects/toxicities and observe for late effects of the treatment.
- Help them to live a normal life as much as possible.
- Help them cope with emotional aspects of the disease.
- Prepare the child and family for diagnostic and therapeutic procedures.
  - From the time of diagnosis till the end of treatment, the child needs to undergo many traumatic investigative procedures (e.g. bone marrow aspiration, lumbar puncture, biopsy, multiple finger sticks, venipuncture).
  - It takes several years for the cessation of treatment.
  - The child along with the family members needs explanation why it is being done and what is to be expected.
  - The child's level of understanding needs to be assessed to provide adequate explanation as per the stage of development.
  - Information given should be age-appropriate.
  - Explain what he/she will hear, see, smell and feel rather than merely specifying what will happen.
- Use conscious and unconscious sedation when it is needed.
- Help relieve pain.
  Uncontrolled malignant process produces pain. Children need to be given adequate analgesia by pharmacological or nonpharmacological methods. A child with leukaemia has severe bone pain. Proper assessment of pain and quantification of pain and prescription of adequate analgesics are essential.
- Help prevent complications of myelosuppression.
  Leukaemic process and most of the chemotherapeutic agents cause myelosuppression. As a result,

neutropenia, thrombocytopenia and anaemia occur. This causes infection, sepsis and bleeding. The child will be susceptible to infection during three phases of the disease:

At the time of treatment and relapse, when leukaemic process has replaced normal leucocytes; during immunosuppressive therapy; and after prolonged antibiotic therapy that predisposes to the growth of resistant organisms.

- Prevent infection and sepsis through meticulous handwashing; limit the child's exposure to infectious persons, especially with potentially lethal infections such as varicella, and maintain reverse isolation.
- Administer granulocyte colony-stimulating factor (GCSF), as prescribed, to combat infection. It reduces the incidence and duration of infection in children receiving treatment for cancers.
- Employ all measures to control infection, such as following reverse isolation, provide private room for children with leukaemia, restrict visitors, allow only healthy health personnel to provide care to these children and follow strict handwashing technique with antiseptic solution as per hospital policy.
- Evaluate children for potential sites of infection (e.g. mucosal ulceration, skin abrasion or tear and broken nails and observe for any elevation of temperature).
- Prevention of infection after discharge is also important. Check for satisfactory WBC count and absolute neutrophil count (ANC). It must be greater than 500/m³. ANC can be calculated as follows:
  Determine the percentage of neutrophil count (poly or SEGS and bands). Multiply WBC count by the percentage of neutrophils.

For example, if WBC count is 2000, neutrophils = 7% and neutrophil bands = 7%, then total neutrophils + bands = 7 + 7 = 14%.
ANC = 14% × 2000 = 280/m³

- Isolate the child from infection source, especially viral diseases as mentioned earlier.
- Promote optimum nutrition to maintain and rebuild healthy tissue. Frequent, small feeds are recommended by promoting the child's choices and preferences in selection of foods.
  Adequate protein and calorie intake to be promoted to provide better host defence against infection and increase tolerance to chemotherapy and irradiation. But foods that can lead to infection such as fruits and also foods such as yogurt and curds need not to be given from outside as there is a chance for acquiring infection. See that properly prepared food is given to these children.
- Take measures to prevent haemorrhage by turning children frequently to relieve pressure on bony prominence, and provide meticulous mouth care and good skin care. Use only soft tooth brush for mouth care, measure temperature only by axial route, as rectal and oral routes can produce injury to the mucous membrane.

- Do not give intramuscular injections, as this may promote bleeding in these children as a result of thrombocytopenia.
- Observe children receiving blood transfusions for transfusion reactions.
- Prevent constipation resulting from neutropathic side effects of chemotherapy by providing high-fibre diet, and promote activity as per tolerance of the child and administer stool softeners.
- Take measures to prevent nausea and vomiting resulting from chemotherapy by administering an antiemetic agent 30 minutes to 1 hour before chemotherapy administration and continue the antiemetic every 2–6 hours after chemotherapy, as prescribed.
- Prevent renal damage resulting from chemotherapy by administering allopurinol to prevent uric acid crystal formation and resultant haemorrhagic cystitis. Alkalinize urine with acid-ash diet. Provide adequate hydration by giving frequent fluids and promoting frequent voiding.
- Promote adequate rest by providing calm, quiet environment and by clustering nursing care activities and other procedures to ensure long periods of uninterrupted rest periods.
- Provide adequate explanation and reassurance about alopecia and tell them that this is temporary side effect of chemotherapy and the lost hair will grow after sometime.
- Provide play activities according to the child' stage of development and condition.
- Give health/family education on diagnosis and nature of disorder and treatment, and side effects of chemotherapy and radiation therapy in a nonthreatening way.
- Evaluate the nursing care provided.
  The points to be noted are as follows:
  - The child and parents should verbalize an understanding on the disease process and treatment.
  - The child should not exhibit any side effects of chemotherapy and radiation therapy.
  - The child is consuming adequate nutrition and develops no constipation.
  - Family members should know the schedule of treatment and dates of subsequent treatment.

WILMS TUMOUR

Definition – It is most common intra-abdominal tumour in children and the malignant neoplasm of the kidney. It is also the most curable solid tumour of childhood.

Incidence and aetiology – The exact cause is unknown. The predicted factors include the following:
- Genetic influence: Autosomal dominant trait seems to account for the mode of transmission. Bilateral Wilms tumours have a genetic influence. About 15% of children with Wilms tumour have associated anomalies such as hypospadias, cryptorchidism and ambiguous genitalia.
- Genomic imprinting showed that chromosome 11 has the absence of maternal allele.
- Wilms tumour associated with renal development is called nephrogenic rests (nephroblastomatosis).

Nephrogenic rests developing in the periphery of the lobe are usually found in children with Wilms tumour.
- Familial predisposition is also seen in the occurrence of Wilms tumour. Siblings and identical twins of a child with Wilms tumour have a high risk of developing the disorder.
- Increased incidence of the tumour is observed in children with aniridia.
- Its incidence is about 6% of all childhood tumours in children.
- About 75% of the cases are diagnosed before the age of 5 years.
- Male and females are affected equally.

Pathophysiology

The tumour arises from the immature renoblast cells (blastema, tubules and stroma) located in the renal parenchyma. Classic Wilms tumours are known to be heterogeneous with respect to component proportions and exhibit aberrant differentiation, e.g. adipose tissue, skeletal muscle, cartilage and bone. The tumour is well encapsulated in early stages but may later extend into lymph nodes and renal vein or vena cava and metastasize to the lungs and other sites. Wilms tumour can also occur with only one type of cell and is called monophasic Wilms tumour.

Prognosis of the tumour depends on the type of histology. Anaplastic histology is the most unfavourable in terms of prognosis. Anaplastic tumours are characterized by cells with nuclear enlargement two to three times the diameter of adjacent cells, hyperchromatic nuclei and abnormal mitotic figures. The single most important indicator of a poor prognosis for Wilms tumour is the presence of anaplasia in the tumour.

Treatment is surgical removal of the tumour and affected lymph nodes and selected metastasis. The staging is determined by lymph node sampling and careful examination of the liver and the contralateral kidney.

Chemotherapy is administered at all stages. A total of eight cycles are given as follows: one induction and seven maintenance cycles (3 monthly cycles).
Stages I, II and III (favourable histology):
  Induction
  - Injection vincristine – 0.05 mg/kg weekly × eight doses
  - Injection actinomycin D – 30 mcg/kg on days 1 and 8
  Maintenance
  - Injection vincristine – 0.05 mg/kg weekly × two doses
  - Injection actinomycin D – 30 mcg/kg weekly × 2 doses
Stages IV, V and unfavourable histology – all stages:
  Induction
  Obtain platelet count and an electrocardiogram (ECG).
    - Injection vincristine – 0.05 mg/kg weekly × two doses
    - Injection actinomycin D – 30 mcg/kg on days 1 and 8
    - Injection Adriamycin (doxorubicin) – 45 mg/m^2 at weeks 3 and 9

Maintenance
- Injection vincristine – 0.05 mg/kg weekly × two doses
- Injection actinomycin D – 30 mcg/kg weekly × 2 doses
- Injection Adriamycin – 30 mg/m² on day 1

For stage II and above, administer radiation therapy as well. Radiation therapy may be performed to eradicate residual tumour cells and selected metastatic foci, such as tumour cells that have been left behind in the selected area of the abdomen during surgery.

Assessment Findings

Common clinical features of Wilms tumour include the following:
- Asymptomatic abdominal mass and palpable renal mass of nontender type, deep and confined to the one side, usually left side, are present.
- Early symptoms include microscopic haematuria in one-third of patients and other urinary disturbances, malaise, weight loss and anaemia.
- Occlusion of the left renal vein by tumour extension may obstruct the left spermatic vein with a resultant varicocoele on the left. Urological anomalies such as hypospadias and undescended testis are often seen with Wilms tumour. Aniridia – congenital abnormality of iris, Beckwith–Wiedermann syndrome (BWS) – an overgrowth syndrome characterized by exomphalos, visceromegaly, macroglossia, umbilical defects, hyperinsulinaemic hypoglycaemia, hemihypertrophy and susceptibility to a number of paediatric cancers such as Wilms tumour, adrenocortical carcinoma and hepatoblastoma.
- Hypertension is related to excessive rennin release from the diseased kidney.
- Pallor, anorexia and lethargy are related to anaemia.
- Weight loss is related to anorexia.
- Fever is related to infection.
- Dyspnoea and chest pain are related to lung metastasis.
- Careful palpation of the abdomen and measurement of blood pressure in all limbs are needed as a part of physical assessment.
- Laboratory findings Include the following:
  - Routine blood and urine examination
  - MRI
  - Computed tomography (CT)
  - Biopsy
- Evidence of metastasis can be obtained by radiological examinations.

Nursing Diagnoses

- Anxiety
- High risk for infection
- High risk for injury
- Altered nutrition
- Pain
- Powerlessness
- Altered family process
- Altered tissue perfusion.

Nursing Interventions

- Prepare the child for diagnostic tests and treatments according to the level of development and understanding.
- Address the specific fears and misconceptions of the family and include them in planning the care for their child.
- Provide information appropriate to their level of understanding.
- Help prevent rupture of the encapsulated tumour by avoiding abdominal palpation and by promoting careful bathing and handling.
- Monitor bowel sounds and assess for signs and symptoms of obstruction.
- Prevent infection by proper precautions such as avoiding contact with infected persons and following universal precautions.
- Check for complications of chemotherapy.
- Administer chemotherapeutic agents in time with adequate precautions.
- Prepare the child for radiation therapy, as and when needed.
- Provide family and patient education, as needed.

BRAIN TUMOURS

Brain tumours are the second commonest tumours in children after leukaemia. These are always primary tumours in children, and 60% of them are infratentorial. The common manifestations in brain tumours include:
- Headache that will be worse on lying down
- Vomiting, which is projectile and seen usually on waking from sleep
- Nystagmus
- Squint (secondary to sixth cranial nerve palsy)
- Ataxia
- Personality and behaviour disorders

The common types of brain tumours are as follows:
- Astrocytoma (40%)
- Medulloblastoma (20%)
- Ependymoma (8%)
- Brainstem glioma (6%)
- Craniopharyngioma (4%).

Astrocytoma is the most common type of tumour which is often cystic in nature. It is slow growing in children. It responds very well to surgical intervention. The common site of occurrence is cerebral hemispheres.

Medulloblastoma arises in the midline of the posterior fossa. The tumour spread occurs through cerebrospinal fluid (CSF). Spinal metastasis is common. Treatment includes surgical removal of the tumour and CNS irradiation.

Ependymoma also occurs in the posterior fossa and behaves like medulloblastoma, with presenting symptoms such as headache and vomiting.

Brainstem glioma presents with cranial nerve defects and ataxia, along with pyramidal tract signs.

Craniopharyngioma is a developmental tumour arising from the squamous remnants of Rathke's pouch. It is actually not malignant but locally invasive. The common feature is increased ICP symptoms.

Multidisciplinary Management

Diagnosis is by CT scan and presenting clinical features.

NEUROBLASTOMA

Neuroblastomas are frustrating tumours of childhood. Some of the neuroblastomas may completely regress spontaneously or mature into ganglioneuromas. A neuroblastoma arises from the neural crest tissue in the adrenal medulla and the sympathetic nervous system. Because these tumours arise from the embryonic neural crest, which gives rise to the sympathetic system and the adrenal medulla, it can develop anywhere from the base of the skull to the presacral area. Most of them are found in the retroperitoneal space, where it is not always possible to determine whether a lesion has arisen from the adrenal gland. Approximately 25% of neuroblastomas originate in the mediastinum, pelvis or neck. It is most common before the age of 5 years. Usually, children present with an abdominal mass but the primary tumour lies anywhere in the sympathetic chain. Abdominal neuroblastomas are encapsulated. Paravertebral neuroblastomas may invade the vertebral foramina and compress the spinal cord. Metastasis is common in adjacent lymph nodes, but they also occur in bones, liver and skin. Ganglioneuromas and ganglioneuroblastomas are often encapsulated and do not invade adjoining tissues.

Assessment Findings

Diagnosis is made by the characteristic clinical features (pallor, irritability, anorexia, weight loss, abdominal mass, hepatomegaly, bone pain, limp paraplegia, cervical lymphadenopathy, proptosis, periorbital bruising and skin nodules); radiological studies including CT scan and biochemical studies for urine catecholamines for VMA (vanilmandelic acid) and HVA (homovanillic acid). Confirmatory biopsy is also done, and evidence of metastasis is confirmed by bone marrow samples. Levels of norepinephrine derivative VMA are elevated in 80% of children with neuroblastomas. When determination of VMA, HVA and total catecholamines is performed with 24-hour urine specimens, the diagnostic accuracy approaches 100%. Certain food substances such as vanilla, nuts and chocolates may falsely elevate values.

Other investigative procedures include intravenous pyelogram, a 24-hour urine test for VMA excretion; total catecholamine calcification is more common in neuroblastomas than in Wilms tumours. Blood cell count and bone marrow examination are also indicated because in bone marrow metastasis or clinically inoperable tumours, a bone marrow aspirate which is positive for neuroblastoma cells will confirm the diagnosis.

Staging

When the diagnosis is made, the child is assigned to a presumptive staging classification, which may determine the proper course of treatment.

Stage 1: Tumour is confined to the organ or the structure of origin.

Stage 2: Tumours extending in continuity beyond the organ or structure of origin but not beyond the midline. Regional lymph nodes on the epsilateral side may be involved.

Stage 3: Tumours extend in continuity beyond the midline. Regional lymph nodes may be involved bilaterally.

Stage 4: Remote disease involving the skeleton, organs, soft tissues or distant lymph node groups is present.

Stage 5: This includes patients who would be otherwise be in stage 1 or stage 2 but who have remote metastasis confined to one or more of the following sites: liver, skin or bone marrow, without radiological evidence of bone metastasis.

Multidisciplinary Management

Therapy for neuroblastomas depends on the child's age, tumour location and clinical staging. Complete surgical removal, radiation therapy and chemotherapy may be required.

Nursing Interventions

Nursing interventions are similar to that of any other cancers.

TERATOMAS

Teratomas consist of a mixture of tissues originating from all the three germ layers, which are not usually found at the site of origin of the tumour. These unusual lesions may occur in the ovary, sacrococcygeal area, testicle, anterior mediastinum, face, neck, liver, stomach, brain and retroperitoneum. There are a number of hypotheses on the origin of teratomas, but none of them adequately explain the peculiarities and differing locations of these tumours. There are various explanations regarding the development of teratomas.

- Teratomas represent incomplete attempts to form Siamese twins.
- They are the resting places of totipotential cells left behind during embryogenesis.
- Germ cells may give rise to teratomas by parthenogenesis.

Teratomas are gonadal and extragonadal tumours. Because the gonads develop from retroperitoneal tissues, all the tumours in this area may arise by parthenogenesis of haploid cells, probably by fusion of two such cells. Regardless of their origin, teratomas are regarded as both developmental anomalies and tumours. Cystic teratomas are filled with turbid fluid as well as teeth, hair and sebaceous material, and often a mixture of cystic and solid tissue increases the possibility of malignancy. Microscopically, the three germ layers are represented by skin, skin appendages, glial tissues, cartilage, bone fat and various types of gastrointestinal endothelium and kidney tissue.

Teratomas are seen in various organs such as ovary, testicles, stomach, retroperitoneum, sacrococcygeal area, face, mediastinum, etc.

Multidisciplinary Management

- Surgical removal of the teratomas
- Adjunctive treatment of malignant teratomas

Nursing Interventions

Nursing interventions are the same as that of any other cancers.

LYMPHOMAS IN CHILDREN

Lymphomas are heterogeneous group of lymphoproliferative malignancies resulting from clonal expansion of tumour cells derived from B, T or NK cells. A majority of them are derived from B lymphocytes. Lymphomas are primary tumours of lymph cells called lymphocytes, a type of WBCs. The lymphatic system is a major part of immune system of the body. The two main types of lymphocytes concerned with immunity are B and T lymphocytes. B lymphocytes produce antibodies and protect the body against infections such bacterial and viral infections. There are different types of T lymphocytes; each one has a specific function in protecting the body. Lymphocytes are seen in bone marrow, thymus, adenoids and tonsils, and digestive tract. Lymphoma is the third most common cancer in children.

Clinical presentations vary and range from asymptomatic in routine blood workup to painless adenopathy to an emergent medical problem such as pain and failure to thrive and organ failure.

The two main kinds of lymphomas are as follows:

- **Hodgkin lymphoma** ([HL], also known as **Hodgkin disease [HD]**), which is named after Dr Thomas Hodgkin who first described it.
- **Non-Hodgkin lymphoma (NHL)**

Lymphomas differ in how they behave, spread and respond to treatment, so it is important to know the types of lymphomas. NHL tends to occur in younger children, whereas HL is more likely to affect older children and teens.

Non-Hodgkin Lymphoma

This type of lymphoma is rapidly growing in nature, with the potential doubling time of 16 hours. It has metastatic potential. Two-thirds of NHL cases have already widespread disease at the time of diagnosis. Bone marrow and CNS have most metastatic lesions. Childhood NHL can present many different signs and symptoms, depending on where it is located in the body. Common symptoms include:

- Enlarged lymph nodes (seen or felt as lumps under the skin)
- Swollen abdomen (belly)
- Feeling full after intake of only a small amount of food
- Shortness of breath or cough
- Fever
- Weight loss
- Night sweats
- Fatigue (feeling very tired)

Cell origins are small noncleaved – B cells exclusively; lymphoblastic – T cells predominantly; and large cells have either T or B cells (mostly B cells).

- Nearly all NHLs in children are one of three main types: Lymphoblastic lymphoma (LBL)
- Burkitt lymphoma (small noncleaved cell lymphoma)
- Large cell lymphoma

All three types are high grade (meaning they grow quickly) and diffuse, but it is important to find out which type a child has because each type is treated differently.

The WHO classification of NHLs is based on B-cell malignancies and T-cell malignancies.

B-cell Malignancies

Lymphoblastic Lymphoma. LBL accounts for about 25%–30% of NHLs. Boys are more affected than girls (in 2:1 ratio). Cancer cells are lymphoblasts, and if the bone marrow contains more than 25% of lymphoblasts, then the disease is classified under lymphoblastic leukaemia. In most cases, LBL develops from T cells and usually starts from thymus (thymus contains T lymphocytes). Rarely, LBL is seen in tonsils, too.

Burkitt Lymphoma. Burkitt lymphoma is also known as *small noncleaved cell lymphoma*. It accounts for about 40% of childhood NHLs. It is common among boys 5–10 years of age. Burkitt lymphoma is named after the physician who identified this type of lymphoma among African children. In African children, this lymphoma is mainly seen in the jaw or other facial bones. In other part of the world, it is often seen in the abdomen as a large mass obstructing the passage of food and blocking the intestine. This type of lymphoma develops from B lymphocytes. It can spread to other parts of the body such as brain and is one of the fastest growing tumour of childhood. All B-cell lymphomas have translocation of the c-*myc*-oncogene.

Histopathology shows small and uniform shape and size of the cells, nucleus with chromatin, high ratio of nuclear cytoplasm, lipid vacuoles and two to five nucleoli. It is endemic in the African variety and is associated with Epstein–Barr virus (EBV) infection (20%). It is sporadically seen in other parts of the world.

Diagnosis

- Physical examination
- Complete blood cell (CBC) count
- Serum chemistry – electrolytes, liver, renal panels, lactate dehydrogenase (LDH), uric acid
- LDH is a marker of tumour burden important to determine the outcome of management; uric acid is a measure of tumour lysis
- Imaging – CT chest and abdomen, gallium scan, fluorodeoxyglucose–positron emission tomography (FDG-PET) scan
- Bone marrow
- CSF examination for finding brain metastasis

Multidisciplinary management

- Chemotherapy alone; surgery only for abdominal emergency; radiation therapy for superior vena cava (SVC) obstruction or paraspinal compression

- B-cell involvement – treatment is with high-dose intensive therapy
- T-cell involvement – treatment is similar to ALL therapy

Complications

- Tumour-related complications are SVC syndrome, spinal cord compression, pleural and pericardial effusion, pulmonary embolism, obstructive uropathy, airway/pharyngeal obstruction.
- Metabolic complications are tumour lysis, syndrome of inappropriate antidiuretic hormone secretion (SIADH), hypo/hyperglycaemia.
- Gastrointestinal complications are bleeding and obstruction.
- Cytokine-mediated complications are cachexia and fever and malaise.
- Haematological complications are bone marrow infiltration and pancytopenia.
- Out of all these complications, the most dreaded one is tumour lysis. It needs to be evaluated. Assess serum phosphorus, uric acid, calcium and potassium levels. Adequately hydrate and alkalinize the child.

Large Cell Lymphomas. Large cell lymphomas arise from mature T or B cells and can develop in any part of the body where lymphocytes are there. T-cell lymphoma is seen as anterior mediastinal mass. B-cell lymphoma is mainly manifested as an abdominal mass but less likely to spread to the brain and bone marrow. It is a slow-growing tumour unlike that of lymphoblastic or Burkitt lymphoma and tends to occur more often in older children and teens.

The two main subtypes of large cell lymphoma are:

- **Anaplastic large cell lymphoma (ALCL):** It constitutes 10% of all NHLs in children. It usually develops from mature T cells. It may start in lymph nodes in the neck or other areas and may be found in the skin, lungs, bone, digestive tract or other organs.
- **Diffuse large B-cell lymphoma (DLBCL):** This type accounts for about 15% of all childhood lymphomas. It starts in B cells, as the name implies. These lymphomas sometime grow as large masses in the mediastinum and referred to as **primary mediastinal B-cell lymphomas.**

Risk factors

- Age, gender and race
  NHLs are not common in young children. They are mainly seen in teens and adults. They are more common in boys than in girls and more common in white children than in black children.
- Weak immune system: Children with weak immunity are more prone to develop NHL.
- Congenital immunodeficiency syndrome: Children born with abnormal immune system as a result of genetic syndrome are more affected with NHL. Examples of such syndromes are:
- Wiskott–Aldrich syndrome
- Severe combined immunodeficiency syndrome (SCID)
- Ataxia-telangiectasia
- Common variable immunodeficiency
- X-linked lymphoproliferative syndrome

Other risk factors are:

- Organ transplants
- HIV/AIDS
- Radiation exposure
- EBV infection

According to lymphoma biology, it can be aggressive NHL (has a short natural history – patients die within months if remain untreated; rapid cell proliferation; and potentially curable) and indolent NHL (has a fairly long history – patients live for long if remain untreated, too; disease of slow cellular proliferation and generally incurable). Treatment approach to aggressive type is cure, but for indolent lymphoma, the goal of treatment is control of growth.

In indolent type, immediate treatment does not prolong the overall survival. The treatment starts when constitutional symptoms develop such as compromise of vital organs as a result of compression or infiltration (bone marrow compression), bulky adenopathy, evidence of transformation, etc. Aggressive type is treated with a goal of cure. Administer most effective therapy at diagnosis itself.

Prognosis of NHL is not rewarding, as it has many histological subtypes.

Hodgkin Lymphoma

Out of lymphomas, HL constitutes 40% and is 5% of all paediatric malignancies. Its incidence is bimodal. In developed industrialized countries, its peak incidence is seen in late 20s and after 50s. But in developing countries, early peak is before adolescence. Three distinct forms are seen. Childhood form (<14 years), young adult form (15–34 years) and older form (55–74 years). It is rarely diagnosed in children younger than 10 years, and male children are more affected. But in adolescence, the male and females are equally affected. It is more common in children with congenital acquired immunodeficiency, ataxia-telangiectasia and AIDS. Familial tendencies are noted in concordance with first-degree relatives. So, genetic predisposition is suspected. There is an increased association with certain HLA types and its incidence is higher among monozygotic twins.

Aetiology

- EBV infection
- Human herpes virus 6
- Cytomegalovirus (CMV)
- High EBV titres and the presence of EBV genomes in Reed–Sternberg cells
- Surface markers show T-cell or B-cell linkage

Clinical Features

- Most common feature is asymptomatic cervical lymphadenopathy.
- Nodes are painless, firm and noninflammatory.
- Extension is seen from one lymph node group to another.

- Two-thirds of patients have mediastinal adenopathy with cough and breathing difficulty as a result of compression.
- Rarely, inguinal and axillary lymph node enlargement is present.
- Extranodal metastasis are seen in pleura, pericardium, lung, liver, bone and brain.
- Paraneoplastic syndrome is seen in relapsing patients and involves haematological, skin, nervous system and kidneys.

Diagnosis

- Histopathological examination of the tissue from the most accessible node
- Physical examination with careful attention and measurement of lymph nodes
- Laboratory investigations include CBC count, erythrocyte sedimentation rate (ESR), renal function, alkaline phosphatase, ferritin, copper; cytokines
- Staging workup: Gallium scan/ PET scan
- Staging laparotomy (rarely done)
- Bone marrow biopsy
- Bone scan
- CT chest

Histological Subtypes

Rye's classification:
- Nodular sclerosing (most common) accounts for 50%–75% of all HDs and is seen in 40% of young people.

- Mixed cellularity accounts for 15%–30% of all cases and most common in children and patients with HIV/AIDS. Many Reed–Sterberg cells are seen.
- Lymphocyte depletion is rare in children; many Reed–Sterberg cells, few lymphocytes diffuse fibrous and necrosis are seen.
- Lymphocyte predominance shows B-cell lineage and accounts for 10%–15% of children with HD. More in boys than in girls (in 2:1 ratio).

Ann Arbor classification:
  Stage I – Involvement of single lymph node region or of a single extralymphatic region
  Stage II – Involvement of two or more regions on the same side of the diaphragm or localized involvement of extralymphatic organ or site and one or more node regions on the same side of the diaphragm
  Stage III – Involvement of lymph node regions on both sides of the diaphragm accompanied by involvement of the spleen or by localized involvement of extra-lymphatic organ or both
  Stage IV – Diffuse or disseminated involvement of one or more extralymphatic organs or tissue with or without lymph node involvement

B symptoms:
- Fever of 38 consecutive days, drenching night sweats, unexpected loss of 10% or more of body weight in the 6 months preceding diagnosis
  A symptoms – Absence of all the aforementioned symptoms

Differentiation between Hodgkin Lymphoma and Non-Hodgkin Lymphoma

Hodgkin Lymphoma	Non-Hodgkin Lymphoma
HL	NHL
• Characterized by the presence of Reed–Sternberg cells	• NHL is a heterogeneous group of B- and T-cell malignancies, with diverse growth patterns and responses to therapy
• Stage more important than that of the histological subtype	• NHL cure rate mediocre
• Often limited stage (stage I or II)	• Many histological subtypes
• Spreads to contiguous nodes	• Histological subtype often more important that the stage
• Often affects younger patients	• Indolent vs. aggressive
• Very responsive to therapy	• Function of underlying biology
• Approach to the patient	• Indolent:
• Staging evaluation	• Often asymptomatic
• History and physical examination (H & P)	• Less responsive to treatment
• CBC, differential, platelet counts	• Approach dictated mainly by histology
• ESR, LDH, albumin, liver function tests (LFTs), creatinine (Cr)	• Reliable haematopathology crucial
• CT scans of chest/abdomen/pelvis	• Aggressive:
• Bone marrow evaluation	• Cure is often the goal
• PET scan in selected cases	• Indolent:
B-cell lymphoma	• Cure is rarely the goal
• Several histological subtypes	• Control is the goal
• Generally does not affect the approach to the patient	• Treatment is less responsive
• Reed–Sternberg cells	• 30 histological subtypes identified
• Tends to occur in young adults	• B cell (85%), T cell, NK cell
• Mediastinal disease common	• Histological subtype dictates the approach to treatment
• Spreads to contiguous nodes	• Median age at diagnosis 60 years
• Common to have a 'localized' presentation	• Often widespread disease at diagnosis
• Highly curable with current treatment	• Wide variation in outcome
	• Some cases rapidly fatal
	• Some cases readily curable
	• Some cases incurable, but patients can live for many years with good quality of life

Multidisciplinary Management

- Chemotherapy ± irradiation of the involved area
- Multiagent chemotherapy is preferred with ABVE-PC, ABVD-OPPA/COPP
- Adriamycin, bleomycin, vincristine, etoposide, cyclophosphamide (CTX)
- The number of courses depends on the stage of the disease: two to four for early stage, four to six for advanced stage
- Early relapse – bone marrow transplant
  Prognosis dependent on the stage, response to treatment, presence of metastasis and B symptoms
  - Early-stage prognosis is favourable
  - Advanced stage it is unfavourable.

Nursing Diagnoses

- **High-risk for altered family process/high-risk for ineffective coping**
- Risk for injury
- **Deficient knowledge**
- Risk for infection

Nursing Management of Children with Lymphoma

Assess the child's health status.
  Assess the patient's knowledge of disease and treatment plan.
  Assess for coping mechanisms used in previous illnesses or prior hospitalizations.
Evaluate resources and support systems available to the patient at home and in the community.
  Explain the need for diagnostic procedures and treatment.
  Prepare the child, specifically for procedure such as lymphangiography.
Encourage the child to sleep, or provide diversions as far as possible.
Provide opportunities for the child and parents to openly express their feelings, fears and concerns. Provide reassurance and hope as indicated.
  Introduce new information about disease treatment, as available.
  Observe the child for complication of diagnostic procedure such as pulmonary embolism.
  Reassure the child and family.
  Assess knowledge of disease, treatment strategies and prognosis.
Describe the function of the lymphatic system and the abnormalities associated with lymphoma.
  Clarify the needs of the diagnostic process:
  - Peripheral blood analysis
  - Lymph node biopsy
  - Bone marrow biopsy
  - Lymphangiogram
  - X-ray study
  - CT scan
  Clarify the similarities and differences between HD and NHL.
Common presenting symptoms include fever, weight loss, night sweats, pruritus, nontender enlarged lymph nodes, and possibly enlarged spleen and liver.

Explain the expected reaction of the contrast medium.
Explain treatment protocol and side effects.
  Discuss common treatment approaches:
  - Radiation therapy
  - Combined chemotherapy
  - Biological response modifier therapy
  - Bone marrow and peripheral stem cell transplantation
Explain common complications of the therapy.
  Auscultate the lungs for respiratory infections such as crackles, diminished air entry and breath sounds.
  Observe the child for coughing spells and character of sputum.
  Inspect body sites with a high infection potential (mouth, throat, axilla, perineum, rectum, etc.).
  Inspect intravenous central catheter sites for redness, tenderness, pain and itching.
  Observe for changes in colour, character and frequency of urine and stool.
  Monitor temperature as indicated. Report if the temperature is higher than 38° C (100.4°F).
  Obtain cultures as indicated.
  Explain the cause and effects of leucopenia.
  Instruct parents to provide and maintain personal hygiene, especially at home.

Prevention

Most of the cancers can be prevented up to an extent if precautions are taken. NHL has no risk factors that can be prevented; hence, preventing NHL is not easy. The best way to reduce the risk for NHL is to improve the immune system, as one of the major risk factors is the weakened immune system. Prevent HIV infection in children through education of parents and children; e.g. treating the pregnant women with HIV with anti-HIV drugs and advising HIV-positive mothers not to breastfeed their baby. NHL can also develop as a consequence of treating other cancers with chemotherapy, immune-suppressing drugs and radiation therapy. Caution may be taken while treating children with cancers and find better ways to treat children with cancers for not raising the risk for NHL.

CHEMOTHERAPY IN CHILDREN

Essential Concepts

- Chemotherapeutic agents work on the dividing cells.
- Tumour location and cell type affect the choice of drugs.
- Most chemotherapeutic drugs are metabolized in the liver and excreted by the kidneys; so, they must be functional to prevent toxicity.

Nurses' Responsibility

- Identify the number of chemotherapeutic agents administered.
- Identify potential side effects of each drug.

- Monitor fluid–electrolyte balance and be vigilant about potential imbalances.
- Assess for adequate urine output.
- Monitor laboratory values.
- Assess oral cavity for irritation and bleeding gums.
- Assess and establish a baseline data of the following:
  - Nutritional status
  - Oral condition
  - Skin condition
  - Degree of mobility
  - Psychological status
  - Neurological condition
- Observe for side effects of cell breakdown
  - Elevated blood urea nitrogen (BUN)
  - Stone formation in the urinary tract
- Maintain a chemotherapy flow sheet.

- Observe for side effects on rapidly dividing cells.
  - Gastrointestinal mucosa: diarrhoea, nausea and vomiting
  - Administer antiemetics.
  - Provide mouth care with hydrogen peroxide every 4 hours. Do not use toothbrush or glycerine.
  - Administer anaesthetic spray to mouth prior to meals.
  - Provide frequent cold, high-calorie beverages.
  - Hair follicles: loss of hair – Prepare the client for hair loss; suggest wig or scarf.
  - Reassure the client that hair will grow back in 6 weeks.
  - Apply tourniquet around the scalp during chemotherapy and in 2–3 hours following chemotherapy to lessen the amount of hair loss.
- Monitor administration of common drugs.

Common Drugs	Side Effects	Nurse's Responsibility
Prednisolone – an immunosuppressive agent	Increased appetite, change in fat distribution, retention of fluid, hirsutism, occasional hypertension, psychological disturbances	Monitor side effects such as infection, monitor serum blood sugar level and monitor tapering of medication.
6-Mercaptopurine – interrupts the synthesis of purines essential for the structure and function of nucleic acids	Less toxic to children – kidney excrete increased amount of uric acid	Observe intake and output and increase fluid intake.
Methotrexate – folic acid antagonist that suppresses the growth of abnormal cells enough to permit regeneration of normal cells	Ulceration of oral mucosa, vomiting, diarrhoea and abdominal pain	Observe for ulceration – discontinue drug temporarily at the appearance of ulcers. Observe renal function as the drug is excreted through kidneys.
Cytoxan – alkylating agent that suppresses cellular proliferation	Haemorrhagic cystitis	Monitor uric acid/urea clearance level. Provide increased amount of fluid. Observe colour of urine.
Vincristine – alkylating agent used to induce remission rapidly	Insomnia, severe constipation, peripheral neuritis or paralysis	Provide symptomatic management, and once remission is achieved, administer the patient with the toxic drugs.

RADIATION THERAPY

Essential Concepts

- Radiation affects all cells of the body but is particularly lethal to rapidly multiplying cells.
- It is used for treating tumours to eradicate or relieve symptoms of pressure.
- It is usually used along with chemotherapeutic agents.

Common Problems

- Easy fatigability
- Fluid–electrolyte imbalances as a result of vomiting, diarrhoea and increased urine output associated with radiotherapy
- Decreased blood cell count – Monitor haemoglobin and haematocrit
- Skin breakdown at the site of irradiation
- Oral ulcers, gum diseases
- Loss of hair
- Infection as a result of bone marrow depression

Nurses' Responsibility

- Monitor for radiation sickness such as nausea, vomiting and malaise.
- Offer high-calorie feeds (milkshakes with extra protein and vitamins).
- Provide feeds in attractive and palatable ways.
- Observe side effects of cell breakdown.
- Monitor elevation of BUN, accumulation of uric acid and stone formation in the urinary tract.
- Treat side effects of cell breakdown by:
  - Increasing fluid intake
  - Monitoring intake and output
- Treat skin breakdown.
- Check the client regularly for any redness or irritation at the radiation site.
- Notify the physician immediately.

- Apply lotion to the area following termination of radiation therapy.
- Avoid any irritation to the area from clothing, soap or weather extremes.
- Treat bone marrow depression.
- Watch laboratory values carefully.
- Isolate client because of susceptibility (low leucocyte count).
- Avoid intramuscular injections, as it causes bleeding as a result of a low platelet count.
- Administer antibiotics.

ISSUES OF CANCER SURVIVORSHIP

A brief history of cancer therapy in children showed that cure was possible for most cancers by 1970s. Effective multimodality protocols have been evolved with randomized control trials in 1980s. In 1990s, therapy risk was tailored, late effects defined and radiation dosage and substituted effective drugs for radiation reduced. By 2000, the health care workers identified the dose-related effects of drugs and started educating the survivors of cancer on surveillance of late effects based on risks, interventions to reduce risks and transition to adult health care. In the United States, one in 1000 population is a childhood cancer survivor. One in 570 is a childhood cancer survivor in those aged 20–34 years. Survival rates of childhood cancer have increased greatly during the last 25 years. In developed countries such as the United States, 80% of children live more than 5 years after diagnosis and treatment. Out of these, two-thirds will experience at least one late effect. One-third will experience a severe or life-threatening late effect. In India, too, survivors of childhood cancers are on the increase, especially children with lymphoblastic leukaemia, Wilms tumour and certain types of brain tumours. The increase in long-term survival has brought quality-of-life issues after comprehensive treatment of childhood cancer. This trend in survivability has made a shift in management from psychological issues of cancer to caring children with life-threatening chronic illnesses after treatment. During childhood, life-threatening complications can be especially destructive for the child's psychological growth and development. During this growing age, children with cancer face harsh treatment such as chemotherapy and radiation therapy, contradicting the normal developmental needs such as play.

Survivors of cancer may be trained to live healthy, with normal or near normal activities such as exercise, balanced diet, maintaining a healthy weight and adequate follow-ups. Regular exercise increases sense of well-being after cancer treatment and can speed the recovery. Survivors of childhood cancer who exercise may experience:

- Increased strength and endurance
- Fewer signs and symptoms of depression
- Less anxiety
- Reduced fatigue
- Improved mood
- Higher self-esteem

A balanced diet with vegetables, fruits and whole grains will help improve health and well-being. Excess amount of any diet can be harmful. Consulting a dietician for selection of food is important, as certain types of food items may aggravate cancer symptoms. Maintaining normal weight and preventing obesity are also very important, as obesity is a late effect that may lead to metabolic syndrome.

Survivors face psychological or societal barriers, such as posttraumatic stress disorders. Children surviving after haemopoietic stem cell transplantation require long-term follow-up. Patients undergoing allogeneic bone marrow transplant can experience graft versus host disease (GVHD) and autoimmunity.

Late Effects

Late effects of childhood cancer treatment are most devastating, leading to many quality-of-life problems from children through adulthood. The late effects are defined as persistent and adverse changes that are directly related to disease process, treatment process, or both.

Late effects of cancer occur as a result of:
- Disease – the type of cancer
- Location of tumour
- Treatment
  - Surgery
  - Chemotherapy
  - Radiation therapy

Risk factors for late effects are:
- Age and developmental stage
- Gender
- Comorbidities
- Family history and/or genetic predispositions
- Location of tumour
- Types and dose of chemotherapy agents
- Site, dose and type of radiation
- Extend of surgical treatment

Types of Late Effects

Physical
- Head and neck
- Endocrine
- Neurocognitive
- Second malignancies
- Psychosocial
- Emotional
- CNS
- Pulmonary
- Cardiovascular
- Gastrointestinal
- Genitourinary
- Musculoskeletal
- Renal
- Integumentary
- Haematopoietic

Head and neck
Head and neck is widely affected because of sensitive structures and is the common site for soft tissue tumours. Development of brain during childhood is essential to maximum health and quality of life in adulthood.

Common late effects:
1. Hypoplasia of bone as a result of >30 Gy radiation
2. Skin necrosis/ulceration as a result of >70 Gy radiation
3. Growth disturbances as a result of radiation therapy and chemotherapy
4. Xerostomia when given a dose >30 Gy radiation
5. Sensorineural hearing loss as a result of radiation therapy and chemotherapy

Ocular late effects
- Hyperkeratosis
- Chronic injection of conjunctiva and sclera
- Cataracts
- Glaucoma with prolonged steroid use
- Retinopathy
- Deformities in orbital bone growth

Effects on hearing
- Conductive hearing loss
- Sensorineural hearing loss
- Chronic otitis externa
- Stenosis or necrosis of ear canal
- Excess cerumen

Dental late effects
- Delayed dentition
- Missing or underdeveloped permanent teeth
- Increased caries
- Blunting, thinning and shortening of roots
- Hypocalcification

CNS late effects
Age at diagnosis and during treatment is an important factor in CNS late effects:
- Paralysis
- Neuropathies
- Seizures
- Neurocognitive problems
- Shunt function

Pulmonary late effects
- Obstructive, restrictive, interstitial or combination lung disease
- Pneumonitis
- Pulmonary fibrosis
- Frequent pneumonias
- Noncardiogenic pulmonary oedema

Cardiovascular late effects
- Coronary artery disease
- Pericarditis
- Cardiomyopathy
- Congestive heart failure (CHF)
- Valve damage
- Arrhythmias

Gastrointestinal late effects
- Hepatitis/hepatic dysfunction/cirrhosis
- Feeding disorders
- Chronic GVHD
- Oesophageal strictures
- Oesophagitis/gastroesophageal reflux disease (GERD)
- Adhesions
- Enteritis

Genitourinary late effects
- Renal function
- Urethral strictures or fibrosis
- Bladder and/or bowel dysfunction
- Vaginal fibrosis, malformation, fistulas
- Testicular/prostate dysfunction

Musculoskeletal late effects
- Hypoplasia
- Leg length discrepancies
- Prosthetic devices
- Scoliosis
- Amputation
- Rhabdomyolysis
- Slipped capital femoral epiphysis
- Exostosis
- Osteonecrosis
- Fibrosis/contractures
- Bone density changes – Osteopenia/osteoporosis

Integumentary late effects
- Pigment changes
- Alopecia
- Melanoma/skin cancers
- Skin necrosis
- Telangiectasia spidery blood vessels beneath the skin surface
- Fibrosis/contractures/scarring/striae
- Acceleration of skin ageing

Hematopoietic immune reconstitution
- Reimmunization
- Chronic anaemia
- Chronic thrombocytopenia
- Eosinophilia, especially after stem cell transplantation
- Bone marrow depression

Endocrine late effects
- Thyroid dysfunction
- Growth problems
- Fertility dysfunction
- Gonadal dysfunction
- Pituitary dysfunction
- Adrenal insufficiency
- Diabetes
- Osteopenia
- Hypothalamic obesity

Thyroid late effects
- Hypothyroidism
- Hyperthyroidism
- Thyroid nodules
- Silent thyroiditis

Effects on growth
- Growth hormone deficiency
- Microcephaly
- Catch-up growth after completion of therapy

Effects on gonads and fertility
Precocious or delayed puberty
Ovarian dysfunction of primary/secondary: Egg harvest or donation is practiced before starting treatment itself

Testicular dysfunction
Primary/secondary requires sperm banking or donors

Adrenal insufficiency and diabetes
- Adrenocorticotropic hormone (ACTH) deficiency
- SIADH/salt wasting syndrome
- Diabetes mellitus
- Diabetes insipidus

Osteopenia may be asymptomatic with risks for fractures. Bone density screening **and** calcium and vitamin D supplements are required.

Hypothalamic obesity
Unrelenting weight gain that does not respond to diet or exercise modifications.

Risk is greater for brain tumour survivors:
- Age <6 years at diagnosis
- Radiation
- Tumour location
- Risk greater with the presence of other endocrinopathies

Neurocognitive late effects
- Learning disabilities
- Loss of IQ points
- Developmental delay
- Attention deficit
- Behavioural abnormalities
- Fine and gross motor coordination difficulties
- Decrease in processing speed
- Memory loss
- Leucoencephalopathy

Second malignancies
- Thyroid carcinoma
- Leukaemia or myelodysplastic syndrome (MDS)
- Bone tumours
- Meningiomas
- Brain tumours
- Skin cancers
- Breast cancer

Psychosocial/Emotional effects
- Posttraumatic stress
- Quality of life
- Social functioning
- Functional impact
- Depression
- Anxiety
- Fatigue
- Sleep disorders
- Body image

Challenges for Survivors

- Medical
- Educational
- Social/emotional
- Employment
- Legal
- Financial

Medical Challenges

Survivors of childhood disease need to be integrated into adult health care. This requires specific guidelines as they have been treated for cancer and there should be definite criteria for identifying their problems for providing health care. Health professionals must be cognizant about the late effects of treatment to provide needed health care to the survivors. Getting medical insurance for them is another problem. In India, no agencies have come with insurance scheme for treatment of late effects. Health insurance for pregnant ladies, neonates and children has not been implemented so far. So, their care mainly depends on the capacity to pay by the family and the free medical care available in the government sector. These places may not have adequate facilities for caring such children with cancer.

Educational Challenges

Right to education for all can be applied in these cases. But how many children can cope with schooling during the treatment period? Home-based education system should be developed for these children to continue their schooling. They may need cognitive remediation, neurocognitive testing and need to readjust personal goals.

Social/Emotional Challenges

These children exhibit many high-risk behaviours such as smoking, alcohol abuse, drug use and sexual promiscuity. Difficulty finding peer group, forming intimacy and experiencing anxiety, depression and sleep disturbance are other social and emotional problems faced by these children.

Challenges with Employment

They may have certain physical disabilities that pose problem for employment. This is common after treatment with surgery, radiotherapy and certain chemotherapy. They may also have psychosocial disabilities, neurocognitive issues and chronic fatigue that result in problem for maintaining employment. They may also face job discrimination.

Financial Challenges

- Income
- Lower paying job as a result of disabilities
- Job discrimination leading to lower salary and promotions

Medical reimbursement problems may arise. ESI benefits are derived only when they are employed by established companies and registered firms. Debt from treatment may be a big financial crisis they may face. Costs incurred from medical care for late effects and follow-up are real burden, as treatment is very costly and not affordable by common men.

Care of Survivors

Challenges faced by caretakers of survivors are as follows:
- Lack of knowledge of primary care providers
- Long-term follow-up programmes need to be available in paediatric cancer centres and adult cancer centres

Role of a Paediatric Nurse

- Program coordination
- Screening
- History and physical examination, and preparing follow-up guidelines
- Educating survivors on treatment summaries and recommendations for long-term follow-up. They may

be assisted to find special schooling program to complete education. The side effects of treatment and therapy need to be informed to the child and family so that they may go for neurocognitive tests and decide on the type of schooling. They may be directed to medical facilities specifically available for cancer patients. Nurses need to help children and parents to mobilize social resources to manage financial crisis. Anticipatory guidance to parents and children is one of major responsibilities of paediatric oncology nurses who provide care to children with cancer. Empowering patients and families, integrating chronic/late effects in teaching, being an advocate for these children and their family, and promoting transition to adult care are other major roles of nurses working with childhood cancer programmes.

STUDY QUESTIONS

- What is leukaemia?
- What are the types of leukaemia and their clinical features?
- What is Wilms tumour?
- Describe the medical and surgical management of a child with Wilms tumour.
- What are the common types of brain tumours?
  What is Hodgkin lymphoma?
  Differentiate between Hodgkin and non-Hodgkin lymphomas.
- Write short notes on the following:
  a. Hodgkin lymphoma
  b. Neuroblastoma
  c. Retinoblastoma
  d. Rhabdomyosarcoma
  e. Teratomas
  f. Reverse barrier technique
- What are the nurse's responsibilities in the following situations:
  a. Leukaemic child receiving intrathecal methotrexate
  b. A child with Wilms tumour receiving chemotherapy

c. A leukaemic child undergoing CNS irradiation
d. A leukaemic child preparing for bone marrow transplantation
e. A child with retinoblastoma undergoing nucleation
- Prepare a nursing care plan for a child admitted with ALL using the nursing process.

BIBLIOGRAPHY

1. Allen CE, Kamdar KY, Bollard CM, Gross TG. Malignant non-Hodgkin lymphomas in children. In: Pizzo PA, Poplack DG, eds. *Principles and Practice of Pediatric Oncology*. 7th ed. Philadelphia, Pa: Lippincott Williams & Wilkins; 2016:587–603.
2. Ashely, D.J.B. (1973). Origin of Teratomas. Cancer, 32, pp. 390–394.
3. Beckwith, J.B., Martin, R.F. (1968). Observation on the Histopathology of Neuroblastomas. Journal of Pediatric Surgery, 3, pp. 106–110.
4. Beevi A. (2012) Paediatric Nursing Care Plans. Jaypee Publishers. New Delhi.
5. Bohoun, C. (1968). Catecholamine Metabolism in Neuroblastomas. Journal of Pediatric Surgery, 3, pp. 114–118.
6. Crump C, Sundquist K, Sieh W, et al. Perinatal and family risk factors for non-Hodgkin lymphoma in early life: A Swedish national cohort study. J Natl Cancer Inst. 2012;104:923–930.
7. Kamdar KY, Sandlund JT, Bollard CM. Malignant lymphomas in childhood. In: Hoffman R, Benz EJ, Silberstein LE, Heslop HE, Weitz JI, Anastasi J, eds. *Hematology: Basic Principles and Practice*. 6th ed. Philadelphia, Pa: Elsevier; 2013:1255–1266.
8. Nandy, A.D., Sengupta, Chatterjee, S.K., et al. (1974). Teratoma of the Stomach. Journal of Pediatric Surgery, 9, pp. 563–564.
9. National Cancer Institute Physician Data Query (PDQ). Childhood Non-Hodgkin Lymphoma Treatment. 2016. Accessed at www.cancer.gov/types/lymphoma/hp/child-nhl-treatment-pdq on May 22, 2017.
10. Poplack DG, ed. Principles and practices of paediatric oncology. 4th ed. Philadelphia, Pa: JB Lippincott; 2002.
11. Rabin KR, Margolin JF, Kamdar KY, Poplack DG. Leukemias and lymphomas of childhood. In: DeVita VT, Lawrence TS, Rosenberg SA, eds. *DeVita, Hellman, and Rosenberg's Cancer: Principles and Practice of Oncology*. 10th ed. Philadelphia, Pa: Lippincott Williams & Wilkins; 2015:1500–1510.
12. Sandlund JT, Onciu M. Childhood lymphoma. In: Niederhuber JE, Armitage JO, Doroshow JH, Kastan MB, Tepper JE, eds. *Abeloff's Clinical Oncology*. 5th ed. Philadelphia, Pa: Elsevier; 2014:1873–1889.
13. Wilson, J.W., Gehweiler, J.A. (1970). Teratomas of the Face Associated with a Patent Canal Extending into the Cranial Cavity (Rathke's Pouch) in a 3-week-old child. Journal of Pediatric Surgery, 5, pp. 349–358.

UNIT 8

SPECIAL TOPICS

443

ADMINISTRATION OF MEDICATIONS IN CHILDREN

LEARNING OBJECTIVES

At the end of the chapter, the learner will be able to:

- Describe the steps and processes of medicine administration in children.
- Describe the assessment and management of common traumas in children.
- Describe neonatal resuscitation.
- Describe paediatric pain management.
- Discuss various parasitic infestations and their management.

Administration of medications to children requires utmost care from the part of paediatric nurses. Though the physician orders drugs and their route, dose and schedule, it is the nurse who administers the drugs. It is the legal and ethical responsibility of the nurse to know about each drug he/she administers to a paediatric patient and its implications.

Children's ward should have a friendly, welcoming atmosphere conducive to the alleviation of stress. Normal childhood activities are encouraged, and as a result, a children's ward may not always have the safest environment when it comes to the giving of drugs. Meticulous checking should be undertaken by two nurses – one with paediatric nursing experience so that when a calculation for the quantity of drug is needed, his/her independent calculations might serve as safeguard. The child's identity must be confirmed before administration, preferably with the name band, which includes a hospital identity number, and with prescription.

It is not uncommon for children to have the same or similar names; they may change beds and pretend they are another patient on the ward or even swap name bands if they are not of the approved type. If doubt exists, the parent, guardian or a third nurse should confirm the identity of the child. When medications are given from a trolley in the ward, there is possibility of children taking medicines without the nurse's knowledge. So, be careful of the little hands that may reach the trolley.

FIVE RIGHTS

The most useful set of guidelines for administering drugs in any setting includes the '**FIVE RIGHTS**'.

Five Rights of Medicine Administration	
Five Rights	**Nurse's Responsibility**
Right patient	Check identification band. Verify identity with verbal children or parents of nonverbal children.
Right drug	Check the container label against orders or Kardex – Follow the three checks (taking from the cupboard or medicine cabinet, before reconstituting and before administering with the order).
Right dose	Check concentration per capsule, tablet, cubic centimetre and container.
Right route	Check the physician's order for specific administration procedure: oral, intramuscular, intravenous, subcutaneous, topical, per oculus dexter (OD, right eye), oculus sinister (OS, left eye), oculi unitas (both eye), etc.
Right time	Ensure that the medication is administered within 30 minutes before or after it is scheduled.

A nursing assessment must be done before administering any drug to children. The important factors to be considered are as follows:
- Age of the child
- Stages of physical, social, intellectual and emotional development
- The family's culture, attitudes and previous experiences in relation to the use of drugs

- How medications are taken at home
- Child's preference of form, flavour, known drug allergies, etc.
- Nature and severity of the child's current illness

Most of the teaching hospitals will not permit nursing students to administer medications. This safeguards the children but will not permit learning. The students can administer medication under the supervision of a nurse teacher/clinical instructor or qualified staff nurse. The drugs that can be particularly dangerous to children need to be checked by two qualified paediatric nurses. A few minutes of double-check may avoid serious drug error and may save the child, the nurse and the hospital or agency employing the nurse from possible litigation and incalculable hours of regret and pain.

Drugs that Need Double-Checking

Class of Drugs	Types	Names of Drugs
Vasoactive drugs	Cardiac glycosides	Digoxin, propranolol (Inderal), diazoxide, hydralazine
Respiratory depressants	Narcotics	Morphine, codeine, meperidine (Demerol)
	Sedatives Barbiturates	Pentobarbital (Nembutal)
	Benzodiazepines	Phenobarbital Valium
Central vaso-pressors	Catecholamines	Epinephrine, norepi-nephrine (Levo-phed), isoproterenol (Isuprel), dopamine (Intropin), dobuta-mine (Dobutrex)
Miscellaneous	Insulins	Insulin – all types
	Heparin	Heparin
	Intravenous methylxanthine	Aminophylline

PAEDIATRIC PHYSIOLOGY

Physiological parameters that affect drug activity in children are as follows:
- Immature organ system
- Increased concentration of body water
- Increased tissue response
- Rapid metabolism of drugs

The physiology of children varies in many aspects from that of adults; the younger the child, the more marked the differences. At birth, the renal tubules have structural and functional immaturities that prolong glomerular filtration and tubular absorption. These functional limitations, which are further handicapped by illness, have particular consequences on drug therapy during the first 5 months of life, though the adult rate of glomerular filtration is not reached until 1–2 years of age. The liver may be inadequate in detoxification, and target organs have differing sensitivities.

Because of the physiological parameters, drug activities are different in relation to absorption, distribution, metabolism and excretion of drugs in children. At birth, renal tubules have structural and functional immaturities that prolong glomerular filtration rate (GFR) and tubular absorption. Thus, functional capacities are further deteriorated with illness and have particular consequences on drug therapy during the first 5 months of life. The liver may be inadequate in detoxification, and target organs have differing sensitivities. For this, drug dosage is carefully calculated.

Children have more rapid heart rate, causing fast metabolism of drug. Periods of rapid growth and development (neonatal, infancy, toddlerhood and adolescence) are sensitive that may cause negative side effects of drugs.

Negative side effects in preverbal children are difficult to recognize such as ringing in the ears, pain or laryngeal oedema in preanaphylactic reactions.

SPECIAL MONITORING OF CERTAIN DRUGS

Some drugs require special monitoring of vital signs, both before and after administration.
- Thus, ensure that emergency airway and other advanced life support equipment are ready for function when administering any dangerous drugs to children.
- No narcotics should be given to children with head trauma or increased intracranial pressure (ICP). Brain does not feel pain, and administration of narcotics masks symptoms of deteriorating neurological status.
- When giving barbiturates to children with brain injuries, caution must be exercised. Phenobarbitone as an anticonvulsant may be given to put the child in a protective coma stage.
- When administering catecholamines, even as inhalant, keep ready advanced monitoring equipment.
- Antihypertensives given by infusion (e.g. nitroprusside) require arterial line monitoring.

DESIRABLE APPROACH FOR ADMINISTRATION OF MEDICATIONS

- Provide developmentally appropriate explanation to children.
- Be honest about expected hurts.
- Provide distractions.
- Permit expression of anger.
- Praise cooperation.
- Accept reactions.
- Never treat medications as candy, rewards or punishment.

Age and Stages of Development

Infants

- The nurse in charge and the prescribing doctor should work together with the parent to coordinate the times for nursing care, feeds and medications to avoid undue disturbances to an ill baby.

- Milk affects the absorption of some drugs, so care with timing of medication is needed for both breastfed and formula-fed babies.
- Until the baby has got head control (about 3 months), it is a good idea to cradle the baby with his/her head slightly positioned backwards to give medications.
- Once head control is achieved, the baby may be made to sit on the lap with support to give medication. But if the medicine is unpleasant, cradling or swaddling may be required.
- Drugs should not be mixed with feeds.
- Transfer medicine in small amounts with a plastic spoon as far as possible to ensure quantity.
- Volume a baby is able to swallow may be as little as 2 mL (200 mL in adults).
- Provide oral medicines through the sides of the mouth to ensure proper administration and swallowing by the baby.
- Syringes are best used for ensuring the exact amount, but see that the baby is not choking.
- Nasogastric (NG) routes are used in very sick babies. See that gravity drainage is used and no pushing of medications through NG tubes is done.
- Instil sterile water after giving medications through NG tubes, with precautions taken in fluid administration.
- Absorption of intramuscular medications is erratic in newborns, and the injection site needs to be rotated to promote absorption and to prevent muscle atrophy.
- Buttocks are contraindicated as an injection site because of the risk of nerve damage.
- When giving injections, a second person is preferred to restrain the baby.

Toddlers and Preschool-aged Children

- These children are masters of habits and respond best to familiar routines.
- Parental involvement is best in sorting such concerns while administering medications to these children.
- A positive approach and a strong command are essential to making these kids to take their medications.
- Choices may prove unsuccessful.
- The approach must be firm and without hesitancy so that children do not have a way out.
- Toddlers are best held in security of their parent's lap or failing that a nurse or other person in the ward with whom he/she is familiar.
- Preschool-aged children may be managed to drink from the medicine measure on their own.
- Self-poisoning is a feature of this group, and safety precautions must be instituted at the hospital as well as at home.

Primary School Children

- They are cooperative and eager to be helpful to the nurse.
- But sometimes they may not obey instructions.
- Injections should be prepared separately and not in front of these children.

- Gain children's cooperation before attempting painful injections.
- Involve parents in giving medications as their presence help children face difficult situations with much comfort.
- Restraining a child while giving injection is very important, as the distressing child may react violently, causing breaking of needles and harming himself/herself.

Secondary School Children

- They are more understanding and obey the instructions.
- Adolescents manifest noncompliance to medications. So, they need to be monitored and instructions may be repeated to ensure compliance.

Medication Documentation Basics
What, When and How and Consequences

No matter what kind of drug regimen your patient receives, you will need to document the following:
- What he/she receive?
- When he/she receive it?
- How he/she receive it?
- What happens as a result?

Documenting Single-Dose Medications

A single-dose medication, such as supplemental dose or a stat dose, should be documented not only in the patient's medication record but also in your progress notes.

Documenting Narcotics

Any time you administer a narcotic, you are required to document its administration according to narcotic law regulations of the country. These requirements may differ somewhat depending on what storage system your facility uses. If your facility uses an automated storage system, you will use an ID and password to obtain narcotics (and other drugs and floor stocks for nursing units).

Documenting p.r.n. Medications

For drugs given as whenever necessary (p.r.n.), document what you gave and when and how you gave them. For example, when trichloryl is given for sedation in children, document the amount of medication given, the date and time you gave it and the strength of the drug.

Go to the Extra Step. You will also need to include any other clinically relevant information. For example, include additional information about the patient's behaviour (such as nonstop crying and refusing feeds, etc.) and vital signs. Also note his/her response to the medication. You might write, 'Child is resting after 15 minutes of administration and not crying'.

If Something Goes Wrong, you Should Have a Safety Belt. If your facility does not use an automated storage and dispensing system, you will need to take a couple of additional steps. Before giving a narcotic, verify the amount of drug in the container and sign out the medication on the appropriate form, usually a narcotic sheet. Someone will need to count the remaining narcotics at the end of each shift.

Incidentally. Whether your facility has an automated system or not, you may need to have another nurse observe and document your actions if you have to discard all or part of a narcotic dose. If you discover a discrepancy in the narcotic count, follow your facility's policy for reporting it. Also, file an incident report. An investigation will follow. And you have a responsible witness as your observer.

Reporting Adverse Reactions. If you think a medication has caused an adverse reaction in your patient, follow your hospital's policy for reporting it internally.

A Med Watch form is required when you suspect that a drug, medical device, nutritional product or any Drug Control Act (DCA)-regulated product causes the following:
- A death
- A life-threatening illness
- An initial or prolonged hospitalization
- A disability
- A congenital anomaly
- The need for medical or surgical intervention to prevent a permanent impairment or an injury

Just the Facts. When filling out a Med Watch form, remember that you are not expected to establish a connection between the product and the problem.

You do not have to include copious details; simply describe the adverse event or problem that you observed with a drug or product. Send your completed form to the DCA through your quality control department.

Do not Double Up. File a separate Med Watch form for each patient. Attach additional pages, if needed. Also, remember to comply with your facility's protocols for reporting adverse events. Your supervisor should keep a copy of your report and the product lot number in case the DCA needs to identify, track or recall the product.

Also, promptly inform the DCA of product quality problems, such as a defective device, an inaccurate or unreadable product label, packaging or product mix-ups, intrinsic or extrinsic contamination or stability problems, particulates in injectable drugs or product damage.

ORAL MEDICATIONS

- Pills or tablets are not given to children younger than 5 years as a result of possible aspiration.
- Choose an appropriate article for delivery of oral medication such as spoons, syringes, cups, droppers, etc.
- Medications should not be mixed with a large amount of fluids or formula, as it may result in inadequate dosage owing to incomplete consumption.

- Never administer oral medications while the child is in the supine position, as it causes aspiration.
- Do not force oral medication, as it causes aspiration.
- Restrain infants and small children.
- Administer oral medication through the corner of the mouth to the cheek pouch.
- Use carefully calibrated vehicles (articles) for administration of dangerous oral drugs, e.g. digoxin, elixir.
- Powder tablets to be divided as per dose and mixed with a small amount of syrup or fruit juice if permitted for administration. (Tablets can be crushed by rolling a hard object, such as a bottle of sterile water.)
- Scored tablets can be broken. Others need to be crushed, mixed in liquid and given as the appropriate portion of the solution.
- Timed release medications should not be crushed or divided.

TOPICAL MEDICATIONS

- Usually, such drugs include antifungal and antibiotic creams and ointments.
- Medications must be applied in thin layers.
- Instruct family members about application as a large amount of medication application may cause toxic effects.
- Nose and eye drops can be applied as that in adults.
- Apply eardrops to children younger than 3 years by gently pulling the pinna downwards and straight back. In children older than 3 years, the pinna is pulled upwards and back.

RECTAL ADMINISTRATION

- As far as possible, do not give medications rectally.
- If it needs to be given, position the child on the left side; assess the length of time required for administration.
- Suppository may be divided length-wise to promote maximum contact with the rectal mucosa. Hold the buttocks or tape them together firmly for 5–10 minutes to minimize the urge to expel the suppository. Dilute liquid medications before administration as that for retention enema.

AEROSOL MEDICINE ADMINISTRATION

- Nebulization is aimed at providing medications directly to the tracheobronchial tree. It can be continuous or intermittent. It is delivered via tent, collar or mask or intermittent ventilation via electric air compressor or positive pressure apparatus.
- Sophisticated apparatus provide smaller droplets so that greater effect will be obtained by reaching the tracheobronchial tree and alveoli. In hospitals, the mode of delivery of aerosol medications is usually propulsion with oxygen. Oxygen itself is a drug, and the nurse must be vigilant about the hazardous effect of oxygen. A written presentation must be obtained before propelling aerosol medications with oxygen,

especially in premature babies and neonates as a result of the possible complication of retrolental fibroplasia. Compressed inhalers create psychological dependence, rebound bronchospasm, asthma and even fatal dysrhythmias from overuse of bronchodilators.

Specific Nursing Responsibilities for Aerosol Administration

- Use sterile, distilled water to replenish delivery system reserve to prevent mineral build-up and bacterial colonization.
- Be sure that percussion and segmental bronchial drainage follow minutes of intermittent nebulization treatment.
- Measure blood pressure (BP) and pulse prior to and every 2 minutes during treatment with isoproterenol because dramatic cardiovascular changes may result within seconds of administration. Use cardiorespiratory monitor and Dinamap, if available.

INTRAMUSCULAR INJECTIONS

Now intramuscular injections are rarely used in children. They are used for giving certain vaccines and few drugs, which can be given only through intramuscular routes. The following points are important for the nurse to remember while giving intramuscular injections:

- The sites used for intramuscular injections are vastus lateralis and the outer aspect of the rectus femoris muscle are the safest sites for all ages, particularly for children.
- Anterolateral thigh muscles may be used with care in infants and children.
- Use of buttock muscles in children younger than 2 years is not allowed because of close proximity to the sciatic nerve.
- Aspirate before injecting into any muscle to ensure that the medicine is not given to blood vessels.
- Properly restrain the child before administering medication to avoid unintentional trauma and injury to the child.
- Assess the child's muscle mass and needle size before administering medications. (An intradermal needle may be too big for a preterm baby. A 5/8 needle is enough for a term infant.)

INTRAVENOUS MEDICINE ADMINISTRATION

Nowadays, most of the paediatric parenteral medications are given through intravenous routes. This is the most preferred route of administration for antibiotics that are given in divided doses. This route spares a child from repeated pocking and trauma of intrusive procedure. This is a part of atraumatic care. A cannula kept on-site can be maintained safely for a period of 48–72 hours without harm if inserted with sterile precautions. This creates a positive attitude outcome towards hospitalization, too. If there is no additional fluid administration, children can move about freely with a cannula flushed with heparin or bacteriostatic normal saline (NS) as per the hospital's policy. There are certain important points to be kept in mind while giving intravenous medications, such as:

- Do not inject into a site that may be infiltrated.
- Do not administer caustic medications into tiny surface or scalp veins.
- Administer intravenous medications slowly over the longest safe amount of time; e.g. aminophylline injections or aminoglycosides require 30 minutes.
- Avoid flushing of clots.
- If heparinization is followed, permit the heparin flush to remain in the catheter.
- Flush lock every 2–4 hours to ensure patency if medications are given at a wide interval.

Intravenous absorption is very fast, and adverse effects may start within few minutes. If mixing medications, check for compatibility. It is better to have an incompatibility chart. Most antibiotics are incompatible when given at the same time. When medications are given through intravenous tubings, see that the whole medication is flushed from the chamber to the vein. Partial emptying of medications may happen and the desired effect of the same will not be obtained.

Documenting Intravenous Therapy

At least eight of 10 hospitalized patients receive some form of intravenous therapy. You may use intravenous therapy to deliver fluids, electrolytes, total parenteral nutrition (TPN) or drugs.

In all cases, document all facets of intravenous therapy carefully and completely, including not only administration but also any complications that arise. You may need to use a special intravenous therapy sheet or a nursing flow sheet.

Do Not Round the Corner

Whenever you insert an intravenous line, remember to document the following:

- Date
- Time
- Venipuncture site
- Equipment used, such as the type and gauge of catheter or needle

Always chart the exact time you performed a procedure rather than charting on the hour or half hour.

A-one and a-two ... and Done

The Infusion Nurses Society (INS) recommends making only two attempts to start an intravenous line. Document the number of attempts you made and the type of assistance you needed to start the line. Follow your facility's policy.

Using a Flow Sheet to Document Intravenous Therapy

This sample shows some typical features of an intravenous therapy flow sheet. To document, use the flow sheets' key to abbreviations and numbers.

Documenting an Infusion Therapy Procedure. Precise, accurate documentation of infusion therapy is critical for effective communication among staff members caring for the child. The list summarizes the information that should be contained in each notation about initiating, monitoring and discontinuing an intravenous line.

Initiating
- Site chosen
- Condition of the insertion site before and after inspection (bruising, burns and other observations)
- Type of cannula used
- Length and gauge of the cannula
- Time and date of insertion
- Number of attempts at cannulation
- Name and title of person responsible for insertion
- Type of medication administered
- Flow rate

Monitoring
- Condition of the insertion site and the surrounding area
- Flow rate
- Type of medication being administered
- Intake and output
- Description of any complications as well as what action was taken
- Name and title of person making the assessment

Discontinuing
- Condition of the site and the surrounding area
- Condition of the cannula upon removal (documented only if a problem occurred)
- Reason for discontinuation
- Date and time of discontinuation
- Name and title of person removing the infusion device

DESIRED DOSE CALCULATION

Before administering the drug, the nurse should ensure whether the ordered dose of medication is safe. For verifying the dose accuracy, the following formula can be used:
- Body surface area (BSA) of child × Adult dose = Estimated child dose
  BSA of an adult,
- BSA (m²) × Dose/m² = Child dose
  BSA can be calculated by the following norms:

Weight in kg	Approximate BSA
0–5 kg	(0.05 × kg) + 0.05
6–10 kg	(0.04 × kg) +0.1
11–20 kg	(0.03 × kg) = 0.2
21–40 kg	(0.02 × kg) = 0.4

Verifying dose accuracy using recommended dose per kg.

Example 1: *An order reads:* Give ampicillin 175 mg i.v. q6h. The infant's weight is 3.5 kg. The recommended dose given as per formulary is 150–200 mg per 24 hours.

Find out the dose accuracy by identifying the low and high ends of dose.

Answer

Low end of dose = 150 mg × 3.5 kg = 525 mg per 24 hours

Divide this amount 525 mg into four doses = 131.25 mg per dose

High end of dose = 200 mg × 3.5 kg = 700 mg per 24 hours

Divide this amount 700 mg × 4 doses = 175 mg per dose

So, the dose ordered for the infant falls on high end of the normal range.

Metric Calculations

It is a safe and simple method to determine a therapeutic dose. The formula is based on the recommended paediatric dosage per kilogram of body weight. Drugs prescribed in mg/kg body weight are in terms of simplicity and efficacy. It is most suitable for a paediatric dose regimen. There is little evidence that the BSA method is any more effective than the body weight method. Different children receiving the same drug invariably require differing dosages. The use of several preparations and/or the need to make frequent calculations of the same drug necessitate extra care.

The following table lists some approximate solid equivalents among the avoirdupois, apothecaries and metric systems:

Avoirdupois	Apothecaries	Metric
1 g	1 g	0.065 g
15.4 g	15 g	1 g
1 ounce (oz)	480 g	28.35 g
0.75 pound (lb)	1 lb	373 g
1 lb	1.33 lb	454 g
2.2 lb	2.7 lb	1 kg

Fraction Method

The fraction method for conversion requires an equation made up of two fractions.

First, set up a fraction by placing the ordered dose (the one you need to convert) over x units of the available dose. For example, the doctor orders 300 mg of aspirin, and the bottle is labelled 'aspirin g v per tablet'. The 'mg dose' is the ordered dose, and the 'g dose' is the available dose. Because the amount of the available dose is unknown, it is represented by an x. So, the first fraction in the equation is:

$$\frac{300 \text{ mg}}{x \text{ g}}$$

Next, set up a second fraction that includes standard equivalents between the ordered and available measures. Because 60 mg equals 1 g, the second fraction is:

$$\frac{60 \text{ mg}}{1 \text{ g}}$$

The same unit of measure appears in the numerator of both fractions, and the same unit of measure appears in both denominators. The entire equation appears as:

$$\frac{300 \text{ mg}}{x \text{ g}} = \frac{60 \text{ mg}}{1 \text{ g}}$$

Finally, to solve x, cross-multiply and follow these steps:

$$300 = 60x$$
$$5 \text{ g} = x$$

Based on this conversion equation, your patient should receive 5 (g v) of aspirin, which in this case equals one aspirin tablet.

$$300 \text{ mg} \times 1 \text{ g} = 60 \text{ mg} \times x \text{ g}$$

Ratio Method

When using the ratio method to make conversions, first express the ordered dose and available dose as a ratio. For example, the doctor's order calls for Tylenol elixir (acetaminophen) 2.5 mL for a paediatric patient. You want to tell the child's mother how many teaspoons to give at home. As a result, the first ratio appears as 2.5 mL: x tsp. The x represents the standard equivalents between the ordered and available measures. Because 5 mL equals 1 tsp, the second ratio appears as 5 mL: 1 tsp. Note that the same unit of measure (mL) appears in the first half of each ratio, and the same unit (tsp) appears in the second half.

The equation should appear as:

$$2.5 \text{ mL} : x \text{ tsp} :: 5 \text{ mL} : 1 \text{ tsp}$$

To solve x, multiply the means of the ratio (inner portions) and the extremes (outer portions):

$$x \text{ tsp} \times 5 \text{ mL} = 2.5 \text{ mL} \times 1 \text{ tsp}$$
$$x = 0.5 \text{ tsp}$$

Based on this calculation, you would tell the child's mother to give ½ tsp, which equals the ordered 2.5-mL dose.

Delivering into Dimensional Analysis

Dimensional analysis is an alternative way of solving mathematical problems. It is a basic and easy approach to calculating drug dosages because it eliminates the need to memorize formulas.

Key Factors

When using dimensional analysis, a series of ratios called factors are arranged in a fractional equation.

Each factor, written as a fraction, consists of two quantities of measurement that are related to each other in a given problem. Dimensional analysis uses the same terms as fractions, specifically the terms 'numerator' and 'denominator'.

Here's how it works: A patient is ordered 70 mg of enoxaparin (Lovenox). It is available in vials that contain 30 mg per 0.3 mL. How much quantity should be prepared?

- *Begin by identifying the given quantity:* 70 mg
- *Then isolate what you are looking for:* X mL
- *Next, know your conversion factor:* 30 mg = 0.3 mL
- *Now set up your equation:* 70 mg 0.3 mL 30 mg
- *Finally, multiply the numerators and denominators and divide the products:*
  $70 \times 0.3 \text{ mL} = 21 \text{ mL}$
  $1 \times 30 = 30$

The patient would receive 0.7 mL of Lovenox.

Make the Difference 10% Less

Keep in mind that converting drug measurements from one system to another and then determining the amount of drug form to be given can be easily produced in exact doses. You may determine a precise drug amount to be given, such as 0.97 tablets, only to find it impossible to administer that amount.

Follow this general rule to help prevent calculation errors and discrepancies between theoretical and real doses: Allow no more than a 10% variation between the dose ordered and the dose given. According to this rule, if you find that the patient should receive 0.97 tablets, you may safely give the patient a full tablet.

Calculating per Dose Medications

Most of the time medications are prepared as adult dose. So, nurses need to calculate the amount/quantity of medication per dose for administration. For example, if the physician's order is 125 mg of ampicillin and stock available is 500 mg in 2 mL, the nurse can calculate the dose using the following formula:

$$\frac{\text{Prescribe dose}}{\text{Stock available}} \times \text{Strength of solution} = \text{Required dose}$$

OR

$$\frac{\text{What we want}}{\text{What we have}} \times \text{Amount in mL} = \text{Required dose}$$

Using the formula, the dose for the aforementioned problem can be calculated:

$$\frac{125 \text{ mg}}{500 \text{ mg}} \times 2 \text{ ml} = 0.5 \text{ ml}$$

The nurse has to take 0.5 mL of medication to deliver 125 mg.

Calculation of Gravity Drip Rates
Drops per Minute

$$\frac{\text{Total volume/hour} \times \text{gtts/ml}}{\text{Total infusion time in min}} = \text{gtts/min}$$

Example: An order reads 1000 mL i.v. D5NS at 100 mL per hour. The drop factor is 60 drops/mL.

$$\frac{100 \text{ ml/hour} \times 60 \text{ gtts/ml}}{60 \text{ min/hour}} = 100 \text{ gtts/min}$$

Infusion Time

$$\frac{\text{Total volume to be delivered}}{\text{mL delivered/hour}} = x \text{ hours}$$

$$\frac{100 \text{ mL}}{100 \text{ mL/hour}} = 10 \text{ hours}$$

Calculating an Intravenous Drip Rate

The doctor's order is 1000 mL of dextrose 5% in half-normal saline solution to infuse over 12 hours. The administration set delivers 15 drops/mL. What should the drip rate be?

- *Use the equation:*

$$\frac{\text{Total no. of mL}}{\text{Total no. of min}}$$

- *Set up the equation using the given data:*

$$\frac{1000 \text{ mL}}{12 \text{ hours} \times 60 \text{ min}}$$

- *Multiply the elements in the denominator:*

$$\frac{1000 \text{ mL}}{720 \text{ min}}$$

- *Divide the fraction:*

$$1.39 \text{ mL/min} \times 15 \text{ gtts/mL} = X \text{ gtts/min}$$

The final answer is 20.85 gtts/min, which can be rounded to 21 gtts/min. The drip rate is 21 drops per minute.
- *Multiply the elements in the denominator:* $\frac{1000 \text{ mL}}{720 \text{ min}}$
- *Divide the fraction:*

$$1.39 \text{ mL/min} \times 15 \text{ gtts/mL} = X \text{ gtts/min}$$

The final answer is 20.85 gtts/min, which can be rounded to 21 gtts/min. The drip rate is 21 drops per minute.

Quicker Drip Rate Calculations

Here is a quicker way to compute an administration rate for an intravenous solution. If you are using a micro drip set, which has a drip rate of 60, you can simply set the flow rate in millilitres (mL) to match the drip rate (because it is 60 drops per minute).

If you were using an equation, you would divide the flow rate by 60 minutes and multiply by the drip factor, which in this case also equals to 60. For example, if you need to administer 125 mL of fluid per hour, the equation would be: $\frac{125 \text{ mL}}{60 \text{ min}}$.

When Flow Equals Rate

Because the flow rate and drip factor are the same, mathematically they cancel each other out. So, rather than taking time to set up and solve the equation, you can simply use the number assigned to the flow rate as the drip rate. If your administration set delivers 15 drops/mL, divide the flow rate by 4 to get the drip rate. If your administration set has a drip factor of 10, divide the flow rate by 6 to find the drip rate.

Ages and Stages

Calculating Paediatric Dosages. The doctor orders 150 mg of a drug to be given every 6 hours to an 18-kg child. (Remember that 1 kg equals 2.2 lb). The package insert indicates that the safe dosage range for the drug is 30–35 mg/kg per day to be given in divided doses. Can you safely administer the ordered dose?
- *Use the ratio method to determine the lower limit of the safe dosage range:*
  30 mg: X mg:: 1 kg: 18 kg
- *Cross-multiply the means and the extremes to find that $X = 540$ mg, which represents the low dosage. Use the same method to calculate the upper limit of the safe dosage range:*
  35 mg: X mg:: 1 kg: 15 kg
- *Cross-multiply the means and the extremes to find that: $X = 630$ mg, the high dosage.*

The safe dosage range for the child is 540–630 mg per day. Because the doctor ordered 150 mg to be given every 6 hours, the child would receive four doses per day or a total daily dose of 150 mg $\times$ 4 doses per day = 600 mg per day. This daily dose falls within the safe range, so the nurse can safely administer 150 mg q6h.

$$\frac{\text{Child's BSA}}{1.73 \text{ m}^2} \times \text{Average adult dose} = \text{Child's dose}$$

Crunching with Numbers. Here is an example. You know that your patient weighs 25 lb and is 33 inches (84 cm) tall.

Using a nomogram, you find that he has a BSA of 0.52 m². You also know that the average adult dosage is 100 mg. To determine the appropriate drug dose, set up the equation in the following way:

$$\frac{0.52}{1.73 \text{ m}^2} \times 100 \text{ mg} = 30.06 \text{ mg (child's dose)}$$

Based on your calculation, you know that your patient should receive 30 mg of the drug.

Your knowledge of measurement systems, understanding of conversion procedures and ability to perform dosage calculations accurately are crucial to delivering appropriate drug dosages.

ASSESSMENT AND MANAGEMENT OF TRAUMA VICTIMS

Paediatric trauma is the leading cause of death in children from 1 to 14 years of age. The six most common

types of fatal childhood injuries amenable to prevention strategies are as follows:
- Motor vehicle injuries as passengers
- Pedestrian injuries
- Bicycle injuries
- Drowning
- Burns
- Firearm injuries

Early and effective support of airway, ventilation, oxygenation and perfusion is vital for survival from out-of-hospital cardiac arrest.

Epidemiology

Two out of three accidents occur with male children. Peak incidence is at 8 years of age (parents allow some amount of freedom to school-aged children).

Pattern of injury – The most common injuries are blunt injuries compared with penetrating ones (80%). In total, 80% of blunt injuries are caused by rapid deceleration that occurs from automobile injuries or from child abuse/contact sports. Blunt injuries are complicated, as they are associated with multiple injuries including head injuries. The outcome from cardiopulmonary collapse and cardiopulmonary arrest associated with blunt injuries constitutes 20% of trauma. Blunt injuries are difficult to evaluate, but penetrating ones are not so difficult. Other factors that constitute difficulty in evaluation are the stages of development of the child, semi-comatose child and poor language development, leading to limited feedback.

The nurse must understand certain factors in evaluating a paediatric trauma victim. The nurse should have clear understanding of the anatomical, physiological and psychological differences of the different age group of children as compared with an adult.

Anatomical Impact of Injury

The head is proportionally larger in children than the body mass. Hence, head injury occurs in up to 70% of paediatric trauma and it accounts for the highest mortality rate (6%–7%). Chest injuries are relatively uncommon (9%) as compared with adults, as the chest wall of infants and children is extremely compliant. A child may sustain severe blunt chest trauma; for this reason, the nurse must suspect injury to the underlying thoracic and abdominal organs whenever a child experiences blunt injuries/force to the chest.

The common chest injuries that impede initial stabilization in paediatric trauma victim are tension pneumothorax and open pneumothorax. Out of this, tension pneumothorax is common and can result from blunt as well as penetrating injuries. Rib fracture and flail chest are uncommon. Pulmonary contusion is more common. Kidneys are more involved than bladder and urethra.

The ABCs of Paediatric Emergencies

Paediatric triage requires the understanding of concepts related to paediatric emergencies. The important concepts are as follows:
- Anatomic, physiological and developmental differences between children and adults
- Recognition of conditions leading to paediatric arrest
- Dealing with parents

Paediatric Difference in ABC

Factor	Nursing Considerations
Airways Large tongue	Airway easily gets obstructed by a large tongue; proper positioning is often all that is necessary to open the airway.
Smaller diameter of all airways – The internal diameter of the trachea is less than the diameter of the little finger in a 1-year-old child. Division of the trachea to a smaller airway further reduces the diameter. Cartilage of the larynx is softer than that of adults; cricoid cartilage is the narrowest portion of larynx.	Small amounts of mucus or swelling easily obstruct the airways; the child normally has increased airway resistances. Nasal congestion in infants creates big problems, whereas it creates only minor irritation in an adult.
	Airways of infant can be compressed if neck is flexed or hyperextended; it provides a natural seal for the endotracheal tube; cuffed tubes are not necessary in children younger than 8–10 years. If a child must be incubated, use a regular endotracheal tube. Choose one that fits comfortably into the child's nostril. It will be about the same size as the narrowest part of the airway through which the tube must pass. If you are not skilled in paediatric intubation, use a bag or mask to ventilate the child until you can get help. Intubation is not a first resort in opening the airway. Proper positioning, suctioning and oral airway all that are needed.
Breathing Sternum and ribs are cartilaginous; chest wall is soft; intercostal muscle are poorly developed; infants are obligate nose breathers for the first 3 months of life; increased metabolic rate (about twice that of adults) increased respiratory demand for oxygen consumption and carbon dioxide elimination.	The infant's chest wall may move inward instead of outward during inspirations (retractions) when lung compliance is decreased. Greater intrathoracic pressure is generated during inspiration; anything causing nasal obstruction can produce respiratory distress; respirations increases oxygen demand as does any condition that increases metabolic rate, such as fever.
Tachypnoea causes children to blow off excessive carbon dioxide, which can lead to respiratory alkalosis.	Respiratory rate and pattern need to be assessed. Respiratory muscles are underdeveloped. Diaphragm plays an important role in breathing.

Continued

Paediatric Difference in ABC—cont'd

Factor	Nursing Considerations
Fever is one cause of tachypnoea. Other causes are hypoxia, metabolic acidosis (e.g. diabetic ketoacidosis or salicylate poisoning).	Chest auscultation and observation of rise and fall of the abdomen are the best method for assessing the respiratory rate in patients younger than 2 years.
Bradypnoea is usually associated with a severe head injury or injection of depressants. It can also occur in children with severe respiratory distress from asthma or croup.	Respiratory rate is irregular and should be assessed for full 1 minute. There is an increase in the respiratory rate in the initial period with respiratory distress.
Work of breathing increases in respiratory distress and also the use of accessory muscles.	A resting respiratory rate faster than 60 bpm is a sign of respiratory distress in a child regardless of age.
Tell-tale sign of respiratory distress includes:	Normal inhalation/exhalation ratio is 1:1, but in respiratory distress it is 1:2 or 1:3.
• Nasal flaring	When auscultating for breath sounds, listen over the entire chest area. Small chest in children leads to breath sounds to be referred from one part to other.
• Retraction of sternum and intercostal muscles and infra- and supra sternal muscles.	Ask for colour of the baby to find out the preexisting congenital heart diseases.
Breath sounds	
• Croup like stridor – upper respiratory tract obstruction	
• Wheeze – lower respiratory tract obstruction (asthma, aspiration)	
• Wet rales – congestive heart failure	
• Cyanosis	
Circulation	Blood loss considered minor in an adult may lead to shock in a child; decreased fluid intake or increased fluid loss quickly leads to dehydration.
Child's circulating blood volume is larger per unit of body weight, but absolute volume is relatively small; 70%–80% of a newborn's body weight is water (50%–60% in an adult). About one-half of this volume is extracellular.	Do not depend on BP to assess for shock. Children can maintain their BP until they lost a large volume of blood. Instead, monitor for such signs of tachycardia, decreased perfusion and a decreased level of consciousness. Tips for accurate circulation checks are capillary refill, colour, temperature and mottled experience of the extremities.
Frequent exhalation causes the child to lose fluids, leading to the risk of dehydration. Sick children often refuse to drink, compounding fluid loss.	Tachycardia is the child's most efficient method of increasing cardiac output if the heart rate is greater than 180–200 bpm.
Increased heart rate decreases stroke volume; cardiac output is higher per unit of the body weight.	
Tachycardia in children is overlooked, as their heart rate is faster than that of adults.	
Causes of tachycardia – heart failure, shock, fever, fear, hypoxia and acute infection.	
Bradycardia – The most common cause is hypoxia. Other causes include head injury, poisoning and vagal stimulation such as suctioning.	
If hypoxia not corrected, it leads to cardiac arrest.	
Bradycardia with widened pulse pressure often indicates an increase in ICP.	
Hypertension	It is not a very common. It can be a sign of increase ICP, renal disease or coarctation of aorta. Normally, infants younger than 1 year have higher BP in their upper extremities. Abnormal high pressure in the upper extremities indicates coarctation. If the assessment shows the need of fluid replacement, start an intravenous line. Try to avoid starting an intravenous line in the lower extremities for children 3 months to 6 years of age.
Arrhythmias are usually caused by underlying congenital heart diseases, poisoning or hypoxia.	Assess rhythm by connecting to a cardiac monitor. Premature ventricular contraction in a child needs to be checked to evaluate this respiratory status. PVC – the main cause is hypoxia.
Temperature – high or low? Usual cause is viral infection. Children with fever will be tachypnoeic and tachycardiac.	Fever itself is not harmful unless above 106°F for a long time.
	Children from 3 months to 6 years of age are prone to convulsion.
	For older children, antipyretics and increased fluid intake are recommended.
	Tepid sponge if temperature is above 40°C.
	No alcohol sponge.
Hypothermia – metabolic acidosis, decreased respiration, bradycardia and cardiac arrest. Even leaving a baby uncovered on a cold table leads to heat loss through conduction.	Rewarming and warmed humidified oxygen, peritoneal dialysis with warm fluid. Rewarming if core temperature is lower than 90°F.
	Warm intravenous fluids and blood before infusing them.
	Recommended temperature of 39.3°C (102.7°F).
Head-to-toe examination	Examine the mucous membrane and assess turgor. Check the hydration status of a child younger than 18 months.
Look at the entire hydration status of the child	Anterior fontanel will be depressed or bulged in increased ICP.
	Decreased urine output in dehydration.
	Infants usually wet 6–8 diapers a day.

Paediatric Difference in ABC—cont'd	
Factor	**Nursing Considerations**
Neurological status	Level of consciousness, shock and hypothermia, hypoxia, sepsis, metabolic abnormalities, suspected poisoning
Condition of extremities	Check colour, movement, perfusion and sensation.
	Check for fracture, sprains and strains.
	Examine the skin for rashes and bruising.
	Purpura/petechiae may indicate bacterial or viral or haematological problem.
	Look for lacerations – bleeding point suturing.
Evidence of abuse	Examine for bruises, bleeding, small burns, lashes and haematoma.
	Look for signs of sexual abuse.

Initial Approach to Paediatric Trauma Victim

The principle of resuscitation for the seriously injured child is the same as those for any other paediatric patient. But there are chances of making errors during resuscitation. The four common errors are as follows:
- Failure to open and maintain airway with concurrent spinal stabilization
- Failure to provide appropriate oxygenation and ventilation
- Failure to provide appropriate fluid resuscitation
- Failure to recognize and treat haemorrhage

The two major causes of early death in paediatric trauma victims are airway compromise and inadequate fluid volume resuscitation.

ABCDE Approach

Stabilization of the trauma victim involves two surveys – initial primary survey and secondary survey.

Primary survey is the initial assessment that consists of the initial cardiopulmonary arrest and stabilization of the patient. It is designed to identify and treat life-threatening injuries unique to trauma victim. Components of primary survey include assessment of stabilization of airway, breathing, circulation, disability and exposure (ABCDE).

Primary Survey

- Initial rapid assessment
- Does the child look good or bad?
- Respiratory rate
- Work of breathing
- Skin colour (pallor, mottling and cyanosis)
- Response to the environment

A = Airway – Open the airway using a jaw thrust with cervical spine stabilization.

B = Breathing – Provide effective ventilation and oxygenation. Assess for and treat pneumothorax and haemothorax.

C = Circulation – Control obvious bleeding. Obtain vascular access for delivery of fluid or blood products.

D = Disability – Evaluate neurological response.

E = Exposure and environment – Look for external signs of injuries. Control bleeding and maintain normothermia.

Primary Assessment
- Evaluate ABCDE.
- Are the ABCs within normal limits?
- Assess D = Disability (neurological status).
- E = Exposure and environment – Look for injuries and check body temperature.
- A full set of all vital signs may be taken if ABCs are not normal; start immediate interventions.

Environment
- Undress the patient fully by cutting garments to facilitate thorough examination and assessment.
- Protect from hypothermia.

Airway

Maintain patient airway – Suction blood, mucus and dental fragments.

Potential indications for tracheal intubations are as follows:
- Respiratory arrest or failure
- Actual or potential airway obstruction
- Coma or significant alteration in mental status – Glasgow Coma Scale (GCS) score
- To facilitate acute hyperventilation when appropriate (e.g. transtentorial herniation)
- Anticipated need for prolonged ventilatory support (e.g. thoracic injuries, pulmonary contusion or intrahospital transport)
- Decomposed shock
- Avoiding use of nasotracheal intubation, especially if there is cervical spine injury or maxillofacial injury

Modified Glasgow Coma Scale for Children (Simpson & Jelly, 1982)	
Eye Response	**Best Motor Response in the Upper Limb**
4. Spontaneous	6. Obeys commands >2 years
3. Speech	5. Localized pain 6/12 – 2 years
2. Pain	4. Normal flexion to pain >6/12
1. None	3. Spastic flexion to pain <6/12
	2. Extension to pain
	1. None

Continued

Modified Glasgow Coma Scale for Children (Simpson & Jelly, 1982)—cont'd

Eye Response	Best Motor Response in the Upper Limb
Best verbal response	
5 Oriented to place	>5 years
4 Words	>12 months
3 Vocal sounds	>6/12
2 Cries	<6/12
1 None	

Other Coma Scales
- Brussels Coma Grade (1976)
- Grady Coma Grade (1976)
- Ommaya's Scale
- Innsbruck Coma Scale

Severe Head Injury
1. When the postresuscitation GCS score is <8
2. Unequal pupils
3. Unequal motor response
4. Open head injury with cerebrospinal fluid (CSF) leak or exposed brain
5. Neurologically deteriorating patient
6. Depressed fracture skull

Breathing

Causes of respiratory failure are as follows:
- Central neurological injury leading to a depressed level of consciousness
- Transections of the upper cervical spinal cord leading to respiratory paralysis
- Midbrain or medullary contusion

Support of Breathing
- Routine use of hyperventilation does no good to a child with head injury.
- Be alert to life-threatening intrathoracic injuries even if there is no chest trauma.
- Consider gastric decompression using an NG tube.

Circulation

- Asses for signs of hypovolaemic shock.
- Control bleeding with direct pressure.
- Suspect internal bleeding and consider early administration of blood products.

Potential Causes of Cardiopulmonary Deterioration
- 4Hs–4Ts–4Cs
  - 4H – Hypoxia, hypovolaemia, hypothermia and hyperkalaemia
  - 4T – Tamponade, tension pneumothorax, toxins and thromboembolism
  - 4Cs – Central neurological injury or cervical spinal cord transection
- Cardiovascular injury
- Chest wall injury
- Comorbid condition

Fluid Resuscitation
- Signs of inadequate systemic perfusion
- Rapid infusion (20 minutes) 20 mL/kg NS or Ringer's lactate (RL)
- Continued signs of inadequate perfusion
- Second rapid infusion 20 mL/kg NS or RL
- Continued signs of inadequate perfusion
- Third rapid infusion 20 mL/kg NS or RL
- OR packed red blood cells (RBCs) mixed with NS at 10–15 mL/kg bolus
- Repeat every 20–30 minutes as needed or whole blood at 20 mL/kg bolus and repeat every 20–30 minutes

Child with Severe Trauma and Life-threatening Condition
- Type and cross-match urgently.
- Consider giving O −ve blood without cross-match.
- Consult trauma service at once.

Disability
- Rapid assessment of critical neurological functions by GCS, Adelaide Coma Scale and AVPU paediatric response scale
  A – Alert
  V – Verbal response
  P – Pain response
  U – Unresponsive

Secondary Survey

- Obtain a brief history: Is there any underlying illness or psychosocial issues? Use abbreviated trauma-specific history.
- Conduct detailed head-to-foot examination for injuries.
- Conduct laboratory studies.
- Perform radiological investigations.
- Use AMPLE mnemonic to recall the components of the focused history.
  A – Allergies
  M – Medications
  P – Past medical history
  L – Last meal
  E – Events leading to current injury

Cervical Spine Immobilization

Cervical spine immobilization can be done with a semi-rigid collar, which immobilizes the head and maintains cervical immobilization throughout resuscitation.

Common Paediatric Emergencies

- Status epileptics
- Acute severe asthma
- Shock
- Coma
- Acute upper gastrointestinal bleeding
- Lightening injury
- Drowning
- Poisoning
- Anaphylaxis

- Acute liver failure and hepatic coma
- Congestive cardiac failure (CCF)

Status Epilepticus

- *Definition:* When seizure lasts for more than 30 minutes
- Aetiology
- Simple febrile seizure
- Traumatic head injury
- Nontraumatic ICP
- Central nervous system (CNS) infections
- Poisoning/toxic exposures
- Anoxia
- Fluid and electrolyte imbalances
- Metabolic disorders
- Idiopathic epilepsy

Assessment Parameters

- Time: Initial onset of seizure activity
- Duration of each phase of seizure
- Total duration
- Movement: Part of the body affected first
- Progression to other body parts
- Type: Spastic, tonic, tremors
- Postseizure tone: Flaccid, hypertonic
- Lack of movement in any body parts

Respiratory Status

- Airway patency
- Respiratory effort
- Apnoea: Presence and duration
- Secretions: Amount, colour and need for suctioning
- Mental status
- Total loss of consciousness
- Other changes
- Postictal status
- Pupil: Size, equality
- Behaviour: Autonomous, bizarre, postictal status
- Elimination: Incontinence – bladder and bowel
- Oral condition: Presence of loose teeth or dentures; tongue, mucous membrane injury, presence of bloody saliva or sputum

Risk Factors for Epilepsy

- Neurological or developmental abnormality before seizure
- Infantile febrile seizures/focal or multiple in nature or greater than 15 minutes of duration
- History of nonfebrile seizures in one or both parents

Characteristics of Febrile Seizures

- Seizures usually occur between 3 months and 5 years of age
- Seizure associated with a fever of less than 24 hours of duration
- No history of neurological problems
- No intracranial injury or CNS diseases
- Usually nonfocal

- Seizure activity less than 15 minutes of duration
- Positive family history

Nursing Priorities

- Ensure a patent airway: Position the patient on sides; prepare to suction if necessary; insert oropharyngeal airway if possible but avoid placing potentially occlusive objects into the mouth.
- Provide supplemental oxygen.

Protect from Physical Injury

- Do not restrain.
- Remove the patient immediately from the dangerous environment.
- Loosen restrictive clothing.

Continuous Monitoring During and after Seizure

- Observation of seizure activity
- Mental status
- Vital signs
- Injuries secondary to seizures

Prepare and Administer Anticonvulsants

- Anticonvulsants are highly indicated if seizure duration is greater than 15 minutes or airway becomes compromised.
- Prepare to start an intravenous line.
- Determine accurate dose of anticonvulsants.
- Administer anticonvulsants for control of seizures.

Paediatric Anticonvulsant Therapy

- Diazepam: 0.25–3 mg/kg; intravenous push – 1 mg/min
- Onset of action within seconds – half-life = 20 minutes; can repeat the dose every 5–15 minutes to a maximum dose of 10 mg
- Lorazepam: 0.05–0.1 mg/kg; intravenous push – 1 mg/min
- Onset of action within seconds: half-life = 9 hours; can repeat the dose every 5–15 minutes to a maximum dose of 4 mg

Drugs

- Phenobarbitone: 10–20 mg/kg – slow intravenous push – 1 mg/min; onset of action within 20 minutes – half-life = 48 hours; can repeat the low dose every 20 minutes to a maximum dose of 300 mg
- Phenytoin (Dilantin): 10–20 mg/kg – slow intravenous push – 1 mg/min; onset of action within 20 minutes – half-life = 48 hours; can repeat the minimum dose every 20 minutes to a maximum dose of 100 mg.
- Caution: Large doses of any of these drugs as well as a combination of these drugs may precipitate respiratory distress

If Convulsions are Still not Controlled

- Give Phenobarbitone: 20 mg or 1 mg/kg with a maximum dose of 40 mg.
- If again not controlled, diazepam drip should not be mixed with glucose. Use NS. Initial 1 drop/kg/min.

If not controlled, add 1.5 drops/kg micro drops. Usual dose is 0.5 drops/kg. For a 10-kg child, 5 drops/min is required, with a maximum of 2.5 drops/kg/min.
- Other method: Retention enema of sodium valproate (ratio 1:1) with NS. Dose is 20 mg/kg. For a 10-kg baby, 200 mg is required.
- If still not controlled: Mannitol 2.5 mL/kg to rescue the child without neurological damage.

Febrile Convulsions
- Keep the baby in a low-lying head position with head turned to one side.
- Suck secretions to prevent aspiration.
- Give oxygen: Keep airway patent.
- Examine the cause of fever and provide treatment.
- If sensorium alteration, lumbar puncture (LP) is indicated.
- Administer appropriate antibiotics.
- Advise preventing further attacks.
- Provide intermittent prophylaxis at home.

Status Asthmaticus (Acute Severe Asthma)
- If a child continues to have significant respiratory distress despite administration of drugs and other supportive measures for 4–6 hours, the following is required:
- Management
- Intensive care unit (ICU) admission
- Airway clearance by suction
- Position
- Intravenous fluids if not dehydrated; paediatric maintenance 100 mL/kg per 24 hours (4–6 hours)
- If dehydrated: RL 30 mL/kg in 2 hours, followed by 40 mL/kg in 4 hours
- Oxygen supplementation: 3–5 L/min

Drugs
- β_2 sympathetic agonists are the drug of choice
- Theophyllines: Aminophylline 3–5 mg/kg per dose every 6 hours (3–5 mg/kg in 50 mL 5% or 10% glucose or NS in 20 minutes as intravenous drip
- If no cardiac problem, adrenaline is useful: dose 0.01 mL/kg s.c.
- Corticosteroids: Hydrocortisone 5 mg/kg i.v. every 6 hours
- Sodium bicarbonate: 1–3 mEq/kg every 4–6 hours
- Antibiotics
- Mucolytic agents

Anaphylaxis
- Flushing, urticaria, angioedema, stridor, wheeze, decreased BP, abdominal cramps
- Any drug with the potential to cause anaphylaxis
- Syringe loaded with adrenalin 1:100 and 1:10,000 solutions
- Various drugs: Intravenous fluids, oxygen, bag and mask, equipment for intubations
- Stop administration of the offending drug or allergen
- Injection of adrenalin 0.01 mL/kg 1:1000 solution up to a maximum 0.3 mL s.c.
- If the child is pulseless, the dose may be repeated after 5 minutes by the intramuscular route.

- If intravenous 1:10,000 solution – 0.1 mL/kg
- Oxygen administration by face mask
- Elevate foot end of the bed
- Start intravenous line. Run NS 10 mL/kg in 5 minutes
- Injection of hydrocortisone: 5–10 mg/kg
- Antihistamines: Benadryl 1 mg/kg i.v./i.m. or chlorpheniramine maleate 0.1 mg/kg per dose
- If hypotension, start dopamine by intravenous infusion.

Snake Bite
- Reassure the child.
- Clean the wound with water.
- No local application of ice.
- Apply a wide band for venous obstruction; only the little finger can be inserted.
- Incision and section not recommended.
- Immobilize the patient.
- Identify the snake.
- Decision on treatment depends on the clinical features of venomation and not on the identification of snake.
- Neutralize the poison before 6 hours.
- After 6 hours, poison goes enters the vital organs.
- Maximum dose 50, ASB, ADB – 1–20 vials. 10 mL. 1:3 dilution NS.
- 15–20 vials required.

Shock
- Acute circulatory insufficiency. Failure of delivery of sufficient oxygen and nutrients to meet the metabolic demands of the body
- Types: Hypovolaemic, cardiogenic, distributive and neurogenic
- Clinically: Compensated, decompensated and irreversible

Look For
- Tachycardia
- Delayed capillary refill
- Altered sensorium
- Decreased urine output (<1 mL/kg per hour)
- Undue pallor
- Low BP

Remember
- An anxious child with cold extremities and tachycardia is in compensatory shock unless otherwise proved.
- Normal BP (systolic) over 1 year of age is 90 + (2 × age in years).
- Low BP = 70 + 2 × age in years.

Treatment
- Clear airway.
- Supplement oxygen.
- Provide vascular access: Packed cell Volume (PCV), blood count grouping and matching.

Drugs
- Dopamine: Body weight × 6 = amount of drug (mg) to be added to the total volume of 100 mL i.v. fluid
- Infusion rate: 1 mL/hour = 1 mcg/kg/min
- For example, to deliver 10 mcg/kg/min, run infusion at 10 mL per hour

- Epinephrine
- Norepinephrine: Body weight in kg × 0.6
- Milrinone:
- 1 mL/hour = 0.1 mcg/kg/min
- For example, to deliver 0.3 mcg/kg/min, run infusion at 3 mL per hour.

Dosages
- Dopamine: 5–10 mcg/kg/min (inotropic dose); 10–20 mcg/kg/min (vasopressive dose)
- Epinephrine: 0.1–0.3 mcg/kg/min (inotropic dose); 0.3–2 mcg/kg/min (vasopressive dose)
- Norepinephrine: 0.5–1 mcg/kg/min
- Dobutamine: 2–20 mcg/kg/min
- Milrinone: 50–75 mcg/kg/min (loading dose); 0.5–1 mcg/kg/min (infusion dose)

NEONATAL RESUSCITATION

Transition from fetal circulation to neonatal circulation makes marked changes in the cardiovascular and respiratory systems. After birth, the fluid-filled lung is rapidly filled with air to increase oxygenation and prepares the lung to assume the role of placenta before birth. Lung expansion with air requires higher ventilation pressure. Expansion of lungs with air and increased alveolar oxygen tension mediates a critical decrease in pulmonary vascular resistance that results in increased pulmonary blood flow after birth. Failure to normalize pulmonary vascular resistance may result in persistence of right-to-left intracardiac and extracardiac shunts into persistent pulmonary hypertension in newborns.

Newborn resuscitation is required to reverse asphyxiated conditions and to restore and support cardiopulmonary support. Approximately 5%–10% of newborns require active resuscitation. Most neonates respond to administration of oxygen and ventilation with bag and mask.

After drying, stimulation, airway opening and bag and mask ventilation, further interventions are based on the triad of clinical characteristics as respiration, heart rate and colour.

Respiration – The newborn infant should have regular respiration that is adequate to improve colour and maintain a heart rate greater than 100 bpm. Grasping respiration and apnoea after brief stimulation are signs that indicate the need for positive-pressure ventilation. Heart rate is a critical determinant of the resuscitation sequence. The heart rate may be evaluated by palpation of the pulse at the base of the umbilical cord. Auscultate apical heart sounds with a stethoscope.

Colour – Most newborns are centrally cyanotic at birth, as normal fetal PO$_2$ is quite low. At birth, colour should rapidly become pink. Central cyanosis is detected by examining the face, trunk and mucous membrane. Acrocyanosis (blue hands and feet) is common in the first few minutes of life.

Other way of assessing neonates is by Apgar 1- and 5-minute assessment. The most crucial action is establishment of ventilation. A very small percentage of neonates may require chest compression and medications. A majority of infants respond to simple measures.

Resuscitative measure for newborns is essentially the same. But modifications are necessary for newborns with meconium aspiration.

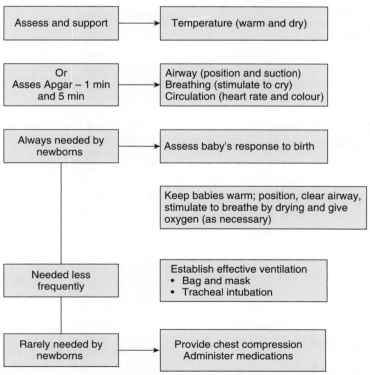

Essential interventions recommended for resuscitation in newborn except in meconium aspiration.

Maternal Risk Factors

Antepartum Risk Factors	Intrapartum Risk Factors
Maternal diabetes	Emergency caesarean section
Pregnancy-induced hypertension	Forceps or vacuum-assisted delivery
Chronic hypertension	Breech or other abnormal presentation
Chronic maternal illness	Premature labour
• Cardiovascular diseases	Precipitous labour
• Thyroid dysfunctions	Chorioamnionitis
• Neurological abnormalities	Prolonged rupture of membrane (18 hours before delivery)
• Pulmonary diseases	
• Renal diseases	Prolonged second stage
Anaemia or isoimmunization	Fetal bradycardia
Previous fetal or neonatal death	Irregular fetal heart
	Uterine tetany
Bleeding in the second or third trimester	Narcotics administration
Maternal infections	Meconium-stained amniotic fluid
Polyhydramnios	
Oligohydramnios	Prolapse cord
Premature rupture of membrane	Abruptio placenta
	Placenta previa
Post-term gestation	Diminished fetal activity
Multiple-fetus gestation	
Drugs such as lithium or narcotics	
Maternal substance abuse	
Fetal malformations	
Age <16 or >35 years	

In an anticipated high-risk delivery, the team should get prepared for neonatal resuscitation. For this, better communication should be maintained between professionals. The obstetrical team should convey the details of antepartum and intrapartum maternal medical conditions and treatment and specific indicators of fetal conditions, fetal heart rate monitoring, lung maturity, prenatal diagnosis and certain features of the perinatal history and clinical course that may alert the resuscitation team to these special factors.

Conditions Pertaining to Newborns who Require Resuscitation

Mechanical blockage of airway:
- Choanal atresia
- Pharyngeal airway malformation

Impaired lung function:
- Pneumothorax
- Pleural effusion/ascites
- Congenital diaphragmatic hernia
- Pneumonia/sepsis

Impaired cardiac function:
- Congenital heart disease
- Fetal/maternal haemorrhage

Steps of Neonatal Resuscitation

It is essentially similar to that of a child.

Initial assessment – Look for complex signs (presence of meconium in amniotic fluid or on the skin, cry or respiration, muscle tone, colour, term or preterm) along with visual inspection. Once intervention begins, the sequence of intervention is determined by findings of the triad of evaluation (respiration, heart rate and colour). Conduct a rapid assessment to find out the following:
- Whether the amniotic fluid is clear of meconium
- The baby is breathing or crying
- There is good muscle tone
- The colour is pink
- The infant is term.

If answer to any of these findings is yes, then the newborn receives routine care such as:
- Provision of warmth
- Position of newborn infant on his/her back or the side with the neck in a neutral position

If there is no meconium-stained amniotic fluid, clear the airway by suctioning the mouth. Meconium-stained amniotic fluid is a risk factor for meconium aspiration syndrome. Meconium aspiration produces respiratory distress and hypoxaemia, aspiration pneumonia, pneumothorax and persistent pulmonary hypertension.

If meconium is present in the amniotic fluid, suction the mouth, nose and posterior pharynx with a large-bore catheter or a bulb syringe. If the newborn with meconium aspiration is distressed after suctioning (respiratory effort, decreased muscle tone or heart rate less than 100 bpm), suction the trachea before taking other resuscitative steps. Place the infant in the prewarmed environment and conduct the following interventions:
- Examine the hypopharynx with a laryngoscope and suction any residual meconium in the hypopharynx.
- Intubate the trachea and suction the lower airway (mechanical suction with no higher than 100 mm Hg can be used).

Ventilation

Key to successful neonatal resuscitation is adequate expansion of the lungs with gas, followed by effective ventilation.

Indications for positive pressure ventilation are as follows:
- Apnoea
- Gasping respirations
- Heart rate less than 100 bpm
- Persistent central cyanosis despite administration of 100% oxygen

When a newborn is born outside the hospital, it is difficult to maintain body temperature, airway patency and vascular access during transport.

The ideal bag volume for neonatal resuscitation is approximately 500 mL. A volume more than 750 mL makes it difficult to judge the small tidal volumes (6–8 mL/kg) administered to neonates and may cause hyperinflation and possible barotraumas. A flow-inflating bag (anaesthetic bag) requires a well-modulated flow of gas into the inlet port and correct adjustment of the flow control valve.

Ventilation of the neonate is provided at a rate of 40–60 breaths/min. To prevent barotraumas, all neonatal ventilation bags should be equipped with a pressure release valve or manometer to limit respiratory pressure.

If the heart rate is less than 60 bpm despite adequate ventilation with 100% oxygen, continue positive-pressure ventilation and initiate chest compression.

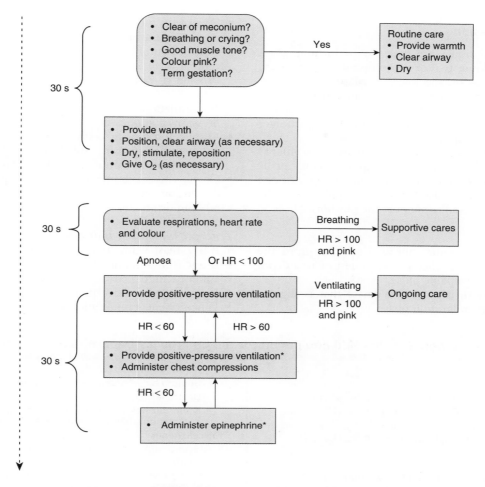

*Tracheal intubation may be considered at several steps.

Overview of resuscitation in the delivery room.

Medications Used in Resuscitation of a Newborn

Medications	Dose/Route	Concentration	Weight (kg)	Total Volume (mL)	Precautions
Epinephrine	0.001–0.03 mg/ kg tracheal, i.v. or i.o.	1:10,000	1	0.1–0.3	Give rapidly
			2	0.2–0.6	Repeat every 3–5 minutes
			3	0.3–0.9	
			4	0.4–1.2	
Volume expand- ers Isotonic crystalloid (NS or RL or blood)	10 mL/kg i.v., i.o.		1	10	Give over 5–10 minutes
			2	20	Reassess after each bolus
			3	30	
			4	40	
Sodium bicarbonate	1–2 mEq/kg i.v., i.o.	0.5 mEq/mL 4.2% solu- tions	1	2–4	A slow push over at least 2 minutes will require dilution with 8.4% solution
			2	4–8	
			3	6–12	Give only if the infant is effectively ventilated
			4	8–16	
Naloxone	0.1 mg/kg tracheal, i.v., i.m., i.o., s.q.	0.4 mg/mL 1 mg/mL	1	0.25	Establish adequate ventilation; first, give rapidly and then repeat every 2–3 minutes as needed
			2	0.50	
			3	0.75	
			4	1.0	
			1	0.1	
			2	0.2	
			3	0.3	
			4	0.4	
10% Dextrose	0.2 g/kg i.v., i.o.	0.1 g/mL	1	2	Check beside glucose, it may require dilution with 25% or 50% dextrose using sterile water
			2	4	
			3	6	
			4	8	

Chest Compression

Two rescuer techniques are used for performing chest compressions. When two or more rescuers are present, place both thumbs on the lower third of the sternum, with the finger encircling the chest and supporting the back. Position the thumbs side on the sternum just below the nipple line. Avoid compressing the xiphoid portion of the sternum, as it damages the liver.

If the rescuer's hands could not encircle the infant's chest (too small hand), two-finger compression can be done using the ring finger and the middle finger of one hand on the sternum just below the nipple line. The other hand can be used to support the newborn's back.

Technique
• Compress the sternum approximately one-third the anterior–posterior diameter of the chest or to a depth that generates a palpable pulse.
• Provide a smooth compression phase that is slighter shorter than the relaxation phase.

• Do not lift the thumbs or fingers off the sternum during the relaxation phase.
• Deliver compression at a ratio of 3:1 with interposed ventilations.
• Provide a rate of compression and ventilation to deliver 132 events per minute (90 compressions and 30 ventilations) or one complete cycle of three compressions and one ventilation every 2 seconds.
• Always accompany compressions with positive-pressure ventilation using 100% oxygen because ventilation is of primary importance in neonatal resuscitation.
• Check the spontaneous pulse rate periodically and discontinue compressions when the heart rate reaches 60 bpm or greater.

Tracheal Intubation Indications
• If bag–mask ventilation is ineffective
• If tracheal suctioning is required in meconium-stained amniotic fluid
• If prolonged positive-pressure ventilation is necessary
• When tracheal medication is needed (epinephrine)

Neonatal Resuscitation Supplies and Equipment for the Emergency Department

Suction equipment
• Bulb syringe
• Mechanical suction and tubing, manometer
• Suction catheters, 5F or 6F, 8F, and 10F or 12F
• 8F feeding tube and 20-mL syringe
• Meconium aspirator (for attachment to mechanical suction)

Bag-mask equipment
• Self-inflating or flow-inflating bag with pressure release valve or pressure manometer (200–750 mL); self-inflating bag must have an oxygen reservoir
• Face masks, premature and newborn sizes
• Oxygen with a flowmeter (rate up to 10 L/min) and tubing

Intubations equipment
• Laryngoscope with straight blades, No. 0 (preterm) and No. 1 (term)
• Extra bulbs and batteries for laryngoscope
• Tracheal tubes 2.5, 3.0, 3.5, 4.0 mm
• Stylet (optional)
• Scissors
• Tape or securing device for tracheal tube
• Exhaled CO_2 detector (optional)
• Laryngeal mask airway (optional)
• Medications
  · Epinephrine 1:10,000
  · Isotonic crystalloid
  · Naloxone hydrochloride 0.4 mg/mL

• NS for volume expansion
• Sodium bicarbonate 4.2% (5 mEq/10 mL)
• Dextrose 10%
• NS for flushes and sterile water if dilution of bicarbonate or hypertonic glucose solutions is necessary

Miscellaneous
• Gloves and other appropriate personal protection equipment
• Feeding tube, 5F (optional for administration of tracheal medications)
• Radiant warmer
• Towels and warmed blankets
• Clock (timer optional)
• Stethoscope
• Tape, ½ or ¾ inch
• Syringes 1, 3, 5, 10, 20, 50 mL
• Needles 25-, 21-, 18-gauge or puncture device for the needless system
• Alcohol sponges

Umbilical vessel catheterization supplies
  Sterile gloves
• Scalpel or scissors
• Umbilical tape
• Umbilical catheters, 3.5F, 5F
• Three-way stopcock
• Cardiac monitor and electrodes (optional)
• Oropharyngeal airways
• Pulse oximeter and probe (optional)

Confirmation of Tracheal Intubation
• Symmetric chest movement
• Auscultation of equal and adequate breath sounds in the axillae and absent breath sounds over the stomach
• Improvement in the neonates colour, heart rate and activity
• Detection of exhaled CO_2

Depth of insertion of the tracheal tube = Weight in kg + 6 cm = tracheal tube insertion depth at lip in centimetres.

PAEDIATRIC PAIN MANAGEMENT

Pain is an unpleasant sensory and emotional experience associated with actual or potential tissue damage or described in terms of such damage. This definition explains the subjective nature of pain and avoids linking it to specific stimulus. The subjective experience of pain describes sensory discriminative, cognitive evaluative and affective motivational dimensions.

Pathophysiology

Pain causes may adverse effects and physiological consequences in children. In neonates, the development of CNS is extremely vulnerable to environmental influence and can be altered by external events. No distinction is given to acute or chronic pain in children. They are unable to distinguish quality of pain (e.g. stinging, burning) or even location. Assessment of pain focuses only on the measurement of pain intensity.

Neurodevelopment of Pain Mechanism

Contrary to previous belief, research has proved that infants and children can perceive and feel pain. Infants have neurological capability to feel pain before birth, even premature birth. The peripheral, spinal and central structures necessary for pain information transmission are present and functional early in gestation (between the first and second trimesters). Rapid synaptogenesis begins in the cortex with demonstrated functional maturity by 20–24 weeks of gestation. Infants possess a well-developed hypothalamic–pituitary–adrenal axis and can mount a fight or flight stress response with release of catecholamines and cortisol. Neuropeptides, which mediate analgesia (inhibit or amplify), are also present and functional before birth. Cortisol and endorphin levels have been shown to increase during intrahepatic transfusion in 23–34 weeks old fetuses, demonstrating an appropriate hormonal response to needling of the abdomen.

Immediate Effects

Pain causes adverse physiological effects in all major organ systems as follows:
- Reduced tidal volume
- Decreased vital capacity in lungs
- Increased demands of cardiovascular system (CVS)
- Hypermetabolism resulting in neuroendocrine imbalances
- Increased metabolic demands on the CVS and the respiratory system caused by pain lead to increased oxygen consumption, which, in turn, causes hypoxaemia and myocardial ischaemia
- Mobilization of endocrine and metabolic resources results in changes in BP ($\neq$ or $\emptyset$)
- Changes in skin colour and temperature.

Immature cerebral vascular bed is particularly vulnerable to injury because of lack of autoregulation, and any stimuli that increase cerebral vascular congestion or result in hypoxaemia (e.g. crying) may increase the risk of intraventricular haemorrhage. Endorphin release may also affect BP and respiration.

Long-term effects of environmental manipulation can permanently alter behaviour, brain function and even brain structure, particularly when events occur during critical periods of development. The amount and frequency of painful stimuli inflicted on the infant receiving intensive care would possibly result in a reallocation of cortical resources and permanent alteration in cerebral neuroanatomy. Pain experience in the intensive care neonates may alter the normal course of development of pain

behaviour in toddlers. It is also found from animal studies that pain and stress in the neonatal period result in altered pain sensitivity, decreased weight gain, decreased ability to learn mazes, body temperature instability and even immunosuppression in the adulthood. It was found that arousal resulting from painful events may be overwhelming for the infant who then may attempt to shut out all stimuli and alter interactions with caregivers and sleep patterns.

Stress Responses to Surgical Trauma

Hormonal metabolic changes seen in infants after surgical stress are greater in magnitude but shorter in duration than those in adults. Immature enzyme processes and decreased lipid stores result in an even greater degree of tissue breakdown in preterm infants after surgery. It has also been demonstrated that anaesthesia can reduce the magnitude of the hormonal metabolic stress response. Anand and Ansely-Green (1988) demonstrated prolonged catabolic reactions as well as circulatory and metabolic complications after patent ductus arteriosus (PDA) ligation when anaesthetic agents were not administered in inadequate doses.

Measurement of Pain in Infants and Children

Pain assessment tools are useful for measuring pain in children as young as 3–4 years of age. Some use pictures for children to select; some use a variety of techniques to assess pain. But these are useful in verbal children. In nonverbal children and neonates, behavioural observations are made. The common behaviours that are assessed include crying, change in facial expression, palmar sweating, etc. Some use a combination of behavioural and physiological parameters to assess pain in neonates and infants. In infants, pain cries show spectrographically distinct acoustic frequency and pitch from overstimuli. Infants also form a cry face characteristics of pain. The facial expression in response to heelstick is different from other tactile stimuli such as rubbing or cleaning the heel and is a sensitive measure of pain. Measurement of neonatal physiological response to painful stimuli includes changes in heart rate, BP, transcutaneous oxygen and carbon dioxide levels, oxygen saturation, ICP, cardiac vagal tone and palmar sweat. Heart rate variability (HRV) has been established as a promising physiological measure of pain in infants that measures the amplitude of beat-to-beat change in the heart rate.

The neuroendocrine response of pain results in the release of catecholamines, cortisol, endorphins and other chemicals, which, too, cause physiological changes. Changes in plasma, urinary and salivary cortisol levels have also been observed in response to painful stressors in infants.

On the basis of the findings of the study conducted by Assuma (2004), the investigator proposes the use of a common tool for assessing pain in children from 0 to 5 years of age. This tool was prepared using pain characteristics that had been manifested in more than 90% of infants under study (n = 150) and children (n = 150) with postoperative pain. Because it contains only 10 items and the scoring is simple, it can be incorporated along with any postoperative assessment format. Pain assessment may be included as the fifth vital sign along with other vital signs. This tool contains the portion of major vital signs; the assessment of other parts will not take much time in a nurse's routine.

Developmental Overview of Children's Responses to Pain

Age	Nonverbal Behaviour	Verbal Behaviour	Child's Description of Pain
Toddler	Withdrawal of extremity, nonspecific aggression (hitting, biting, kicking); use of entire body to resist; regression	Crying, screaming	Identifies location; 'arm hurts', points to the abdomen; touches the area
Preschool-aged	Goal-directed aggression; active physical resistance (pushes the nurse away, hides); regression	Attempts to postpone; pretends to be another person; uses aggressive statements ('I hate you'; 'Go away')	Locates and express intensity ('My leg hurts a lot')
School-aged	Passive resistance (rigid body, clenched teeth or fists); regression	Denial of pain	Identifies location and intensity in more detail; progress from physical to psychological aspects

Recommended APAT for Children

Sl. no.	Criteria	Score		
		0	1	2
1	Respiratory rate	Normal	>5/min	>10/min
2	Respiratory secretion	Normal	Slight increase	Marked increase
3	Pulse rate	Normal	>10/min	>15/min
4	Temperature	Normal	>1°C–2°C	>2°C
5	Diaphoresis	No increase	Minimal; increase	Marked increase
6	Lacrimation/tearing/cry	No tearing/no crying	Tearing inside the cantus/moaning	Tears come out/crying continuously
7	Rigidity	No rigidity	Rigidity in extremities	Whole-body rigidity
8	Facial expression	Face composed	Face distorted	Facial grimace
9	Sleep disturbances	Normal sleep	Wakes up easily	Not able to sleep
10	Touching painful area/pulling the site	No touching/no pulling	Touching/pulling	Guarding and crying when approached
	Total score	0	10	20

Age-appropriate postoperative pain assessment tool (APAT) is a scoring tool that combines both physiological and behavioural indices and demonstrates initial validity and reliability in infants and children from 0 to 5 years of age. The simplicity of the scale and inclusion of quantitative physiological parameters increase its acceptance and use as a pain scoring tool.

Recommended pain assessment tool for routine pain assessment is given as follows:

Maximum score will be 20.

This tool can be used for any children with postoperative pain. But self-report or vocalization about pain can be included for older children who can verbalize their pain.

Implementation of a standardized pain assessment protocol improves pain management for patients. The nurse must be vigilant to make pain visible by incorporating pain assessment in routine care, using standardized terms and including discussion of pain issues into medical and nursing rounds. Use the slogan 'Just do it' in pain assessment even if you do not have a very precise tool.

Effective management of pain decreases suffering and may speed up recovery after surgery and shorten hospital stay. Children's pain experiences have long been of concern to nurses, who assume primary responsibility for assessing and managing children's pain when they are hospitalized. Systematic pain assessment should become part of the postoperative routine as measuring other physiological variables. The nurse must become familiar with the physiological changes and behavioural observations that may indicate pain in infants and children. A silent, apparently quiescent infant who manifests a pain face, is tense and hard to comfort needs to be assessed for pain.

Nursing Management of Infants and Children with Pain

The major goals of pain management are as follows:
- Minimize intensity, duration and physiological cost of the pain experience.
- Maximize the child's ability to cope with and recover from painful experience.

The twofold management regimens are pharmacological and nonpharmacological management. The nonpharmacological management is age dependent. In neonates, the major nonpharmacological interventions include minimal handling and minimization of the physiological cost of pain with various interventions.

Minimal handling can be achieved by the following nursing interventions:

- Protect from noise.
  - Do not talk over the infant.
  - Do not allow telephone to ring in the room.
  - Close Isolette doors softly.
  - Do not set bottles or other objects on top of Isolette.
  - Remove all sources of low jarring noises such as trash receptors with lids that bang.
- Protect from over-stimulation.
  - Cluster nursing care activities.
  - Allow the infant 2–3 hours of undisturbed rest.
  - Do not routinely suction or perform postural drainage.
  - Contain the infant's limb during suctioning or other procedures.
- Protect from light.
  - Shade the infant's eyes with blanket over Isolette or table or use cut-out box over the infant's head.
- Provide boundaries.
  - Place the infant in a prone or side-lying position.
  - Cover, wrap and swaddle the infant.

Minimize the physiological cost of pain by the following measures:

- Provide containment to reduce excessive and immature motor responses.
- For bigger infants, utilize distraction with oral, visual/auditory or tactile stimulation.
- Swaddle and assist the infant with hand-to-mouth contact or non-nutritive sucking pacifiers.
- Provide contralateral tactile stimulation to increase functional response time (FRT).

Interventions for Pain Management in Preschool- and School-aged Children

- Prepare by providing sensory and procedure information to allow the child to prepare self for procedure.
- Provide relaxation exercise (focused breathing, blow out like a kiss, etc.) to decrease muscle tension.
- Use guided imagery to provide distraction.
- Use soft touch and soft talk that give distraction/decrease muscle tension.
- Provide progressive relaxation (contract/relax different muscles) to decrease muscle tension.
- Use hypnosis that alters perception of pain.
- Use music/videos to provide distraction.
- Use storytelling ('Once upon a time…') to provide distraction.
- Use positive self-talk ('I can make it') that promotes mastery.

Interventions that Help Children during Painful Procedures

- Let parents remain with the child so as to relieve fear of separation and reduce stranger anxiety.
- Allow the child to hold an object or keep it in sight to provide security.
- Keep explanations simple and use nonthreatening language, as children have limited cognitive and comprehensive skills.
- Use firm but gentle restraining to prevent attempts to escape by kicking, biting, etc.
- Reassure family and gain their trust; talk calmly, quietly and confidently to reduce the parental upset, thereby reduce child upset.
- Examine/treat the child in an upright position whenever possible, as the child feels vulnerable and out of control in a lying down position.

Pharmacological Management

Pharmacological agents are often required to alleviate the pain caused by invasive procedures or surgery. There are narcotic and non-narcotic analgesics. The gold standard is the use of opioids. Opioids acts at mu receptors (mu1 and mu2) to hyperpolarize the cell membrane and reduce neuronal excitability.

Narcotic analgesics that are commonly used are as follows:

- Morphine
- Meperidine
- Fentanyl
- Sufentanil and alfentanil
- Methadone
- Epidural
- Local anaesthetics
- Topical applications
- Nerve blocks

Nonopioid Analgesics

Acetaminophen is useful in treating mild to moderate pain in children. The use of acetaminophen in neonates is limited, as it is usually administered orally or intrarectally. Although acetaminophen is metabolized by liver, hepatic toxicity is not a concern in neonates if standard doses are used.

PARASITIC INFESTATIONS

Roundworm Infestation (Ascariasis)

It is the infestation caused by roundworms (*Ascariasis lumbricoides*). Eggs are laid by the worm in the gastrointestinal tract of a host and passed out in faeces. Transmission is by the faeco-oral route. The eggs hatch out into larvae. These larvae in the host invade lymphatics and venules of the mesentery and migrate to the liver, lungs and heart. Larvae from the lungs reach the host's epiglottis and are swallowed. Once it reaches the gastrointestinal tract, larvae mature and mate and females lay eggs. This infestation manifests as light infection which is asymptomatic, whereas heavy infections manifest as anorexia, irritability, nervousness, enlarged abdomen, weight loss, fever and intestinal colic. The severe infections may have intestinal obstruction, appendicitis, perforation of intestine with peritonitis, obstructive jaundice, lung involvement and pneumonitis.

Assessment Findings

- Signs of atypical pneumonia
- Gastrointestinal symptoms such as nausea, vomiting, anorexia and weight loss
- Manifest pica, insomnia, irritability
- Severe cases show signs and symptoms of intestinal obstruction as a result of worm mass

Multidisciplinary Management

- Examination of stool for the presence of ova
- Treatment with anthelminthics, e.g. piperazine citrate

Nursing Diagnoses

- Knowledge deficit
- Alteration in growth and development
- Complication potentials

Nursing Interventions

- Provide immediate care as per the condition of the child.
- Provide hygiene education to the family.
- Prevent infection through the use of sanitary toilet.
- Dispose infected stools carefully.
- Demonstrate environmental sanitation in health education.

Pinworm Infestation

Ingested eggs mature in the caecum and then migrate to the anus. Worms exit at night and lay eggs on the host's skin. Itching is the common problem that leads to reingestion of eggs.

Assessment Findings

- Loss of weight and anorexia
- Irritability
- Insomnia
- Itching in the perianal region
- Signs and symptoms of acute or subacute appendicitis

Multidisciplinary Management

- Diagnosis by tape test (place a transparent adhesive tape over the anus and examine for evidence of worms)
- Administration of anthelminthics

Nursing Diagnoses

- Knowledge deficit
- Parental anxiety
- Complication potential

Nursing Interventions

- During treatment, maintain meticulous cleansing of the skin, particularly the anal region, hands and nails.
- Instruct not to bite nails.

- Ensure bed linen and clothing are boiled.
- Use anti-itching cream for itching.
- Teach preventive measures to parents and children.
- Instruct importance of treating everyone at home simultaneously.

Hookworm

Eggs of hookworm are evacuated from the human bowel and are left in soil and hatch to larvae within 5–10 days. These larvae are infective and invade the host when come in contact with the skin (barefoot) or handling the soil. The worms live in the upper gastrointestinal tract of the host and suck blood from the interstitial wall. Light infections in well-nourished individuals have no problems. Heavier infections show mild to moderate anaemia, malnutrition and burning and itching of the area of migration, leading to redness and papule formation.

Assessment Findings

- Disturbed digestion
- Unformed stool containing undigested food
- Stools tarry with decomposed blood
- The child will have pallor – microcytic anaemia
- Dull hair, increased pulse and mental apathy

Multidisciplinary Management

- Check signs and symptoms of blood smear.
- Treat with anthelminthics – tetrachloroethylene.
- Avoid fat, oil and alcohol.
- Keep the child NPO (nothing by mouth) the evening preceding treatment.

Nursing Diagnoses

- Knowledge deficit
- Complication potential

Nursing Interventions

- Administer medication by following strict instruction.
- Prevent infection by maintaining hygiene, wearing shoes, preventing nail-biting, disposing stools carefully, etc.
- Administer blood if anaemia is severe, as per directions.

General Instructions to Family to Prevent Parasitic Infestations

- Always wash hands and finger nails properly with soap and water before handling food and eating and after going to toilet.
- Avoid nail-biting and sucking fingers.
- Discourage children scratching the bare anal area.
- Change diapers as soon as soiled and dispose diapers properly.
- When using clothes as diapers, adequate care must be taken while cleaning and drying.

- Properly disinfect potty when using the same.
- Use only safe water for drinking.
- Wash all raw fruits and vegetables before eating.
- Use slippers/shoes having proper protection.
- Keep cats and dogs/pets away or also protect them from infestations so that they will not transmit infestation to human beings.
- Wash children's hands and feet frequently, especially when playing in the soil.

Medications Used for Treating Common Parasitic Infections

- Mebendazole (Vermox)
- 100 mg b.i.d. × 3 days
- 100 mg × 1 dose (repeat in 2 weeks' time for pinworm)
- Piperazine citrate (Antepar)
- 75 mg/kg per day (maximum 3.5 g) × 2 days (repeat in 2 weeks' time for pinworm)
- Pyrantel pamoate (Antiminth)
- 11 mg/kg × one dose (maximum of 350 mg) (repeat in 2 weeks' time for pinworm)

STUDY QUESTIONS

1. What are the age-specific approaches to paediatric medicine administration?
2. Why is it important for a paediatric nurse to understand the paediatric physiology in relation to medicine administration?
3. Why is it important to document medicine administration?
4. How will you calculate paediatric per dose medications?
5. What are the precautions to be taken while giving intravenous medications to children?
6. How will you calculate gravity drip rates?
7. How will you assess a paediatric trauma victim?
8. What is triage? What are its principles?
9. What is neonatal resuscitation?
10. What are the maternal risk factors that make requirement for neonatal resuscitation?
11. What are the common parasitic infestations seen in children?
12. How will you prevent pinworm infestations?

BIBLIOGRAPHY

1. Abu-Saad, H. (1984). Assessing Children's Response To Pain. Pain, 19(3), pp. 163–171.
2. Abu-Saad, H. (1994). Pain In Children. Developing A Programme of Research. Disability Rehabilitation, 16, pp. 44–50.
3. Adams, J. (1989). Paediatric Pain Assessment Trends and Research Directions. Paediatric Oncology Nursing, 6, pp. 79–85.
4. Anand, K. (1990). The Biology Of Pain Perception In Newborn Infants. Advances in Pain Research and Therapy, 15, pp. 113–122.
5. Anand, K.J.S., Craig, D.B. (1989). The Neuroanatomy, Neurophysiology And Neurobiochemistry Of Pain, Stress And Analgesia In Newborn And Children. Paediatric Clinics of North America, 36(4), pp. 795–822.
6. Anand, K.J.S., Plotsky, P.M. (1995). Neonatal Pain Alters Weight Gain And Pain Threshold During Development. Pediatric Research, 4(2), p. 57A.
7. Apgar, V. (1953). A Proposal For New Method Of Evaluation Of The New Method Of Evaluation Of The Newborn Infant. Current Research in Anesthesia and Analgesics, 32, pp. 260–267.
8. Assuma Beevi, T.M. (2004). Development Of A Tool To Assess Postoperative Pain In Children And Assess Parental Coping Towards Postoperative Pain In Children. Unpublished Doctoral Thesis. University of Calicut [Submitted].
9. Berde, C., et al. (1991). Patient Controlled Analgesia In Children And Adolescents, A Randomised Prospective Comparison With Intramuscular Administration Of Morphine For Postoperative Analgesia. Journal of Paediatrics, 118(3), pp. 460–466.
10. Bonadio, M. (1993). Defining Fever And Other Aspects Of Body Temperature In Infants And Children. Paediatrics Annals, 22(8), p. 467.
11. Brazy, J.E., Goldstein, R.F., Oehler, J.M., Gustafson, K.E., Thompson, R.J. (1993). Nursery Neurobiologic Risk Score: Levels Of Risk And Relationships With Nonmedical Factors. Journal of Developmental and Behavioural Pediatrics, 14, pp. 375–380.
12. Cantor, R., Learning, J. (Feb 1998). Evaluation And Management of Pediatric Major Trauma. Emergency Medicine Clinics of North America, 16(1), pp. 229–256.
13. Cortiella, J., Marvin, J. (June 1997). Management of Pediatric Burn patient. Nursing Clinics of North America, 32(2), pp. 311–329.
14. Duffy, T.E., Kohle, S.J., Vannucci, R.C. (1975). Carbohydrate And Energy Metabolism In Perinatal Rat Brain: Relation To Survival In Anoxia. Journal of Neurochemistry, 24, pp. 271–276.
15. Foster, R., Hester, N. (1989). The Relationship Between Assessment And Pharmacological Interventions For Children In Pain. In: Funk, S., Torquist, E., Champague, M., et al. (Editors). Key Aspects Of Comfort: Management of Pain, Fatigue and Nausea. New York: Springer.
16. Fuller, B.F. (1991). Acoustic Discrimination Of Three Types Of Infant Cries. Nursing Research, 40, pp. 137–145.
17. Fuller, B.F., Conner, D.A. (1991). The Effect Of Pain In Infant Behaviours. Clinical Nursing Research, 4, pp. 235–273.
18. Gill, D., O'Brien, N. (1998). Paediatric Clinical Examination. 3rd Edn. Edinburgh: Churchill Livingstone.
19. Gunau, R.V., Johnston, C.C., Craig, D. (1990). Neonatal Facial And Cry Responses To Invasive And Non-Invasive Procedures. Pain, 42, pp. 295–305.
20. Grunau, R.E., Whitfield, M.F., Petrie, J.H. (1994). Pain Sensitivity And Temperament In Extremely Low-Birth-Weight Premature Toddlers And Preterm And Full-Term Controls. Pain, 58, pp. 341–346.
21. Grunau, R.E., Whitfield, M.F., Petrie, J.H. (1998). Children's Judgements About Pain At Age 8–10 Years: Do Extremely Low Birthweight (≤1000 g) Children Differ From Full Birth-weight Peers? Journal of Child Psychology, Psychiatry and Allied Disciplines, 39, pp. 587–594.
22. Grunau, R.E., Whitfield, M.F., Petrie, J.H., Fryer, E.L. (1994). Early Pain Experience, Child And Family Factors As Precursors Of Somatization: A Prospective Study Of Extremely Premature And Fullterm Children. Pain, 56, pp. 353–359.
23. Harper, V.A., Rutter, N. (1983). Sweating In Preterm, Thermoregulation In Term And Preterm Newborn Babies. Archives of Disease of Childhood, 58, pp. 504–508.
24. Haszinski, M.F. (1992). Nursing Care Of The Critically Ill Child. St. Louis: Mosby.
25. Herzog, L., Coyne, L. (1993). What Is Fever? Normal Temperature In Infants Less Than Three Month Old. Clinical Paediatrics, 32(3), p. 142.
26. Hood, C. (1989). Enterobius Vermicularis. Practitioner, 233 (1466), p. 503.
27. Hotez, P. (1989). Hookworm Disease In Children. Paediatric Infectious Diseases Journal, 8(8), pp. 516–520.
28. Kattwinkel, J. (2000). Textbook of Neonatal Resuscitation. Elk Grove, IL: American Academy of Pediatrics and American Heart Association.
29. Katzman, E.M. (1989). What Is The Most Common Helminthic Infection In The USD? MCN, 14(3), pp. 193–195.
30. Kelley, S.J. (1994). Paediatric Emergency Nursing. 2nd Edn. Norwalk, CT: Appleton and Lange.
31. Malseed, R. (1982). Pharmacology: Drug therapy and nursing considerations. Lippincott: Philadelphia.

32. Masoorli, S., Perry, S. (1984). A Step-By-Step Guide To Trouble-Free Transfusions. RN, 47(5), pp. 34–42.
33. Merskey, H. (1979). On The Development Of Pain. Headache, 10, pp. 116–123.
34. Rossi, E.M., Philipson, E.H., Williams, T.G., Kalhan, S.C. (1989). Meconium Aspiration Syndrome: Intrapartum And Neonatal Attributes. American Journal of Obstetrics and Gynaecology, 161, pp. 1106–1110.
35. Sporing, E., Walton, M., Cady, C. (1984). The Children's Hospital Manual Of Paediatric Nursing Policies, Procedures And Personnel. NJ: Medical Economics.
36. Stevens, B.J., Johnston, C.C., Grunau, R.V.E. (1995). Issues Of Assessment Of Pain And Discomfort In Neonates. Journal of Obstetrics, Gynecology, and Neonatal Nursing, 24, pp. 849–855.
37. Thomas, D.O. (1996). Assessing Children – It's Different. RN, pp. 38–42.
38. Todres, I.D., Rogers, M.C. (1975). Methods of External Cardiac Massage In The Newborn Infant. Journal of Paediatrics, 86, pp. 781–782.
39. Wong, D.L., Baker, C.M. (1986). Pain In Children. Comparison Of Assessment Scales. Paediatric Nursing, 14(1), p. 9.

CHAPTER 41

PLANNING VARIOUS TYPES OF PAEDIATRIC UNITS (PCUs)

CHAPTER OUTLINE

This chapter is arranged with three important topics: planning of a paediatric unit, paediatric intensive care unit and a neonatal intensive care unit. Each topic is started with content outline. At the end of the chapter, study questions and references for each topic are given separately with separate numbers and names. This is for easy understanding of the reader.

LEARNING OBJECTIVES

At the end of the chapter, the learner will able to:
- Understand the impact of proper design for PCU.
- Discuss the prerequisite for PCU design.
- Describe in detail the various factors affecting design of PCU.
- Identify the harmful effects of noise and sound.
- Understand the beneficial effect of having natural lights in PCU.
- Understand the concept of going green.
- Identify the importance of PICU in a tertiary hospital.
- Understand the basic requirement for planning a PICU.
- State the physical facilities.
- List the manpower requirements of various categories of professional required for PICU.
- List the equipment, drugs and other stationaries required for PICU.

LEARNING OBJECTIVES—cont'd

- Understand the humanized care concept in PICU along with family-cantered care.
- Understand the quality protocol in PICU.
- Identify the need for NICU care for sick neonates and preterm and Small for gestational age (SGA) babies.
- Describe an NICU.
- Describe the various parameters to be considered while planning an NICU.
- List the various categories of manpower required for an NICU.
- List the equipment needed for an NICU.
- Explain various quality control measures to be followed.
- Describe the common ethical issues confronted in NICU and how to take precautions.
- Explain in detail the developmentally supportive care to be provided in an NICU.

A. PAEDIATRIC CARE UNIT (PCU) PLANNING

TOPICAL OUTLINE

- Introduction
- Prerequisites for Paediatric Care Unit
- Determining Optimal Number of Beds
- Care Delivery Models
- Cost to Construction
- Schematic Design and Design Decision
- Construction Documents
- Space Planning
- Occupancy Planning
- Space Planning for Ancillary Services
- Technical Planning
- Single Room
- Healing Environment
- Safety
- Noise and Lighting
- Single Room Design
- Distance and Space
- Influence of Design on Patient Care LEED and Green

INTRODUCTION: PAEDIATRIC CARE UNIT PLANNING

Paediatric health care unit should be planned to promote an environment of healing. The design should depict an environment that promotes patient safety, satisfaction and quality patient care.

If we go back to the history, eighteenth century facilities were like almshouse where indigent, destitute, orphans and sick who had no place to go had been taken care. It took 100 years to develop children's hospital even in develop countries like the USA. The Institute of Medicine (IOM), Agency for Healthcare Research and Quality (AHRQ) and the Joint Commission have all indicated that the work environment impacts not only patient and nurse satisfaction but also patient outcomes. Florence Nightingale, in her notes on nursing, wrote about the impact of environment on patient care and safety long back. Keeping and maintaining a clean and healthy environment in a hospital stays as the prime part of providing quality nursing care. Patient room design is extremely important because it is duplicated numerous times throughout the hospital environment. Decisions made about hospital design today will have an impact on how care can be delivered for decades. So, careful planning and design of a hospital is very important. This is particularly true about a children's hospital. A hospital for children should be child friendly and of one that reduces trauma and promotes psychological well-being of children.

Nurses are in a unique position to impact design decisions as advocates for patients and families and professionals who have an understanding of the processes that support patient care which are influenced by the built environment.

Prerequisite for paediatric care unit design includes:
The people who are involved in designing paediatric care unit should have knowledge base on the common childhood disorders/ailments that need hospitalization, common trends in admission decision, common types of investigations and treatment options. It is also important to have an understanding of the operational sense, patient and family focus, and familiar with care space needs. The nurse also should use evidence-based principles to address high priorities such as emergency preparedness, noise, lighting and transport. It is vital to include design flexibility, incorporate green principles and address practice implications.

PLANNING PHASE

Usually, the planning phase includes the following:
- Strategic plan 3–5 years
- Operational plan: What will we do with available resources – man, money, material?
- Financial plan: What will it cost?
- Approval phase
- Resource allocation, i.e. operating versus bonds

Space plans are essential to meet the programmatic needs and allocation of square footage to each space. The usual requirements are as follows:
- 200 square feet – medical–surgical areas
- 250 square feet – critical care areas
- 300–600 square feet – operation room areas
- 15%–20% allocation for support space – low

The clinical area should be planned in such a way that it should be flexible to accommodate different ratios and adaptable to accommodate levels of acuity, multiple diagnosis/ages and growth – surge capacity – flex up/down, etc.

Determining Optimal Number

It is a difficult task to determine the optimal number of beds in a specific unit. If it is too large, walking distance will make the staff burn out **and** if too small, it will isolate staff and will be inefficient for providing care. The recent trend is to have **32**-bed units. It is found to be cost and space effective.

Care Delivery Models

This is very important as it definitely affects the care provided. The usual models are as follows:
- Centralized
- Decentralized
- Both centralized and decentralized models, it is better to have family support areas and with visitor amenities like coffee bar.

Efficiency

Targeted census: Productivity target at a rate of 80% occupancy determines the number of beds needed:
- That is, a unit with a targeted occupancy of 22 patients a day at 80% occupancy would need 28 beds (28 × 80% = 22.4). Largest recommended number of beds in a unit is 54 beds.

Cost to Construction

Critical care at 250–300 square feet – Rs 2500/square feet
- Or at 350 square feet – Rs 3000/ square feet
- Medical–surgical unit at 150–200 square feet – Rs 2000/ square feet
- These figures include support space at 10%–20% of total square feet

This will vary according to inflation and market fluctuations.

Schematic Design

Floor plans for each clinical area to be prepared in advance to identify the defects.

Design Development

Room detail and surfaces in each room need to be determined to develop a proper design. Otherwise after construction, making changes will be difficult and lots of resource wastage will occur. So before starting the work, a final decision should be made on needs of the unit to guide the design and construction.

Construction Documents

It is important to have the following design documents clearly made before starting construction:
- Architectural design
- Plumbing
- Electrical layout
- HVAC (heat, ventilation and air conditioning)
- Proper government sanction orders for construction
- Statutory documents to prove sanctions from government and building development authority and electrical, pollution control and water authority

Occupancy Planning

It should have a move plan that includes:
- Begins months before occupancy
- Multidisciplinary
- Sequencing of patients
- Process for the move
- Ancillary support
- Tracking system

Space Planning – Ancillary Services

Most difficult task is to plan and fix the following:
- IT
- Equipment
- Floor plan – facilities
- Rooms
- Decentralized stations
- Medication and treatment rooms

Technology planning
- Phones
- Computers
- Tracker devices
- GetWellNetwork
- White boards
- Monitor alarms – tracking responses
- Electronic Medical Records (EMR) impact

How Space Impacts Care

Nurses are patient advocates. They need to think how space and architecture of a hospital impact patient care. She/he should see that unit should provide a *healing environment that promotes safety and satisfaction to patients and their relatives.*

Healing Environment

The notion that the physical environment has the potential to impact healing is not new – it is as old as antiquity. Florence Nightingale insisted on environment and her theory of nursing is based on providing comfortable environment to promote patient safety and rapid recovery. She had emphasized the need for natural light. This includes:
- Airiness
- Cleanliness
- Order
- Quietness
- Proper nutrition

Hippocrates referred to the environment as the fourth factor following disease, patient and physician as contributing to healing (J.M. Currie, *The Fourth Factor: A Historical Perspective on Architecture and Medicine*)

Plant a Tree and Get Beautiful World Free of Cost

A recent concept raised in Western world is Planetree. It emerged from the unpleasant hospital experience of Angelica Thieriot in the 1970s. She founded the nonprofit organization called Planetree to transform health care experiences. Planetree is relationship-based care facilitating efforts to create patient centered care in healing environment. Patient is the centre of the relationship. Most of the hospitals in the USA have alliance with Planetree. When we consider the natural light, we need to include elements of nature – stone, wood and plants. Home-like features and culture need to be impregnated for holistic and atraumatic care of children. So planning an environment that is green with natural trees is important. It is important to remember the dictum – 'Plant a tree and get all seasons free of cost'.

Access to Nature

Exposure to nature has been demonstrated to have calming restorative effect on paediatric patients and their families. Views or images of nature and natural light are associated with reduced stress and increased pain tolerance in children. Exposure to view of nature positively affects caregivers, on a daily basis and it can improve alertness. Providing natural paintings and aquarium inside the hospital with adequate safety has been proved to be beneficial in reducing trauma due to hospitalization in children. This promotes distraction in children from pain and such experiences.

Safety

The factors that need to be considered in safety are as follows:
- Noise
- Lighting
- Infection
- Single-patient rooms
- Distance and space

Sound

Sound has many different manifestations from disturbing and stressful to soothing and calming. Nurse must remember that speech is sound. Noise is unwanted sound. Hospitals are generally extremely noisy. Playing soft Indian classical music in the unit is soothing to children.

Hospital Noise

World Health Organization (WHO) has defined values for background hospital noise in patient rooms.
- Daytime – 35 dB
- Night-time – 30 dB

Busch-Vishniac (2005) reviewed 35 published studies over 45 years – not one reported noise levels that were within the WHO values. The following sounds in decibels will give a picture to the nurse in considering noise pollution in hospital premises:

- Peak level in hospitals often reaches 85–90 dB
- Motorcycle at 25 feet – 90 dB
- Diesel train at 45 miles/hour at 100 feet – 83 dB
- Spoken language between 40 and 60 dB
- Normal breathing – 10 dB
- Busy traffic – 70 dB

Noise and Patients

Exposure to excessive noise in NICUs impacts short-term and long-term auditory development (NACHRI and The Center for Health Design). It can lead to:

- Annoyance and sleep disturbance
- Decreased oxygen saturation
- Elevated blood pressure
- Increased heart rate and respiration
- Decreased rate of wound healing

Many studies have been conducted on sensory overload in intensive care units in different parts of the world and all of them reported the harmful effects of noise and sensory overload.

Noise and Staff

Increased stress and annoyance due to sensory overload interferes with ability to work effectively and evidence suggests that reduced noise levels result in more effective recall and communication of information and reduction in perceived work demand and pressure (Benjamin SE, De witty S, 2008).

Effective Methods to Reduce Noise

- Sound-absorbing ceiling tiles and flooring.
- Single-patient rooms.
- Staff and family education related to effects of noise and lighting. It has been found that patients exposed to brighter natural sunlight took 22% less medication for pain per hour. Exposure to natural light reduces vitamin D deficiency in patients and hospital staff.
- **Sufficient lighting** for caregivers when completing complex tasks, such as preparing medications, reduces errors.
- There is increased need for illumination with increased age.
- Average age of the practicing nurse is above 40 years which necessitates good illumination.

Single-Patient Rooms

JACHO, in 2008, in its *Health Care at the Crossroads: Guiding Principles for the Development of the Hospital of the Future* stated that single-patient rooms may have the single most important impact on patient safety and protect patients' health.

Benefits of single-patient rooms can reduce the number of transfers and handoffs and improve patient flow. It was identified that 85 beds in single-patient rooms function as the same bed capacity as 100-multipatient bedrooms (Detsky, Etchells 2008)

Benefits of Single-Patient Rooms

Infection Control

- Decreases spread of infectious agents between patients sharing a room
- Increases visual cue for caregivers to wash hands prior and after contact with patients
- Easier to decontaminate empty single-patient room than shared-patient room
  - It is quieter.
  - It provides privacy.
  - It decreases interruptions – promotes rest and recovery.
  - It supports family participation in care.
  - It facilitates private consultations with care.

Distance and Space

It is imperative to think about distance and space the staff need to spend in caring patients. A 1996, time and motion study conducted by IOM, of more than 1000 hours on a medical–surgical nursing unit over 18 months demonstrated that total time all health care workers (not just nurses) spent in patient rooms ranged from 1.1 to 3.3 hours in a 12-hour shift. Majority of time was spent walking between patient rooms, nurse's stations or other supply areas (medication room, supply room). Older hospitals have racetrack or single or double corridor with a central nursing station. This configuration locates nursing staff away from patients. Decentralized work stations and supply and medication rooms facilitate nurses being closer to patients and increase in direct care activities.

Teamwork and Collaboration

Caring for patients is a team activity requiring official and unofficial collaboration with other nurses and other members of the multidisciplinary team. Teamwork and communication are critical to providing safe patient care. Decentralized work stations must be combined with flexible spaces for interactive team collaboration and social interaction.

Influence of Design on Patient Care

Health care environment must be designed for the caregiving processes. This has direct correlation between staff performance and patient safety. Poorly designed environments force workaround and 70% of hospital preventable errors or potential errors are the result of process errors.

No involvement of nurses or other health professionals in design may lead to disastrous openings of hospitals. Commonly seen defects of such hospital planning are as follows:

- ED and ICU rooms too small
- Resuscitation room in ED does not allow staff access to head of patient
- Patients in mental health unit have access to roof and courtyard leading to 20-m drop
- Paediatric patients have access to roof with a three-storey drop
- Maternity assessment room doorway too narrow for stretchers

Standardization

Current trends
- Rooms and units organized in an identical manner
- Standardization fosters 'force functioning' of routine tasks by designing the environment in such a way that it guides caregiver processes in the most efficient and safe manner
- Supports unit adaptability to adjust to change in volumes or acuity

Same-Handed Design

- Beds – oriented against the same wall in every room
- Rooms – identical, so use becomes intuitive and therefore safer
- Can be more expensive to build because each room requires its own plumbing and medical gas drops

Mirror-Reverse Design

- Beds – oriented against opposite walls
- Headwall can be standardized to decrease variation
- No conclusive evidence that supports same-handed rooms are safer

Whatever may be the designs, it is better to reduce the number of room types to decrease variation. Standardize same-handed rooms where chances of critical events are high (ED, ICU) and standardize placement of medical gases in headwall so that use becomes more intuitive.

It has been found that design of space impacts the quality of nurses' work life, job satisfaction, stress and productivity. Nurses' job satisfaction has been shown to be a more important predictor for patient satisfaction than nursing skill (Berry, Parish 2008). Environments that support active involvement by families in the care process demonstrate higher levels of satisfaction among patients and families.

LEED and Green

This is a current trend adopted by the US hospitals for designing hospitals. LEED is Leadership in Energy and Environmental Design. Certification is done by the US Green Building Council.

Creation of LEED to:
- Establish common standard of measure for a 'green building'
- Promote integrated whole building design practices
- Stimulate green competition
- Raise consumer awareness
- Transform building market (Healthcare Informatics, 2008)

Going Green – What is it?
- Hospitals are major contributors to toxic waste.
- Intravenous bags and tubings – polyvinyl chloride (PVC) – when incinerated release dioxin and other toxic substances.
- Wastes from body fluids, toxic cleaning supplies and medication waste move into water supply.

The R's of going green
- Recycle – to reduce environmental impact
- Reuse – cleanable materials
- Renew – use sustainable building materials
- Refuse – to purchase supplies that are not biodegradable
- Reduce – use of fossil fuels (promote carpools, public transportation, high-efficiency bulbs, solar or wind energy to supplement energy supplies, rainwater collection)

Going Green – why?
- Cost savings – to reduce energy demands.
- Water consumption through rainwater storage and drought-resistant landscaping can reduce consumption by 30%.
- Natural lighting reduces energy use.
- This helps hospitals to align their actions with their mission to improve the health of the community they serve.

Now in India too, we are considering these aspects, though violations of laws and rules are there. The activists of environmental groups are propagating the need for going green in constructions of all hospitals and waste management. The experience that comes with age and leading multidisciplinary teams, nurse is in a unique position to provide proper information to the designers about how to consider these items in architectural planning of paediatric facility.

B. PAEDIATRIC INTENSIVE CARE UNIT (PICU) PLANNING

INTRODUCTION: PRINCIPLES AND PLANNING A PAEDIATRIC INTENSIVE CARE UNIT

The field of paediatric intensive care is rapidly growing in India. The number of intensive care units providing care to infants and children is also progressing at a rapid pace. Currently, there are no well-defined guidelines for paediatric intensive care units (PICUs) in Indian context. The Indian Academy of Pediatrics and Indian Society for Critical Care Medicine, paediatric section jointly took the initiative to develop such guidelines for PICU.

The planned facility should provide comprehensive medical and surgical care for children from birth through adolescence with acute or chronic system failure, multisystem trauma, organ transplantation, and so on.

Paediatric critical care population consists of patients who range in age from full-term neonates to adolescents and their families. So in PICU, nurses have to care for this wide age group ranging from congenital disorders to common medical and surgical problems. In PICU, a wide spectrum of illnesses is found unlike system-specific adult critical care units. Extremes in age and illness require paediatric critical care nurses to function as generalists within a subspecialty area.

Paediatric critical care practice had undergone dramatic changes for the last 3 decades. Increase in understanding of the pathophysiology of life-threatening diseases and the technologic capacity to monitor and treat paediatric patients had contributed to this advancement. There are different levels of PICU care that are usually patient based and are applied to describe a unit.

Level I: These Cater children needing greater attention than can be provided on the ward, and are generally classed as a high-dependency unit (HDU). This is usually available in secondary hospitals. Nurse–patient ratio is 1.5:1.

Level II: These facilities are provided to the children who need more intensive care including certain levels of monitoring. Level I PICUs provide multidisciplinary definitive care for a wide range of complex, progressive, rapidly changing medical, surgical, and traumatic disorders, occurring in paediatric patients of all ages, excluding premature newborns.

Level II PICUs provide stabilization of critically ill children before transferring to another centre or to avoid long-distance transfers, provide care for disorders of less complexity or lower acuity. Here, children require continuous nursing supervision who are intubated and ventilated and also children who are recently extubated requiring nursing supervision. Nurse–patient ratio is 1:1. For a child in a cubicle in level II PICU, nurse–patient ratio is 0.5:1.

Level III: A child requiring intensive supervision at all times, who needs additional complex therapeutic procedures and nursing. For example, unstable ventilated children on vasoactive drugs, inotropic support or multiple organ failure and organ transplant such as renal replacement and Extracorporeal membrane oxygenation (ECMO) therapy. This is usually available in quaternary hospitals. The nurse–patient ratio is 1:1.

Planning a PICU requires cooperation between hospitals and professionals within a given region. This will ensure the design and construction of an appropriate number of level I and II units. Duplication of services leads to underuse of resources and inadequate development of skills by clinical personnel and are costly.

Planning of a PICU requires
- Planning the administrative structure
- Planning the staffing
- Planning the protocols

PLANNING THE ADMINISTRATIVE STRUCTURE

Physical Design and Facilities

The physical facilities for PICU vary according to differences in hospital architecture, size, type of hospital (community, district, state headquarters, tertiary referral hospitals or quaternary hospitals) space and design.

The PICU should be located in proximity to:
- Elevators for patient transport, to the physicians' on-call room, and to family waiting and sleep areas.

- The emergency department, operating room, and recovery room is desirable.

The design of the PICU should reflect a patient- and family-centred approach and policies. (The psychological, spiritual, cultural and social needs of the patient and family should be taken into consideration.)

It is also important to see that the access to the PICU should be monitored to maintain patient and staff safety and confidentiality. It is also desirable to have the offices of medical and nursing directors located near the PICU.

Floor Plan

In a PICU, several distinct room types are required:
- Rooms for patient isolation
- Separate rooms for clean and soiled linens and equipment.
- A laboratory area for rapid determination of blood gases and other essential studies is desirable, assuming compliance with national, state and local regulations. There should be rapid and reliable system to obtain laboratory results to PICU through computerized links.
- Space need to be allocated for a medication station (including a refrigerator and a narcotics locker)
- A feed preparation station, counters and cabinets.
- It is always better to have a satellite pharmacy within the PICU that is capable of providing routine and emergency medications at the point of ordering.
- A reception area is ideal to control visitation, so that all visitors must go by this area before entering PICU. This area should be monitored by security personnel or surveillance cameras.
- A family counselling room is necessary for private discussions between the staff and the family.
- An area for storing patients' personal belonging and a conference room for staff personnel are essential.
- Toilet facilities for staff and patients' families must be provided separately. Parents/relatives rest room should be made available.

Size of PICU

- The ideal size of PICU cannot be stated, but 6–10 beds are desirable.
- PICU with less than 4 beds is inefficient and greater than 16 beds may be difficult to manage.
- The number of ICU beds should be 5–10% of total children beds in the hospital.

Bedside Facilities

- PICUs with individual patient rooms should allow at least 250 square feet per room (assuming there is one patient per room), and ward-type PICUs should allow at least 225 square feet per patient.
- The head of each bed or crib should be rapidly accessible for emergency airway management. In most cases, 12 or more electrical outlets and a minimum of two compressed air outlets, two oxygen outlets and two vacuum outlets are necessary per bed space.
- Reserve emergency power and gas supply (oxygen, compressed air) are essential.
- All outlets, heating, ventilation, air conditioning, fire-safety procedures and equipment, electrical grounding, plumbing and illumination must adhere to appropriate statutory regulations (Ministry of Health and Family Welfare Department regulations).
- Walls or curtains must be provided in between patients to ensure patient privacy.

Power Supply and Temperature Control

- Units should be centrally air conditioned and should have central heating for temperature control.
- In case of lack of central heating system, overhead warmer should be available. Units should have an uninterrupted power supply by means of backup power sources such as inverters and generators in accordance with load of various equipment.
- Adequate lighting, child-friendly wallpaper or paintings with soothing colours and curtains are desirable.

PLANNING THE STAFF PATTERN

Medical Director/Head of PICU

A medical director should be in charge of the PICU who should usually be:
- Medical Council of India (MCI)-approved paediatric intensivist or paediatric anaesthetist with paediatric critical care experience
  Or
- Paediatric surgeon with added qualification in paediatric critical care or paediatric critical care physician (paediatrician)

A letter of official appointment should be kept in ICU for inspection purpose with necessary certification documents. A paediatric intensivist/surgeon/paediatrician with critical care experience should be appointed as codirector or coordinator.

Job Specification

The medical director, in conjunction with the nurse manager will:
- Develop policies related to functioning of PICU
- Formulate admission and discharge policies
- Develop protocols for treatment and management of common conditions
- Prepare budget
- Procure equipment and supplies
- Coordinate staff education programme
- Maintain database of unit experience and performance
- Ensure communication between the intensivists and referring physicians
- Supervise resuscitation techniques
- Coordinate with the nurse manager, lead quality-improvement activities and coordinate medical research

In the absence of medical director, his deputy or in charge will perform all the responsibilities of the medical director. The medical director or designated substitute should serve as the attending physician on patients in the unit.

Medical Staff

The number of physicians depends on the number of admissions in the unit. This should be based on MCI requirements. (In hospitals where a postgraduate course in critical care is available, there will be adequate postgraduate students in all shifts to take care of patients.) In addition, all hospitals with PICUs must have a physician in-house 24 hours per day who is available to provide bedside care to patients in the PICU. A physician must be available within 30 minutes to assist with patient management.

Desirable Medical Staff

For level 1 PICUs, it is desirable to have a craniofacial (plastic) surgeon, an oral surgeon, a paediatric pulmonologist, a paediatric haematologist/oncologist, a paediatric endocrinologist, a paediatric gastroenterologist and a paediatric allergist or immunologist available on short notice. These physicians should be available for patients in level 2 PICUs within a 24-hour period. It is desirable to have paediatric subspecialty experts on request to attend critically ill children.

Nursing Staff

A nurse manager with substantial paediatric expertise should be appointed in PICUs. A master's degree in paediatric nursing or an additional qualification in nursing administration after basic degree with paediatric intensive care experience is desirable. In collaboration with the nursing leadership team, the nurse manager is responsible for assuring a safe practice environment consisting of appropriate nurse staffing, skill-level mix, and supplies and equipment. The nurse manager should participate in the development and review of written policies and procedures for the PICU; coordinate multidisciplinary staff education, quality assurance and nursing research; and prepare budgets together with the medical director. These responsibilities can be shared or delegated to other paediatric nurses, but the nurse manager has responsibility for the overall programme. The nurse manager should name qualified substitutes to fulfil his/her duties during absences. All nurses working in PICUs should complete a paediatric critical care orientation before assuming full responsibility for patient care. Paediatric advanced life support (PALS) or an equivalent course should be required. Nurse–patient ratios should be based on patient acuity, usually ranging from 1:1, 1:2 to 1:3. National Accreditation Board for Hospitals and Healthcare Providers (NABH) is also recommending this ratio.

Respiratory Therapy Staff

There should be a specified respiratory therapist designated and assigned to the PICU for 24 hours per day. All respiratory therapists who care for children in PICUs should have clinical experience managing paediatric respiratory failure and paediatric mechanical ventilators and should have training in PALS or an equivalent course.

Ancillary Support Staff

- An appropriately trained and qualified clinical pharmacist should be assigned to the PICU. Staff pharmacists must be in-house 24 hours per day in hospitals with PICUs.
- Biomedical technicians must be available within 1 hour, 24 hours per day in PICUs.
- A radiology technician (preferably with advanced paediatric training) must be in-house 24 hours per day in hospitals with PICUs.
- In addition, social workers; physical, occupational and speech therapists; nutritionists; child life specialists; clinical psychologists; and clergy must be available.

REQUIREMENT OF HOSPITALS WITH PICU

A hospital with PICU should have an emergency department with a separate entrance for paediatric emergencies. The emergency department should have two or more areas within the capacity and equipment to resuscitate paediatric patient with medical, surgical or traumatic illness.

The department of surgery in hospitals with PICU will have at least one operating room available within 30 minutes, 24 hours per day, and a second room available within 45 minutes. Capabilities in the operating room in hospitals with PICUs must include cardiopulmonary bypass, paediatric bronchoscopy, endoscopy and radiography.

The blood bank must have all blood components available 24 hours per day. Unless unusual cross-matching issues are encountered, blood typing and cross-matching should allow transfusion within 1 hour.

Paediatric radiology services must include portable radiography, fluoroscopy, computerized tomography scanning and ultrasonography.

Nuclear scanning angiography and magnetic resonance imaging should be available at all times. Facilities must be able to provide for the age-adjusted needs of paediatric patients (thermal homeostasis, sedation).

The availability of radiation therapy is desirable for PICUs.

Clinical laboratories should have microspecimen capability and 1-hour turnaround time for complete blood cell, differential and platelet counts; urinalysis; measurement of electrolytes, blood urea nitrogen, creatinine, glucose, and calcium concentrations and prothrombin and partial thromboplastin time; and cerebrospinal fluid analysis. Blood gas values must be available within 15 minutes. Results of drug screening and levels of serum ammonia, serum and urine osmolarity, phosphorus and magnesium should all be available within 3 hours for PICUs. Results of Gram stains and bacteriologic cultures should be available 24 hours per day.

The hospital pharmacy must be capable of dispensing all necessary medications for paediatric patients of all types and ages, 24 hours per day. A satellite pharmacy close to the unit is desirable. A pharmacist with paediatric experience is highly desirable. At each bedside, there should be a reference that lists urgent and resuscitation drugs with dosages appropriate for the individual patient.

Diagnostic cardiac and neurologic studies are preferred for infants and children in hospitals with PICUs.

Technicians with special training in paediatrics should be available to perform these studies. Electrocardiograms, two-dimensional echocardiograms with colour Doppler and electroencephalograms should be available 24 hours per day for PICUs.

A catheterization laboratory or angiography suite equipped to perform studies in paediatric patients should be present. Doppler ultrasonography devices and evoked potential monitoring equipment are desirable in hospitals with a PICU.

Haemodialysis equipment and technicians with paediatric experience should be available 24 hours per day.

Hospital facilities should include a comfortable waiting room, private consultation areas, dining facilities and resting rooms with telephone, for patients' families. Facilities and personnel should also be available to meet the psychological and spiritual needs of patients and their families. Medical staff, patients and patient families must have 24-hour-a-day access to competent, nonfamily member who can understand the common language used as spoken or written.

DRUGS AND EQUIPMENT

Drugs for resuscitation and advanced life support must be present and immediately available for any patient in the PICU. These drugs should be available in accordance with advanced cardiac life support and PALS guidelines, and should include all those necessary to support the patient population that the PICU serves. The life-saving, therapeutic and monitoring equipment detailed in the following text should be available at all time.

Portable Equipment

Portable equipment will include an emergency ('code' or 'crash') cart; a procedure lamp; paediatric-sized blood pressure cuffs for systemic arterial pressure determination; a Doppler ultrasonography device; an electrocardiograph; a defibrillator or cardioverter with paediatric paddles and preferably with pacing capabilities; thermometers with a range sufficient to identify extremes of hypothermia and hyperthermia; an automated blood pressure apparatus; transthoracic pacer with paediatric pads; devices for accurately measuring body weight; cribs and beds with head access; infant cooling devices; lights for photograph therapy; temporary pacemakers; a blood-warming apparatus; and a transport monitor. A suitable number of infusion pumps with microcapability (0.1 mL/h) must be available. Oxygen tanks are needed for transport and backup of the central oxygen supply. Similarly, portable suction machines are needed for transport and backup.

Additional equipment that must be available include volumetric infusion pumps, air-oxygen blenders, an air compressor, gas humidifiers, bag-valve-mask resuscitators, an otoscope and ophthalmoscope, and isolation carts. A portable electroencephalography machine must be available in the hospital for bedside recordings.

Televisions, radios and chairs should be available for patients and families who would benefit from their use.

Small Equipment

Certain small equipment appropriately sized for paediatric patients must be immediately available at all times. Such equipment include suction catheters; tracheal intubation equipment (laryngoscope handles, sizes and types of blades adequate to intubate patients of all ages, and Magill forceps); endotracheal tubes of all sizes (cuffed and uncuffed); oropharyngeal and nasopharyngeal airways; laryngeal mask airways; central catheters for vascular access; catheters for arterial access; pulmonary artery catheters; thoracostomy tubes; transvenous pacing catheters; and surgical trays for vascular cut-downs, open-chest procedures, cricothyroidotomy and tracheostomy.

Respiratory Equipment

Mechanical ventilators suitable for paediatric patients of all sizes must be available for each PICU bed. Equipment for chest physiotherapy and suctioning, spirometers and oxygen analysers must always be available for every patient. Oxygen monitors (pulse oximeters and transcutaneous oxygen monitors) and CO_2 monitors (transcutaneous and end-tidal) are required; portable (transport) ventilators are desired.

Bedside Monitors

Bedside monitors in all PICUs must have the capability for continuously monitoring heart rate and rhythm, respiratory rate, temperature, haemodynamic pressure, oxygen saturation, end-tidal CO_2 and arrhythmia detection. Bedside monitoring in PICUs must be capable of simultaneously monitoring systemic arterial, central venous, pulmonary arterial and intracranial pressures. The capability for a fifth simultaneous pressure measurement is desirable but not essential.

Monitors must have high and low alarms for heart rate, respiratory rate and all pressures. The alarms must be audible and visible. A permanent hard copy of the rhythm strip must be available in PICUs. Hard copy for all monitored variables is desirable. All monitors must be maintained and tested routinely.

PREHOSPITAL CARE

Often, patients requiring admission to a PICU are transported from the scene of an injury or from another hospital. Accordingly, PICUs shall be integrated with the regional Emergency Medical Services (EMS) system. The method of communication may vary, but a standard written approach to emergencies involving the EMS system and the PICU should be prepared.

All PICUs must have multiple telephone lines so that outside calls can be received even at very busy times.

Rapid access to a poison control centre is essential.

A fax machine is essential for PICUs.

There must be facilities for transfer in and out in PICUs. Policies should describe mechanisms that achieve smooth and timely exchange of patients between the emergency department, operating rooms, imaging facilities, special procedure areas, regular inpatient care areas and the PICU.

QUALITY IMPROVEMENT

The PICU must use a multidisciplinary collaborative quality assessment process. Objective methods should be used to compare observed and predicted morbidity and mortality rates for the severity of illness in the population examined. Benchmarking methods should be used to compare outcomes between similar PICUs.

TRAINING AND CONTINUING NURSING EDUCATIONS (CNEs)

Each PICU should train health care professionals in basic aspects of, and serve as a focus for, continuing education programmes in paediatric critical care. In addition, all health care providers working in the PICU should routinely attend or participate in regional and national meetings with course content pertinent to paediatric critical care.

Nurses, respiratory therapists and physicians, all must have basic life support certification and participate in resuscitation practice sessions and should be encouraged and supported to attend appropriate on-site or off-site educational programmes. Successful completion and current reaffirmation of PALS or a similar course should be required.

It is desirable for PICU personnel to participate in regional paediatric critical care education for EMS providers, for emergency department and transport personnel, and for the general public.

Research is essential for improving the understanding of the pathophysiology affecting vital organ systems as well as appropriate symptom management and psychosocial supportive interventions for the patient, family and bereaved survivors. Such knowledge is a vital component in improving patient care techniques and therapies, thereby decreasing morbidity and mortality. PICUs must stay as a laboratory for clinical research for physicians, nurses and paramedics.

PLANNING THE PROTOCOL FOR ADMISSION, DISCHARGE AND TRANSFER OUT

Admission procedure
- Prepare the necessary equipment.
- Prepare the patient bed.
- Take the initial vital signs and assess patient immediately.

- Notify physician.
- Immediately execute all stat orders.
- Inform dietary department.
- Enter patient's name in census book.
- Record the nursing interventions.
- Provide information to family.

Patient transfer to ward
- Confirmation by attending physician.
- Inform patient and family.
- Inform the nurse in the ward regarding the transfer.
- Notify the admitting and billing section and dietary department.
- Proper recording and documentation of transfer out.

Transfer to another hospital
- A discharge summary must be secured from the resident physician.
- Inform the nursing supervisor on duty.
- Secure consent of transfer to hospital of choice.
- Arrange ambulance for transfer.
- Discharge clearance must be got.

Discharge procedure
- Written order from physician.
- Settle the discharge clearance and return of medication.
- Forward two copies of discharge clearance slip – one to billing section and other to patient's relatives.
- Sign of discharge consent by patient or relatives.
- Complete documentation by the nurse on duty.

Conclusion

Patients admitted to the PICU are those who are unstable and need specialized personnel and equipment available in the PICU. The main goal of PICU is to provide optimum care for critically ill infants and children. So when we plan a PICU, there should be good design on physical facility, equipment and staff. It is also important to give specialized training for the critical management of the children.

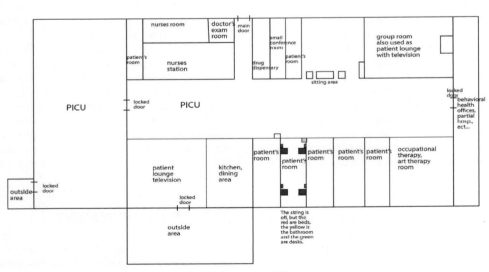

Physical Layout of PICU.

C. NEONATAL INTENSIVE CARE UNIT PLANNING

INTRODUCTION: PLANNING OF A NEONATAL INTENSIVE CARE UNIT

Newborn intensive care is defined as care for medically unstable or critically ill newborns requiring constant nursing, complicated surgical procedures, continual respiratory support or other intensive interventions. Intermediate care includes care of ill infants requiring less constant nursing, but does not exclude respiratory support. When an intensive care nursery is available, the intermediate nursery (step down neonatal intensive care unit [NICU]) serves as a 'step down' unit from the intensive care area. But all hospitals will not have this facility. Any hospital that has birthing unit, it is always better to have a facility to care for critically ill neonates. The cases of premature labour, complicated pregnancies, babies born after infertility treatment are all in the increase. This contributes a major session of precious babies. All these factors warrant the requirements of NICU in hospitals. NICU plan is a teamwork and the team should include, among others, health care professionals, families (whose primary experience with the hospital is as consumers of health care), administrators and design professionals.

Nurse is an important person in the planning team of NICUs. Nurse should have working knowledge of the requirements and statutory regulations guiding the plan of any intensive care unit. The nurse is responsible for planning nursing service in NICU. There are set criteria and standards for designing and developing a neonatal ICU. An NICU design should facilitate excellent health care for infants in a setting that supports the family needs and the needs of the staff.

For the last decade, remarkable changes have occurred in the 'landscape' of NICU design. The designing team should take into consideration the following requirements of the hospital and the availability of newer technology and advanced treatments. The people concerned should look into current evidence to make it affordable. The programme and design process should consider many factors such as vision and mission of the institution. The team should learn and carefully do the space planning, operations planning including traffic patterns, functional locations and relations to ancillary services, interior planning, surface material selection, building construction, postconstruction verification and remedying before actual occupation. When considering the type of design, private or family room design are preferred as such designs are practical, popular with families and justified by increasing awareness of the impact of sensory input (emotional bonding) on premature and ill newborns.

UNIT CONFIGURATION

The NICU design should be based on the vision, mission, philosophy, goals and objectives that define the purpose of the unit, service provision, space utilization, projected bed space demand, staffing requirements and other basic information related to the mission of the unit. The design should allow for flexibility and creativity to achieve the stated objectives. The NICU environment should be configured to provide individualized care for the infant and the family.

NICU LOCATION WITHIN THE HOSPITAL

The NICU should be planned at a distinct area of the hospital with controlled access and a controlled environment. NICU should provide effective circulation of staff, family and equipment. Traffic to other services shall not pass through the unit. The NICU should be in close proximity to labour rooms for easy transport of neonates. When obstetric and neonatal services are on separate floors of the hospital, an elevator with priority call and controlled access by keyed operation should be provided for service between the birthing unit and the NICU. This is to provide safe and efficient transport of infants while respecting their privacy. This facilitates transport of infants within the hospital without using public corridors.

SIZE OF THE UNIT

As a general rule, the intramural requirement is three beds for every 1000 annual deliveries. For extramural deliveries (deliveries taking place outside the hospital), number of beds in NICU will be 30% of the estimated beds. If a hospital has 3000 deliveries per year that hospital should have 9 beds for NICU (intramural) and for outside neonates, 30% of this will be 3 beds and the hospital may need 12 beds all together. But for planning size and equipment one has to consider sustainability of the unit.

SPACE REQUIREMENTS

Each infant space shall contain a minimum of 100–120 square feet (9.9–11.2 m^2) of clear floor space, excluding handwashing stations, columns and corridors. Out of this, 100–120 square feet half space should be utilized for baby care area and half for general support and ancillary areas. There should be corridor adjacent to each infant space with a minimum width of 4 feet (1.2 m) in multiple bedrooms. When single-infant rooms or fixed cubicle partitions are utilized in the design, there should be an adjacent corridor of not less than 8 feet (2.4 m) in clear and unobstructed width to permit passage of equipment and personnel. In multiple bedrooms, there shall be a minimum of 8 feet (2.4 m) between infant beds. Ideally, each infant space should be designed to allow privacy for the infant.

Baby care area may be divided into two interconnected rooms separated by transparent observation windows with nurse's workplace in between. This even promotes the purpose of isolation, if required.

General Support Space

Distinct facilities should be provided for clean and soiled utilities, medical equipment storage and unit management services.

Clean utility/holding area(s): For storage of supplies frequently used in the care of newborns.

Soiled utility/holding room: Essential for storing used and contaminated material before its removal from the NICU. The ventilation system in the soiled utility/holding room should be engineered to have negative air pressure with air 100% exhausted to the outside. The soiled utility/holding room should be placed to allow removal of soiled materials without passing through the infant care area. A designated area for collection of recyclable materials used in the NICU should be established. This area should measure at least 1 square feet per patient bed and be located outside the patient care area.

The handwashing station should have hot and cold running water that is turned on and off by hands-free controls, soap and paper towel dispensers, and a covered waste receptacle with foot control.

Charting/staff work areas: Provision for charting space at each bedside should be provided. An additional separate area or desk for tasks such as compiling more detailed records, completing requisitions and telephone communication should be allowed in an area acoustically separated from the infant and family areas. Dedicated space should be allocated as necessary for electronic medical record keeping within infant care areas. A clerical

area should be located near the entrance to the NICU so that personnel can supervise traffic into the unit. Newborn charts, computer terminals and hospital forms can be located in this space. In addition, there should be one or more staff work areas, each serving 8–16 beds. These areas will allow groups of 3–6 caregivers to congregate immediately adjacent to the infant care area for report, collaboration and socialization.

Storage areas: A three-zone storage system is desirable. The first storage area should be the central supply department of the hospital. The second storage zone is the clean utility area.

Routinely used supplies such as diapers, formula, linen, cover gowns, charts and information booklets may be stored in this space. There should be at least 8 cubic feet (0.22 m^3) for each infant for secondary storage of syringes, needles, intravenous infusion sets and sterile trays.

There should also be at least 18 square feet (1.7 m^2) of floor space allocated for equipment storage per infant in intermediate care, and 30 square feet (2.8 m^2) for each infant bed in intensive care. Total storage space may vary by unit size and storage system. The third storage zone is for items frequently used at the infant's bedside. Bedside cabinet storage should be at least 16 cubic feet (0.45 m^3) for each infant in the intermediate care area and 24 cubic feet (0.67 m^3) for each infant in the intensive care area. Bedside storage should be designed for quiet operation.

Use of electric medical record system will help to reduce the space consumption by avoiding files and papers. Design considerations include ease of access for staff, patient confidentiality, infection control and noise control, both with respect to that generated by the devices and by the traffic around them.

Laundry room: If laundry facilities for infant materials are provided, a separate laundry room can serve the functions of laundry and toy cleaning within the NICU. Infant clothing and the cloth covers or positioning aids should be laundered on a regular schedule and as needed. In addition, toys utilized by infants or siblings (while visiting if permitted) are required to be cleaned on a regular basis for each infant and between infants. Space for an automatic washing machine with dryer promotes the aseptic cleaning process.

Staff Support Space

Space should be provided within the NICU to meet the professional, personal and administrative needs of the staff. Locker, lounge, private toilet facilities and on-call rooms are required at a minimum. These areas should include doctors' and nurses' changing rooms and support staff's changing rooms, etc.

Step Down Area (Rooming-in Facility or Family Transition Rooms)

Family–infant room(s) should be provided within or immediately adjacent to the NICU, which allow(s) families/mothers and recovering neonates to stay together. This will release the pressure off NICU partially. The room(s) should have direct, private access to sink and toilet facilities, emergency call and telephone or intercom linkage with the NICU staff, sleeping facilities for at least one parent, and sufficient space for the infant's bed and equipment. The additional space requirement should be about 40–50 square feet per bed for this step down NICU.

Family Support Space

Space should be provided in or immediately adjacent to the NICU for the following functions: family lounge area, lockable storage, telephone(s) and toilet facilities. Separate, dedicated rooms should also be provided for lactation support and consultation in or immediately adjacent to the NICU. A family library or education area is preferred within the hospital.

Support Space for Ancillary Services

Ancillary services such as (but not necessarily limited to) respiratory therapy, laboratory, pharmacy, radiology, developmental therapy and specialized feeds preparation are common in the NICU. Distance, size and access are important considerations when designing space for each of these functions. Satellite facilities (intranet) may be required to provide these services in a timely manner. A specialized feeding preparation area or room should be provided in the NICU. In some hospitals, this facility may be at or near central supply or pharmacy area. They supply the prepared formula to NICU according to requisitions. Feed preparation area should be equipped with a hands-free handwashing station, counterwork space and storage areas for supplies, formula and both refrigerated and frozen breast milk.

Isolation Facilities

An airborne infection isolation room should be available for NICU infants. A hands-free handwashing station for hand hygiene and areas for gowning and storage of clean and soiled materials should be provided near the entrance to the room. Ventilation systems for isolation rooms should be engineered to have negative air pressure with air 100% exhausted to the outside. The perimeter walls, ceilings and floors, including penetrations, should be sealed tightly so that air does not infiltrate the environment from the outside or from other airspaces. Airborne infection isolation rooms should have self-closing devices on all room exit doors. An emergency communication system and remote patient-monitoring capability should be provided within the airborne infection isolation room. These rooms need to have observation windows with internal blinds or switchable privacy (opaquing) glass for privacy. Placement of windows and other structural items should allow for ease of operation and cleaning. It should have a permanently installed visual mechanism to constantly monitor the pressure status of the room when occupied by a neonate with an airborne infectious disease (example meningococcal meningitis). There should be facility to monitor the direction of the airflow continuously. These rooms should have a minimum of 150 square feet of clear floor space, excluding the entry work area, family entry

and reception area. This part of NICU should have a clearly identified entrance and reception area for families. Families should have immediate and direct contact with staff when they arrive at this entrance and reception area, and handwashing stations.

Handwashing Facility

Where a single-infant room concept is used, a hands-free handwashing station should be provided within each infant room. In a multiple bedroom, every infant bed should be within 20 feet (6 m) of a hands-free handwashing station. Handwashing stations should be no closer than 3 feet (0.9 m) from an infant bed or clean supply storage. Handwashing sinks should be large enough to control splashing and designed to avoid standing or retained water. Minimum dimensions for a handwashing sink are 24 inches wide, 16 inches front to back, 10 inches deep (61 cm × 41 cm × 25 cm) from the bottom of the sink to the top of its rim. Space for pictorial handwashing instructions shall be provided above all sinks. There should be no aerator on the faucet. Walls adjacent to handwashing sinks should be constructed of nonporous material. Space should also be provided for soap and towel dispensers and for appropriate trash receptacles. Towel dispensers should operate so that only the towel itself needs to be touched in the process of dispensing. Separate receptacles for biohazardous and nonbiohazardous waste should be available. Sinks for handwashing should not be built into counters. Sink location, construction material and related hardware (paper towel and soap dispensers) should be chosen with durability, ease of operation, ease of cleaning and noise control in mind. Nonabsorbent wall material should be used around sinks to prevent the growth of mould on cellulose material.

Administrative Space

Administrative space shall be provided in the NICU for activities directly related to infant care, family support or other activities routinely performed within the NICU.

Electrical needs: The unit should have 24-hour uninterrupted power supply. Backup power supply is a must.

ELECTRICITY SUPPLY, GAS SUPPLY AND MECHANICAL NEEDS

Mechanical requirements at each infant bed, such as electrical and gas outlets, shall be organized to ensure safety, easy access and maintenance. There shall be a minimum of 20 simultaneously accessible electrical outlets. The minimum number of simultaneously accessible gas outlets is air – three, oxygen – three and vacuum – three and others for power supplies.

There should be a mixture of emergency and normal power for all electrical outlets per current.

To handle equipment, six to eight central voltage–stabilized outlets are required per bed: four of them should be of 5 amperes and other four should be of 15 amperes. Two alternate sockets for mobile bedside X-ray equipment or USG machine need to be planned.

Lighting of the unit should be well illuminated with adequate daylight. Panel of lights with cool white fluorescent tubes, preferably CFL or LED (light-illuminating diodes) will be required for adequate illumination.

AMBIENT LIGHTING IN INFANT CARE AREAS

Ambient lighting levels in infant spaces need to be adjustable through a range of approximately 1–60 foot candles, as measured at each bedside. Both natural and electric light sources should have controls that allow immediate darkening of any bed position sufficient for transillumination when necessary. The lighting system should avoid unnecessary ultraviolet or infrared radiation by the use of appropriate lamps, lens or filters. Control of illumination should be accessible to staff and families, and capable of adjustment across the recommended range of lighting levels. Use of multiple light switches to allow different levels of illumination is one method helpful in this regard. A master switch may help when rapid darkening of the room is required to permit transillumination. Perception of skin tones is critical in the NICU; light sources should be capable to provide accurate skin-tone recognition. Light sources should be as free as possible of glare or veiling reflections. No direct light source or sun should be permitted in the newborn space as this does not exclude direct procedure lighting.

PROCEDURE LIGHTING IN INFANT CARE AREAS

Separate procedure lighting should be available to each infant bed. The luminaire should be capable of providing adequate illumination at the plane of the infant bed. It must be framed in such a way that no more than 2% of the light output of the luminaire extends beyond its illumination field. This lighting should be adjustable. Temporary increase in illumination is necessary to evaluate a baby or to perform a procedure. It should be possible without increasing lighting levels for other babies in the same room. Every effort should be made to prevent direct light reaching infant's eyes, as intense light may be unpleasant and harmful to the developing retina. For this, procedure lights should be with adjustable intensity, field size and direction. It will help to protect the infant's eyes from direct exposure and provide the best visual support to staff.

ILLUMINATION OF SUPPORT AREAS

Illumination of support areas within the NICU, including the charting areas, medication preparation area, the reception desk and handwashing areas, should conform to statutory specifications. Illumination should be adequate in areas of the NICU where staff performs important or critical tasks.

DAYLIGHTING

At least one source of daylight should be visible from infant care areas, either from each infant room itself or from an adjacent staff work area. When provided, external windows in infant care rooms should be glazed with insulating glass to minimize heat gain or loss, and should be situated at least 2 feet (60 cm) away from any part of an infant's bed to minimize radiant heat loss. All external windows should be equipped with shading devices that are neutral in colour or opaque to minimize colour distortion from transmitted light.

AMBIENT TEMPERATURE AND VENTILATION

The NICU should be designed to provide an air temperature of 78.8–82.4°F (26–28°C) and a relative humidity of 30%–60%. A minimum of six air changes/hour is required, with a minimum of two changes being outside air. **The ventilation** pattern should inhibit particulate matter from moving freely in the space, and intake and exhaust vents should be placed to minimize drafts on or near the infant beds.

Air delivered to the NICU should be filtered. Filters should be located outside the infant care area so that they can be changed easily and safely. Fresh air intake should be located at least 25 feet (7.6 m) from exhaust outlets of ventilating systems, combustion equipment stacks, medical–surgical vacuum systems, plumbing vents or areas that may collect vehicular exhausts or other noxious fumes. Prevailing winds or proximity to other structures may require greater clearance. The airflow pattern should be at low velocity and designed to minimize drafts, noise levels and airborne particulate matter. A 'high efficiency particulate air' or 'high efficiency particulate arrestance' (HEPA) filtration system may provide improved infection control for immunocompromised patients. Supply and exhaust ventilation is a good choice for units with heating or cooling ducts, as it is an inexpensive way of providing fresh air.

ACOUSTIC ENVIRONMENT

Infant bed areas (including airborne infection isolation areas), staff work areas, family areas, and staff lounge and sleeping areas and the spaces opening onto them should be designed to produce minimal background noise and to contain and absorb much of the transient noise that arises within them. The combination of continuous background sound and transient sound in any of these areas should not exceed an hourly Leq of 45 dB and an hourly L10 of. The acoustic conditions of the NICU should favour speech intelligibility, normal or relaxed vocal effort, acoustic privacy for staff and parents, and physiologic stability, uninterrupted sleep and freedom from acoustic distraction for infants and adults. Speech intelligibility ratings in infant areas, parent areas and staff work areas should be 'good' to 'excellent' as defined by the International Organization for Standardization (ISO) 9921:2003. Fire alarms in the infant area should be restricted to flashing lights without an audible signal. The audible alarm level in other occupied areas must be adjustable. Noise-generating gadgets and activities should be acoustically isolated. Telephones audible from the infant area should have adjustable announcing signals.

MECHANICAL NEEDS

The type of water supply and faucets in infant areas should be selected so as to minimize noise, and should provide instant warm water to minimize time 'on'.

Floor Surfaces

Floor surfaces should be easily cleanable and should minimize the growth of microorganisms.

Flooring material with a reflectance of no greater than 40% and a gloss value of no greater than 30 gloss units shall be used. This will minimize the possibility that glare reflected from a bright procedure or work area light will impinge on the eyes of infants or caregivers. Floors should be highly durable to withstand frequent cleaning and heavy traffic. Flooring materials should be free of substances known to be teratogenic, mutagenic, carcinogenic or otherwise harmful to human health. Although ease of cleaning and durability of NICU surfaces are of primary importance, consideration should also be given to their glossiness (the mirror-like reflectivity of a surface), their acoustical properties and the density of the materials used. Reduced glossiness will reduce the risks from bright-reflected glare; acoustic and density properties will directly affect noise and comfort.

Materials suitable to these criteria include resilient sheet flooring (medical grade rubber or linoleum) and carpeting with an impermeable backing, heat-welded or chemically welded seams and antimicrobial and antistatic properties. Big floor tiles are suitable. Additional efforts should be made to exclude persistent, bioaccumulative toxic chemicals (PBTs) such as PVC from health care environments. Dioxin releases are not associated with materials such as polyolefin, rubber (latex) or linoleum. Infants should not be moved into an area of newly installed flooring for a minimum of 2 weeks to permit complete off-gassing of adhesives and flooring materials. In India, majority of hospitals use vitrified titles. Other preferred flooring materials are Kota Stone or chip flooring, but requires thorough polishing.

Wall Surfaces

Wall surfaces should be easily cleanable and provide protection at points where contact with movable equipment is likely to occur. Surfaces should be free of substances known to be teratogenic, mutagenic, carcinogenic or otherwise harmful to human health. Specify low- or no-volatile organic compounds in paints (VOC paints) and coatings. Wall should be glazed up to 7 feet height.

Furnishings

Built-in and freestanding furnishings such as cabinets and carts, especially those in the infant care areas, should be easily cleanable with the fewest possible seams in the integral construction. Exposed surface seams shall be sealed. Furnishings should be of durable construction to withstand impact by movable equipment without significant damage. The ceiling construction should not be friable. As sound abatement is a high priority in the NICU, acoustical ceiling systems are desirable, but must be selected and designed carefully to meet this standard.
Safety/infant security

The NICU should be designed as part of an overall security programme to protect the physical safety of infants, families and staff in the NICU. The NICU shall be designed to minimize the risk of infant abduction.

Access to Nature and Other Positive Distractions

When possible, views of nature should be provided in at least one space that is accessible to all families and one space that is accessible to all staff. Other forms of positive distraction should be provided for families in family spaces, and for staff in staff spaces. Culturally appropriate positive distractions provide important psychological benefits to staff and families in the NICU to avoid sensory deprivation as well as sensory overload.

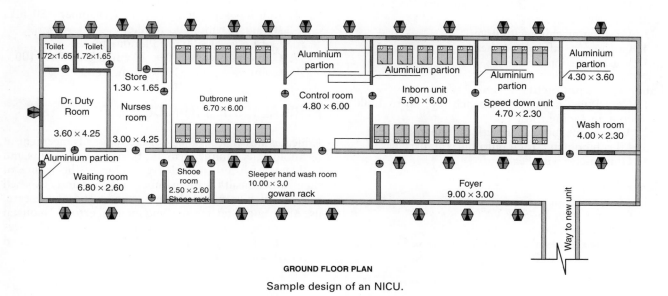

GROUND FLOOR PLAN

Sample design of an NICU.

EQUIPMENT REQUIRED FOR NICU

1. Open care system: Radiant warmer, fixed height, with trolley, drawers, O_2 bottles
2. Phototherapy unit, single head, high intensity
3. Resuscitator, hand-operated, neonate, 250 mL
4. Resuscitator, hand-operated, neonate, 500 mL
5. Laryngoscope set, neonate
6. Pump, suction, portable, 220 V, w/access
7. Pump, suction, foot-operated
8. Surgical instrument, suture/SET
9. Syringe pump, 10, 20, 50 mL, single phase
10. Oxygen hood, S and M, set of three each, including connecting tubes
11. Oxygen concentrator
12. Thermometer, clinical, digital, 32–43°C
13. Scale, baby, electronic, 10 kg <5g>
14. Pulse oximeter, bedside, neonatal
15. Stethoscope, binaural, neonate
16. Sphygmomanometer, neonate, electronic
17. Light, examination, mobile, 220-12 V
18. Hub cutter, syringe
19. Tape, measure, vinyl-coated, 1.5 m
20. Basin, kidney, stainless steel, 825 mL
21. Tray, dressing, ss, $300 \times 200 \times 30$ mm
22. Stand, infusion, double hook, on castors
23. Indicator, TST control spot/PAC-300
24. Irradiance meter for phototherapy units
25. Monitor, vital sign, NIBP, HR, SpO_2, ECG, RR, Temp
26. Monitor, vital sign, NIBP, HR, SpO_2, ECG, RR, Temp
27. ECG unit, 3 channel, portable/SET
28. Infantometer, plexi, 3½ feet/105 cm
29. X-ray, mobile
30. Transport incubator, basic, with battery and O_2, w/o ventilator
31. Autoclave, steam, bench top, 20 L, electrical
32. Laundry washer dryer, combo, 5 kg

Equipment for disinfection
1. Drum, sterilizing, 165 mm diameter
2. Electric sterilizer
3. Washing machine with dryer
4. Gowns for staff and mothers
5. Washable slippers

Laboratory equipment
1. Centrifuge, haematocrit, bench top, up to 12,000 rpm, including rotor
2. Microscope, binocular, with illuminator
3. Bilirubinometer, total bilirubin, capillary based
4. Glucometer with dextrostix

General equipment
1. AC (1.5 Tonne)
2. Generator set 25–50 KVA
3. Refrigerator, hot zone, 110 L
4. Voltage servo-stabilizer (three phase): 25–50 KVA
5. Room heater (Oil)

6. Computer with printer
7. Spot lamps
8. Wall clock with second hand

Renewable and consumable items
1. Adaptor, meconium aspirator, disposable (for suction pump)
2. Line, infusion pump, sterile, disposable
3. Multistix, urine, 5 parameter, Glu, Prot, Eryt, Spc Grav, pH
4. Cuvettes, Glu, box of 200
5. Cuvettes, Hb, box of 200
6. Vacuum tube, EDTA, 3 mL, set of 100
7. Vacuum tube, EDTA, 6 mL, set of 100
8. Vacuum tube, serum, 3 mL, set of 100
9. Vacuum tube, holder, set of 100
10. Vacuum tube, needle, 22 G set of 100
11. Lancet, safety, sterile, single-use/PAC-200 (1.8 mm)
12. Capillary tubes, box 1000
13. Sealing compound, capillary tubes, pck 500 g
14. Mask, surgical, disposable, box 100
15. Cap, surgical, disposable, box 100
16. Cord clamp, disposable, set of 10
17. Extractor, mucus, 20 mL, ster, disp Dee Lee
18. Tube, suction, CH10, L50 cm, ster, disp
19. Tube, suction, CH12, L50 cm, ster, disp
20. Tube, feeding, CH05, L40 cm, ster, disp
21. Tube, feeding, CH06, L40 cm, ster, disp
22. Tube, feeding, CH07, L40 cm, ster, disp
23. Syringe, dispos, 1 mL, ster/BOX-100
24. Syringe, dispos, 2 mL, ster/BOX-100
25. Syringe, dispos, 5 mL, ster/BOX-100
26. Syringe, dispos, 10 mL, ster/BOX-100
27. Syringe, dispos, 20 mL, sterile/BOX-80
28. Needle, disp, 22 G, ster/BOX-100
29. Needle, disp, 24 G, ster/BOX-100
30. Needle, disp, 26 G, ster/BOX-100
31. Needle, scalp vein, 21 G, ster, disp
32. Needle, scalp vein, 25 G, ster, disp
33. Gloves, exam, latex, medium, disp/BOX-100
34. Gloves, surg, 7, ster, disp, pair
35. Infusion set, paediatric, with chamber 150 mL, ster, disp, with 22 G needle
36. Cotton wool, 500 g, roll, non-ster
37. Compress, gauze, 10×10 cm, n/ster/PAC-100
38. Compress, gauze, 10×10 m, ster/PAC-5

ETHICAL ISSUES IN NICU

Ethical issues arise as a part of the rapid advancement of technology, economic changes, resource constraints and problems of health care delivery. Due to the nature of their career, health team members are constantly exposed to ethical issues and challenges such as end-of-life care, use of advanced technology and medical errors. Neonatal wards are filled with moral conflicts. Amazing advances in care of critically ill neonate challenge the established standards and clear procedures.

Essential Aspects of Care and Ethical Constraints

Skilled professional care: Do we have a trained team of professionals to give the skilled professional care? Skilled professional care in NICU is the simple application of critical care technology such as ventilators/monitors, medications, invasive devices and a multiplicity of lab measurements to the sick and premature newborn. Effective team is essential as no single person can do this.

Physical constraints: Care is extended over a necessarily limited time period. The developmental needs of growing infant cannot be met in NICU environment from the standpoint of staffing, time use and patient access and interaction throughout the passing months.

Conclusion of care: The care provides starts with stabilization of the newborn, facilitation of the transition to normal extrauterine neonatal physiology. This transition takes longer times in some neonates and requires specific intervention and support. The reversal of acute disease process is considered as end, e.g. Respiratory Distress Syndrome (RDS), Meconium Aspiration Syndrome (MAS) and infection.

Iatrogenic effects: This includes minimizing chronic or debilitating sequelae of applied neonatal intensive care. The potential for negative iatrogenic effects needs to be identified, such as effects resulting from:
- Environment in which baby is managed (light, noise, touch)
- Mode of ventilation (conventional, synchronized, high frequency); types, doses and results of medication used
- Short- and long-term effects of certain painful procedures
- Foreign bodies or devices used
- How nutritional needs are met (enteral or parenteral nutrition)

Expected Outcome of Ethical Care

Providing care that is reasonable for steady improvement is essential.
- Such care should be with absence of pain and avoidable suffering.
- Develop care towards a capacity for the newborn to experience and enjoy human experience over a life prolonged beyond infancy.

Parents:
Maintain focus upon best interest of the child.
Parents are considered as spokespersons: Seek their opinions and provide care negotiated for the best interest of the child by the parents.
Shared decision-making is commonly used process among relevant care providers, and a willingness and capability to communicate effectively with the parents.
Medical futility of care must be determined in the context of goals and the likelihood as well as appropriateness

of applied intervention achieving the desired ends. Availability of ethical guidelines for practice is essential in deciding on certain type of treatments. For example, do-not-resuscitate orders developed and promulgated by professional societies and ethicists have assisted in day-to-day management of numerous difficult issues; including determining brain death and withdrawal or withholding of life-sustaining therapy.

Positive Aspects of Ethical Guidelines

- Ethical guidelines reflect expert's thoughts on different aspects. A group of experts will be involved in preparation of guidelines. They examine all positive and negative aspects of any intervention before reaching a conclusion of a guideline. So a guideline shows expertise.
- Ethical guidelines enable health care professionals from constraints of what to do in a particular situation.
- It encourages health care team to make appropriate decisions, promote teamwork, best strategies for communication and in confronting issues.
- It empowers the health care team and parents involved in a particular case.
- It is educative to all, especially novice, and help people to mentor the novice by the experts or seniors.

Negative Aspects of Ethical Guidelines

- They are incomplete in nature. Not all health care cases fall under the general guideline parameters. Consistency may not result in every case, even with the best-intended guidelines.
- Guidelines are sometimes imperfect. It stays as a starting point only. It requires much expertise and clinical judgement from the part of users, as it appears as simple anecdotes of experience. One must remember that one cannot resolve the hurt associated with the emotional investment made towards patient care when outcomes are dismal.

Important Points to be Remembered while Preparing Guidelines

- It should be based on facts and experience.
- It should be updated frequently to base on currency of issues based on current political and sociocultural practices. It should reflect the new paradigm (social, political, technological and fiscal influences).
- It should hold the responsibility to public when disclosure is necessary. Guidelines should stem from the principles of respect for persons, patient autonomy, avoidance of harm and maximizing benefit. This will keep the guidelines with its true nature of fiduciary, or trust-based, relationships between health care professionals and their patients.
- The guidelines should have the capacity for patient advocacy.

- It hold the concept of good and beneficence. So what is good for the critically ill neonate must be addressed in the guidelines. Health care people are considered as healers. So the guideline should reflect faith, share cultural heritage and image of health and health care.
- It should based on best interest of the patient and family.

Ethics and Communication Process at NICU

All hospitals have protocols for practice. It is advised to have guidelines for ethical practice too. Parents look upon health professionals as experts; they would like to get the opinion and explanation for any care provided to their newborns. So in communicating the care needs to parents of neonates in NICU, it is essential to develop consensus on care protocol between professionals before communicating them to the parents. The health care professionals should be able to discuss pros and cons of particular intervention to the parents in a clear and understanding manner without using jargons. The health care members should be aware that parents may have difficulty in communicating though they have their wishes about their neonate, but the timing of premature deliveries may not afford them to express their wishes properly. The guideline on communication should not dictate medical care but facilitate the parents for decision-making process. They need to be **empowered** in decision-making.

Health care professionals should **use a cautious approach** and should be aware that the resource they use for a very serious neonate may compromise the care of other less serious neonates such as late preterm or term infants who have better prognosis. **Allocating scarce resources** to provide the needs of all babies is difficult. The professionals should use such resources **judiciously**, so that better use of resources could be done to benefit the most. One must remember that what is used for one neonate is unavailable to the other. While using available technologies and interventions, one should be aware that valuing the technology over human nature of the neonate, family and clinical staff should be curtailed. This may create burden of pain, suffering and moral angst among them.

DEVELOPMENTALLY SUPPORTIVE CARE AT NEONATAL INTENSIVE CARE UNIT (DSC-NICU)

Developmentally supportive care is a bunch of practices incorporated into the care of neonatal intensive care to reduce the harmful effects of neonatal intensive unit on the developing baby and their family by promoting optimal neurological and behavioural development.

Components of DSC

There are seven core components for DSC.

They are partnering with parents, healing environment, minimizing stress and pain, safeguarding sleep, optimal nutrition, protecting skin and positioning and handling.

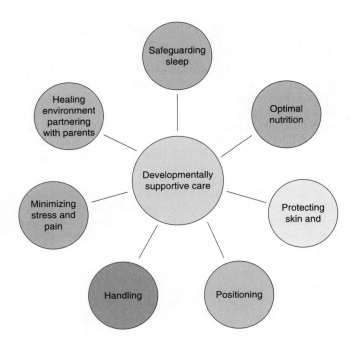

1. **Partnering with parents**

   This is part of family-centred care. Strategies and interventions used in this process facilitate bonding and parent–infant interaction. Parents are not shunted away and they are the partners in provision of care as the infant belong to the family and not to NICU. The main advantages of this concept are parental involvement, parental participation, partnership with parents (families) and shared care (collaboration). This will reduce the stress of negative experiences of preterm birth and NICU experiences such as:
   - Heightened parental stress
   - Negative parent–infant interaction
   - Adverse child developmental and behavioural outcomes

   Health care professionals have a vast range of knowledge and skills that are essential to help a neonate to survive. For better outcomes, infants require their parents and parents need to know their babies. So the nurses need to share the responsibility of taking care of these neonates admitted at NICU with their parents through involving them in the care of neonates. These parents are worried and they are scared to take care of their fragile little ones. Nurses can start with simple gestures such as:
   - Being welcoming and respectful of their role as a parent
   - Giving information freely and truthfully and communicating the medical and developmental needs in a culturally appropriate and understandable manner
   - Involving them in decision-making about the health care of their baby
   - Involving the mother in care
   - Mother-based NICU, need of hour (Cisler, Cahill et al., 2002)

Co-bedding for twins; parent-focussed care (COPE) and spiritual and cultural care are important in DSC.
- Actively teaching parents about their baby and how to gently handle it and be involved with physical caregiving such as temperature taking, nappy changing, bathing and weighing. This will aid parents to be competent in taking care of their baby even after discharge.

2. **Healing environment**

   The healing environment includes the physical environment (space, privacy and safety) and the sensory environment (tactile vestibular, olfactory, gustatory, auditory and visual systems). When considering physical environment, space area is very important and it is stipulated to have 120 square feet per neonate. Environmental manipulation and modification is essential to provide a healing environment for the sick babies in NICU. It is clearly identified that neonatal environment is critical and has big impact on babies and has the potential short-term and long-term outcomes for development. These neonates do not have the capability to deal with the environmental stress of the neonatal intensive care environment. There should be lots of environmental manipulation to avoid the mismatch. Management of the neonatal environment is a core element in 'developmentally supportive care'.

   Environmental management involves a broad range of interventions and strategies designed to modify the physical and caregiving environment of the NICU to reduce the stress.

   In environmentally supportive care, the caregivers need to understand the behavioural cues of the babies and how they are coping with what is going on in and around them. The environmental aspects affecting neonate in NICU requiring manipulation are as follows:

   Noise
   Light
   Smell
   Taste
   Touch
   Handling
   Positioning
   Pain management

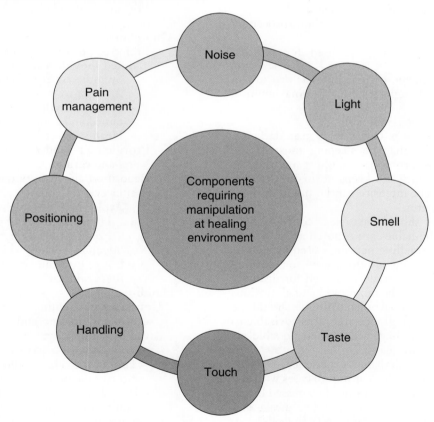

Components of healing environment in DSC.

Noise:
   In utero, the noise level is 40–60 dB. Usual noise levels in NICU are 50–80 dB. Noise levels >90 dB for long times, will lead to hearing loss. Preterm infants on aminoglycosides should be kept at lower decibel levels, as the side effect of aminoglycosides is ototoxicity. Monitor sound levels to maintain sound levels of <50 dB. Turn off alarms as quickly as possible.

Sources of noise in NICU are as follows:
   - Incubator, inside noise level should be 55–88 dB with a peak of 117 dB

- Additional 10–40 dB can be there with surrounding equipment
- Routine care activities have 58–76 dB
- Loud, sharp sound produces 100–200 dB
- 90% of peak noises are due to human-related factors

Interventions to reduce noise:
- Move equipment quietly, repair noisy ones.
- Decrease staff-generated noises.
- Prepare medications and feedings away from the bedside.
- Gently open doors and drawers.
- Follow the sound limit recommendations.

In NICU environment, sound should be monitored through decibel readings and kept at a level <45 dB. Playing Indian classical music is advisable to reduce environmental distractions.

Light:
In NICU environment, there should be light reduction. This is a very important practice and is inherently an inbuilt concern. Safe level of light is not yet established. Useful activities include:
- Shade head of crib/incubator.
- When required, use spotlight/procedure light.
- Eye covers must be used for preterm infants.
- Use available natural light or provide an adjustable light level up to a maximum of 60 ftc.

Light reduction strategies:
Cycled lighting is better than near darkness. The babies may be sleeping most of the time, this promotes weight gain, reduces motor activity and keeps normal heart rate. NICU light intensity can be monitored using lux meter.

Smell: Nurses should have clear concept about the smell the babies are exposed at an NICU. The strong smelling perfumes used by staff or even the cleaning solutions used for cleaning the floor or the disinfectant used for disinfection, etc. need to be monitored and all noxious smell should be avoided. NICU should be scent-free and fragrance-free. It is advisable to provide the mother's scent when possible via breast pad or soft cloth.

Taste: What tastes do babies experience? Do they get any oral medicines or mouth cares with any solutions; do they get drops of expressed breast milk (EBM) in their mouths when awake and receiving Nasogastric Tube (NGT) feeds?

Touch/handling: Who touches/handles the babies? How often? What for? These question are important. The caregivers should provide soft, gentle touch in all caregiving interactions. It is important to teach the parents about the importance of skin-to-skin care by either parent. This will promote the neutral thermal environment too.

3. **Positioning and handling:**
Therapeutic positioning in the NICU is important for neuromotor and musculoskeletal development. It also helps in physiologic function and stability, skin integrity, thermal regulation, bone density, sleep facilitation and brain development. Therapeutic positioning promotes rest, supports optimal growth and helps to normalize neurobehavioral organization. The nurse in NICU can use the validated and reliable positioning assessment tool (The Infant Position Assessment Tool (IPAT) is a six-item tool with . . . developmentally supportive positioning practices in the NICU.) routinely according to hospital protocol.
Educate parents about the principles and techniques of positioning, containment and handling.
Positioning: What positions are babies nursed in? Do you use nests or boundaries to help maintain them in position and keep them calm?
Positioning has effect on:
* Respiratory physiology
* Body alignment
* Preventing postural deformities
* Promoting self-soothing activities
* Position is decided by GA, degree of illness, paralytic agents

Guidelines
Preferred position is prone/side lying to ensure flexed shoulders and hips
- Swaddle/cover to keep in flexed position
- Attempt to 'nest' the infant
- Promote midline alignment that is contained and comfortable
- Head support
Provide four-handed support during positioning and caring
Reposition the baby after care or minimally after every 4 hours.
- Avoid the following:
- Hyperextension of neck
- Frequent head turning to side
No sudden movement while changing positions
- Lower extremity frogging
- Bigger diaper

Handling:
Unnecessary handling must be avoided, as it causes physiologic and behavioural stress. It can be possible by:
- Pacing the care according to baby.
- Timing the care around sleep/wake cycles.
- No routine procedure during sleep hours.
- Provide 2–3 hours of uninterrupted sleep.
- Watch for symptoms of stress. Follow 'minimal handling' or 'quiet hour' protocol by reducing noise, decreasing lights, allowing 2 hours of rest, clustering care activities and sensitizing nursing staff.

Stimulation:
This should begin in the womb. Evidence showed that fetuses are known to respond to mother's heartbeats and voice. Any stimulation through special senses during fetal/neonatal life is

beneficial. Thus, supplementary stimulations help neonates and preterm babies to achieve good developmental outcomes.

Supplemental stimulations can be in the form of: Kangaroo mother care (KMC): It is described Chapter 15 in this textbook.
- Non-nutritive sucking (NNS)
- Massage therapy
- Multimodal stimulation
- Breastfeeding – described Chapter 15 in this textbook.
- Pain management
- Neonatal Individualized Developmental and Assessment Program **(NIDCAP)**

Non-nutritive sucking

- It is different from nutritive sucking and usually permitted to suck on empty breast or pacifier. It provides comfort and promotes physiological organization. Other advantages are pain relief, suck–swallow coordination, facilitates transition to breastfeeding, better weight gain and shorter hospital stay.

Massage Therapy

Stimulation of tactile and pressure receptors through massage therapy is important. The hypothetical mechanisms of benefits are as follows:
- Touch – growth gene interaction
- Increased vagal tone
- Increased insulin levels
- Increased growth hormone secretion

Proposed benefits of massage therapy are better weight gain, more alert and active neonate and better sleep. Issues of massage therapy include collapse/disorganization due to over-stimulation.

Neonatal Individualized Developmental and Assessment Program

This is developed by Als et al. NIDCAP is a model that provides education and specific training for individual health professionals with the goal of an altered developmental approach to care in the NICU and special care nursery. There are four standards of care namely:
- Structuring the environment
- Timing, organizing and giving direct care
- Working collaboratively
- Supporting and strengthening family relationships

Care is provided to neonates through individualized plan for each baby. It decreases oxygen requirement and improves outcome at 12 months.

4. **Safeguarding sleep:**
Nurses in NICU should have clear awareness on infant sleep–wake states, cycles and transitions. They should individualize all caregiving activities by clustering cares based on this sleep–wake states. Nurse should identify infant cues and signs of stress during clustered cares. While raising a sleeping infant, use a soft voice followed by gentle touch. NICU personnel should educate parents regarding the need for safeguarding sleep and infant cues on sleep–wake states. Promote a quiet and comfortable environment for uninterrupted sleep.

5. **Minimizing stress and pain:**
Neonatal stress causes increased energy expenditure, decreased healing and growth, impaired physiologic stability and altered brain development. Stressors and painful interventions may raise cortisol levels, limiting neuroplastic reorganization and therefore, learning and memory of motor skills. Nurses should provide individualized care according to priority that supports the needs of infants to minimize stress and pain. Pain can be monitored using validated pain assessment tools. Teach parents regarding pain management by both pharmacological and nonpharmacological methods and their role in supporting neonate during painful procedures.

6. **Protecting skin:**
Skin helps in thermoregulation, fat storage and insulation, fluid and electrolyte balance, barrier protection against penetration and absorption of bacteria and toxins, sensation of touch, pressure and pain, and conduit of sensory information to the brain. In NICU, nurses should be proficient in skin care practices such as bathing practices, emollient usage, humidity practices and use of adhesives for babies in each stage of development. There should be clear-cut instructions/protocols for such practices.

7. **Optimizing nutrition**
Look for feeding readiness cues and observe for coordinated suck/swallow/breathing (SSB) throughout breastfeeding or bottle-feeding. NICU professionals should support mother's EBM supply. They also should minimize negative perioral stimulation (adhesives, suctioning, etc.). When using gavage feeding, prefer indwelling NG tube rather than intermittent tubes. Promote NNS at mother's pumped breast during gavage feeds. Even if the baby is on gavage feeding, provide the taste and smell of breast milk with gavage feedings. Promote side-lying position close to parent/caregiver when bottle-feeding. Provide family education regarding feeding techniques.

STUDY QUESTIONS

A. Study questions on paediatric unit planning
1. What are the prerequisites for paediatric care unit design?
2. Why is it important to plan paediatric care unit with adequate thought?
3. What are the care delivery models used for PCU?
4. What are the statutory documents required before constructing a PCU?
5. Discuss the various factors affecting in terms of cost, documents, space, noise and light in planning a PCU.

6. What is go green concept?
7. How is go green concept affect patient care in PCU?

B. Study questions on paediatric ICU planning
1. Why is it important to have a PICU in a tertiary care hospital?
2. Who are the critical care population cared in a PICU?
3. What are the levels of care provided in PICU?
4. Explain the levels of care provided in each level with nurse–patient ratio.
5. What are the important points to be kept in mind while planning physical facilities in relation to location, size, floor plan, flooring, bedside facilities and power supply?
6. Explain the requirement of manpower required in a PICU.
7. How will you plan the nursing manpower with proposed ratio?
8. What are the ancillary staff required in PICU?
9. What are the common equipment required for a PICU?
10. How will you prevent infections in PICU?
11. What infection control protocols need to be followed in PICU?
12. What are the quality control measures in PICU?
13. What are the common strategies followed in PICU for family-centred care?

C. Study question on neonatal ICU planning
1. Develop model design for an NICU with a bed capacity of 15 neonates.
2. How will decide the manpower for an NICU with 15 beds?
3. What are the equipment required in an NICU?
4. What is DSC?
5. What are the core components of DSC?
6. What are the components of healing environment in NICU?
7. Explain the components of healing environment with examples and nurse's role in maintaining these components.
8. How will you promote non-nutritive sucking in neonates and what are its benefits?
9. What is multimodal stimulation? State its advantages.

BIBLIOGRAPHY

A. References for Paediatric Unit planning

1. Anthony D. Slonim, Murray M. Pollack. Integrating the Institute of Medicine's six quality aims into pediatric critical care: Relevance and applications. *Pediatr Crit Care Med.* 2005;Vol. 6, No. 3.
2. Institute of Medicine Committee on Quality of Health Care in America: Crossing the Quality Chasm: A New Health System for the 21st Century. Washington DC: National Academy Press, 2001.
3. Institute for Healthcare Improvement: Idealized Design of the ICU. Available at: http://www.ihi.org/idealized/idicu/index.asp. Accessed November 9, 2003.
4. Boat TF: Improving health outcomes for children. *J Pediatr.* 2003;143:559–563.
5. Aiken, L. H., Sermeus, W., Van den Heede, K., Sloane, D. M., Busse, R., McKee, M., et al. (2012). Patient safety, satisfaction, and quality of hospital care: cross sectional surveys of nurses and patients in 12 countries in Europe and the United States. *British Medical Journal*, 344:e1717. doi:10.1136/bmj.e1717.
6. American Academy of Pediatrics. (1994). Staffing patterns for patient care and support personnel in a general pediatric unit. *Pediatrics*, 93(5), 850-854.
7. American Academy of Pediatrics. (1998). Facilities and equipment for the care of pediatric patients in a community hospital. *Pediatrics*, 101(6), 1089-1090.
8. Bowden, V. R., & Greenberg, C. S. eds. (2014). Children and their families: The continuum of nursing care. 3rd ed. Philadelphia: Lippincott Williams & Wilkins.
9. Broome, M., & Rollins, J. eds. (1999). Core curriculum for the nursing care of children and their families. Pittman, NJ: Jannetti Publications.
10. Currie, J. M., American Institute of Architects., & AIA Academy of Architecture for Health. (2007). The fourth factor: A historical perspective on architecture and medicine. Washington, D.C: American Institute of Architects, Academy of Architecture for Health.
11. Ilene J. Busch-Vishniac, James E. West, Colin Barnhill, Tyrone Hunter, Douglas Orellana, Ram Chivukula. (2005). Noise levels in Johns Hopkins Hospital. *The Journal of the Acoustical Society of America*, 118, 3629. https://doi.org/10.1121/1.2118327.
12. NACHRI Facilities Design. The Center for Health Design. December 3, 2012 to December 5, 2012.
13. JACHO. Health care at the crossroads: guiding principles for the development of the hospital of the future. 2008.
14. Michael E. Detsky, MD; Edward Etchells, MD, MSc. Article Information. Single-Patient Rooms for Safe Patient-Centered Hospitals. *JAMA*. 2008;300(8):954-956.
15. LEED v4 ID+C rating system PDF/LEED v4 ID+C scorecard/Reference guide overview.

B. References for Paediatric ICU planning

1. American Academy of Pediatrics. (2004). Guidelines and levels of care for pediatric intensive care units. *Pediatrics*, 114(4), 1114-1125.
2. American Academy of Pediatrics. (2006). Child life services. *Pediatrics*, 118(4), 1757-1763.
3. American Academy of Pediatrics. (2012). Levels of neonatal care. *Pediatrics*, 130(3), 287-597.
4. Bowden, V. R., & Greenberg, C. S. eds. (2014). Children and their families: The continuum of nursing care (3rd ed.). Philadelphia: Lippincott Williams & Wilkins.
5. Epstein David, Brill, Judith E. (2005). A History of Pediatric Critical Care Medicine. *Pediatric Research*, 58(5): 987–996. doi:10.1203/01.pdr.0000182822.16263.3d. ISSN 1530-0447.
6. Frankel, Lorry R; DiCarlo, Joseph V. (2003). Pediatric Intensive Care. In: Bernstein, Daniel; Shelov, Steven P, eds. Pediatrics for Medical Students (2nd ed.). Philadelphia: Lippincott illiams & Wilkins. p. 541. ISBN 978-0-7817-2941-3.
7. Guidelines and levels of care for pediatric intensive care units. Committee on Hospital Care of the American Academy of Pediatrics and Pediatric Section of the Society of Critical Care Medicine. *Pediatrics*. 1993;92(1):166–175. ISSN 0031-4005. PMID 8516070.
8. Hodkinson, Peter; Argent, Andrew; Wallis, Lee; Reid, Steve; Perera, Rafael; Harrison, Sian; Thompson, Matthew; English, Mike; Maconochie, Ian. (2016). Pathways to Care for Critically Ill or Injured Children: A Cohort Study from First Presentation to Healthcare Services through to Admission to Intensive Care or Death. *PLOS ONE*, 11(1):e0145473. doi:10.1371/journal.pone.0145473. ISSN 1932-6203.
9. Morton, Neil S. (1997). Paediatric Intensive Care. Oxford University Press. ISBN 978-0-19-262511-3.
10. Pronovost, P. J., Dang, D., Dorman, T., et al. (2001). Intensive Care Unit Nurse Staffing and the Risk for Complications after Abdominal Aortic Surgery. *Effective Clinical Practice. American College of Physicians–American Society of Internal Medicine*, 4(5): 199–206. PMID 11685977. Retrieved 2009-01-08.
11. Schmalenberg, Claudia; Kramer, Marlene. (2007). Types of intensive care units with the healthiest, most productive work environments. *American Journal of Critical Care: An Official Publication, American Association of Critical-Care Nurses*, 16(5):458–468; quiz 469. ISSN 1062-3264. PMID 17724243.

C References for neonatal ICU planning

1. Philbin MK. Planning the acoustic environment of a neonatal intensive care unit. *Clin Perinatol.* 2004;31(2):331-52, viii. PMID: 15289037. DOI: 10.1016/j.clp.2004.04.014.

2. Damato EG. Discharge planning from the neonatal intensive care unit. *J Perinat Neonatal Nurs.* 1991;5(1):43-53. PMID: 2027087.

3. B Purdy, J W Craig, & P Zeanah. NICU discharge planning and beyond: recommendations for parent psychosocial support. *J Perinatol.* 2015;35(Suppl 1):S24–S28. Published online 2015 Nov 24. doi: 10.1038/jp.2015.146.

4. Judy Smith,Kathleen Bajo, & Judy Hager. Planning a developmentally appropriate neonatal intensive care unit. *Clinics in perinatology.* 2004;31, Issue 2, 313–322.

5. Hack M. Care of preterm infants in the neonatal intensive care unit. *Pediatrics.* 2009;123:1246-47.

6. Luyster RJ, Kuban KC, O'Shea TM, et al. Paediatr Perinat Epidemiol. 2011;25(4):366-76. ISSN: 1365-3016.

7. Hack M, Youngstrom EA, Cartar L, et al. Pediatrics. 2004;114 (Supplement Part 2):932-40. p9.

8. Moster D, Lie RT, Markestad T. Long-term medical and social consequences of preterm birth. *New England Journal of Medicine.* 2008;359:262-73.

9. Hack M. Young adult outcomes of very-low-birth-weight children. *Semin Fetal Neonatal Med.* 2006;11:127-37.

10. Bhutta AT, Anand KJ. Vulnerability of the developing brain: neuronal mechanisms. *Clin Perinatol.* 2002;29:357-72.

11. Aylward GP. Neurodevelopmental outcomes of infants born prematurely. *J Dev Behav Pediatr.* 2014;35:394-407.

12. Johnson S, Marlow N. Early and long-term outcome of infants born extremely preterm. *Arch Dis Child.* 2016.

13. Browne JV, Talmi A. Developmental supports for newborns and young infants with special health and developmental needs and their families: the BABIES model –body function, arousal and sleep, body movement, interaction with others, eating, and self-soothing. *Newborn Infant Nurs Rev.* 2012;12:239-47.

14. Butler S, Als H. Individualized developmental care improves the lives of infants born preterm. *Acta Paediatr.* 2008;97:1173-75.

15. Constable RT, Ment LR, Vohr BR, et al. Pediatrics. 2008;Vol. 121 (2):306-16. ISSN:1098-4275.

16. Altimier L. Mother and child integrative developmental care model: a simple approach to a complex population. *Newborn Infant Nurs Rev.* 2011;11:105-8.

17. Altimier L, Phillips R. The neonatal integrative developmental care model: seven neuroprotective core measures for family centered care. *Newborn Infant Nurs Rev.* 2013;13:9-22.

18. Altimier L. Neuroprotective core measure 1: the healing environment. *Newborn Infant Nurs Rev.* 2015;15:89-94.